MW00837875

MAYO CLINIC PRINCIPLES OF SHOULDER SURGERY

MAYO CLINIC SCIENTIFIC PRESS

Mayo Clinic Atlas of Regional Anesthesia and Ultrasound-Guided Nerve Blockade
Edited by James R. Hebl, MD, and Robert L. Lennon, DO

Mayo Clinic Preventive Medicine and Public Health Board Review
Edited by Prathibha Varkey, MBBS, MPH, MHPE

Mayo Clinic Infectious Diseases Board Review
Edited by Zelalem Temesgen, MD

Mayo Clinic Antimicrobial Handbook: Quick Guide, Second Edition
Edited by John W. Wilson, MD, and Lynn L. Estes, PharmD

Just Enough Physiology
By James R. Munis, MD, PhD

Mayo Clinic Cardiology: Concise Textbook, Fourth Edition
Edited by Joseph G. Murphy, MD, and Margaret A. Lloyd, MD

Mayo Clinic Electrophysiology Manual
Edited by Samuel J. Asirvatham, MD

Mayo Clinic Gastrointestinal Imaging Review, Second Edition
By C. Daniel Johnson, MD

Arrhythmias in Women: Diagnosis and Management
Edited by Yong-Mei Cha, MD, Margaret A. Lloyd, MD, and Ulrika M. Birgersdotter-Green, MD

Mayo Clinic Body MRI Case Review
By Christine U. Lee, MD, PhD, and James F. Glockner, MD, PhD

Mayo Clinic Gastroenterology and Hepatology Board Review, Fifth Edition
Edited by Stephen C. Hauser, MD

Mayo Clinic Guide to Cardiac Magnetic Resonance Imaging, Second Edition
Edited by Kiaran P. McGee, PhD, Eric E. Williamson, MD, and Matthew W. Martinez, MD

Mayo Clinic Neurology Board Review: Basic Sciences and Psychiatry for Initial Certification
Edited by Kelly D. Flemming, MD, and Lyell K. Jones Jr, MD

Mayo Clinic Neurology Board Review: Clinical Neurology for Initial Certification and MOC
Edited by Kelly D. Flemming, MD, and Lyell K. Jones Jr, MD

Mayo Clinic Critical Care Case Review
Edited by Rahul Kashyap, MBBS, J. Christopher Farmer, MD, and John C. O'Horo, MD

Mayo Clinic Internal Medicine Board Review, Eleventh Edition
Edited by Christopher M. Wittich, PharmD, MD

Mayo Clinic Medical Neurosciences, Sixth Edition
By Eduardo E. Benarroch, MD, Jeremy K. Cutsforth-Gregory, MD,
and Kelly D. Flemming, MD

MAYO CLINIC PRINCIPLES OF SHOULDER SURGERY

Joaquin Sanchez-Sotelo, MD, PhD

Consultant, Department of Orthopedic Surgery
Mayo Clinic, Rochester, Minnesota
Professor of Orthopedics
Mayo Clinic College of Medicine and Science

MAYO CLINIC SCIENTIFIC PRESS   OXFORD UNIVERSITY PRESS

MAYO
CLINIC

The triple-shield Mayo logo and the words MAYO, MAYO CLINIC, and MAYO CLINIC SCIENTIFIC PRESS are marks of Mayo Foundation for Medical Education and Research

OXFORD
UNIVERSITY PRESS

Oxford University Press is a department of the University of Oxford. It furthers the University's objective of excellence in research, scholarship, and education by publishing worldwide. Oxford is a registered trade mark of Oxford University Press in the UK and certain other countries.

Published in the United States of America by Oxford University Press
198 Madison Avenue, New York, NY 10016, United States of America.

© 2018 by Mayo Foundation for Medical Education and Research

All rights reserved. No part of this publication may be reproduced, stored in a retrieval system, or transmitted, in any form or by any means, electronic, mechanical, photocopying, recording, or otherwise, without the prior permission of Mayo Foundation for Medical Education and Research. Inquiries should be addressed to Scientific Publications, Plummer 10, Mayo Clinic, 200 First St SW, Rochester, MN 55905.

You must not circulate this work in any other form and you must impose this same condition on any acquirer.

Library of Congress Cataloging-in-Publication Data
Names: Sanchez-Sotelo, Joaquin, author.
Title: Mayo Clinic principles of shoulder surgery / Joaquin Sanchez-Sotelo.
Other titles: Principles of shoulder surgery | Mayo Clinic scientific press (Series)
Description: Oxford ; New York : Oxford University Press, [2018] | Series:
Mayo Clinic scientific press | Includes bibliographical references and index.
Identifiers: LCCN 2017027128 | ISBN 9780190602765 (alk. paper)
Subjects: | MESH: Shoulder—surgery | Shoulder Joint—surgery | Shoulder
Injuries—surgery | Orthopedic Procedures—methods
Classification: LCC RD557.5 | NLM WE 810 | DDC 617.5/72044—dc23
LC record available at https://lccn.loc.gov/2017027128

Mayo Foundation does not endorse any particular products or services, and the reference to any products or services in this book is for informational purposes only and should not be taken as an endorsement by the authors or Mayo Foundation. Care has been taken to confirm the accuracy of the information presented and to describe generally accepted practices. However, the author, editors, and publisher are not responsible for errors or omissions or for any consequences from application of the information in this book and make no warranty, express or implied, with respect to the contents of the publication. This book should not be relied on apart from the advice of a qualified health care provider.

The author, editors, and publisher have exerted efforts to ensure that drug selection and dosage set forth in this text are in accordance with current recommendations and practice at the time of publication. However, in view of ongoing research, changes in government regulations, and the constant flow of information relating to drug therapy and drug reactions, readers are urged to check the package insert for each drug for any change in indications and dosage and for added wordings and precautions. This is particularly important when the recommended agent is a new or infrequently employed drug.

Some drugs and medical devices presented in this publication have US Food and Drug Administration (FDA) clearance for limited use in restricted research settings. It is the responsibility of the health care providers to ascertain the FDA status of each drug or device planned for use in their clinical practice.

9 8 7 6 5 4 3 2 1

Printed by Sheridan Books, Inc., United States of America

Foreword

The author and book have a clear aim and goal: to express in a compact manner the fundamentals of shoulder surgery upon which knowledge and experience can be built. There is so much to learn in orthopedic surgery when one is in educational programs, including the substance of the divisions within the field (for example, pediatric orthopedics), basic sciences (including anatomy), health care systems, general aspects of inpatient care, ethics and professionalism, and details about each anatomic region (for example, the shoulder). Time is of the essence, and texts for early exposure within the field must be comprehensive—yet compact. This book easily accomplishes those needs with crystal clear organization, key points stated throughout, high-quality and abundant illustrations, and classic plus up-to-date referencing.

The book begins as it should with evaluation, making the structural diagnosis. Last, the concluding chapter tells the truth about the principles and practice of immobilization and rehabilitation that can be adapted to almost any shoulder injury, whether nonoperative or postoperative sequence of care. After the initial chapter, the author gets right to the point with the practical explanation of surgical exposures and the details about doing arthroscopic shoulder surgery. These are supplemented with videos of the common surgical procedures. Orthopedics is orthopedic surgery! Compressing technical material is the profound core of an introductory text in this field.

The other essential is recognizing that there are 4 areas of knowledge one must master to understand diagnosis and treatment. These are rotator cuff and related issues, instability, fractures, and shoulder arthritis. There

is a chapter on each of these topics. The material in each of them is compressed but enough. This is accomplished through expert organization, explaining the material so it is easily understandable. Lesser, yet important, topics are here too. Treatment for clavicle injuries, acromioclavicular dislocations, and sternoclavicular dislocations has been changing in profound manners. The reader will grasp the knowledge needed to apply the newer concepts and surgical techniques. Shoulder stiffness has been a great concern after injury, surgical treatment, or idiopathic causes; this is focused upon in a separate chapter. The final topic is salvage procedures, encompassing arthrodesis or major resections. This limiting definition very well defines these surgical choices.

If each orthopedic subspecialty had a text such as this, educational programing would become clear as a bell. Read each basic, well-organized, yet comprehensive subspecialty text, then supplement that with the material from key journals. It seems so straightforward. Hopefully, other areas within the field will take note of this book and copy its method of delivering the substance of their field to students and practicing surgeons.

Robert H. Cofield, MD

Professor of Orthopedics, Mayo Clinic College
of Medicine and Science
Emeritus Chair, Department of Orthopedic Surgery
Mayo Clinic
Past President, American Shoulder
and Elbow Surgeons

Foreword

Mayo Clinic Principles of Shoulder Surgery is a fantastic tool for teaching and learning! The author, Dr Joaquin Sanchez-Sotelo, has thoroughly thought of everything needed in a book covering basic principles:

- The book is divided into 12 chapters that cover nicely all conditions and possible treatments currently needed in clinical practice: fractures, instability, rotator cuff tears, arthritis, and others.
- The outline of each chapter is very similar throughout the book, very well organized, making reading and learning very easy.
- Analysis of the treatment algorithms and techniques is very precise and objective, without bias. Everything is explained and reported very clearly. The reader will find all the needed information, options, indications, and techniques to determine the best treatment.
- The illustrations, drawings, radiographs, intraoperative photographs, and videos are remarkable; the quality of these materials is simply amazing, making reading this book a very pleasant experience.

Joaquin Sanchez-Sotelo was recognized in Europe as one of the best shoulder surgeons. He was then attracted by the very prestigious Mayo Clinic, in Rochester (Minnesota, USA). We are proud to witness that he has become as successful in the United States as he was in Spain and Europe.

The content of this book is the result of Joaquin's huge experience; each topic is approached in a practical way, which reflects the knowledge and personality of the author: objective, honest, brilliant, skillful surgeon, passionate teacher, and very hard worker. It was a pleasure to have the opportunity to read this book. I have no doubt that many shoulder surgeons around the world, both novice fellows and known experts, will read this book and keep it close in their library. Dr Joaquin Sanchez-Sotelo must be commended for his incredible efforts to put together such a wonderful book.

Gilles Walch, MD

Consultant and Professor of Orthopedic Surgery Centre Orthopédique SANTY, Lyon, France Past President, European Society of Shoulder and Elbow Surgery (SESEC) Past President, French Orthopedic Society (SOFCOT)

Preface

Orthopedic surgery is such a wonderful profession! Many components are necessary to become a good orthopedic surgeon. Knowledge and skills are both extremely important, although it takes several more competencies (including professionalism, ethical values, and systems management) to become a good doctor. Access to information has grown exponentially over the past few years, largely due to availability of content in electronic format that can be obtained almost instantly with modern devices via the internet. Some of this information may be vetted through a peer-review process, but some is made public without much review and may contain mistakes. In parallel, research activities lead to a constantly growing body of knowledge, and the information contained both in classic articles and in the most current literature is equally important to improving the health of our patients. In this setting of an expanding body of easily accessible knowledge, there is 1 question for many overwhelmed trainees in the medical field: Where do I start?

If you are just starting to learn about shoulder surgery, I would love for you to use *Mayo Clinic Principles of Shoulder Surgery* as your introduction. The idea of writing this book came after a number of observations. Teaching orthopedic surgery is 1 of my passions. After years of training medical students, residents, and fellows, I have noticed that most will randomly review a given topic (often selected on the basis of an interesting case) by pulling a review article from the internet or browsing a few papers identified with use of a search engine. Although any reading has the potential to be useful, I get the impression that many of our trainees dive into these sources without having had the opportunity to learn basic principles. I may be wrong, but I believe that reading a book on the principles of shoulder surgery from cover to cover provides a better foundation upon which to build.

There are many excellent books in the field of shoulder surgery. Why another one? In my opinion, most books on shoulder surgery suffer from 1 of the following problems: they are comprehensive but too dense or long to be tackled by our younger trainees, or they are extremely specialized in one small aspect of shoulder surgery (such as instability or arthroplasty). *Mayo Clinic Principles of Shoulder Surgery* was written for individuals just starting to learn about shoulder surgery, or health care providers who need a clear understanding of the basics when they occasionally evaluate a patient with a shoulder condition (i.e., family practitioners, physician assistants, physical therapists, nurses, operating room personnel). If you are a shoulder expert, you will find this book too simple because you already know the basic principles.

Currently, most shoulder books are authored by multiple contributors under the guidance of 1 or more editors; however, I believed that the kind of book I had in mind would best be written by a single author. Summarizing the principles of shoulder surgery in only 12 chapters is not easy, but becomes easier if a single person creates the content for the whole book. Although I am the sole author of this book, you will find that I often use "we," in my discussion of procedures. I use the plural to reflect the team approach used at Mayo Clinic and the general philosophy of the orthopedics practice here. One possible risk of a single-author book is bias. I am sure some will disagree with various aspects of this book when the topics discussed are still unclear or controversial. Also, since the field of medicine is constantly evolving, some content included in this book will become obsolete. However, the basic principles of shoulder surgery will remain fairly consistent, and new content will be added in future editions to replace whatever becomes outdated or is replaced by new discoveries.

Adult learning is fascinating. Did you know that most people listening to a lecture will only retain 10% of the content? Learning by practicing and by teaching others helps us retain the most information; other learning tools fall somewhere in between the 2. Visual content definitely facilitates learning; that is why we made an effort to create original, high-quality illustrations and video recordings of the most common shoulder surgical procedures.

The field of shoulder surgery is quite unique. Physical examination is very important. A number of ancillary tests are used very commonly. Most shoulder surgeons perform open surgery as well as arthroscopic procedures. We take care of a wide range of problems: traumatic injuries, sports-related conditions, joint degeneration, scapular dysfunction, and the list goes on and on. In addition, physical therapy is extremely important for the shoulder, and injections in various locations are performed very commonly. There is so much to learn, and we need a place to start! This book is organized as a starting place to cover many of these basic aspects of shoulder surgery.

What's a book without a reader? A purposeless stack of paper? Probably, yes. This book will have no purpose without you, the reader. I really hope it will help you start to establish a solid foundation in the field of shoulder surgery. And who knows? Maybe you will fall in love with this portion of the human body as much as I did!

Joaquin Sanchez-Sotelo, MD, PhD

Acknowledgments

I have so many people to thank that I might need to write another book just for the acknowledgments part. My teachers, mentors, and partners; my patients; my residents, fellows, and other students; Mayo Clinic and its support personnel; and my family, you all own this book with me.

I was born in Madrid, Spain. I am very grateful to all my teachers and mentors at Universidad Autonoma de Madrid and Hospital La Paz, where I completed my medical school program, PhD program, and residency; however, I am most grateful to my dad, mom, and brother. My dad was a very good orthopedic surgeon; he would take me on Sunday morning rounds, found a way for me to get into the operating room at a very early age, and gave me the inspiration to become the surgeon I am. He left this world way too early, but my mom found strength—I do not know how—to support and guide my brother and me through difficult times. She is still one of my rocks, a person I go to for advice all the time. And so is my brother—Juan you are always there!

I moved to the United States to first learn, then practice, at Mayo Clinic. I am forever indebted to my mentors, and in particular to Dr Robert H. Cofield, in the field of shoulder surgery. I was lucky to interact with other giants in the field of shoulder and elbow surgery: Bernard Morrey and Shawn O'Driscoll. I also work with an amazing team of surgeons now: John Sperling, Scott Steinmann, Mark Morrey, Bassem El Hassan, Aaron Krych, Diane Dahm, Mike Torchia, Chris Camp (and of course Shawn). I cannot thank you all enough for teaching me and supporting me as your student, partner, and friend. The chairs of our department, Dan Berry and Mark Pagnano, have always been so supportive as well!

I have worked on this book very closely with a number of individuals at Mayo Clinic. Mike King has suffered all my painful attention to detail when it comes to illustrations. Jan Case created all the animations for the videos. Our photography department is responsible for surgical pictures and video recording. Kenna Atherton coordinated with Craig Panner to establish layouts and publishing as a joint effort between Mayo Clinic Scientific Press and Oxford University Press.

My patients are part of the inspiration for this book. I love what I do largely because I can help people who are suffering from painful shoulder conditions, have lost function, or cannot practice their favorite sports. Thanks to all of you for letting me be your doctor. My students are also part of my inspiration: generations of residents, fellows, and medical students (from the United States and abroad). Thank you for challenging me with questions and for your constant stimulation.

My 3 children know that I am a workaholic; writing this book, and everything I do for work, has taken so much away from them. I am very grateful to have you in my life. You make me proud and happy every day. Pablo is now starting medical school and plans to become an orthopedic surgeon, Marta is a super-smart young woman who always listens to me, provides me with great advice, and will become a very good lawyer and businesswoman (she loves to litigate), and Alexis is the sweetest, smartest, kindest, fun little girl. But the person who has given me the most during the time it has taken to write this book is my better half and love of my life, Lori. Thank you for making me happy every day, for giving me time to complete this book, and for everything you do every day to support me and help me fulfill my dreams. I do not deserve you, and I love you very much.

Digital Media Accompanying the Book

Individual purchasers of this book are entitled to free personal access to accompanying digital media in the online edition. Please refer to the access token card for instructions on token redemption and access.

These online ancillary materials, where available, are noted with iconography throughout the book.

 Video

A table of contents for video files available with this book appears on p. xvii. The corresponding media can be found on *Oxford Medicine Online* at: http://www.oxfordmedicine.com/mayoclinicshouldersurgery

If you are interested in access to the complete online edition, please consult with your librarian.

Contents

Video Files

1 Evaluation of the Shoulder

Establishing an accurate diagnosis and understanding the severity of the underlying condition are critical in order to provide the best possible treatment for patients presenting with a painful and/or dysfunctional shoulder. Shoulder surgeons need to acquire the knowledge and skills necessary to integrate elements of the patient's history, physical examination findings, imaging, and other studies in order to understand where the pain is coming from and how to improve shoulder function.

The evaluation of the shoulder joint is a great example of medicine as a blend of art and science. Although certain history traits, physical examination tests, and imaging findings have been scientifically analyzed, many diagnoses are established based on a general understanding of the shoulder joint and on reliance on bits and pieces of information that make sense only as a whole.

Before diving into the specifics of how to evaluate the patient with a painful or dysfunctional shoulder, a few facts should be taken into consideration (Table 1.1). Our intention, as physicians, is to identify the structural pathology that is bothering each patient. However, surgeons oftentimes rely on physical examination findings that are not scientifically validated; in addition, certain imaging studies (specifically, magnetic resonance) may reveal structural changes that may or may not be responsible for the patient's symptoms. It is extremely important to avoid reaching a diagnosis based only on advanced imaging studies, without correlation with the history and physical examination findings. As a general rule, it is better to interview and examine the patient first, then analyze any complementary studies.

There are portions of the physical examination that should be assessed in every patient. However, some physical examination tests are useful only in patients with certain conditions: it does not make sense to perform a test

Table 1.1 • Evaluation of the Shoulder Joint: General Principles

Purpose of evaluation
Identify structural pathology that explains patient's symptoms
    Several areas of structural pathology may coexist
    Not all structural changes are symptomatic
    Referred shoulder pain is not uncommon
        Cervical spine
        Chest and abdomen
Determine severity of symptoms

Physical examination maneuvers are not always scientifically validated

Elements of the shoulder evaluation fall into 2 categories
General (to be assessed in most patients, [e.g., pain, motion])
Specific or focused (e.g., tests for labral tears)

Advanced imaging studies may show asymptomatic structural changes

Outcome tools are useful to
Understand severity and
Monitor changes over time

for multidirectional instability in patients with end-stage osteoarthritis. For those reasons, I distinguish between *general* examination maneuvers to be performed on everyone, and *focused* maneuvers directed to specific conditions. Many of the specific maneuvers used to evaluate these conditions are discussed as well in other chapters. This chapter does not intend to provide a comprehensive review of all tests described to examine the shoulder, but to present an organized approach to shoulder evaluation using my preferred maneuvers.

Outcome tools have gained popularity over the past 2 decades (1–4). Although a comprehensive discussion of these tools exceeds the scope of this book, I will provide some information useful for those individuals starting to immerse themselves in the field of shoulder surgery.

History

Most patients with shoulder problems complain of pain; stiffness, weakness, and instability are also present in various shoulder conditions. Excluding patients with a clearly traumatic shoulder injury, and patients with instability, most individuals complain of progressive onset of shoulder pain. Typically, arthritis, capsulitis, and cuff pathology are associated with pain over the deltoid region; patients will grab the side of the shoulder with their opposite hand to explain where their pain is. When patients complain of "shoulder" pain over the trapezius and side of the neck, special care should be taken to *exclude cervical spine disease* (Table 1.2). However, shoulder conditions can hurt around the neck. More commonly, pain is also felt in the periscapular region, indicative of primary or secondary scapular dyskinesis (see chapter 10, The Scapula).

Once the nature and location of the pain have been assessed, patients should be asked about motion loss, subjective weakness, or instability. When evaluating patients with instability, it is important to determine if they have sustained true dislocation episodes, in which positions the shoulder is unstable, and if there is evidence of generalized ligamentous laxity (see chapter 7, Shoulder Instability and the Labrum).

Other important elements of the history to be documented include age, sex, dominance, prior injuries, prior surgeries, and conditions known to be associated with certain shoulder problems (i.e., diabetes mellitus in patients with adhesive capsulitis; see chapter 8, Adhesive Capsulitis) and factors that could negatively affect bone or soft-tissue healing (e.g., lack of compliance, smoking, and others).

Physical Examination

Inspection, accurate localization of pain, motion, and strength should be assessed in all patients with shoulder problems. Additional examination maneuvers are specifically performed for patients with arthritis, cuff disease, acromioclavicular joint symptoms, instability, biceps and labral pathology, or scapular conditions. The examination should be completed with evaluation of possible associated distal neurovascular abnormalities (⦿ Video 1.1).

Both shoulders should be examined in all patients in order to compare the symptomatic shoulder with the opposite one. It is extremely important to examine both shoulders *uncovered*. Examination of the shoulder with the clothes still on does not allow assessment of scars, deformity, or atrophy; it also makes it more difficult to pinpoint the location of pain, and to examine the scapula.

Inspection

Deformity and scars should be noted. Most common deformities include prominence of the clavicle in patients with hypertrophic osteoarthritis or traumatic injuries of the acromioclavicular joint, as well as an abnormally low, bulging biceps muscle belly ("Popeye" sign) when the long head of the biceps is ruptured (Figure 1.1). Ecchymosis may be present initially after a rupture of the long head of the biceps as well as after a proximal humerus fracture.

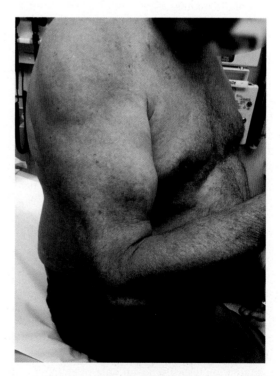

Figure 1.1 *Rupture of the long head of the biceps results in an abnormally low, bulging biceps, producing the "Popeye" deformity.*

Table 1.2 • Cervical Spine Pathology Is the Most Common Reason for Referred Shoulder Pain

Pain located over the side of the neck and trapezius

Cervical spine motion is painful and/or limited

Radicular symptoms (pain radiates along the upper extremity in a dermatomal fashion)

Neurologic deficits (hypoesthesia or weakness)

Positive Spurling test (The examiner turns the patient's head to the affected side while extending and applying downward pressure to the top of the patient's head; the test is positive when the pain arising in the neck radiates in the direction of an ipsilateral dermatome.)

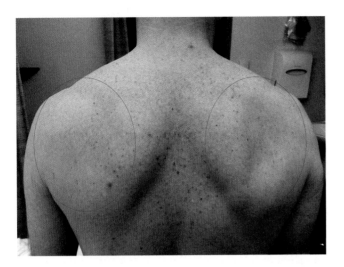

Figure 1.2 Infraspinatus atrophy can be appreciated by comparing both shoulders from the posterior view.

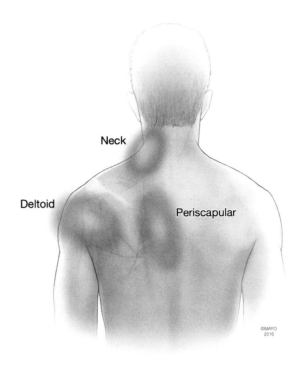

Figure 1.3 Most shoulder conditions generate pain in the deltoid region. Pain in the neck region should prompt careful evaluation of the cervical spine. Periscapular pain can be seen in glenohumeral or scapular conditions.

Ganglion cysts over the acromioclavicular joint may be seen in patients with cuff tear arthropathy. Pectoralis major ruptures may be missed if the contour of the affected pectoralis is not compared with the opposite side.

Muscle atrophy should also be noted. Deltoid atrophy should prompt exclusion of an associated injury to the axillary nerve or surgical muscle damage. Atrophy at the supraspinous and infraspinous fossae is observed in long-standing cuff tears, suprascapular nerve compression at the suprascapular notch, and brachial plexus injuries; isolated infraspinatus atrophy almost always indicates suprascapular nerve compression at the spinoglenoid notch or an isolated infraspinatus rupture at the myotendinous junction (Figure 1.2). Isolated atrophy of the trapezius is seen in injuries to the spinal accessory nerve, or rarely in traumatic ruptures. Inspection will also reveal scapular winging when present (see Scapular Position later).

Location of Pain

Accurate localization of pain is extremely helpful in diagnosing shoulder conditions (Figure 1.3). I first ask patients to point with a single fingertip of the opposite hand where they feel their pain to be the most intense, realizing that sometimes they feel pain over a somewhat larger area. Next, I try to identify painful spots in a specific order not to miss any structures. Specific areas palpated for pain include the sternoclavicular joint, acromioclavicular joint, greater tuberosity region (or cuff insertion site), bicipital groove and tendon, posterior glenohumeral joint line, and periscapular musculature. Pain in multiple locations not corresponding with specific joint locations may be indicative of fibromyalgia.

Motion

Accurate assessment of shoulder motion is an essential element of the evaluation of any patient with shoulder

problems (5). My preference is to assess active motion prior to passive motion. Lack of active motion with normal passive motion is most commonly seen in rotator cuff tears. Patients with capsulitis or arthritis will have similar ranges of active and passive motion.

Although many experienced shoulder surgeons are able to visually estimate arcs of motion with some accuracy, at the beginning of my practice I found it very useful to use a goniometer in order to train myself and understand how to measure motion accurately. It is important to realize that normal shoulder motion tends to decrease with age: patients in their 80s are unlikely to demonstrate 170° of active elevation, even if their shoulder has no abnormalities. To understand what is normal and abnormal for a given patient, it is best to compare with the opposite side.

Shoulder surgeons differ regarding which planes of motion are assessed, the starting position of the upper extremity, and scapular constraint during motion assessment. My preference is to allow patients to show me their best motion without maintaining the upper extremity in a specific position and without constraining the scapula, since I want to understand their functional abilities and limitations. However, true measurement of glenohumeral motion requires blocking scapular motion to some degree. As detailed in the following, small variations in how motion is measured will lead to angle discrepancies; after reading this textbook, pick the methods that will work best for you and stay consistent so that your intraobserver variation is minimized.

Forward Flexion, Abduction, and Elevation

One of the main functions of the shoulder is to position the hand up in space. Three terms are commonly used to describe this motion (Figure 1.4). *Forward flexion* refers to raising the upper extremity in the parasagittal plane (straight forward). *Abduction* refers to raising the upper extremity in the coronal plane (straight lateral). *Elevation* (or scaption) refers to raising the upper extremity in the plane of the scapula (approximately at the bisector between the parasagittal and the coronal planes, or at a 30° to 45° angle) (5).

Most healthy individuals are able to reach the highest with their hand when the shoulder is elevated, as compared with flexed or abducted (Figure 1.5). This is attributed to easier clearance of the greater tuberosity respective to the acromion (in flexion the tuberosity impinges the front of the acromion, and in abduction it impinges the side of the acromion); it may also be related to greater scapulothoracic excursion and positioning of the scapula extended and abducted, which facilitate acromial clearance.

My preference is to assess elevation, but many surgeons and researchers prefer to measure flexion, abduction, or all 3.

To measure elevation or flexion, the patient is observed from the side and the angle between the axis of the arm and the patient's trunk is measured. To measure abduction, the patient is observed from the front. It is important to ensure that the patient does not compensate for lack of shoulder motion by arching the spine. Table 1.3 summarizes normal motion averages in various planes (6). Motion changes with age, gender, and dominance; and there is a wide range of normal ranges of motion reported, probably based on variations in subjects included and interobserver concordance.

It is important to realize that when these 3 motions are performed, the final position of the upper extremity in space is the result of the combination of gliding of the scapula on the chest wall (i.e., scapulothoracic motion) and rotation of the humeral head on the glenoid (i.e., glenohumeral motion). The term *scapulothoracic rhythm* refers to the relative contribution of scapulothoracic and glenohumeral motions.

The scapulothoracic rhythm is 2:1 for abduction (7); this means that when the shoulder is abducted, two-thirds of the final motion is provided by glenohumeral rotation and one-third by scapulothoracic motion. The values for elevation and flexion are 1.6:1 and 1.1:1, respectively (7). Thus, motion loss in elevation, abduction, or flexion may be due to loss of glenohumeral motion and/or scapulothoracic

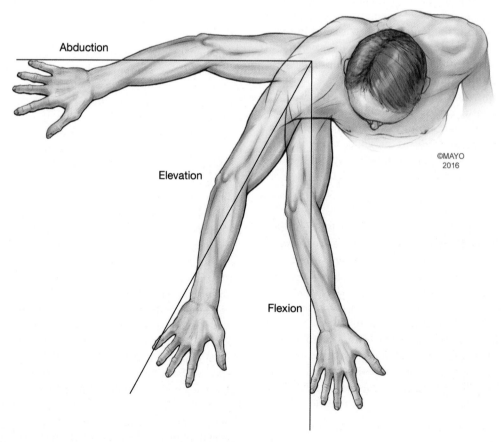

©MAYO
2016

Figure 1.4 *Planes of motion for flexion, abduction, and elevation.*

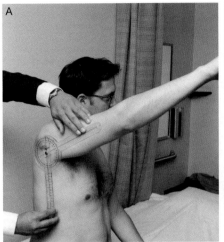 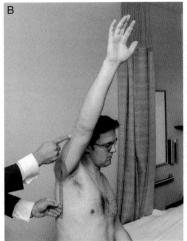 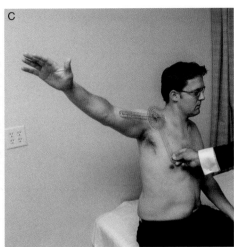

Figure 1.5 *Range of motion in flexion* **(A)**, *elevation* **(B)**, *and abduction* **(C)**.

motion. Patients with a very flexible scapulothoracic articulation can compensate better for glenohumeral stiffness.

External and Internal Rotation

External rotation is most commonly measured with the arm at the side (Figure 1.6A). When measured with the patient supine or with the arm in complete adduction, scapulothoracic motion is limited, allowing measurement of isolated glenohumeral external rotation. The goniometer is placed so that one arm is facing straight forward in the parasagittal plane and the other arm is parallel to the forearm. By convention, 0° (neutral) means that the forearm is facing straight forward; negative and positive values indicate the shoulder can or cannot be rotated beyond 0°, respectively. Alternatively, external rotation at the side can be measured with the shoulder in slight abduction, which allows some scapulothoracic retraction and provides higher values of

rotation; this is my preference, since I am interested in overall function.

Internal rotation is typically evaluated with the patient standing or sitting, and measured according to the highest vertebral level reached by the thumb (Figure 1.7). However, this method has low intra- and interobserver agreement (8): vertebral levels may be difficult to identify by the observer, and elbow range of motion affects the observation, especially for higher degrees of internal rotation. A few practical reference points include C7 at the level of the most prominent spinous process, T3 at the level of the spine of the scapula, T7 at the inferior pole of the scapula, and L4 at the top of the iliac crest. Lower degrees of internal rotation are referenced to the sacroiliac joint or trochanter.

External and internal rotation may also be measured with the arm in 90° of abduction (Figure 1.6B). The patient is observed from the side. By convention, 0° (neutral) means that the forearm is parallel to the ground. Shoulder rotation (so that the hand is raised) is measured as external rotation, whereas lowering the hand is measured as internal rotation.

Strength

Manual testing of strength in various planes is another essential component of shoulder evaluation. Table 1.4 summarizes the most commonly accepted grading system (5). There are specific maneuvers described to isolate specific muscles of the shoulder region as well as periscapular muscles, detailed as follows (see also chapter 6, The Rotator Cuff and Biceps Tendon and chapter 10, The Scapula). I do not include all those maneuvers in the general evaluation of the shoulder but do try to assess strength in flexion, extension, abduction, external rotation, and internal rotation in every patient to scan for unexpected weakness, regardless of my working diagnosis.

Table 1.3 • Average Active Shoulder Motion

Plane	Degrees
Elevation	170
Flexion	150
Abduction	150
External rotation	
At the side	75
At the side in adduction or supine	50
At 90° of abduction	90
Internal rotation	
At the side	T7 level
At 0° of abduction	70

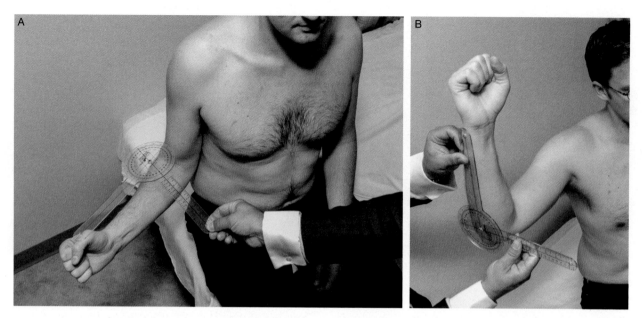

Figure 1.6 *Measurement of shoulder external rotation with the arm at the side* **(A)** *and with the arm in abduction* **(B)**.

Flexion and Extension Strength

The patient is asked to hold the hand of the examiner and push forward (to test flexion strength) and then pull back (to test extension strength). These tests mostly evaluate the deltoid muscle, which can be felt to contract with the examiner's opposite hand.

Abduction Strength

The patient is asked to position the shoulder in approximately 45° of elevation with the elbow flexed at 90°

(Figure 1.8). The examiner applies progressive resistance by pushing down on the side of the elbow. Weakness with this maneuver may be related to the deltoid or the supraspinatus muscle. By testing strength at a low angle of elevation with the elbow flexed, pain is less likely to interfere with strength testing. If strength is tested with the elbow extended and pushing down on the wrist and hand, the examiner has a much larger lever arm; however, smaller supraspinatus tears will not be detected with this maneuver (see Supraspinatus Testing later).

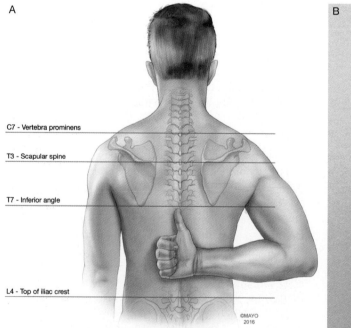

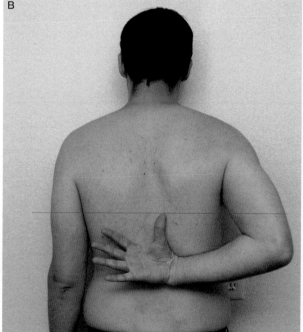

Figure 1.7 **A** *and* **B.** *Internal rotation is measured as the highest vertebral level the patient can reach with the thumb.*

Table 1.4 • Strength Grading Scale for Manual Testing

Grade 0	No contraction
Grade 1—Trace	Contraction without effective motion
Grade 2—Poor	Motion with gravity eliminated
Grade 3—Fair	Motion against gravity
Grade 4—Good	Motion against resistance
Grade 5—Normal	Normal strength

External Rotation Strength

The patient is asked to position the shoulder in approximately 20° of external rotation (Figure 1.9). The examiner resists the patient's distal forearm while the patient attempts to push out, assessing the strength of the posterior deltoid and posterior rotator cuff (infraspinatus and teres minor). The opposite hand may be used to feel for contraction of the infraspinatus.

Internal Rotation Strength

The patient is asked to position the shoulder the exact same way, and the examiner holds the patient's distal forearm while the patient attempts to pull away from the examiner. This maneuver assesses the strength of the pectoralis major and subscapularis.

Arthritis

Evaluation of the arthritic shoulder will vary depending on the underlying diagnosis (see chapter 9, Shoulder Arthritis and Arthroplasty). However, there are a few

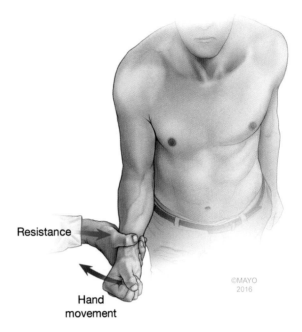

Figure 1.9 Initial assessment of strength in external rotation with the arm at the side.

specific findings that may be helpful. General examination of the shoulder will demonstrate pain along the posterior joint line and stiffness in several planes. Strength will be normal in patients with an intact rotator cuff (common in primary osteoarthritis) and decreased in patients with cuff dysfunction secondary to inflammatory arthritis, cuff tear arthropathy, or sequelae of trauma. Not uncommonly, crepitus can be felt, or even heard, as motion or strength is tested.

Pain related to loss of articular cartilage is thought to be reproduced by forced motion of the preloaded joint in order to induce a shear stress at the joint surface. This can be done by asking the patient to hold the shoulder in external rotation and forcefully moving the shoulder into internal rotation while the patient is asked if motion against resistance in the mid arc replicates pain (articular shear test, Figure 1.10).

Bumping of osteophytes and pinching the inflamed synovium and capsule are also painful in many patients with an arthritic joint; these may be elicited by taking the shoulder to the maximum extent of passive external rotation and then jerking the shoulder in a little more rotation.

Rotator Cuff, Biceps, and the Acromioclavicular Joint

Many patients presenting in the office with shoulder pain may have a combination of subacromial impingement with or without associated pathology at the acromioclavicular joint and biceps. Some will also have a torn rotator cuff. These structures are typically all assessed in the typical rotator cuff patient.

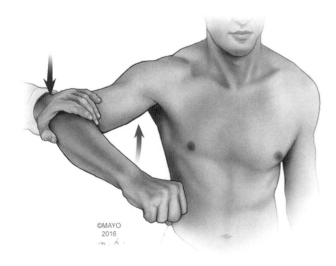

Figure 1.8 Initial assessment of strength in abduction is best performed with the elbow flexed. The shorter lever arm of the examiner makes this maneuver less likely to be painful, but will not detect smaller cuff tears.

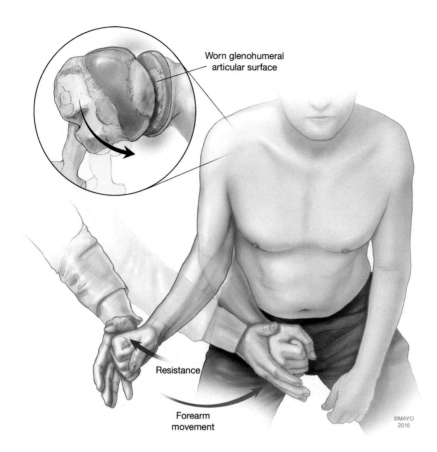

Figure 1.10 In the articular shear test, pain from the articular surface is reproduced by forcing the joint to move under load (resistance).

Subacromial Impingement

Although there is controversy about the relationship between subacromial impingement and rotator cuff disease, most shoulder surgeons do evaluate for impingement when pain is judged to be somewhat related to the subacromial region and rotator cuff. The most commonly used maneuvers are those described by Neer and Hawkins. The rationale behind these tests is to reproduce in the office forced impingement between the proximal humerus and the coracoacromial arch. The reported sensitivity and specificity of these tests has been variable (9).

Neer Sign and Test

The examiner stabilizes the scapula with 1 hand and places the shoulder in forced flexion with the other hand until there is contact between the proximal humerus and the acromion (Figure 1.11). The Neer sign is positive if this maneuver is painful. The Neer test is positive if subacromial injection of a local anesthetic will turn a painful Neer sign pain free. For impingement to be reproduced with the Neer sign, the patient needs to have full passive forward flexion: this test cannot be performed in patients with stiffness in flexion.

Hawkins (Hawkins-Kennedy) Sign

The shoulder is placed in 90° of forward flexion and 90° of internal rotation (Figure 1.12). The test is positive when further passive internal rotation applied by the examiner reproduces the patient's pain.

Yocum Test

The patient places the hand of the affected extremity on top of the contralateral shoulder. Then the patient attempts to raise the elbow, moving the shoulder against downward pressure by the examiner. The test is considered to be positive if the patient feels pain during the test.

Biceps

Biceps tendinopathy, tenosynovitis, hourglass deformity, subluxation, or dislocation may contribute to shoulder symptoms as isolated entities, or in the setting of rotator cuff disease or labral tears. Over the past few years, more and more patients with shoulder pain are having their biceps tendon addressed surgically, but the tests commonly used to determine whether the biceps tendon is painful have not been clearly validated (10–12). As already mentioned, a "Popeye" deformity is consistent with complete rupture of the long head of the biceps (Figure 1.1).

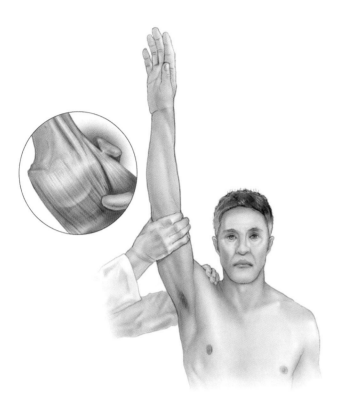

Figure 1.11 Neer sign.

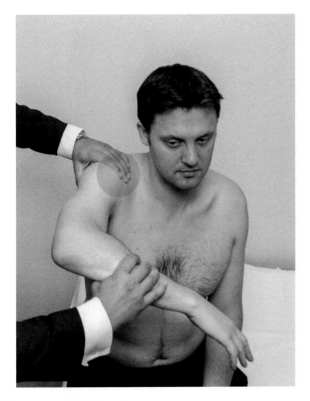

Figure 1.12 Hawkins sign.

Pain on Direct Palpation Over the Biceps Location
The biceps tendon faces directly anteriorly when the shoulder is placed in approximately 30° of external rotation. It can also be visualized in line with the patient's thumb with the forearm in neutral rotation; the thumb points to the biceps with the elbow flexed. In thin, nonmuscular individuals, it may be possible to feel the biceps tendon. However, in most patients the biceps cannot be felt. The anterior aspect of the shoulder is pretty sensitive, so it is difficult to determine that the presence of anterior shoulder pain with deep palpation in the anticipated location of the biceps tendon correlates with symptomatic biceps pathology. I try to determine if the anterior shoulder pain elicited in patients with possible biceps pathology is highest with the shoulder in approximately 30° of external rotation and diminishes as the rotation of the shoulder is changed while pressure is still applied.

Speed Test
The shoulder is placed in 60° of flexion and external rotation, with the forearm supinated and the elbow extended so that the palm of the hand is facing up (Figure 1.13). The test is positive when pain at the bicipital groove is reproduced as the examiner applies downward pressure at the distal forearm. Multiple studies have shown that this test has relatively high sensitivity but very low specificity.

Yergason Test
The arm is placed at the side, with the elbow flexed 90° and the forearm pronated (Figure 1.14). The examiner places 1 hand over the bicipital groove and uses the other hand at the patient's forearm to resist supination. Some surgeons also ask the patient to attempt elbow flexion and shoulder external rotation as they supinate the forearm. The test is positive if there is pain or subluxation at the bicipital groove.

Upper Cut Test
The shoulder is placed in a neutral position, with the elbow flexed to 90°, the forearm supinated, and the patient making a fist. The patient is asked to rapidly bring the hand up and toward the chin—a boxing "upper cut" punch (Figure 1.15). The examiner places his or her hand over the patient's fist and resists the motion as the hand comes up to the chin. The test is positive when there is pain or a painful pop over the anterior portion of the involved shoulder during the resisted movement. This test has been reported to have a relatively high positive likelihood ratio (10).

Acromioclavicular Joint
Distal clavicle osteolysis and acromioclavicular joint osteoarthritis are characterized by pain on deep palpation over the acromioclavicular joint with or without deformity secondary to osteophytes and bone enlargement (Figure 1.16). Pain originating from the acromioclavicular joint increases with cross-body adduction, the acromioclavicular resisted

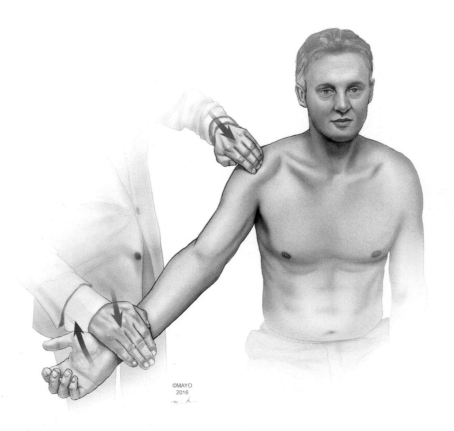

Figure 1.13 Speed test.

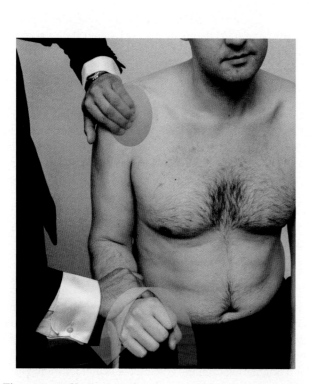

Figure 1.14 Yergason test.

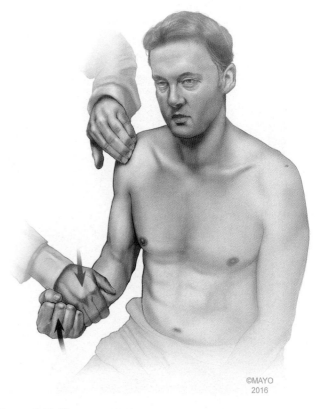

Figure 1.15 Upper cut test.

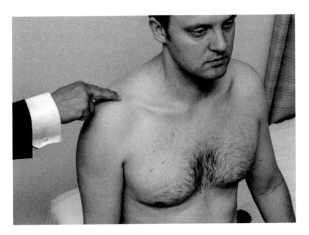

Figure 1.16 Pain on direct palpation over the acromiocla-vicular joint.

extension test, and the acromioclavicular horizontal translation test; in addition, the active compression test, designed for the diagnosis of superior labral tears (see section later in chapter) may also elicit pain at a pathologic acromioclavicular joint (13,14).

Cross-Body Adduction

The shoulder is placed in 90° of flexion and moderate internal rotation, with the elbow extended. The examiner stabilizes the scapula with 1 hand and places the other hand on the elbow or forearm, forcing the shoulder in adduction across the body (Figure 1.17). A positive test is indicated by pain over the acromioclavicular joint.

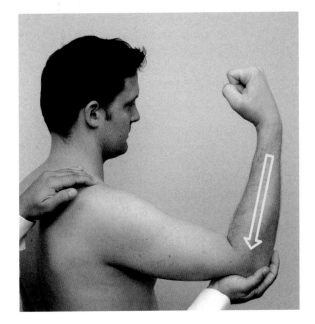

Figure 1.18 Acromioclavicular resisted extension test.

Acromioclavicular Resisted Extension Test

The patient's shoulder is elevated to 90° with the elbow flexed 90°. The examiner places 1 hand behind the distal arm and the patient is asked to extend the arm against resistance (Figure 1.18). Again, this test is considered positive if pain is created at the acromioclavicular joint.

Acromioclavicular Horizontal Translation Test

The examiner's hand is placed over the affected shoulder such that the thumb rests under the posterolateral aspect of the acromion and the index and long fingers of the same or contralateral hand are placed superior to the midpart of the ipsilateral clavicle (Figure 1.19). The

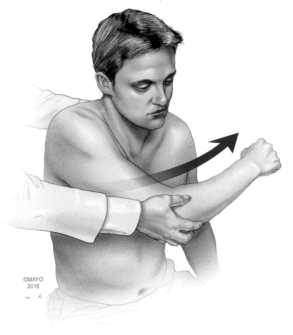

Figure 1.17 Cross-body adduction test.

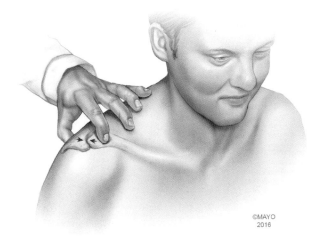

Figure 1.19 Acromioclavicular horizontal translation test.

examiner then applies pressure to the acromion with the thumb, in an anterosuperior direction, and inferiorly to the midpart of the clavicular shaft with the index and long fingers. The test is considered positive if pain is felt or increased in the region of the acromioclavicular joint.

Cuff Integrity and Lag Signs

As mentioned before, many individuals with a rotator cuff tear will present evidence of pain with impingement maneuvers, pain at the acromioclavicular joint, and/or biceps pathology. However, the integrity of the rotator cuff is mostly evaluated through strength testing. The findings on the physical examination will be determined by the size and chronicity of the tear, the severity of any associated pain, and the ability of the patient to compensate with other muscles. The goal of the examiner is to try to isolate the different rotator cuff muscles to understand the location and extent of the tear.

Painful Arc and Drop Arm Sign

These tests are not very specific and do not discriminate tear extent or location, but are classically described and observed for patients with cuff disease. A positive subacromial painful arc exists when the patient performs maximum active elevation and then brings the arm down through the same arc, experiencing pain on the way up and/or down, most often between 60° and 120° of elevation (i.e., pain starts at 60° and resolves beyond 120°). In the drop arm sign, the shoulder is placed in 90° of abduction passively or actively; as the patient tries to bring the shoulder down to the resting position, the arm suddenly drops, typically accompanied by pain.

Supraspinatus Testing

Large supraspinatus tears will be detected by the presence of weakness in abduction, assessed as described before (Figure 1.8). However, patients with high-grade, partial-thickness tears, small full-thickness tears, or a strong deltoid may demonstrate almost normal strength with the shoulder at 45° of abduction and the elbow flexed. In these circumstances, strength can be tested in 90° of elevation and with the elbow straight; the examiner pushes downward on the distal forearm, using the lever arm of the whole upper extremity (Figure 1.20).

Controversy remains regarding the relative value of performing this test in forced internal rotation ("empty can" Jobe test) or moderate external rotation ("full can" test). Although the "empty can" was introduced as a more specific test for supraspinatus weakness, some studies seem to indicate similar value for both tests, with the empty can test having the potential for more false

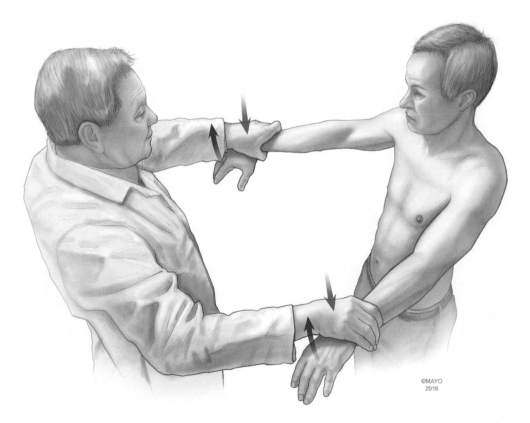

©MAYO 2016

Figure 1.20 Strength testing in abduction with the elbows extended and the thumbs pointing down (Jobe or "empty can" test).

A

B

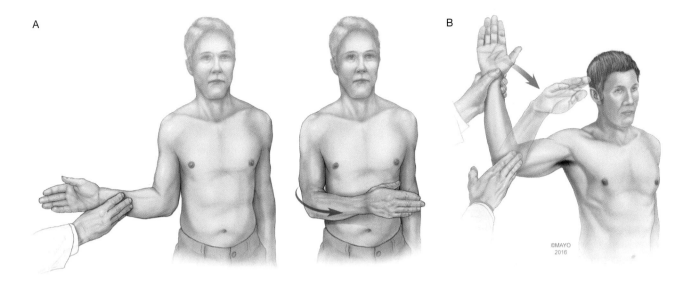

Figure 1.21 **A,** *External rotation lag sign.* **B,** *External rotation drop sign.*

positives, since it is more painful (15). Supraspinatus weakness may also be detected using the Whipple test. The Whipple test is positive when the patient demonstrates weakness with the arm in 90° of flexion and the elbow flexed with the palm down at the level of the opposite shoulder.

Infraspinatus and Teres Minor Testing

Resisted strength in external rotation with the arm at the side is a good first test to evaluate for posterior cuff insufficiency (Figure 1.9); as noted before, atrophy (Figure 1.2) and muscle contraction at the infraspinatus fossa can be evaluated with the patient actively contracting. It is very useful to test both upper extremities at the same time to compare. Additional testing as described in the following sections may be used to fine tune the evaluation; it is not completely clear if these tests assess mostly the infraspinatus, mostly the teres minor, or both (16).

Resisted External Rotation in Elevation (Patte Test)

The shoulder is supported by the examiner in 90° of elevation and some external rotation. Strength in external rotation is resisted with the opposite hand of the examiner on the patient's forearm or hand.

External Rotation Lag and Drop Signs

These 2 tests demonstrate inability by the patient to actively keep the shoulder in external rotation. In the external rotation lag sign (Figure 1.21A), the examiner places the shoulder in 20° of abduction and passive external rotation; the patient is asked to maintain this position of the shoulder actively, and the arm drops into internal rotation toward the abdomen when there is posterior cuff

insufficiency. The drop sign is identically performed with the shoulder in 90° of abduction (Figure 1.21B) (16).

Hornblower Sign

This sign is thought to indicate insufficiency of the teres minor. The patient is asked to bring both hands to the mouth; on the side where there is teres minor insufficiency, the only way the patient can get the hand to the mouth is by abducting the shoulder, typically over 90° (Figure 1.22) (17).

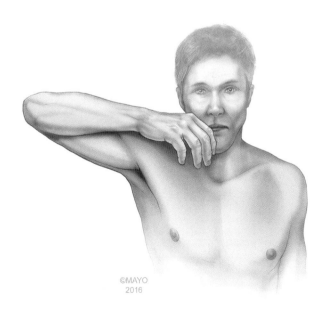

Figure 1.22 *Hornblower sign.*

Active External Rotation with the Upper Extremity
Supported in Shoulder Abduction
Some argue that this test also isolates the teres minor. The examiner supports the shoulder in 90° of abduction and neutral rotation; the patient is asked to actively externally rotate the shoulder until it contacts the opposite hand of the examiner.

Subscapularis Testing
Subscapularis insufficiency should be suspected during the general physical examination of the shoulder when patients are found to have *abnormally increased passive external rotation* compared with the opposite side (the torn subscapularis does not limit external rotation of the shoulder) and when there is weakness in internal rotation. The following tests are commonly used to assess the subscapularis.

Lift-off Test (Gerber Test) and Internal Rotation Lag Sign The patient is asked to place his or her hand behind the back, with the dorsum of the hand resting in the mid-lumbar spine. For the lift-off test, the patient is asked to separate the hand off the spine. For the internal rotation lag sign, the examiner places the hand separated off the spine and asks the patient to maintain that position (Figure 1.23). The main potential problem with these tests is that they may be impossible to perform if the patient has painful or

limited internal rotation. Also, patients may try to separate their hand by extending their elbow, as opposed to internally rotating their shoulder (18).

Belly-Press Test The patient is asked to place the palm of the hand on the affected side flat on the abdomen just below the xyphoid process and move the elbow forward as much as possible while pressing back on the abdomen (Figure 1.24). Patients with subscapularis insufficiency are unable to place the elbow forward, and they try to press on their belly by flexing their wrist and extending their shoulder (19).

Bear-Hug Test The bear-hug test is performed with the palm of the involved side placed on the opposite shoulder and the fingers extended (so that the patient could not resist by grabbing the shoulder) and the elbow positioned anterior to the body (Figure 1.25). The patient is then asked to hold that position (resisted internal rotation) as the physician tries to pull the patient's hand off the shoulder with an external rotation force applied perpendicular to the forearm. The test is considered positive if the patient cannot hold the hand against the shoulder or if he or she shows weakness of resisted internal rotation of greater than 20% compared with the opposite side (11,20).

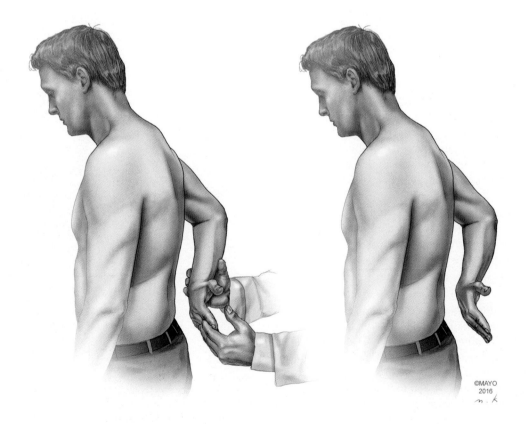

Figure 1.23 Internal rotation lag sign.

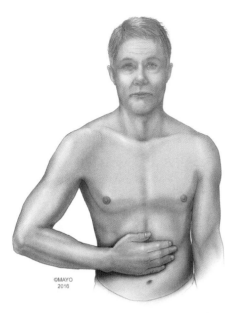
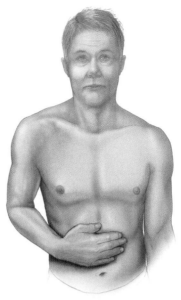

Negative test: Pressure is applied to the abdomen with the elbow forward.

Positive test: As the patient tries to press on his/her belly, all he/she can do is extend the shoulder and the elbow moves backwards.

Figure 1.24 Belly-press test.

Pseudoparalysis

The term *pseudoparalysis* is used to describe those patients with such an extensive rotator cuff tear that they are unable to elevate the shoulder against gravity (pseudoparalysis in elevation), unable to externally rotate the shoulder against gravity (pseudoparalysis in external rotation), or both (combined pseudoparalysis) (Figure 1.26).

Instability

Translation of the humeral head on the glenoid occurs to some extent in all individuals. As described in detail in chapter 7 (Shoulder Instability and the Labrum), *laxity* is a term used to describe those individuals with larger translation excursions without symptoms, whereas instability is used for those individuals who complain of pain and/

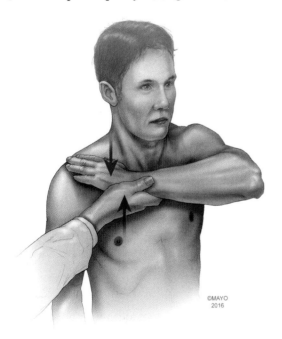

Figure 1.25 Bear-hug test.

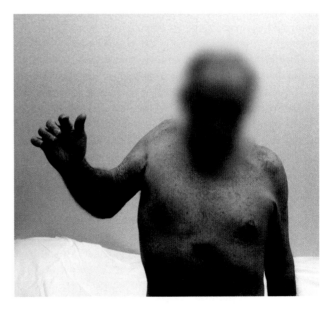

Figure 1.26 Massive cuff tears with or without arthropathy can result in pseudoparalysis.

or dysfunction with excessive translation, resulting in sub-luxation or dislocation. The examination of a complete anterior or posterior dislocation is reviewed in chapter 7, and will not be reviewed in this chapter.

There are a number of well-recognized patterns of insta-bility (anterior, posterior, and multidirectional). In most of them, there is structural pathology affecting the labrum and/or capsule, with or without bone involvement. Most tests for anterior and posterior instability stress the glenohumeral joint at the terminal range of motion; in those positions, the static stabilizers are tightened and, when intact, avoid excessive symptomatic translation. Tests that assess trans-lation in the resting position or the mid range of motion are more difficult to interpret, since in these positions normal shoulders with laxity will have a fair amount of translation; the distinction between laxity and instability can solely be made based on how translation correlates with symptoms.

Anterior Instability

Anterior instability occurs with excessive anteroinferior translation of the humeral head. This is best reproduced by placing the shoulder in abduction and external rota-tion. When any of the tests described later are performed, care must be taken to avoid fully dislocating the patient's shoulder in the office.

My preference is to examine for anterior instability with the patient lying supine and the side to be evaluated at the edge of the examining table. Three maneuvers are per-formed sequentially: apprehension, relocation, and release (Figure 1.27). For the apprehension maneuver, the shoulder is placed in combined abduction and external rotation until the patient complains that his or her shoulder is about to dislocate (apprehension test). This apprehension is con-firmed to disappear by displacing the humeral head poste-riorly with the hand of the examiner (relocation test), and confirmed again to create apprehension when the hand of the examiner is suddenly removed (release test).

Multiple authors have reported small variations of the apprehension test by adding an anteriorly directed force to the humerus (augmentation test) or the humeral head (crank test), or using the closed fist of the examiner as a fulcrum posteriorly (fulcrum test). The release test has also been named the surprise test by others. For extremely appre-hensive patients, it may be more useful to first place the shoulder in the relocation position and then perform the release test.

The hyperextension internal rotation (HERI) test is par-ticularly useful to demonstrate insufficiency of the inferior glenohumeral ligament without making the patient feel apprehensive (Figure 1.28). The nonaffected shoulder is placed in elevation to block trunk/spinal motion, and the affected shoulder is placed in as much passive extension as possible, keeping the shoulder in internal rotation. The amount of extension is compared with the opposite side. Insufficiency of the inferior glenohumeral ligament results

in approximately 15° of hyperextension compared with the opposite side (21).

Posterior Instability

Posterior instability occurs when the humeral head experi-ences excessive posterior translation, which is reproduced best by placing the shoulder in flexion (approximately 90°), adduction (approximately 30°), and internal rotation (Figure 1.29). In this position, adding a posteriorly directed force along the axis of the arm will provoke apprehension and may produce posterior subluxation of the humeral head over the glenoid rim (posterior apprehension test). The jerk test may then be perform by slowly extending the shoulder until a "jerk" is felt as the humeral head jumps over the glenoid rim to the reduced position. The Whipple test, described previously for supraspinatus assessment, will also exaggerate posterior subluxation in shoulders with posterior instability.

Multidirectional Instability and Generalized Ligamentous Laxity

Individuals with multidirectional instability (mid-range instability) experience symptoms secondary to abnormal excessive translation of the humeral head anteriorly, pos-teriorly, and inferiorly. Increased soft-tissue elasticity may be limited to the shoulder joint or may be associated with generalized ligamentous laxity. Translation of the humeral head on the glenoid is graded according to the terminol-ogy summarized in Table 1.5 (Figure 1.30). Instability is considered to be present when the tests described below reproduce the patient's symptoms, especially in patients with grade III translations.

Anterior and Posterior Drawer Tests

My preference is to perform these tests with the patient supine. For the posterior drawer, the shoulder is placed in 40° to 80° of abduction; the examiner holds the patient's wrist with 1 hand and uses the opposite hand to grab the humeral head, pushing the humeral head posteriorly with the thumb while feeling posterior translation with the fin-gers. The arm is extended at the same time. For the anterior drawer, the shoulder is placed in 40° to 80° of abduction, 20° of flexion, and neutral rotation. The examiner holds the patient's wrist with 1 hand and uses the other hand to translate the proximal third of the humeral shaft anteriorly. Grade II translation can be normal in many individuals, especially posteriorly; the key is to compare with the con-tralateral side. Grade III translation is more commonly an expression of true instability (11,22).

Load and Shift Test

Again, my preference is to perform this test in the supine position. The shoulder is placed in 40° to 60° of abduction, 20° of flexion, and neutral rotation with the back of the arm resting on the examiner's thigh. Axial load is applied to the

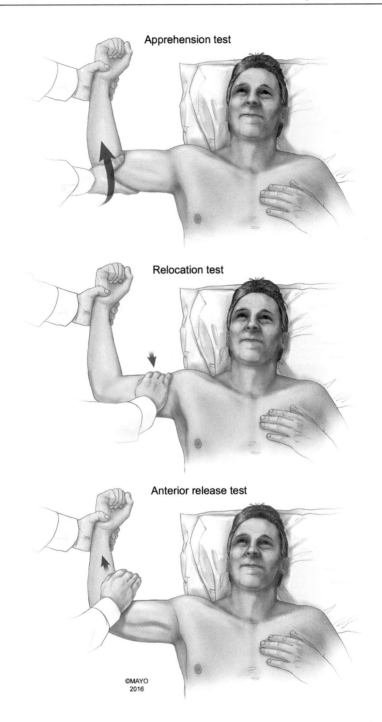

Figure 1.27 *Physical examination maneuvers for recurrent anterior glenohumeral instability.*

arm to "load" the joint and center the humeral head on the glenoid. While maintaining this load, the proximal third of the arm is shifted anteriorly and posteriorly, and translation is graded in each direction.

Inferior Sulcus

With the patient standing or sitting and the shoulder in the resting position, the examiner pulls straight down on the humerus to evaluate the distance between the acromion and the humeral head (Figure 1.31). A distance greater than 1.5 cm is accepted as consistent with inferior laxity; instability in the inferior direction requires a sulcus sign greater than 1.5 cm that replicates the patient's symptoms.

Generalized Ligamentous Laxity

Excessive arcs of motion in multiple joints have been postulated to be a risk factor for shoulder instability and for subsequent failure of surgical treatment, although this has

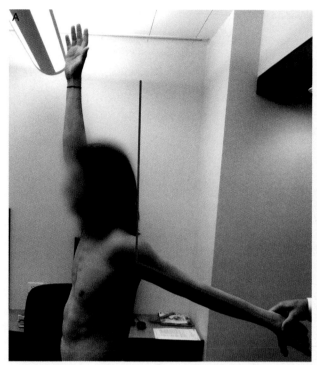
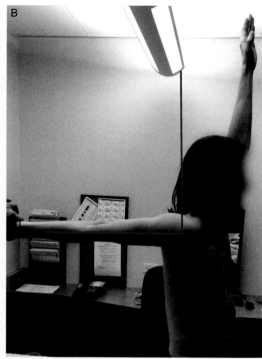

*Figure 1.28 HERI test. The nonaffected side (**A**) hyperextends much less than the affected side (**B**). HERI indicates hyperextension internal rotation.*

not been substantiated by data. Commonly used tests for generalized ligamentous laxity include hyperextension of the fingers parallel to the forearm, ability to place the thumb in the ipsilateral forearm, hyperextension of elbows or knees, and placement of the hands on the floor with the knees extended while standing. Some patients with generalized ligamentous laxity can be formally diagnosed with collagen disorders such as Ehlers-Danlos syndrome (see chapter 7, Shoulder Instability and the Labrum).

Table 1.5 • Glenohumeral Translation Grading (Laxity and Instability Testing)

Grade	Description	% Translation
0	Does not get to the rim	0%–25%
I	To the rim but not over	25%–50%
II	Over the rim, does not dislocate	>50%
III	Dislocates fully	. . .

Voluntary Instability

Some individuals are able to demonstrate their ability to voluntarily sublux their shoulder, most commonly posteriorly. By using specific patterns of muscle activation on a very lax joint, these patients can bring the humeral head to or over the glenoid rim. Most times, these voluntary subluxations are pain free, and patients have no real apprehension anteriorly or posteriorly. Rarely, voluntary instability becomes more symptomatic due to an additional injury or progressive soft-tissue stretching.

Superior Labral Tears

The term *superior labrum from anterior to posterior* (SLAP) tear refers to structural pathology at the superior labrum; it may contribute to instability or manifest itself only with pain with or without mechanical symptoms. Since the

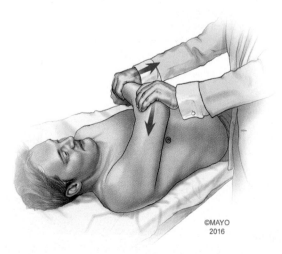

©MAYO
2016

Figure 1.29 Posterior apprehension test.

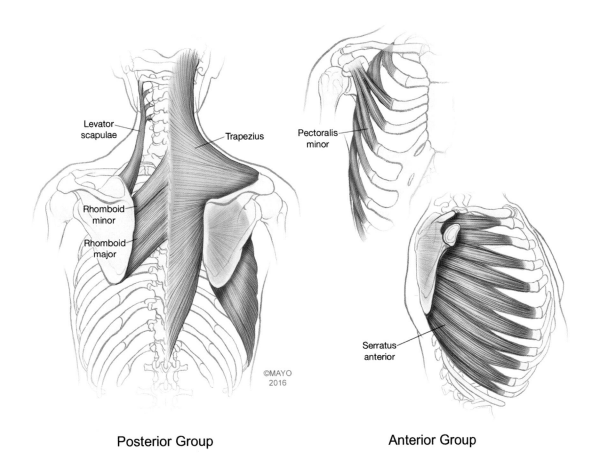

Posterior Group **Anterior Group**

Figure 1.34 *Main periscapular muscles.*

Table 1.6 • Motion of the Scapulothoracic Joint[a]

Motion	Joint Movement	Muscles Used
Adduction or approximation (retraction)	Medial border is brought closer to the midline in the horizontal plane	Middle trapezius Rhomboid major and minor
Abduction (protraction)	Medial border is brought away from the midline in the horizontal plane	Serratus anterior Pectoralis minor
Elevation	The scapula is raised straight up (shoulder shrug)	Upper trapezius Levator scapulae Rhomboid major and minor
Depression	The scapula is moved straight down	Lower trapezius Pectoralis minor Latissimus dorsi
Upward rotation	The scapula is abducted and rotated on the chest wall so that the inferior pole of the scapula is higher and more lateral; the scapula is also extended or tilted posteriorly	Upper and lower trapezius Serratus anterior (lower half)
Downward rotation	The scapula is adducted and rotated on the chest wall so that the inferior pole of the scapula is lower and more medial; the scapula is also flexed or tilted anteriorly	Rhomboid major and minor Levator scapulae Pectoralis minor
Anterior tilt	Forward movement of the superior and backward movement of the inferior scapula	Pectoralis minor
Posterior tilt	Backward movement of the superior and forward movement of the inferior scapula	Trapezius Serratus anterior

[a] Note that the term **lateral or external rotation** is used by some surgeons to define abduction and by others to refer to upward rotation; similarly, some surgeons use the term **medial or internal rotation** as a synonym of either adduction or downward rotation. The term **protraction** is used by some as equivalent to abduction + downward rotation + anterior tilt, while the term **retraction** would combine adduction + upward rotation + posterior tilt.

Table 1.7 • Main Muscles Involved in Scapulothoracic Motion

Muscle Group	Origin	Insertion	Innervation	Function
Posterior group				
Trapezius	Occipital protuberance + spinous processes C1-T12	Lateral clavicle, acromion, scapular spine	Spinal accessory (9th cranial) nerve C2-C4	Superior—elevation and lateral rotation Inferior—depression and lateral rotation Middle—adduction Posterior tilt
Rhomboid major	T2-T5	Medial scapular border below the spine of the scapula	Dorsal scapular nerve	Adduction Elevation Downward rotation Keeps scapula pressed against the thorax
Rhomboid minor	C7-T1, nuchal ligament	Medial scapular border at the level of the spine of the scapula		
Levator scapulae	Transverse processes C1-C4	Superior angle and medial border of the scapula proximal to the spine	C3-C4 and dorsal scapular nerve	Elevation Downward rotation
Anterior group				
Serratus anterior	Ribs 1 to 8 or 9	Anterior portion medial scapular border	Long thoracic nerve	Abduction Upward rotation Keeps scapula pressed against the thorax Posterior tilt
Pectoralis minor	Ribs 3 to 5	Coracoid process	Medial pectoral nerve	Abduction, depression and downward rotation Anterior tilt

a normal or abnormal position in the resting state?), analysis of the overall active motion of the scapula (are there abnormalities when the patient actively moves the shoulder?), changes in patient symptoms when scapular positioning is improved (is there less pain or more motion when the scapula is in a better place?), and specific testing of individual muscles. Since scapular dysfunction may also be secondary to abnormalities at the sternoclavicular joint, clavicle or acromioclavicular joint, or to brachial plexus dysfunction, these structures should be examined as well when evaluating the scapula.

Scapular Position

Scapular examination begins by assessing the resting position of the scapula in comparison with the normal side. The most common abnormal observation is scapular winging (*scapula alata*), which indicates a change in the position of the scapula best appreciated as prominence of the medial border (25).

Severe scapular winging is almost always due to a neuromuscular abnormality, such as injury to the spinal accessory nerve or long thoracic nerve, fascioscapulohumeral dystrophy, congenital absence of the trapezius or other muscles, or a brachial plexus injury (Figure 1.35). Injury to the spinal accessory nerve with trapezius dysfunction results in the unopposed lateral translation of the

prominent medial border of the scapula, most often by the serratus, whereas injury to the long thoracic nerve results in marked prominence of the medial border of the scapula, most often by the trapezius and rhomboids. Bilateral symmetric winging is the hallmark of fascioscapulohumeral dystrophy.

Less obvious alterations of scapular position at rest may accompany acromioclavicular joint separations, clavicle fractures, nonunions or malunions, or represent a poor functional response of the periscapular muscles to chronic shoulder pain or to alterations in any element of the kinetic chain (26). The most common findings in these circumstances are generalized periscapular pain and neck pain, prominence of the inferomedial border of the scapula, and coracoid malpositioning. A measuring tape can be used to determine the distance between the midline and the medial border, superior angle, and inferior angle of the scapular body in the resting position compared with the opposite side.

Scapular Motion, Dyskinesis, and Snapping

Dynamic evaluation of scapular motion is usually performed by observing the medial border of the scapula as the patient performs active elevation and descent. Both shoulders and the back of the patient need to be uncovered. The examiner compares both scapulae as the patient

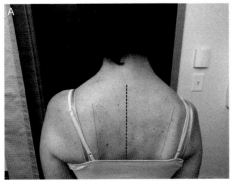 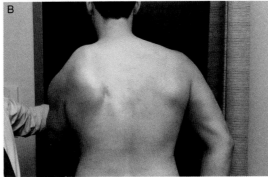 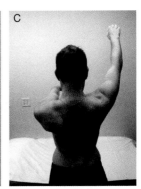

Figure 1.35 A, *Scapular winging secondary to trapezius palsy; note lateral positioning of the right scapula with a stretched atrophic trapezius mass.* **B,** *Scapular winging secondary to dysfunction of the serratus anterior, lifting the medial border of the scapula off the chest wall.* **C,** *Scapular winging secondary to fascioscapulohumeral dystrophy, before surgery on the left and after surgery on the right.*

is requested to bring both shoulders to maximum elevation and back to the starting position. This motion sequence is repeated 3 to 5 times and the patient may be asked to perform the exercise with 3 to 5 pounds of weight in each hand if needed. Prominence of any aspect of the medial scapular border on the symptomatic side is indicative of scapular dyskinesis (26–28). Three patterns of abnormal scapular motion have been described in patients with scapular dyskinesis (Table 1.8).

The acronym SICK scapula has been coined to refer to a relatively common combination of *S*capular malposition at rest, prominence of the *I*nferior medial border of the scapula, *C*oracoid malpositioning with pain, and scapular dys*K*inesis. In some patients, the main complaint will be the presence of palpable or audible noise (crepitus) with active scapulothoracic motion; the term *scapular snapping* is used in these circumstances (29). Snapping of the scapula may or may not be associated with pain or dyskinesis.

Specific Muscle Testing

Once the presence of scapular dyskinesia has been established, the next question is to determine the reasons why. In some circumstances, the cause may be obvious (e.g., clavicle malunion, known iatrogenic injury to the spinal accessory nerve secondary to nerve section). Specific muscle testing helps in establishing a specific diagnosis (25).

Serratus Anterior

Winging secondary to weakness or paralysis of the serratus anterior is accentuated by attempting to perform a push-up on a wall (Figure 1.36A), active elevation, or active forward flexion (Figure 1.36B). The patient may also be asked to place the shoulder in the position of a boxing punch (Figure 1.37); the examiner can then determine whether the patient can resist retraction by grabbing the patient's shoulder and pulling backward.

Trapezius

Winging secondary to weakness or paralysis of the trapezius is accentuated with resisted abduction and also with resisted external rotation (scapular flip sign; Figure 1.38). The scapula is positioned extremely laterally in the resting position and becomes even more lateral with resisted abduction. In some patients with compensatory scapular dyskinesis, there may be differential contracture and weakness of the various portions of the trapezius. Weakness of the superior trapezius is best assessed by asking the patient to shrug the shoulders against resistance. Weakness of the middle trapezius is assessed by asking the patient to approximate the scapula to the midline.

Rhomboids and Levator Scapulae

These muscles are difficult to test because an intact trapezius, which completely covers these muscles, may

Table 1.8 • Types of Scapular Dyskinesis

	At Rest	**With Active Elevation**	**Proposed Structural Pathology**
Type I	Prominence inferior angle scapula	Anterior scapular tilt	Pectoralis minor contracture
Type II	Prominence medial border scapula	Increased dorsal tilt	Weakness of the middle portion of the trapezius, rhomboids, and serratus anterior
Type III	Scapula resting high with a prominent superior border	Abnormally accentuated shrug	Superior trapezius hyperactivity or contracture + inferior trapezius weakness

A

B

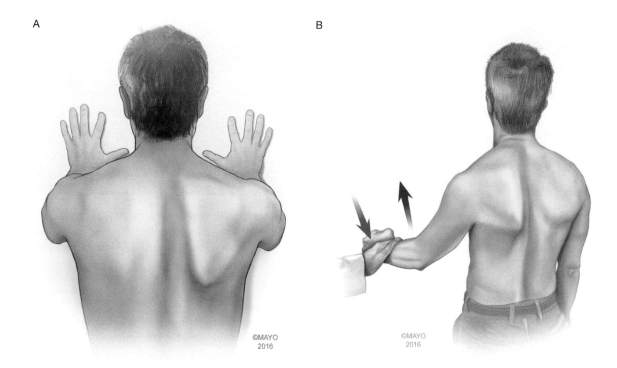

Figure 1.36 A, *Serratus anterior dysfunction can be unmasked by noticing winging when performing a push-up on a wall.* **B,** *Winging also increases with resisted flexion at 45°.*

compensate for their weak function. Rhomboid weakness may lead to a slightly more lateral position of the scapula at rest and subtle winging. Difficulty with scapular approximation to the midline in a patient with completely normal contour of the superior trapezius and a strong shrug is the best indicator of rhomboid weakness.

Pectoralis Minor
Contracture and shortening of the pectoralis minor have been proposed to play an important role in type I scapular dyskinesis, especially in throwers. Palpation of a cordlike pectoralis minor may be attempted, but it is difficult to achieve. The patient may also be placed with the back

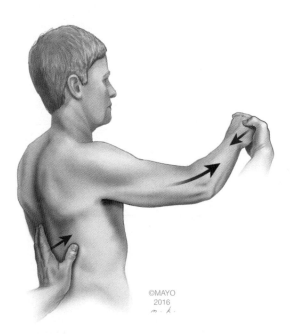

Figure 1.37 *The boxer punch test will also unmask serratus anterior weakness.*

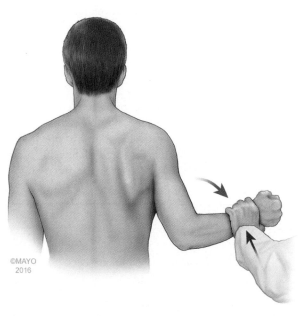

Figure 1.38 *The scapular flip sign demonstrates increased winging with resisted external rotation in abduction in patients with trapezius palsy.*

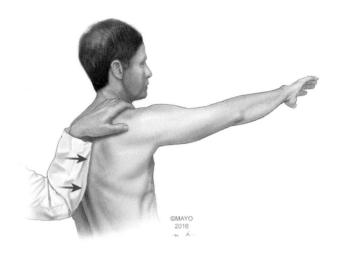

Figure 1.39 *The scapular assistance test.*

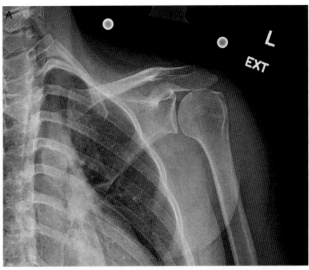

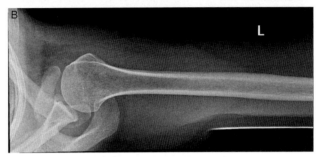

Figure 1.40 *Anteroposterior radiograph in the plane of the scapula* **(A)** *and axillary projection* **(B)**.

resting on a wall, and the distance between the wall and the tip of the coracoid can be measured and compared with the opposite side.

Scapular Assistance and Retraction Tests

A final goal of evaluating the scapula consists in determining whether improved scapular positioning would alleviate the patient's symptoms. This is especially useful in patients with palsies, instability, labral pathology, and impingement (26,30).

Scapular Assistance Test

The examiner stands behind the patient and uses his or her hand and forearm to compress the medial border of the scapula against the chest wall and tilt the scapula posteriorly (Figure 1.39). It is considered positive if patients achieve higher active elevation and/or if pain improves.

Scapular Retraction Test

The examiner instructs the patient to retract the scapula and helps keep the scapula in the retracted position. Supraspinatus and labral testing are repeated before and after scapular retraction to determine if scapular dyskinesis may be contributing to the patient's symptoms. When that is the case, patients have better strength with the empty can test and the dynamic labral shear test becomes negative, respectively.

Imaging Studies

Radiographs and Fluoroscopy

Plain radiographs should be obtained in all patients presenting for evaluation of the shoulder. The 2 basic projections include an anteroposterior radiograph in the plane of the scapula with the arm in external rotation and an axillary radiograph (Figure 1.40). Anteroposterior radiographs are obtained in the plane of the scapula in order to avoid overlapping of the humeral head with the glenoid; the opposite side of the trunk is tilted forward 30° so that the radiographic beam is perpendicular to the glenohumeral joint line. Throughout this book I will mention other radiographic projections of value for specific conditions. Fluoroscopy is mostly used for certain surgical procedures, most commonly internal fixation of proximal humerus fractures. It also can be considered to position radiographs so that the radiographic beam is perfectly perpendicular to the bone–implant interface when assessing arthroplasty components (fluoroscopically positioned patients).

Magnetic Resonance Imaging

Magnetic resonance imaging (MRI) has become 1 of the most useful tools for evaluation of the shoulder joint. As technology continues to advance, MRI will continue to improve. As a shoulder surgeon, it is important to 1) have a general understanding of the basic science of MRI, 2) learn how to read MRIs (through practice, interaction with radiologists, and correlation with surgical findings), and 3) understand that abnormalities on MRI do not always mean symptomatic structural changes.

MRI Acquisition and Processing

Pulse sequences are waveforms of the radiofrequency pulses and gradients applied during MRI acquisition. This is a vast and complicated subject and I will provide a very brief overview to facilitate communication with your radiology partners.

The quality of the images will depend on the quality of the equipment used (mostly the power of the magnetic field, measured in tesla units) and the sequences used. There are only 2 fundamental types of pulse sequences: spin echo (SE) and gradient echo (GRE). SE sequences use a radiofrequency pulse for rephasing; they take longer to acquire but are very efficient in reducing magnetic inhomogeneity, providing true T2 weighting. Variations of SE sequences include fast or turbo SE, conventional inversion recovery, STIR (short T1 inversion recovery), and FLAIR (fluid-attenuated inversion recovery). GRE sequences use a variation of gradients for rephasing, which provides images faster but does not provide true T2 weighting. GRE sequences can be partially refocused, fully refocused, or spoiled. Echo-planar imaging may be applied to either SE or GRE sequences to shorten acquisition time. Fat saturation techniques may be used to null the signal from fat so that the signal from other tissues is more conspicuous.

Echo time (TE) is the time between application of a pulse and acquisition of the maximum echo. Repetition time (TR) is the time in between pulses. T1-weighted images are obtained with short TE and TR. T2-weighted images are obtained with long TE and TR. Proton-density images are obtained with short TE and long TR. The T2-weighted images obtained with GRE sequences are not true T2, and by convention are named T2*. To distinguish tissues on MRI, contrast is required. Contrast is due to differences in signal.

The higher the signal, the brighter the image. Different tissues will provide different signals in T1, T2, and proton density images. Bone, cartilage, muscle, tendon, fat, nerves, vessels, fluid, and other structures can be distinguished accordingly. Contrast can also be obtained by use of solutions of chelated organic gadolinium (gadolinium contrast) that may be injected intra-articularly (magnetic resonance arthrogram) or administered intravenously.

Shoulder MRI

Many MRI protocols are acceptable to evaluate the shoulder joint. A commonly used protocol is a fast-spin echo in the oblique coronal plane using T1-weighted sequences and T2-weighted sequences with fat suppression. Images are provided in 3 planes: oblique coronal, axial, and oblique sagittal. Use of a 3-part Tesla coil, thin slices (≤3 mm), and a small field of view (16–20 cm) provide very detailed, high-quality images (31–33).

Rotator Cuff

Normal cuff tendons typically present with uniformly low signal (dark) on all pulse sequences. However, increased signal can be seen in some normal shoulders at the end of the supraspinatus tendon in T1-weighted images. On the contrary, bright signal in T2-weighted images is abnormal and typically indicates fiber rupture (or partial-thickness tear). In full-thickness tears, fluid accumulated at the tear is seen as bright signal in T2-weighted images (Figure 1.41).

As mentioned in chapter 6 (The Rotator Cuff and Biceps Tendon), muscular atrophy and fatty infiltration are considered good predictors of outcome after rotator cuff repair; these are best assessed in the T1-weighted oblique sagittal view (Figure 1.42). Isolated atrophy of the infraspinatus

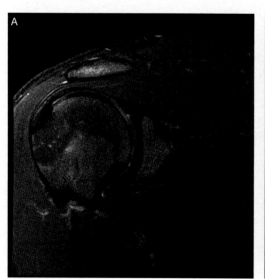
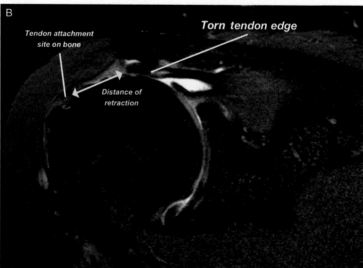

Figure 1.41 *Magnetic resonance image of a normal supraspinatus tendon* (**A**) *and a supraspinatus tendon full-thickness tear* (**B**).

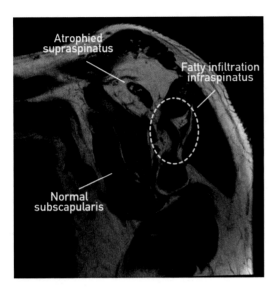

Figure 1.42 Muscle atrophy and fatty infiltration are important predictors of success after rotator cuff repair. They are typically assessed in T1-weighted parasagittal MRI. The cross-section of the supraspinatus is very small in size (atrophy). In addition, there is more fat than muscle inside the infraspinatus outline (fatty infiltration). MRI indicates magnetic resonance imaging.

muscle should prompt assessing for suprascapular nerve entrapment in the spinoglenoid notch or an isolated infraspinatus rupture at the myotendinous junction. Isolated atrophy of the teres minor may be seen in the so-called quadrilateral space syndrome (i.e., axillary nerve compression between teres major and minor, triceps, and humeral shaft).

Labrum
The normal labrum is a triangular-shaped, low-signal structure. The anterior and posterior portions of the labrum are best visualized in axial images, whereas the superior labrum is assessed in oblique coronal images. When there is a labral tear, fluid is seen as a bright line between the labrum and the glenoid rim (Figure 1.43); the labrum may also appear displaced or truncated. As mentioned in chapter 7 (Shoulder Instability and the Labrum), there are a number of anatomical variations that can be confused with true labral tears (e.g., sublabral foramen and Buford complex). Labral tears may facilitate development of paralabral cysts, seen as bright collections of fluid at the posterior or superior aspect of the glenoid on T2-weighted images.

Biceps Tendon
The biceps tendon is best visualized in axial images as a round, low-signal structure in the bicipital groove (Figure 1.44). If no round structure is visualized, the tendon may be ruptured or dislocated. A small amount of fluid around the biceps in the T2 sequences is normal. Larger amounts of fluid and signal changes within

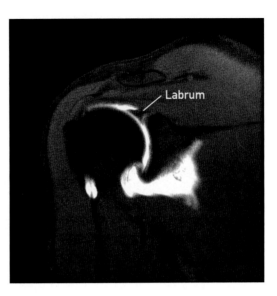

Figure 1.43 Superior labral tear seen on MRI as contrast leaking between labrum and superior glenoid. MRI indicates magnetic resonance imaging.

the tendon may indicate tenosynovitis and tendinopathy, respectively.

Cartilage and Bone
Cartilage is best visualized in proton density images with fat suppression as a gray band of tissue between dark subchondral bone and bright fluid. Cartilage thinning or areas of full-thickness cartilage absence may be visualized. Bone abnormalities most commonly identified on shoulder MRI include an *os acromiale* if present, increased signal change

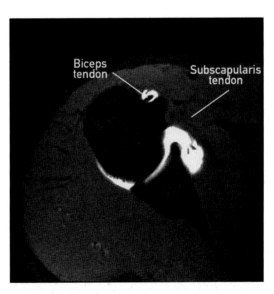

Figure 1.44 Axial MRI cuts show the tendon of the long head of the biceps as a round structure in cross-section. MRI indicates magnetic resonance imaging.

at the acromioclavicular joint in patients with arthritis or osteolysis, intraosseous cysts in patients with cuff disease (greater tuberosity) or arthritis (glenoid), increased intraosseous signal in T2-weighted images in avascular necrosis or after a recent injury (bone contusion), and a posterosuperior impaction defect (Hill-Sachs lesion) in patients with anterior shoulder instability.

Computed Tomography

Computed tomography (CT) uses computer-processed combinations of many radiographs taken from different angles to produce cross-sectional (tomographic) images or virtual slices. CT images are combinations of pixels. A pixel is a 2-dimensional unit with shades of gray proportional to the relative radiodensity or mean attenuation of tissues, measured using the Hounsfield scale (from −1,024 least attenuating to +3,071 most attenuating units). Because of the high dynamic range of the Hounsfield scale, CT datasets need to be reduced for displaying. This is accomplished by "windowing," which maps a range (i.e., the window) of pixel values to a grayscale ramp. Shoulder CT scans are typically visualized using a bone window and a soft-tissue window. CT scan data may be processed further to create 3-dimensional reconstructions, which are achieved by either multiplanar reconstruction or 3-dimensional rendering. Iodinated contrast solutions may be injected in the joint if needed (CT arthrogram).

CT is most commonly used for imaging of traumatic injuries. In my practice, it is commonly used to assess proximal humerus fractures and fractures of the glenoid or other parts of the scapula. It is also very useful to determine bone loss on the anterior rim of the glenoid in patients with recurrent anterior instability (chapter 7, Shoulder Instability and the Labrum). CT arthrograms are a good alternative to evaluate the rotator cuff and labrum when MRI is contraindicated or when metal artifact makes MRI impractical (such as for the evaluation of a painful shoulder arthroplasty) (34). However, ultrasonography is becoming more popular as an alternative to both MRI and CT to assess the soft tissues of the shoulder. Three-dimensional printing of models based on CT data sets is growing in popularity to understand complex deformities and create patient-specific instrumentations.

Ultrasonography

Ultrasonography involves the use of a transducer and transmits high-frequency sound waves into the body through a gel applied on the skin. The transducer also collects the sound waves as they bounce back, and computer processing is used to create an image. Conventional ultrasonography displays the images in thin, flat sections of the body in a gray scale. Doppler ultrasonography evaluates flow through blood vessels. Three-dimensional ultrasonography

formats the sound wave data into 3-dimensional images. Major benefits of ultrasonography include lack of radiation, ease of comparison with the contralateral side, and the possibility of evaluating structures dynamically (i.e., structures may be followed through a long course or assessed while in motion). The main disadvantages include poor evaluation of bone and dependence on the operator's experience.

The use of ultrasonography in the field of shoulder surgery will continue to grow over time (35). Interestingly, shoulder surgeons are learning how to perform ultrasonography in the office without the assistance of a radiologist or technician, which represents a departure compared with other advanced imaging studies. Ultrasonography is most commonly used to assess the rotator cuff and biceps tendon, identify abnormal collections of fluid, and guide needle placement for injections.

Electromyogram and Nerve Conduction Studies

Muscle and nerve abnormalities are a very common source of symptoms around the shoulder. The axillary nerve is particularly prone to injury with proximal humerus fractures or dislocation, as well as complex surgical procedures. Scapular dysfunction is not uncommonly due to nerve injuries. In addition, cervical radiculopathy is a relatively common reason for referred shoulder pain. For all these reasons, electromyography (EMG) and nerve conduction studies (NCSs) are useful tests in shoulder surgery.

EMG records the electrical potential generated by muscle cells. Muscle electrical activity may be recorded using either a surface electrode or inserting a needle intramuscularly; surface EMG provides a more limited assessment. Muscle electrical activity may be recorded at rest, with active muscle contraction, or as a response to electrical stimulation of the corresponding nerve (motor NCSs). Sensory NCSs are performed by electrical stimulation of a peripheral nerve and recording from a purely sensory portion of the nerve, such as on a finger.

Interpretation of EMG and motor and sensory NCSs is best performed with the assistance of a clinical electrophysiologist or a neurologist. Parameters commonly assessed on EMG include insertional activity (electrical activity present as the electrode is inserted into the muscle cells), spontaneous activity at rest (normal muscle should be silent after the needle is inserted), and voluntary muscle recruitment. Parameters commonly assessed in NCSs include motor and sensory conduction velocity (proportional to myelination), amplitude (proportional to axon number or loss), late responses (F waves for polyneuropathies and H reflexes for radiculopathies), and small fiber activity (for chronic regional pain syndrome).

There are 5 key questions to answer and discuss when you receive the EMG and NCS reports: Is there evidence of radiculopathy, neuropathy, nerve injury, or a primary muscle disease? What is the location of the change(s)? Is the process active? What is the severity of the process? and Is there any evidence of reinnervation?

When ordering EMG and NCS, it is important to provide accurate information about the clinical working diagnosis. Standard protocols may not routinely assess the suprascapular nerve or other periscapular nerves. It is also important to understand that EMG and NCS changes do not appear right away after a nerve injury. Abnormal spontaneous activity is typically not seen until week 2, 3, or 4 after nerve injury, and evidence of reinnervation is not seen until week 5 or 6. The diagnostic value of both EMG and NCS depends on the accuracy of needle placement, among other factors. This can be a particular challenge when evaluating

atrophied periscapular muscles, where the muscle thickness may be decreased to the point that it is not possible to insert the needle in the muscle of interest, providing false-negative results.

Diagnostic Injections

Injections of a local anesthetic with or without corticosteroids are very commonly used for the diagnosis and treatment of multiple shoulder conditions. Chapter 12 (Rehabilitation and Injections) provides a review of the indications and methods to perform various injections. Insertion of the needle can be performed based on superficial anatomical landmarks or guided with ultrasonography or fluoroscopy. Areas most commonly injected for diagnostic purposes include the subacromial space, bicipital

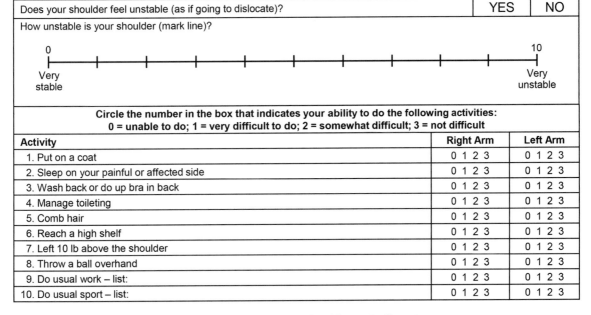

ASES SCORING SYSTEM

Are you having pain in your shoulder?	YES	NO
Do you have pain in your shoulder at night?	YES	NO
Do you take pain medication (aspirin, Tylenol, Advil, etc…)?	YES	NO
Do you take narcotic pain medication (codeine or stronger)?	YES	NO
How many pills do you take each day (average)?	____ pills	

How bad is your pain today (mark line)?

0   10

No pain at all   Pain as bad as it can be

Does your shoulder feel unstable (as if going to dislocate)?	YES	NO

How unstable is your shoulder (mark line)?

0   10

Very stable   Very unstable

Circle the number in the box that indicates your ability to do the following activities:
0 = unable to do; 1 = very difficult to do; 2 = somewhat difficult; 3 = not difficult

Activity	Right Arm	Left Arm
1. Put on a coat	0 1 2 3	0 1 2 3
2. Sleep on your painful or affected side	0 1 2 3	0 1 2 3
3. Wash back or do up bra in back	0 1 2 3	0 1 2 3
4. Manage toileting	0 1 2 3	0 1 2 3
5. Comb hair	0 1 2 3	0 1 2 3
6. Reach a high shelf	0 1 2 3	0 1 2 3
7. Left 10 lb above the shoulder	0 1 2 3	0 1 2 3
8. Throw a ball overhand	0 1 2 3	0 1 2 3
9. Do usual work – list:	0 1 2 3	0 1 2 3
10. Do usual sport – list:	0 1 2 3	0 1 2 3

Figure 1.45 *ASES Shoulder Score. ASES indicates American Shoulder and Elbow Surgeons.*
(Adapted from Michener LA, McClure PW, Sennett BJ. American Shoulder and Elbow Surgeons Standardized Shoulder Assessment Form, patient self-report section: reliability, validity, and responsiveness. J Shoulder Elbow Surg. 2002 Nov-Dec;11[6]:587–94. Used with permission.)

groove, glenohumeral joint, acromioclavicular joint, and suprascapular nerve.

Outcome Tools

Outcome tools are instruments used to determine the severity of conditions and monitor improvement or worsening over time, especially after an intervention. They are also of interest for research, in order to compare different studies. Some outcome tools are based entirely on questions answered by the patient (patient-reported outcome tools), and some require a combination of questions to the patient and assessment by the heath care provider. There are multiple outcome tools used in the field of shoulder surgery. I summarize the ones I find more useful in my clinical practice in the sections that follow.

Subjective Shoulder Value

The subjective shoulder value (SSV) was developed in an effort to provide a simple score reflecting the patient's view of his/her own shoulder in a precise manner (1). The SSV is an example of a single assessment numeric evaluation, or SANE. The SSV is determined entirely subjectively by each patient, who answers the following question: "What is the overall percent value of your shoulder if a completely normal shoulder represents 100%?"; if the patient is unclear, a follow-up question is used: "A completely normal shoulder would cost you 1,000 dollars; how much would you be willing to pay for yours?" This outcome tool has been reported to be valid and useful in various shoulder conditions, including rotator cuff tear, instability, and arthritis (1).

American Shoulder and Elbow Surgeons Score

The American Shoulder and Elbow Surgeons official shoulder score is calculated by adding up to 50 points based on the patient's subjective quantification of pain and up to 50 points based on the ability to perform various activities of daily living (Figure 1.45) (3).

Constant-Murley Score

The Constant-Murley score (4), endorsed by the European Society for Surgery of the Shoulder and the Elbow, provides assessment value based on the patient's subjective assessment of pain (15% of the score), activities of daily living (20%), a physician's evaluation of range of motion (40%), and instrumented measurement of strength in abduction (25%) (Table 1.9). It can be reported as an absolute number (absolute Constant score or C_{abs}) or adjusted by age (adjusted Constant score or C_{adj}). One of the major problems for the practical use of this score is related to difficulties in measuring strength due to lack of equipment or time constraints.

Table 1.9 • Constant-Murley Score

Criteria	Points
Pain	
None	15
Mild	10
Moderate	5
Severe	0
Activities of daily living	
Activity level (10 points possible)	
Full work	4
Full recreation/sport	4
Unaffected sleep	2
Positioning (10 points possible)	
Up to waist	2
Up to xiphoid	4
Up to neck	6
Up to top of head	8
Above head	10
Total	20
Range of motion	40
Power (1 point per pound of weight held in abduction by arm at 90°)	25
Total	100

Oxford Shoulder Score

This score has been very well developed and validated (2). It is simple enough for easy implementation into clinical practice and is completely based on answers provided by the patient (Figure 1.46).

KEY POINTS

✓ Always examine the shoulder joint uncovered; compare both sides and include the scapula and periscapular region in your examination.

✓ Be accurate and use the correct terminology when evaluating and recording shoulder motion and strength.

✓ Arthritic pain is typically present on the posterior aspect of the glenohumeral joint and aggravated by shearing the articular surface with resisted motion.

✓ Most physical examination maneuvers have not been critically analyzed for sensitivity, specificity, or predictive values.

✓ Patients suspected of having rotator cuff pathology should be examined for impingement, symptomatic acromioclavicular joint arthritis, associated biceps pathology, strength, and lag signs.

✓ Laxity and instability are different; always correlate the outcome of physical examination tests for anterior, posterior, and multidirectional instability with the patient's symptoms.

Problems with your shoulder during the past 4 weeks...
✓ Tick ONE box for each question

How would you describe the *worst* pain you had from your shoulder?				
None ☐	Mild ☐	Moderate ☐	Severe ☐	Unbearable ☐

Have you had any trouble dressing yourself because of your shoulder?				
No trouble at all ☐	A little bit of trouble ☐	Moderate trouble ☐	Extreme difficulty ☐	Impossible to do ☐

Have you had any trouble getting in and out of the car or using public transport because of your shoulder?				
No trouble at all ☐	A little bit of trouble ☐	Moderate trouble ☐	Extreme difficulty ☐	Impossible to do ☐

Have you been able to use a knife and fork at the same time?				
Yes, easily ☐	With little difficulty ☐	With moderate difficulty ☐	With extreme difficulty ☐	No, impossible ☐

Could you do the household shopping on your own?				
Yes, easily ☐	With little difficulty ☐	With moderate difficulty ☐	With extreme difficulty ☐	No, impossible ☐

Could you carry a tray containing a plate of food?				
Yes, easily ☐	With little difficulty ☐	With moderate difficulty ☐	With extreme difficulty ☐	No, impossible ☐

Could you brush/comb your hair with the affected arm?				
Yes, easily ☐	With little difficulty ☐	With moderate difficulty ☐	With extreme difficulty ☐	No, impossible ☐

How would you describe the pain you *usually* had from your shoulder?				
None ☐	Very mild ☐	Mild ☐	Moderate ☐	Severe ☐

Could you hang your clothes up in a wardrobe using the affected arm?				
Yes, easily ☐	With little difficulty ☐	With moderate difficulty ☐	With extreme difficulty ☐	No, impossible ☐

Have you been able to wash and dry yourself under both arms?				
Yes, easily ☐	With little difficulty ☐	With moderate difficulty ☐	With extreme difficulty ☐	No, impossible ☐

How much has pain from your shoulder interfered with your usual work (including housework)?				
Not at all ☐	A little bit ☐	Moderately ☐	Greatly ☐	Totally ☐

Have you been troubled by pain from your shoulder in bed at night?				
No nights ☐	Only 1 or 2 nights ☐	Some nights ☐	Most nights ☐	Every night ☐

Figure 1.46 *Oxford Shoulder Score.*
(Adapted from Olley LM, Carr AJ. The use of a patient-based questionnaire [the Oxford Shoulder Score] to assess outcome after rotator cuff repair. Ann R Coll Surg Engl. 2008 May;90[4]:326–31. Used with permission.)

✓ The diagnosis of symptomatic superior labral tears is based on specific tests correlated with the results of imaging studies.

✓ Severe scapular winging typically is secondary to specific neurologic injuries; scapular dyskinesis may also contribute to the clinical presentation of impingement, instability, cuff disease, and labral tears.

✓ Plain radiographs should be obtained and carefully analyzed in all patients presenting for shoulder evaluation.

✓ Evaluation of the soft tissues of the shoulder is best performed with T2-weighted magnetic resonance images or ultrasonography; magnetic resonance tends to overdiagnose structural pathology.

✓ Computed tomography is very helpful to evaluate fractures, bone loss, and when there are contraindications for magnetic resonance.

✓ Diagnostic injections are extremely useful in selected patients.

✓ It is recommended to incorporate one or more outcome tools to a modern shoulder practice.

Acknowledgments

Portions previously published in Villafane JH, Valdes K, Anselmi F, Pirali C, Negrini S. The diagnostic accuracy of five tests for diagnosing partial-thickness tears of the supraspinatus tendon: a cohort study. J Hand Ther.

2015 Jul-Sep;28(3):247–51. Epub 2015 Feb 19; Ben Kibler et al. (10); Walton et al. (13); and Barth et al. (20). Used with permission.

REFERENCES

1. Gilbart MK, Gerber C. Comparison of the subjective shoulder value and the Constant score. J Shoulder Elbow Surg. 2007 Nov-Dec;16(6):717–21.
2. Dawson J, Fitzpatrick R, Carr A. Questionnaire on the perceptions of patients about shoulder surgery. J Bone Joint Surg Br. 1996 Jul;78(4):593–600.
3. Richards RR, An KN, Bigliani LU, Friedman RJ, Gartsman GM, Gristina AG, et al. A standardized method for the assessment of shoulder function. J Shoulder Elbow Surg. 1994 Nov;3(6):347–52. Epub 2009 Feb 13.
4. Constant CR, Murley AH. A clinical method of functional assessment of the shoulder. Clin Orthop Relat Res. 1987 Jan;(214):160–4.
5. McFarland EG. Examination of the shoulder: the complete guide. New York (NY): Thieme Medical Publishers; c2006. 282 p.
6. Barnes CJ, Van Steyn SJ, Fischer RA. The effects of age, sex, and shoulder dominance on range of motion of the shoulder. J Shoulder Elbow Surg. 2001 May-Jun;10(3):242–6.
7. Giphart JE, Brunkhorst JP, Horn NH, Shelburne KB, Torry MR, Millett PJ. Effect of plane of arm elevation on glenohumeral kinematics: a normative biplane fluoroscopy study. J Bone Joint Surg Am. 2013 Feb 6;95(3):238–45.
8. Edwards TB, Bostick RD, Greene CC, Baratta RV, Drez D. Interobserver and intraobserver reliability of the measurement of shoulder internal rotation by vertebral level. J Shoulder Elbow Surg. 2002 Jan-Feb;11(1):40–2.
9. Park HB, Yokota A, Gill HS, El Rassi G, McFarland EG. Diagnostic accuracy of clinical tests for the different degrees of subacromial impingement syndrome. J Bone Joint Surg Am. 2005 Jul;87(7):1446–55.
10. Ben Kibler W, Sciascia AD, Hester P, Dome D, Jacobs C. Clinical utility of traditional and new tests in the diagnosis of biceps tendon injuries and superior labrum anterior and posterior lesions in the shoulder. Am J Sports Med. 2009 Sep;37(9):1840–7. Epub 2009 Jun 9.
11. Jia X, Petersen SA, Khosravi AH, Almareddi V, Pannirselvam V, McFarland EG. Examination of the shoulder: the past, the present, and the future. J Bone Joint Surg Am. 2009 Nov;91 Suppl 6:10–8.
12. King JJ, Wright TW. Physical examination of the shoulder. J Hand Surg Am. 2014 Oct;39(10):2103–12.
13. Walton J, Mahajan S, Paxinos A, Marshall J, Bryant C, Shnier R, et al. Diagnostic values of tests for acromioclavicular joint pain. J Bone Joint Surg Am. 2004 Apr;86–A(4):807–12.
14. Chronopoulos E, Kim TK, Park HB, Ashenbrenner D, McFarland EG. Diagnostic value of physical tests for isolated chronic acromioclavicular lesions. Am J Sports Med. 2004 Apr-May;32(3):655–61.
15. Itoi E, Kido T, Sano A, Urayama M, Sato K. Which is more useful, the "full can test" or the "empty can test," in detecting the torn supraspinatus tendon? Am J Sports Med. 1999 Jan-Feb;27(1):65–8.
16. Hertel R, Ballmer FT, Lombert SM, Gerber C. Lag signs in the diagnosis of rotator cuff rupture. J Shoulder Elbow Surg. 1996 Jul-Aug;5(4):307–13.
17. Walch G, Boulahia A, Calderone S, Robinson AH. The 'dropping' and 'hornblower's' signs in evaluation of rotator-cuff tears. J Bone Joint Surg Br. 1998 Jul;80(4):624–8.
18. Gerber C, Krushell RJ. Isolated rupture of the tendon of the subscapularis muscle: clinical features in 16 cases. J Bone Joint Surg Br. 1991 May;73(3):389–94.
19. Tokish JM, Decker MJ, Ellis HB, Torry MR, Hawkins RJ. The belly-press test for the physical examination of the subscapularis muscle: electromyographic validation and comparison to the lift-off test. J Shoulder Elbow Surg. 2003 Sep-Oct;12(5):427–30.
20. Barth JR, Burkhart SS, De Beer JF. The bear-hug test: a new and sensitive test for diagnosing a subscapularis tear. Arthroscopy. 2006 Oct;22(10):1076–84.
21. Lafosse T, Fogerty S, Idoine J, Gobezie R, Lafosse L. Hyper extension-internal rotation (HERI): a new test for anterior gleno-humeral instability. Orthop Traumatol Surg Res. 2016 Feb;102(1):3–12.
22. Gerber C, Ganz R. Clinical assessment of instability of the shoulder. With special reference to anterior and posterior drawer tests. J Bone Joint Surg Br. 1984 Aug;66(4):551–6.
23. O'Brien SJ, Pagnani MJ, Fealy S, McGlynn SR, Wilson JB. The active compression test: a new and effective test for diagnosing labral tears and acromioclavicular joint abnormality. Am J Sports Med. 1998 Sep-Oct;26(5):610–3.
24. O'Driscoll SW. Regarding "Diagnostic accuracy of five orthopedic clinical tests for diagnosis of superior labrum anterior posterior (SLAP) lesions." J Shoulder Elbow Surg. 2012 Dec;21(12):e23–4. Epub 2012 Oct 26.
25. Srikumaran U, Wells JH, Freehill MT, Tan EW, Higgins LD, Warner JJ. Scapular winging: a great masquerader of shoulder disorders: AAOS exhibit selection. J Bone Joint Surg Am. 2014 Jul 16;96(14):e122. [Epub ahead of print]
26. Kibler WB, Sciascia A, Wilkes T. Scapular dyskinesis and its relation to shoulder injury. J Am Acad Orthop Surg. 2012 Jun;20(6):364–72.
27. Pluim BM. Scapular dyskinesis: practical applications. Br J Sports Med. 2013 Sep;47(14):875–6.
28. Struyf F, Nijs J, Mottram S, Roussel NA, Cools AM, Meeusen R. Clinical assessment of the scapula: a review of the literature. Br J Sports Med. 2014 Jun;48(11):883–90. Epub 2012 Jul 21.
29. Warth RJ, Spiegl UJ, Millett PJ. Scapulothoracic bursitis and snapping scapula syndrome: a critical review of current evidence. Am J Sports Med. 2015 Jan;43(1):236–45. Epub 2014 Mar 24.
30. Rabin A, Irrgang JJ, Fitzgerald GK, Eubanks A. The intertester reliability of the Scapular Assistance Test. J Orthop Sports Phys Ther. 2006 Sep;36(9):653–60.
31. Yu D, Turmezei TD, Kerslake RW. FIESTA: an MR arthrography celebration of shoulder joint anatomy,

variants, and their mimics. Clin Anat. 2013 Mar;26(2): 213–27. Epub 2012 Mar 19.

32. Murray PJ, Shaffer BS. Clinical update: MR imaging of the shoulder. Sports Med Arthrosc. 2009 Mar;17(1):40–8.

33. Chung CB, Corrente L, Resnick D. MR arthrography of the shoulder. Magn Reson Imaging Clin N Am. 2004 Feb;12(1):25–38.

34. Rhee RB, Chan KK, Lieu JG, Kim BS, Steinbach LS. MR and CT arthrography of the shoulder. Semin Musculoskelet Radiol. 2012 Feb;16(1):3–14. Epub 2012 Mar 23.

35. Bouffard JA, Lee SM, Dhanju J. Ultrasonography of the shoulder. Semin Ultrasound CT MR. 2000 Jun;21(3):164–91.

2 Arthroscopic Shoulder Surgery

Arthroscopic surgery involves performing surgical procedures using a camera inserted in the joint for visualization and 1 or more additional access points (or portals) to the joint using stab incisions. Endoscopic surgery uses a camera and portals to complete similar procedures outside of joint cavities. Most shoulder surgeons do not distinguish between endoscopic and arthroscopic procedures, and the term *shoulder arthroscopy* is oftentimes used to refer to both (1).

Arthroscopic shoulder surgery has evolved tremendously over the past few decades. Initially, shoulder arthroscopy was considered mostly a diagnostic procedure. Currently, many shoulder surgeries are largely or exclusively performed arthroscopically. This is due to improvements in equipment, instrumentation, and implants; better surgeon understanding and training in arthroscopic anatomy and techniques; and interest by surgeons and patients in less invasive, more accurate surgeries.

A few general thoughts should be entertained before discussing the specifics of modern arthroscopic shoulder surgery. Certain arthroscopic procedures may require a specific set of skills that are difficult to acquire. Difficulties during arthroscopy may lead to inability to achieve the goals of surgery. However, the patient should not leave the operating room until the goals of surgery have been achieved; shoulder surgeons may feel frustrated when they realize they cannot accomplish the goals of surgery arthroscopically, and fatigue and pride may make any of us avoid conversion to an open procedure. In those circumstances, it is important to place the interests of the patient first, and do whatever it takes to leave the operating room only after adequate completion of the goals of the procedure. When considering if a procedure can be performed arthroscopically, please remember that arthroscopy is a tool, a way to approach the joint or the extra-articular space, not an operation per se. Surgical techniques should not violate surgical principles.

Since arthroscopic shoulder surgery requires a very specific set of skills, along the history of orthopedic surgery some surgeons with experience in arthroscopy for other joints, mostly the knee, migrated into arthroscopic shoulder surgery without proper training in open shoulder surgery or a clear understanding of the shoulder region and its conditions. This amplified problems: patients would be operated on arthroscopically with little understanding of the underlying condition, or surgeons would be hesitant to convert to open surgery when things went wrong due to lack of training in open shoulder surgery.

All these obstacles for the good use of arthroscopy around the shoulder joint have been largely overcome, and arthroscopic shoulder surgery has become an exciting field that allows surgeons to complete some procedures with less morbidity and more accuracy. It is my belief that newer generations of surgeons will only get better in arthroscopic shoulder surgery. In a way, arthroscopy is very much like playing video games, where the controls in your hands translate into action on the screen. Our younger generations of surgeons will have developed better skills to perform procedures looking at a video monitor, and the equipment and technology only continue to get better. Surgeons are already performing certain procedures (e.g., bone block augmentation of the glenoid or tendon transfers) that not even the most expert arthroscopic surgeon of the past could have dreamed of performing.

If you want to become an outstanding, skilled shoulder arthroscopist, you need to excel in four areas: knowledge of the principles of shoulder surgery (i.e., study books like this one), familiarity with the basic elements of shoulder arthroscopy (i.e., equipment, positioning, and portals), use of simulators or cadaver specimens to master general arthroscopic skills, and diligence (i.e., practice, evaluate, improve). Do not let fatigue or pride make you abandon the operating room knowing that you did not accomplish your goals, even if it means conversion to open surgery. If you follow this advice, your arthroscopic shoulder surgical practice will not only be fulfilling but also enjoyable!

Equipment

Arthroscopic shoulder surgery is greatly facilitated by the use of high-quality equipment. Although the operating room personnel and company representatives should be familiar with equipment set-up and troubleshooting, it is in the shoulder surgeon's best interest to have a fair amount of knowledge about equipment pieces at his/her disposal (Figure 2.1).

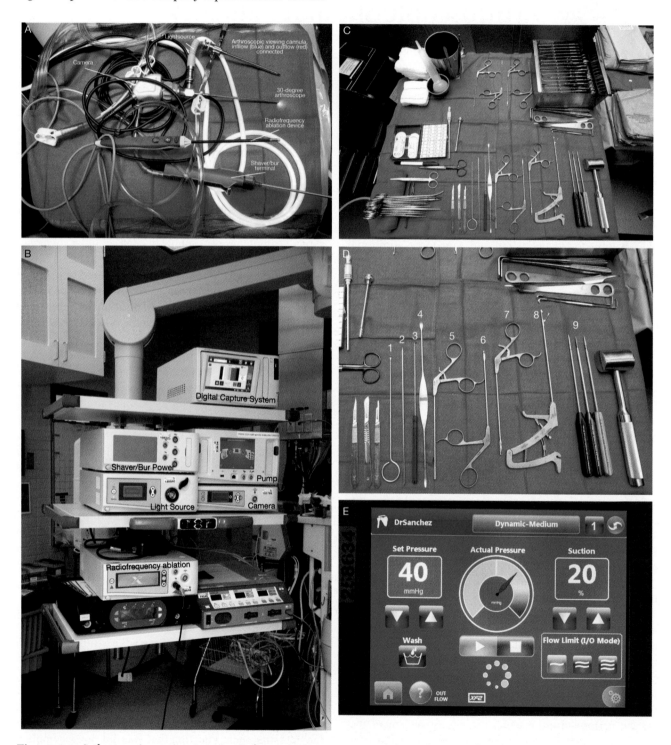

Figure 2.1 Arthroscopic equipment. **A,** *Arthroscope, camera, power intruments and radiofrequency ablation device.* **B,** *Consoles.* **C and D,** *Arthroscopic instrumentation set-up (1, knot pusher; 2, blunt trocar; 3, probe; 4, elevator; 5, closed-ended suture cutter; 6, open-ended suture and tape cutter; 7, tissue grasper; 8, antegrade suture passer; 9, punches and tap for anchor placement).* **E,** *Pump.*

Arthroscopes, Light Source, Camera, Monitors, and Digital Capture System

Arthroscopic visualization requires use of an arthroscope (lens) that receives a fiber optic light source (Figure 2.1A). The arthroscope is introduced into the joint inside a cannula. A camera connected to the base of the arthroscope feeds the signal to a monitor and a digital capture system. Modern cameras and digital capture systems provide high-quality, high-definition imaging. Photographs and video can be captured at any time during the procedure, providing invaluable material that can be shared with the patient afterward or used for education or research (Figure 2.1B).

Most procedures are performed with a 30°, 4.5-mm arthroscope: the lens is angled 30° in reference to the long axis of the camera shaft. Rotation of the lens provides various viewpoints during the procedure. Most arthroscopic shoulder surgeons develop the skills to move the camera and rotate the lens as needed in order to provide the best possible visualization using a 30° arthroscope.

Visualization of certain areas of the shoulder joint is best achieved using a different viewing angle. The most common alternative arthroscope used in shoulder surgery is the 70°, 4.5-mm arthroscope. It allows visualization at almost a right angle past an object (typically past the humeral head). This is particularly useful for arthroscopic instability surgery

(see chapter 7, Shoulder Instability and the Labrum), and assessment and repair of subscapularis tendon tears (see chapter 6, The Rotator Cuff and Biceps Tendon).

Fluid Systems, Pumps, and Hemostasis: Visualization is Key

Saline solution is typically used during arthroscopic shoulder surgery in order to distend the working space, remove debris generated by mechanical instruments, and control hemostasis to some extent. Proper fluid management is paramount for the success of arthroscopic shoulder surgery. Fluid is introduced into the joint under a certain amount of pressure. Although proper fluid management can be accomplished using gravity or gas to provide pressure, use of an automated pump is best (Figure 2.1E). Modern arthroscopic pumps incorporate sensors to measure intra-articular pressure and flow (i.e., velocity).

In order to avoid intraoperative issues with visualization and fluid management, it is important to dedicate some time prior to skin incision making sure the equipment is set up properly (Table 2.1). My preference is to use an arthroscopic cannula that provides both inflow and outflow (Figure 2.1A). Epinephrine added to saline at a dose of 0.3 to 1 mg/L seems to improve local hemostasis without major adverse effects (2). The tubing system for saline to

---

Table 2.1 • Arthroscopic Equipment Checklist

Equipment	Checklist
Arthroscope	30°, 4.5-mm scope available 70°, 4.5-mm in selected cases (subscapularis repair, arthroscopic Latarjet, other)
Cannula for arthroscope	Check adequate fit with the arthroscope Inflow/outflow cannula preferred
Fiber optic light source	Check light intensity
Camera, monitor, capture system	Check image on monitor Adjust focus White balance the camera Take a test picture Check video capture
Pump and saline	Consider adding epinephrine to saline bags (1 mg/L) Calibrate the pump according to the manufacturer's instructions Set preferred starting pressure and flow Monitor pump performance throughout the procedure
Shaver/cutter/bur	Select size and style of terminals Confirm proper function
Radiofrequency ablation devices	Select size and style of terminals Set ablation and coagulation levels Confirm proper function
Switching sticks	Two blunt sticks available Wisinger rod may be helpful in some cases
Cannulas and other instrumentation	Procedure and surgeon specific

circulate from the bags to the shoulder through the pump is connected. The pump is then calibrated and pump settings are selected. A combination of pressure and flow is selected in order to optimize visualization and effectiveness without excessive soft-tissue swelling or other adverse complications secondary to fluid extravasation.

Increasing pressure will lead to more distension and better hemostasis (the pressure of the fluid will lead to collapse of arterioles and veins and will tamponade cancellous bone). However, a high pressure maintained over time will lead to edema of the soft tissues. As the tissues thicken, the working length of arthroscopic instruments is compromised and it may be more difficult to angle them properly. If severe edema is allowed to happen, it could lead to muscle damage, fluid overload, airway compromise, or even compartment syndrome.

Arthroscopic shoulder surgery performed in the confines of a sealed glenohumeral joint (no associated rotator cuff) can usually be performed with a pressure of 20 to 30 mm Hg. Extra-articular (endoscopic) shoulder surgery (i.e., acromioplasty, rotator cuff repair) is typically best performed setting the pump pressure approximately 40 to 50 mm Hg below the systolic pressure (3). Most of the time, I request that my anesthesia team maintain the systolic pressure of the patient around 85 to 95 mm Hg. They set the pump pressure at 40 mm Hg and increase to 50 or 60 mm Hg if I run into trouble with visualization or hemostasis; however, hypotensive anesthesia can be dangerous in some patients, as discussed later.

Flow velocity is adjusted independently. Faster flows are useful when suction is used during removal of debris (i.e., acromioplasty). However, rapid increases in flow can facilitate bleeding according to the Bernouille principle: fluid at high velocity perpendicular to the lumen of a sectioned vessel will create a pressure gradient that will tend to pull blood out of the vessel, increasing bleeding and making visualization more difficult. This is particularly likely to happen when there are unsealed portals that allow quick egress of fluid: the only way the pump can maintain the desired pressure is by using a more rapid flow. Use of cannulas in these portals will help decrease turbulence and improve visualization. Portals that allow too much egress of fluid may also be closed temporarily with suture or a perforating towel clip during parts of the procedure. On the other hand, some outflow will decrease soft-tissue swelling. My preference is to use a flow of 0.5 L/min for most cases, increasing the flow selectively for the débridement portions of the procedure.

You may have already noted that avoidance of uncontrolled bleeding is paramount for arthroscopic visualization. Table 2.2 summarizes actions that can be considered when excessive bleeding impedes visualization and may endanger completing the arthroscopic procedure successfully. Hypotensive anesthesia and hypotensive bradycardic episodes are discussed later.

Table 2.2 • What to Check When Uncontrolled Bleeding Compromises Arthroscopic Shoulder Surgery

Check pump pressure and the patient's systolic blood pressure

Aim for systolic pressure between 85 and 95 mm Hg if possible (if safe)

Consider increasing pump pressure if needed

Avoid uncontrolled high flow (Bernoulli principle)

Consider adding epinephrine to saline unless already done

Coagulate bleeding points with a radiofrequency ablation device

Cannulas

Cannulas can be extremely useful when performing arthroscopic shoulder surgery. We already discussed some details regarding the cannula used for arthroscope insertion, inflow, and outflow. Cannulas inserted in working portals provide a number of benefits, including quick and easy access with instruments, better flow control, and avoidance of soft-tissue entrapment during suture management and knot tying. However, cannulas can also be associated with a number of potential problems, including damage of structures (especially the rotator cuff), and difficulty with instrumentation (cannulas may restrict the overall excursion of an intra-articular instrument, especially when colliding with other cannulas placed too close—cannula overcrowding).

As a general rule, I favor avoiding use of cannulas for débridement procedures (e.g., acromioplasty, biceps tenotomy, cuff débridement, arthroscopic capsular release). When cannulas are necessary for repair or reconstruction, I select the smallest possible cannula that will accommodate instrumentation. A larger cannula is typically used in the main working portal and a smaller cannula is used in an accessory portal if needed, mainly for suture management. Percutaneous portals without cannulas are more and more commonly used to insert anchors at specific locations and to "park" sutures, especially at the time of labral or cuff repair (see chapters 6, The Rotator Cuff and Biceps Tendon, and 7, Shoulder Instability and the Labrum). Currently, some surgeons do not use cannulas at all.

Motorized Shavers, Cutters, and Burs

Multiple styles of motorized shavers, cutters, and burs exist (Figure 2.1A). An arthroscopic shaver or cutter is very commonly used in many arthroscopic procedures to remove soft tissue and occasionally freshen bone. For the shaver to be effective, the correct amount of revolutions needs to be selected. Soft tissue is best removed with the shaver in oscillating mode, whereas freshening of bone surface is best accomplished with the shaver terminal rotating forward. Suction into the shaver can be regulated: more suction will lead to faster but less controlled tissue removal and will increase outflow, leading to worse visualization and potentially bleeding according to the Bernouille principle.

Burs are used on bone surfaces (i.e., acromioplasty, bone preparation for repair of the labrum or rotator cuff, osteophyte removal in arthroscopic débridement for osteoarthritis). The shape and size of the bur is selected based on the goal of the procedure and surgeon preferences. Burs are activated in forward mode most of the time, but they may be used in reverse mode when the bone to be worked on is extremely soft. Burs generate a fair amount of bone debris that may impair visualization. Better visualization may be maintained in 3 ways: increasing flow, using pulses of suction, and approximating the end of the arthroscopic lens close to the bur terminal.

Radiofrequency Ablation Devices

Radiofrequency ablation (RFA) devices are very helpful in arthroscopic shoulder surgery (Figure 2.1A and 2.1B). These devices ablate tissue by delivering heat generated from medium frequency alternating electric current (in the range of 350–500 kHz). RFA probes are designed in several shapes and sizes. The settings can be modified to deliver various levels of heat that are ideal for either removing tissue or coagulating blood vessels. One concern regarding use of RFA devices is the increase in temperature generated in the joint. Excessive heat is chondrotoxic. When RFAs are used intra-articularly, it is best not to use them continuously. Proper outflow also contributes to avoiding excessive heating of the articular space.

Positioning and Anesthesia

Proper patient positioning is paramount for 2 reasons: to successfully perform the arthroscopic procedure and to avoid complications related to positioning. Most arthroscopic shoulder procedures are performed in the beach chair position or the lateral decubitus position (◉ Video 2.1) (4). The prone position is used selectively for endoscopic surgery of the scapulothoracic joint.

Table 2.3 summarizes the relative advantages and disadvantages of the beach chair and lateral decubitus positions for arthroscopic shoulder surgery (1). Most surgeons choose the position of the patient based on their training and personal preferences. Prior to the development of commercially available arm holders for arthroscopic surgery in the beach chair position (◉ Video 2.2), many surgeons preferred the lateral decubitus position to achieve joint distraction with less need for a surgical assistant. My current preference is to place the patient in the beach chair position for most arthroscopic shoulder procedures. However, I prefer the lateral decubitus position for posterior shoulder instability surgery, since this position seems to allow better visualization and access to the posterior and posteroinferior aspects of the labrum and capsule.

Beach Chair Position

In this position, the patient is initially placed supine on an articulated operating room table. Once the patient is under anesthesia, the trunk is flexed to bring the shoulder up, and the hips and knees are slightly flexed to avoid excessive tension on the lumbar spine and postoperative low back pain. The head and trunk are secured to the operating room table, and the nonsurgical upper extremity is secured over the patient's lap (Figure 2.2A and B). The operative upper extremity is draped free and can be left resting on the patient's lap and moved during the procedure. Longitudinal traction may also be applied with a rope and pulley system. More commonly, the operative upper extremity is secured to an articulated arm holder that can provide traction and keep the shoulder in specific positions depending on the phase of the procedure being performed (Figure 2.2C). Surgeons vary in how high they like their patient to sit.

A number of details should be considered when placing the patient in the beach chair position, to minimize iatrogenic complications. The head should be secured so that the neck is not flexed, extended, or laterally bent, as extreme positions of the neck could facilitate compression of cervical nerve roots or the spinal cord. When securing the head, care must be taken to avoid pressure on the ears or eyes

Table 2.3 • Relative Advantages and Disadvantages of the Beach Chair and Lateral Decubitus Position for Arthroscopic Shoulder Surgery

Beach Chair	Lateral Decubitus
Familiar for surgeons and other members of the surgical team commonly involved in open surgery	Better visualization, especially for procedures in the posterior and inferior aspects of the glenohumeral joint
Arm holders facilitate procedures, but are not strictly required (potentially cheaper)	Lower risk of cerebral hypoperfusion
Lower risk of traction-induced brachial plexopathy or distal upper extremity hypoperfusion	
Easier conversion to open surgery using anterior exposures	

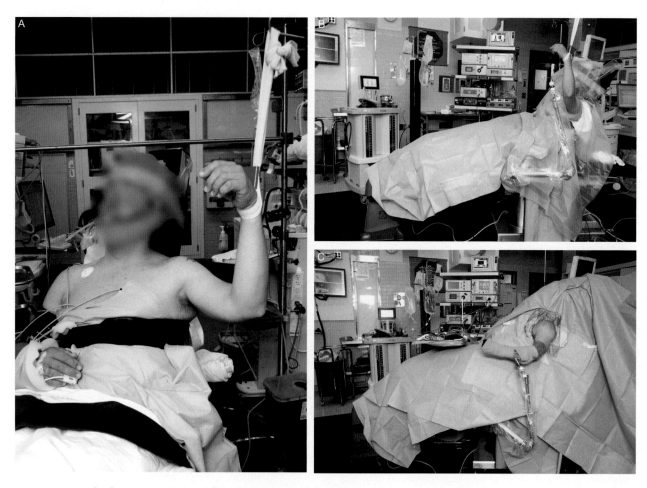

Figure 2.2 *Beach chair position.* **A and B,** *Positioning of the patient prior to draping.* **C,** *Use of a mechanical articulated arm holder.*

with whatever strap system is used. Finally, Trendelenburg inclination of the operating room table should be used so that gravity is directed toward the upper half of the patient's body; otherwise, the body weight is suspended from the head and neck.

Lateral Decubitus Position

The patient is placed laterally lying on the nonoperative side. The table should be padded and the body may be secured to the table using a beanbag or hip rests. The knees are bent and the lateral aspect of the lower knee padded to protect the peroneal nerve. An axillary roll is placed under the nonsurgical arm to protect the neurovascular structures. Care must be taken to avoid placing the nonsurgical arm in a stretched position and to keep the head and neck in neutral alignment. The operating table can be tilted posteriorly 20° to 30° in order to position the face of the glenoid parallel to the floor (Figure 2.3).

The operative upper extremity is then placed under traction using any of the commercially available kits. Typically, longitudinal traction is directed slightly anteriorly (approximately 45°), and lateral traction may be added to the proximal third of the arm. Most surgeons use between 15 and 20 pounds of weight for longitudinal traction. Excessive traction and placing the shoulder in extreme positions can lead to excessive strain on the brachial plexus and postoperative brachial plexopathy. Excessive lateral traction can also markedly reduce local and distal perfusion.

Anesthetic Considerations

Regional Blocks for Arthroscopic Shoulder Surgery

My preference is to request from my anesthesia colleagues use of a regional block of the brachial plexus. The interscalenic space is the preferred location. Since many arthroscopic shoulder procedures are performed without hospital admission, indwelling catheters are uncommonly used, but can be considered for inpatients. Most of the time, a single injection block is used.

Regional blocks have a number of advantages, including the fact that they provide preemptive analgesia, allow for

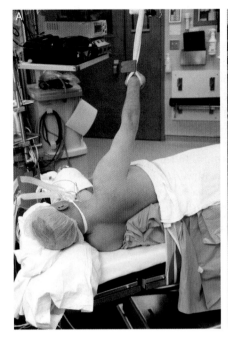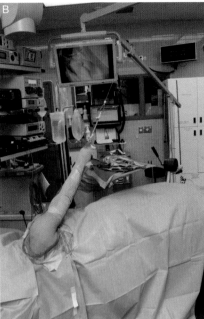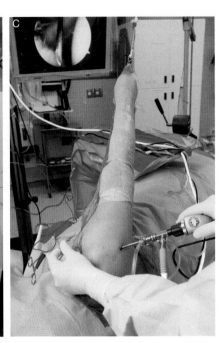

Figure 2.3 *Lateral decubitus position.* **A,** *Position prior to draping the surgical field.* **B,** *Position after draping.* **C,** *Performing arthroscopic surgery.*

more superficial general anesthesia, and help with postoperative pain control (5,6). Currently, many anesthesiologists perform regional blocks under ultrasonographic guidance, which increases the accuracy and effectiveness and decreases possible complications (e.g., permanent nerve injury, central nervous system toxicity, pneumothorax) (6). Interscalenic blocks do lead to blockade of the phrenic nerve, which leads to paralysis of the hemidiaphragm and consequently a 30% reduction in forced vital capacity and forced expiratory volume (7). In patients with substantial pulmonary insufficiency, it may be best to avoid interscalenic blocks or use ultrasonography-guided, phrenic nerve-sparing techniques.

Hypotensive Anesthesia

Hypotensive anesthesia is extremely useful when performing arthroscopic shoulder surgery, especially in procedures with abundant local vascularity such as the subacromial space (i.e., rotator cuff surgery). Low blood pressure decreases intraoperative bleeding, which can really compromise visualization and the ability to complete the procedure.

Most surgeons prefer keeping the systolic blood pressure at no more than 50 mm Hg over the pressure achieved in the working space with use of a pump. As mentioned before, setting the arthroscopic pump at high pressures leads to progressive edema of the surrounding soft tissues with a number of negative consequences. Since the glenohumeral joint is contained, it is typically possible to complete arthroscopic surgery with lower pump pressures around

30 mm Hg. For extra-articular arthroscopic surgery such as cuff repair, many surgeons start with a pump pressure of 40 mm Hg, and may increase the pressure up to 75 mm Hg if needed. That means that ideally the systolic blood pressure should be maintained below 100 mm Hg for most procedures, typically around 90 to 95 mm Hg.

A feared complication of hypotensive anesthesia is hypoperfusion of the brain and heart. The risk of adverse cardiac events is higher in patients with a history of ischemic heart disease. Brain perfusion can be particularly compromised in the beach chair position. When the patient is sitting upright, there is a substantial hydrostatic gradient between the brain and the site of blood pressure measurement, typically the nonoperative upper extremity. The magnitude of this gradient is approximately 2 mm Hg per inch of difference in height. Some studies have documented over 20% of cerebral oxygen desaturation in approximately 80% of patients operated on in the beach chair position (vs. none in the lateral decubitus position) (8). The risk of brain ischemia is higher in patients with underlying carotid stenosis. In these circumstances, consideration should be given to either using the lateral decubitus position instead of the beach chair position if hypotensive anesthesia is still desired, or to perform the procedure with the patient in the beach chair position but without hypotensive anesthesia.

Some studies suggest that holding antihypertensive medications prior to surgery and use of sequential compression devices both help maintain better perfusion when hypotensive anesthesia is performed and the patient is in the beach chair position (9,10).

Hypotensive Bradycardic Episodes

Sudden episodes of unexpected bradycardia and hypotension have also been reported during arthroscopic (and open) shoulder surgery. Risk factors that seem to lead to an increased frequency of these episodes include surgery in the beach chair position, and the use of an interscalenic block, especially if epinephrine is added to the local anesthetic used for the block. These episodes are postulated to happen secondary to sudden reflex autonomic withdrawal of the sympathetic system with vagal hyperactivity through the so-called Bezold-Jarisch reflex. This reflex becomes activated when the heart is in a hypercontractile state (possibly facilitated by the interscalenic block) and low ventricular volume (facilitated by pooling of blood on the lower extremities). Management of a hypotensive bradycardic episode includes administration of a bolus of intravenous fluid and consideration of a β-adrenergic blocker. It is important to realize that these episodes are not related to hypotensive anesthesia, and as long as the episodes do not continue happening during the procedure, they do not justify avoidance of hypotensive anesthesia.

Portals

As mentioned before, an arthroscopic portal is a point of access to the glenohumeral joint or various areas of the extra-articular spaces of the shoulder region. Placing portals in the right location and angle is critical in order to perform arthroscopic surgery safely, accurately, and efficiently. Poor portal placement makes arthroscopic surgery difficult or impossible to complete.

A number of portals are used very commonly in most procedures; other portals are procedure specific (Figure 2.4A–C). As long as the risk of injuring neurovascular structures is known, percutaneous portals can be placed in multiple locations depending on what needs to be done in a specific procedure. In this chapter, I review the most commonly used standard portals (Table 2.4); additional portals will be discussed as needed in other chapters of this book. Portals used for endoscopic surgery in the scapulothoracic space are discussed in chapter 10, The Scapula (11).

Posterior Portal

The posterior glenohumeral portal is the first portal established by most arthroscopic shoulder surgeons. Anatomic references used to create this portal include the posterior corner of the acromion, the glenohumeral joint, and the tip of the coracoid. Most recommend placing a vertical stab incision approximately 2 to 3 cm inferior and 1 to 3 cm medial to the posterior corner of the acromion; however, these distances will vary depending on the patient size and anatomy (12).

My preference is to use one hand to translate the humeral head anteriorly and posteriorly to determine the

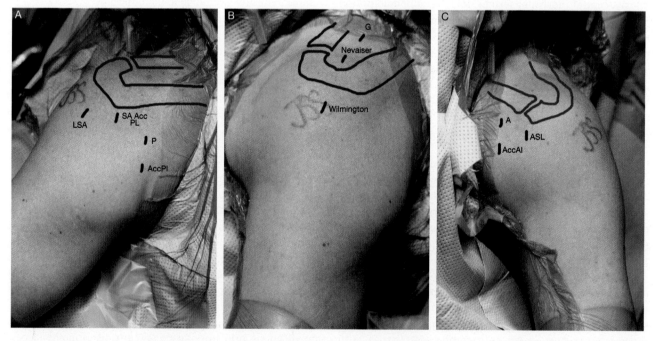

Figure 2.4 *Arthroscopic portals.* **A,** *Posterior. AccPl indicates accessory posterolateral portal; LSA, lateral subacromial; P, posterior; SA Acc PL, subacromial accessory posterolateral portal.* **B,** *Superior. G indicates Lafosse G portal.* **C,** *Anterior. A indicates anterior portal; AccAl, accessory anterolateral; ASL, anterosuperolateral.*

Table 2.4 • Common Arthroscopic Shoulder Portals

Portal	Location	Modifications	Structures at Risk
Posterior	Posterior glenohumeral joint (distal and medial to posterior acromion corner), aiming toward the coracoid	More lateral for posterior labrum/ capsule repair	Suprascapular nerve (too superior and medial) Axillary nerve (too inferior)
Anterior	Interval region, lateral and distal to the coracoid. Enters the joint in space bordered by labrum, humeral head, biceps tendon, subscapularis tendon	More superior for repairs of the superior labrum More inferior for repair of the anteroinferior labrum (anterior instability)	Musculocutaneous nerve (too medial and distal over the conjoined tendon) Brachial plexus and subclavian vessels (medial to the coracoid)
Lateral subacromial	Distal to the lateral rim of the acromion. Can be placed more anterior or posterior depending on the procedure	Anterior and distal for acromioplasty In the center and not as distal for cuff repair Two anterior lateral portals for suprascapular nerve decompression	Branches of the axillary nerve if the portals are placed too distal
Posterolateral	Just inferior to the posterolateral corner of the acromion	Two portals may be placed in this location, one for visualization and a second one for suture management	Branches of the axillary nerve if the portals are placed too distal
Superolateral/ Anterosuperior	At the lateral and superior aspect of the interval region, close to the biceps tendon		
Accessory posteroinferior	2–3 cm distal to the posterior portal, slightly lateral		Axillary nerve, posterior humeral circumflex vessels, branches of the suprascapular nerve
Accessory anteroinferior	Inferior and lateral to the anterior portal, through the subscapularis tendon		Axillary nerve, anterior humeral circumflex vessels, subscapularis tendon
Wilmington portal	1–2 cm anterior and 1–2 cm lateral to the posterolateral corner of the acromion, through the supraspinatus	Can be placed more anterior to provide access through the interval region	Supraspinatus, glenoid articular cartilage
Neviaser portal	Medial to the junction of the clavicle, spine of the scapula and acromion		Suprascapular nerve
Lafosse G portal	2–3 cm medial to Neviaser portal, equidistant between clavicle and scapular spine in the coronal plane	A second more medial portal is used commonly for ligament sectioning	Suprascapular nerve and vessels

deep location of the joint line. After the stab incision is placed (Figure 2.5A), a blunt trocar is introduced through the deltoid until the humeral head can be felt moving forward as it is being gently pushed by the trocar. The tip of the trocar is then moved medially until the step-off between humeral head and glenoid is palpated, and the trocar is then forced into the joint aiming to the tip of the coracoid (Figure 2.5B). Some surgeons prefer to inject the glenohumeral joint with saline in this particular location to distend the joint prior to creating the portal.

Intra-articular placement of the arthroscope is then visually confirmed by identifying synovial vessels, glenohumeral cartilage, the long head of the biceps, and the labrum. Care must be taken to minimize articular cartilage damage with the trocar, especially in patients with glenohumeral stiffness.

The position of the posterior portal may be modified in patients with posterior shoulder instability. The classic location of the posterior portal makes it difficult to approach the glenoid at a steep angle for anchor placement

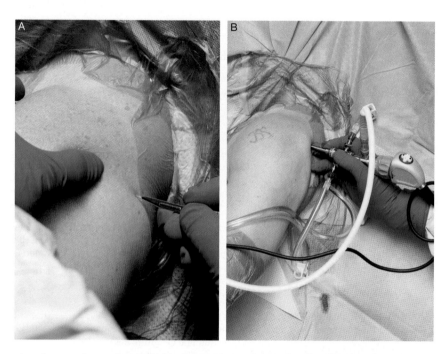

Figure 2.5 Posterior glenohumeral portal. **A,** *Skin incision.* **B,** *Access to the glenohumeral joint.*

and suture management after portals are switched. When posterior labrum and capsule repair is anticipated, the portal is placed more lateral.

The same skin incision used for introduction of the arthroscope into the glenohumeral joint through the posterior portal can also be used to position the arthroscope into the subacromial space posteriorly. The trocar is positioned inside the arthroscopic sheath and directed more superiorly toward the anterior aspect of the acromion. Most surgeons confirm the adequate location of the trocar by feeling the hard undersurface of the acromion. In very obese patients it is possible to place the arthroscope subcutaneously on top of the acromion by mistake. This portal can be used for diagnosis and visualization during subacromial decompression, but it does not provide ideal visualization for cuff repair.

Anterior Portal

This is the second portal typically created for glenohumeral joint arthroscopy (13). Most surgeons establish this portal with an outside-in technique: a spinal needle is inserted through the rotator interval aiming toward the arthroscope (Figure 2.6). Since the base of the coracoid is at the interval region, the tip of the coracoid is a great external landmark; the portal is placed approximately 1 cm lateral and 1 cm distal to the tip of the coracoid, although again these distances will vary from patient to patient. Regarding internal landmarks, the goal is to visualize the needle piercing the space between the labrum medially, the humeral head laterally, the biceps tendon superiorly, and the subscapularis tendon inferiorly.

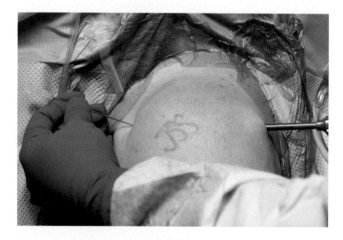

Figure 2.6 Establishing the anterior portal.

In patients with extreme obesity or severe glenohumeral stiffness it may be difficult to establish the anterior portal using an outside-in technique. In these circumstances, the spot on the interval region where the portal needs to be placed can be identified with the arthroscope, the arthroscopic sheath can be pushed anteriorly until it is resting on the rotator cuff interval, and a long switching stick (Wisinger rod) can be pushed through the sheath from posterior to anterior after temporary removal of the arthroscope, establishing the anterior portal with an inside-out technique.

Placement of this portal through the conjoined tendon just distal to the coracoid may injure the musculocutaneous nerve. Placement of this portal even more medial can

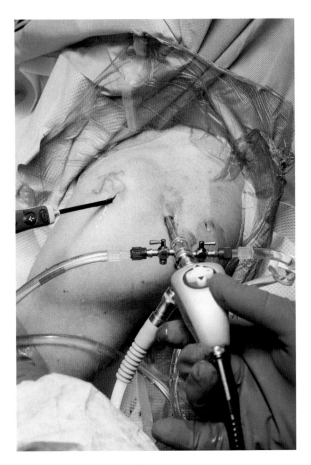

Figure 2.7 Camera through the subacromial accessory posterolateral portal; radiofrequency ablation device through the lateral subacromial portal.

facilitate injury to other branches of the brachial plexus or the subclavian vessels. This portal is placed more superior when repair of the superior labrum is anticipated, and more inferior (just over the edge of the subscapularis) when contemplating repair of the anteroinferior labrum and capsule for anterior instability.

Lateral Subacromial Portals

Procedures performed in the subacromial space (i.e., acromioplasty, rotator cuff repair, suprascapular nerve decompression) are best performed using one or more lateral subacromial portals (14) (Figures 2.4A and 2.7). These portals need to be distal enough to provide the proper angle for the tip of the instruments to work in the subacromial space. However, placing these portals too distally may injure branches of the axillary nerve.

For acromioplasty, the portal is placed in line with the anterior acromion, since bone is removed from the anterior half of the bone. For rotator cuff repair, the portal is placed centered on the tear from anterior to posterior; it can be used for visualization during parts of the procedure (providing the so-called 50-yard line view), and for suture passing and tying for other parts of the procedure. For suprascapular nerve decompression, 2 lateral portals are used, 1 central for the camera and 1 anterior for dissection.

Posterolateral Subacromial Portal

Although posterior visualization of the subacromial space can be accomplished by introducing the arthroscope through the same skin incision used for the posterior

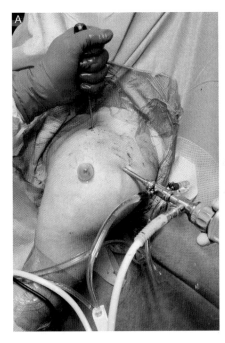

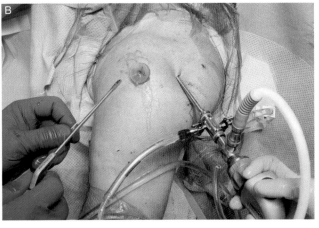

*Figure 2.8 **A,** Use of additional portals as needed for anchor placement in cuff repair. **B,** Suture management through cannulas.*

portal, visualization for rotator cuff repair is much better by placing the arthroscope more lateral and superior than the classic location of the standard posterior portal. This portal is placed just inferior to the posterolateral corner of the acromion (Figures 2.4A and 2.8) (14). Oftentimes, the arthroscope is switched back and forth between the posterolateral subacromial and the lateral subacromial portal.

Superolateral or Anterosuperior Portal (Anterosuperolateral Portal)

This portal is mainly used for repair of the anterior labrum and capsule in patients with anterior instability (13). It is established outside-in at the lateral and superior aspect of the rotator cuff interval (15) (Figure 2.4C). When used for visualization, it provides a panoramic view of the glenoid, labrum, and capsule and facilitates confirmation of complete elevation of the labrum and capsule off the glenoid neck so that the muscular fibers of the subscapularis are visualized. When used for instrumentation and suture management, it avoids overcrowding with a cannula placed in a low anterior portal.

Accessory Posteroinferior Portal

This portal is placed 2 to 3 cm distal to the standard posterior portal. It is mostly used for repair of the posteroinferior labrum and capsule, removal of loose bodies (pieces of debris oftentimes found in arthritis) from the axillary recess, and release of the inferior capsule in patients with frozen shoulder. My preference is to establish this portal under direct vision (Figure 2.4A): the arthroscope is placed in the anterior portal and a switching stick is left at the posterior portal. A spinal needle is then introduced 2 to 3 cm distal to the switching stick, slightly more lateral, and parallel. Placement of this portal lateral enough is critical when used for placement of anchors on the inferior glenoid. Some authors have named this portal the 7 o'clock portal (only valid for a right shoulder) (16). This portal can be risky, as it is close to the axillary nerve, posterior circumflex humeral artery, and lower branches of the suprascapular nerve.

Accessory Anteroinferior Portal

This portal is mostly used for placement of anterior anchors on the lower portion of the anterior glenoid rim in patients with anterior instability. Most surgeons use this as a percutaneous portal without cannulas (Figure 2.4C). The portal pierces the subscapularis tendon (17). Although initially described as an inside-out portal (18), I prefer to place it as an outside-in portal, finding the ideal trajectory of the portal with a spinal needle (19). Some authors have named this portal the 5 o'clock portal (only valid for a right shoulder). The main structures at risk include the axillary nerve, the anterior circumflex humeral vessels, and the subscapularis tendon if a cannula is used.

Superior Portals

Three portals have been described on the superior aspect of the shoulder region (Figure 2.4B).

Wilmington Portal

This portal is commonly used for placement of a superior anchor on the glenoid rim just posterior to the location of the biceps tendon when performing repair of the superior labrum (see chapter 7, Shoulder Instability and the Labrum). The skin incision is made 1 to 2 cm anterior and 1 to 2 cm lateral to the posterolateral corner of the acromion (Figure 2.4B). Instruments are then directed toward the superior glenoid rim, piercing the supraspinatus tendon. As with the accessory anteroinferior portal, my preference is to use this as a percutaneous portal, avoiding use of cannulas to decrease the chance of iatrogenic rotator cuff damage. When inserting sharp instruments through this portal, care must be taken not to inadvertently damage the articular surface of the glenoid. Use of trans-cuff portals does not seem to be associated with symptomatic permanent cuff damage (20).

Neviaser Portal

This portal is placed medial to the confluence of the clavicle and the scapular spine and acromion (Figure 2.4B) (21). A needle is inserted in this location and directed laterally and slightly anteriorly through the capsule. This portal has been used mostly as an outflow portal for repair of superior labral tears and for superior capsular reconstruction. Care must be taken not to injure the suprascapular nerve.

Lafosse G Portal

This portal was described for sectioning of the suprascapular ligament when decompressing the suprascapular nerve (Figure 2.4B; see chapters 6, The Rotator Cuff and Biceps Tendon and 7, Shoulder Instability and the Labrum) (22). The portal is located 2 to 3 cm medial to the Neviaser portal and equidistant between the posterior aspect of the clavicle and the anterior aspect of the scapular spine. A spinal needle is directed anteriorly through the trapezius aiming toward the anterior aspect of the supraspinatus muscle just medial to the base of the coracoid. Commonly, 2 portals are needed in this location, 1 for dissection or retraction and the other to divide the ligament. Obviously, the suprascapular nerve and artery are at risk in this particular location.

Arthroscopic Evaluation of the Glenohumeral Joint and Subacromial Space

Although shoulder arthroscopy is a very powerful diagnostic tool, at the present time most patients undergoing

Table 2.5 • 10-point Diagnostic Arthroscopic Evaluation

Glenohumeral joint
1. Long head of the biceps and superior labrum
2. Glenoid and posterior labrum
3. Inferior axillary recess
4. Humeral head, bare area, posterior cuff
5. Anterosuperior cuff
6. Rotator interval (pulley, long head of the biceps in the groove, superior glenohumeral ligament)
7. Subscapularis, middle glenohumeral ligament, anterior labrum
8. Anteroinferior labrum, inferior glenohumeral ligament

Subacromial space
9. Acromion and coracoacromial ligament
10. Rotator cuff from the bursal side

Adapted from Funk L. Shoulder arthroscopy guide [Internet]. 2008 [cited 2016 Oct 25]. Available from: https://www.shoulderdoc.co.uk/section/858. Used with permission.

Table 2.6 • Southern California Orthopedic Institute 15-point Diagnostic Arthroscopic Evaluation

Viewing from posterior portal
1. Biceps
2. Superior labrum
3. Posterior labrum and posterior capsule
4. Inferior capsule and inferior recess
5. Glenoid cartilage surface
6. Rotator cuff, supraspinatus attachment
7. Posterior cuff attachment, posterior humeral head
8. Humeral head articular cartilage
9. Anterior superior labrum, rotator interval, superior and middle glenohumeral ligament, subscapularis tendon
10. Anterior inferior labrum and inferior glenohumeral ligament, posterior view

Viewing from anterior portal
11. Posterior labrum and posterior capsule
12. Posterior capsule and rotator cuff
13. Anterior inferior labrum and anterior inferior glenohumeral ligament
14. Middle glenohumeral ligament and medial subscapularis and recess
15. Lateral subscapularis tendon and anterior humeral head and biceps

Adapted from Snyder SJ, Fasulo GJ. Shoulder arthroscopy: surgical technique. Surg Technol Int. 1993 Oct;2:447–53. Used with permission.

arthroscopic shoulder surgery should have a firm diagnosis based on their history, physical examination, and imaging studies before they are taken to the operating room. However, the shoulder joint is considered to have many potential pain generators, and a systematic way to assess the glenohumeral joint and subacromial space helps to be efficient without missing anything that may be wrong. At the same time, it is important to remember that some arthroscopic assessments are very subjective, and different surgeons may disagree when evaluating the superior labrum for a tear, assessing the severity of capsular laxity, or determining the extent of a partial thickness rotator cuff tear.

Several authors have suggested a number of structures, or points, of the shoulder that should be systematically assessed in every patient prior to starting the interventional portion of the procedure (Tables 2.5 and 2.6; Figure 2.9). Most surgeons start with the arthroscope in the posterior portal and a probe in the anterior portal to feel and test various intra-articular structures (i.e., biceps, labrum, articular cartilage on both the humeral head and the glenoid, the subscapularis tendon, the inferior axillary recess, and the whole tendinous attachment of the posterosuperior rotator cuff). The long head of the biceps can be pulled into the joint with the probe. Portals can then be switched, and with the arthroscope in the anterior portal and a probe in the posterior portal, the posterior labrum and capsule are assessed as well. The subacromial space is typically assessed with the arthroscope in the posterior portal, looking for bursal thickening, osteophytic formations in the acromion or distal clavicle, the presence of an os acromiale, calcifying tendinitis, or rotator cuff tears.

Commonly Performed Procedures

As mentioned previously, arthroscopic instruments and techniques allow performing procedures in a less invasive, more accurate way. Currently, some procedures are clearly better when performed arthroscopically, some procedures are clearly better performed open, and a number of procedures lie in between. The number of procedures that can be performed arthroscopically will only continue to increase over time. Throughout the pages of this book we will describe the specifics of selected common arthroscopic procedures. In this chapter, they are summarized in Table 2.7.

Arthroscopic Anchor Placement, Suture Passing, Suture Management, and Knot Tying

A number of arthroscopic surgical procedures require a particular set of skills. In addition to being able to maneuver the arthroscope and light source to provide the best possible viewing angles, it is important to develop skills to use instruments inside the joint while looking at the monitor. Many modern arthroscopic shoulder procedures require placing anchors, passing sutures, managing sutures, and tying knots arthroscopically (⬤ Video 2.3).

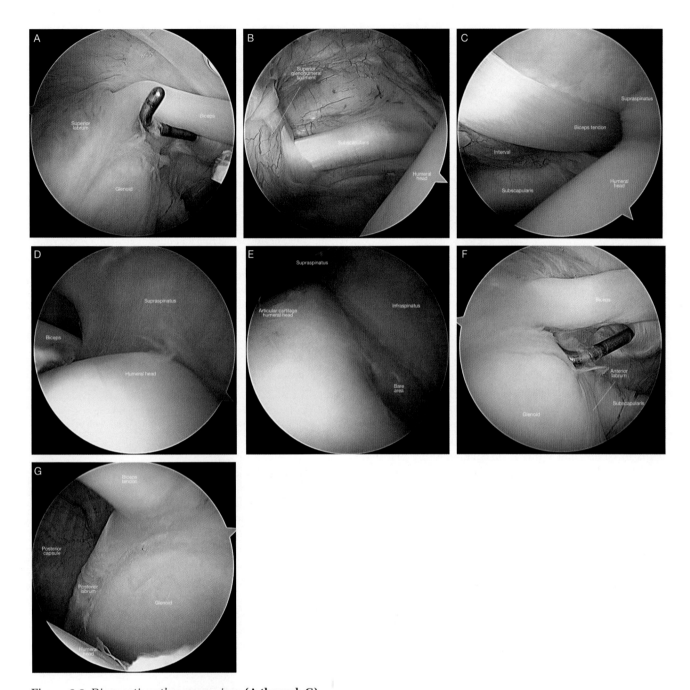

Figure 2.9 Diagnostic arthroscopy views **(A through G)**.

It is extremely important to practice using models, computer simulation, and cadaver specimens so that all these skills are developed prior to operating on patients.

Anchors

Suture anchors are relatively small implants manufactured with an eyelet or similar mechanism to hold suture into bone and can be made of metal or various plastic materials (Figure 2.10). Some have screw-in threads, whereas other are pounded into bone as tacks, and some are made solely of suture with special designs at the very

tip that resist pull-out. Modern anchors oftentimes come loaded with strands of high-tensile nonabsorbable suture or tape. The channel where the anchor will be placed in the bone can be created with a drill or a punch. Harder bone may require taping, whereas soft bone may require use of larger diameter anchors. Each surgeon should make him/herself familiar with the anchors used for various procedures and the instrumentation required to implant them.

The main skills required for successful anchor placement involve finding the right angle of insertion and reproducing

Table 2.7 • Common Arthroscopic Shoulder Procedures

Proximal humerus fractures	Arthroscopically assisted fixation of tuberosity fractures Arthroscopically assisted hardware removal
Clavicle, ACJ, SCJ	Arthroscopic distal clavicle resection Arthroscopic sternoclavicular joint débridement/resection Arthroscopically assisted ACJ reconstruction/repair
Rotator cuff	Acromioplasty Rotator cuff débridement and repair Arthroscopically assisted fixation os acromiale Arthroscopic suprascapular nerve decompression Arthroscopically assisted tendon transfers Superior capsular reconstruction
Biceps	Biceps tenotomy Biceps tenodesis
Instability	Labral repair with or without capsular plication Arthroscopic bone block procedures
Frozen shoulder	Arthroscopic capsular release
Shoulder arthroplasty	Diagnostic arthroscopy Arthroscopic cultures Arthroscopic removal of failed all polyethelene glenoid components
Scapula	Arthroscopic fixation glenoid fractures Arthroscopic scapulothoracic bursectomy Arthroscopic resection of the superomedial border of the scapula Arthroscopically assisted tendon transfers

the exact same angle with the drill/punch and the anchor. It is important to understand that placing anchors at a relatively acute angle in reference to the tissue being repaired maximizes pullout strength. This is particularly important for arthroscopic rotator cuff repair surgery.

Suture Passing

Sutures anchored in bone are used to attach soft tissue (e.g., labrum, capsule, rotator cuff). This requires threading these sutures through the soft tissues similar to what is done with needles in open surgery. Antegrade suture passing involves using an instrument that allows first loading the suture and then piercing the tissue. Retrograde suture passing involves using an instrument that first pierces the tissue and then grabs the suture. Sometimes, sutures are passed through or around tissue using a shuttle made of suture or other material. Efficient and accurate performance of arthroscopic shoulder procedures requiring suture passing requires understanding the modality of suture passing that will be used for each stage of the procedure, and it is largely based on surgeon training and preferences as well as instrumentation available.

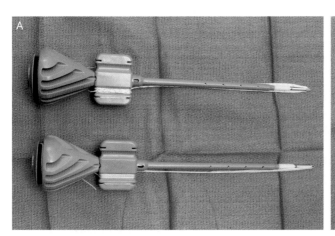
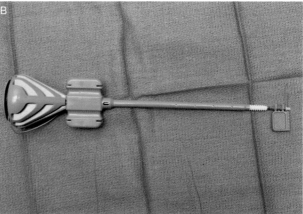

Figure 2.10 Anchors (**A and B**).

Table 2.8 • Preventing Suture Entanglement

- Use sutures of various colors and or patterns to distinguish them.

- Manipulate sutures through cannulas.

- Pass sutures in a specific order and tie them in reverse order.

- Only manipulate 1 suture at a time in your main working cannula, leaving the rest of the sutures "parked" in a different portal.

- Once ready to tie, pass the knot pusher all the way down each of the suture limbs to confirm no issues; alternatively, grab both sutures with an instrument, switching the direction of the mouth of the instrument between the first and the second limb.

Suture Management

Sutures placed in the glenohumeral joint, subacromial space, or other locations can easily get tangled with each other or in the soft tissues, which can compromise the quality of the repair. Table 2.8 summarizes various ways to help prevent suture entangling. If sutures get tangled, take a pause to understand how they are tangled; untangle them by retrieving the tangled suture temporarily in a different portal, or use suture grabbers or the knot pusher to manipulate the suture limbs in the joint.

Another issue that can arise while working with sutures arthroscopically is to unintentionally unload the suture from the anchor. To avoid this problem, try to always keep track of the end of the suture to be manipulated, and visualize the location of the anchor as you are pulling suture ends to confirm that the suture is not "running" through the anchor. If a suture is unloaded, all the work that was done to place the anchor, pass the suture, and so on is wasted, and the surgeon can potentially run out of "real estate" to place more anchors, in addition to the expense implications.

Arthroscopic Knot Tying

There are instruments and devices designed to secure tissue with anchors without tying suture knots (knotless devices). However, many arthroscopic techniques do require tying sutures in the glenohumeral joint or subacromial space under arthroscopic visualization using a knot pusher.

Tying knots arthroscopically may be difficult: fluid makes sutures and the surgeon's hands more slippery, the cannulas do not allow visualization of part of the process, and tying a secure knot requires skillful throws, differential tension on suture limbs, and leaving the knot on the desired location (on the nonarticular side of the labrum, the superior aspect of the cuff, etc). The importance of practicing arthroscopic knot tying cannot be overemphasized: watch videos, understand techniques, practice them with practice ropes and then with real suture, at home or in a laboratory, so that you get "ready for prime time." Knot strength definitely varies widely depending on the surgeon's expertise (23).

Basic Concepts in Arthroscopic Knot Tying

Many of the concepts summarized here are very basic, but still worth remembering to become perfect at arthroscopic knot tying. The 2 limbs of the suture to be tied are called the post (straight limb under tension) and the wrapping limb (wraps around the post). The loop is the portion of the suture that encircles the soft tissue distal to the knot. Secure soft-tissue repair requires both loop security (the loop is maintained tight enough around the soft tissue during the tying process) and knot security (the knot resists slipping back and becoming loose). Loop security is achieved by maintaining the loop tight until the knot is locked, which is difficult because the first throws of the knot may want to back out. Knot security depends mostly on the knot configuration and how well the knot is constructed and tied. The type of suture selected (material and braiding) also impacts the quality of the knot (24).

Table 2.9 summarizes various types of knots commonly used in arthroscopic shoulder surgery. Sliding knots are elegant and useful, but they require suture sliding through the anchor eyelet and tissue. In situations where suture sliding will not happen (somehow the suture is tethered), nonsliding (static) knots are required. I believe that every arthroscopic shoulder surgeon should master nonsliding knot tying using the 6-throw surgeon's knot (Figure 2.11). In addition, it is useful to know how to tie 1 or more sliding knots. There are multiple sliding knots described in the literature; description of each of them exceeds the scope of this book. Pick one that you like, practice it, and stick to it. My preference is to use one particular self-locking sliding knot (the Seoul Medical Center [SMC] knot, Figure 2.12); regardless of the sliding knot selected, it is best to back it up with 3 half-hitches (over-under-over) reversing the post.

Table 2.9 • Knot Classification

Static (nonsliding)	**Multiple individual half-hitches are sequentially thrown and seated using a knot pusher. The direction of the hitch (under or over), and the suture end used as post or wrapping end, can both be alternated to increase knot security**
Sliding	**The wrapping limb is wrapped around the post multiple times in a very specific manner and the knot is dressed outside of the cannula; traction on the post results in the suture sliding through the anchor and tissue and the knot sliding down to the anchor. Sliding knots can be** Self-locking—traction on the post once the knot is seated results in a change inside the knot that avoids backing out Not-self-locking—the knot does not have any features that will lock it in place

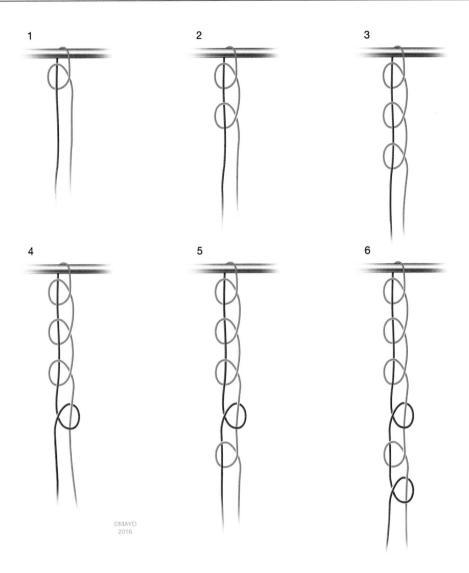

Figure 2.11 *The 6-throw surgeon's knot.*

Alternating the Post
Knot security can be increased by both alternating the direction of the wrapping limb (reversing over and under throws), and alternating which of the 2 suture limbs is used as a post (alternating the post). Reversing the direction of half-hitches and switching the post limb between throws each increase knot security by increasing friction and internal interference (25). There are 2 ways of alternating the post: switching the knot pusher from one suture strand to the other, or applying differential tension to the suture strand. I prefer the second method, which is faster and very reliable: as the knot pusher is sliding a half-hitch along the post, tension is no longer applied to the post, and applied to the wrapping limb instead, while the knot pusher is positioned to past-point. Arthroscopic visualization confirms flipping of the post (the knot flips).

The 6-Throw Surgeon's Knot
This nonsliding knot consists of throwing 3 half-hitches on the same post and then adding 3 reversing half-hitches alternating the post (Figure 2.11). Care should be taken to avoid backing out of any of the first 3 half-hitches to avoid a loose loop. If the knot is tied reversing the post by flipping the knot, care must be taken not to "unflip" the knot inadvertently as the surgeon gets the next throw ready.

The 4-Throw Knot
This nonsliding knot consists of starting with the suture on the left hand as a post, always keeping the knot pusher on that suture strand, and throwing 2 reversing half-hitches alternating the post by flipping the knot, and repeating the same 2 reversing half-hitches with knot flipping again.

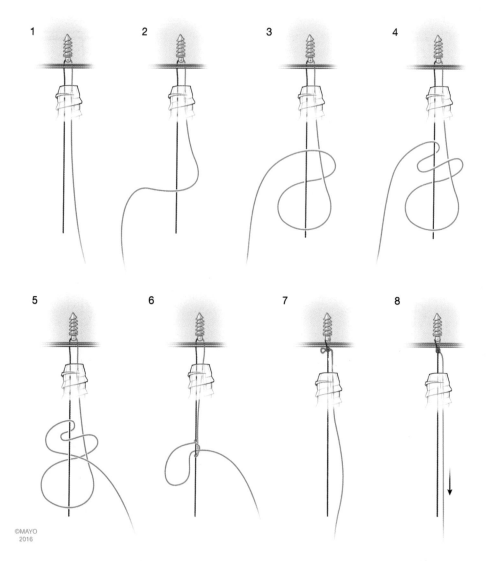

©MAYO
2016

Figure 2.12 *The SMC self-locking sliding knot. SMC indicates Seoul Medical Center.*

The SMC Sliding Self-locking Knot

This knot is sliding, self-locking, and relatively easy to throw and dress (Figure 2.12). As with any sliding knot, it is important to first confirm that the suture does slide through the eyelet and the tissue. The knot starts with a shorter post limb and a longer wrapping limb (Figure 2.12). The wrapping limb is wrapped in 5 places: over the post, over both limbs, in between the limbs, over the post, and in between the limbs. Once the knot is dressed, traction on the post will slide the knot. Once the knot is seated, traction on the wrapping limb will lock the knot. The knot is then backed up with 3 reversing half-hitches alternating the post.

Complications of Shoulder Arthroscopy

Arthroscopic shoulder surgery can be associated with many of the general complications of surgery (e.g.,

infection, hemorrhage, deep venous thrombosis, medical complications, stiffness) (26). However, there are a few complications that are somewhat more specific to arthroscopic shoulder surgery.

Neurologic Injuries

Neurologic injuries complicating arthroscopic shoulder surgery can be devastating. Both patients and surgeons envision arthroscopy as minimally invasive surgery, somewhat minor compared with open surgery. Permanent nerve dysfunction will be seen as a catastrophic complication difficult to accept. There are various mechanisms of neurologic damage with arthroscopy.

Iatrogenic Nerve Injuries

Nerves can be physically damaged at the time of portal placement or when using instruments in the joint or subacromial space (27–29). The axillary, suprascapular, and musculocutaneous nerves are particularly at risk. Prevention requires understanding portal placement along the lines described before, never using instruments blindly, and avoiding use of mechanical instruments or RFA devices in the proximity of nerves.

Traction Plexopathy

As mentioned before, use of traction on the upper extremity with weights in the lateral decubitus position improves visualization but can lead to a stretch injury of the brachial plexus. Meticulous patient positioning and judicious use of weights help avoid this complication. Traditionally, the beach chair position has been associated with traction injuries to the brachial plexus less commonly. However, many surgeons currently use mechanical arm holders that do provide powerful distraction, and can potentially lead to the same problem. As soon as the procedure is finished, remember to release the traction on these holders or remove the weights from the traction system.

Regional Blocks

Permanent nerve injury is a known complication of regional anesthesia attributed to mechanical nerve damage at the time of blockade, or toxicity secondary to a maintained high dose of a local anesthetic. As mentioned, ultrasonographic guidance has decreased the risk of this complication. In patients with a postoperative brachial plexopathy, it may be difficult to tease out if the main culprit was the block or excessive traction.

Brain and Spinal Cord Ischemia

This complication has been reported mostly with the beach chair position. As described earlier, hypotensive anesthesia in the sitting position can easily lead to low oxygen saturation in the brain and spinal cord. This may be further complicated by the development of hypotensive bradycardic episodes. Prevention requires scanning patients for carotid disease and hypertensive vascular disease, selective use of lateral decubitus position for high-risk patients, and good communication with the anesthesia team so that the blood pressure remains stable at 90 mm Hg to 100 mm Hg. There are devices to monitor oxygen saturation at the brain level, and using them may also help prevent permanent neurologic abnormalities.

Air Embolism

Air embolism can also occur when shoulder surgery is performed in the beach chair position if room air finds a way to access the open blood vessels (veins) of the shoulder (30).

Fluid Extravasation

Fluid extravasation occurs to some extent in all arthroscopic shoulder procedures. Substantial fluid extravasation is more likely to occur when pumps are set to maintain very high pressure, as well as with prolonged surgical procedures. The most common issue secondary to fluid extravasation is the inability to complete the procedure properly: soft-tissue edema makes it more difficult to maneuver instruments, maintain cannulas in good position, and reach certain spots. As mentioned before, there have been isolated case reports of skin necrosis, compartment syndrome, and even airway obstruction. Understanding fluid management as well as alternative strategies to control bleeding and maintain visualization are important to prevent excessive fluid extravasation.

Articular Cartilage Damage (Thermal, Pumps)

Unfortunately, rapid joint degeneration has been reported as a complication of shoulder arthroscopy and termed *chondrolysis*. The evaluation and management of this complication is discussed in Chapter 9, Shoulder Arthritis and Arthroplasty. Accelerated destruction of the articular cartilage has been linked to a number of possible culprits, including excessive joint temperature secondary to use of RFAs, prominent anchors or suture material (especially knots on the articular side of the labrum), biochemical adverse effects of biodegradable material, prolonged (24–48 hours) intra-articular infusion of local anesthetics for postoperative pain relief using a pump, or a low-grade infection. Currently, the use of intra-articular pain pumps has been largely discontinued. Remember to avoid uninterrupted use of RFAs inside the glenohumeral joint whenever possible.

KEY POINTS

✓ Arthroscopy and endoscopy have revolutionized the field of shoulder surgery, providing a less invasive, more accurate means to complete certain procedures.

✓ Arthroscopic shoulder surgery can only be performed properly after developing a number of very particular skills.

✓ When difficulties arise while performing arthroscopic shoulder surgery, the overriding principle should be to achieve the goals of surgery without violating surgical principles, even if this requires conversion to open surgery.

✓ Arthroscopic shoulder surgeons need to have a basic understanding of the equipment used, including arthroscopes, light source, camera, monitors, digital capture system, fluid systems, pumps, cannulas, shavers, cutters, burs, and radiofrequency ablation devices.

✓ Careful patient positioning is extremely important. Many surgeons prefer the beach chair position since it is more familiar and facilitates conversion to open surgery. However, the lateral decubitus position may provide better visualization and is not associated with brain hypoperfusion, although it carries a higher risk of traction brachial plexopathy.

✓ Hypotensive anesthesia and regional blocks are commonly used for arthroscopic shoulder surgery. Good visualization is obtained in most patients by setting the pump pressure approximately 50 mm Hg lower than the systolic blood pressure.

✓ Common arthroscopic shoulder portals include the posterior, anterior, and lateral subacromial portals. Other useful portals include the posterolateral subacromial portal for cuff repair, the superolateral portal for anterior instability, accessory posteroinferior and anteroinferior portals for labral repairs, and a number of superior portals.

✓ Most surgeons perform a systematic evaluation of specific structures when performing arthroscopic shoulder surgery. Follow your own.

✓ Arthroscopic repair techniques often require use of suture anchors. Surgeons need to master anchor placement, suture passing techniques, suture management, and arthroscopic knot tying.

✓ The main specific complications of arthroscopic shoulder surgery include neurologic complications, fluid extravasation, and chondrolysis.

REFERENCES

1. Paxton ES, Backus J, Keener J, Brophy RH. Shoulder arthroscopy: basic principles of positioning, anesthesia, and portal anatomy. J Am Acad Orthop Surg. 2013 Jun;21(6):332–42.

2. Jensen KH, Werther K, Stryger V, Schultz K, Falkenberg B. Arthroscopic shoulder surgery with epinephrine saline irrigation. Arthroscopy. 2001 Jul;17(6):578–81.

3. Morrison DS, Schaefer RK, Friedman RL. The relationship between subacromial space pressure, blood pressure, and visual clarity during arthroscopic subacromial decompression. Arthroscopy. 1995 Oct;11(5):557–60.

4. Farmer KW, Wright TW. Shoulder arthroscopy: the basics. J Hand Surg Am. 2015 Apr;40(4):817–21. Epub 2015 Feb 26.

5. Hughes MS, Matava MJ, Wright RW, Brophy RH, Smith MV. Interscalene brachial plexus block for arthroscopic shoulder surgery: a systematic review. J Bone Joint Surg Am. 2013 Jul 17;95(14):1318–24.

6. Singh A, Kelly C, O'Brien T, Wilson J, Warner JJ. Ultrasound-guided interscalene block anesthesia for shoulder arthroscopy: a prospective study of 1319 patients. J Bone Joint Surg Am. 2012 Nov 21;94(22):2040–6.

7. Urmey WF, McDonald M. Hemidiaphragmatic paresis during interscalene brachial plexus block: effects on pulmonary function and chest wall mechanics. Anesth Analg. 1992 Mar;74(3):352–7.

8. Murphy GS, Szokol JW, Marymont JH, Greenberg SB, Avram MJ, Vender JS, et al. Cerebral oxygen desaturation events assessed by near-infrared spectroscopy during shoulder arthroscopy in the beach chair and lateral decubitus positions. Anesth Analg. 2010 Aug;111(2):496–505. Epub 2010 May 27.

9. Trentman TL, Fassett SL, Thomas JK, Noble BN, Renfree KJ, Hattrup SJ. More hypotension in patients taking antihypertensives preoperatively during shoulder surgery in the beach chair position. Can J Anaesth. 2011 Nov;58(11):993–1000. Epub 2011 Aug 24.

10. Kwak HJ, Lee D, Lee YW, Yu GY, Shinn HK, Kim JY. The intermittent sequential compression device on the lower extremities attenuates the decrease in regional cerebral oxygen saturation during sitting position under sevoflurane anesthesia. J Neurosurg Anesthesiol. 2011 Jan;23(1):1–5.

11. Ruland LJ 3rd, Ruland CM, Matthews LS. Scapulothoracic anatomy for the arthroscopist. Arthroscopy. 1995 Feb;11(1):52–6.

12. Totlis T, Natsis K, Pantelidis P, Paraskevas G, Iosifidis M, Kyriakidis A. Reliability of the posterolateral corner of the acromion as a landmark for the posterior arthroscopic portal of the shoulder. J Shoulder Elbow Surg. 2014 Sep;23(9):1403–8. Epub 2014 Feb 28.

13. Wolf EM. Anterior portals in shoulder arthroscopy. Arthroscopy. 1989;5(3):201–8.

14. Ellman H. Arthroscopic subacromial decompression: analysis of one- to three-year results. Arthroscopy. 1987;3(3):173–81.

15. Laurencin CT, Deutsch A, O'Brien SJ, Altchek DW. The superolateral portal for arthroscopy of the shoulder. Arthroscopy. 1994 Jun;10(3):255–8.

16. Davidson PA, Rivenburgh DW. The 7-o'clock posteroinferior portal for shoulder arthroscopy. Am J Sports Med. 2002 Sep-Oct;30(5):693–6.

17. Dwyer T, Petrera M, White LM, Chechik O, Wasserstein D, Chahal J, et al. Trans-subscapularis portal versus low-anterior portal for low anchor placement on the inferior glenoid fossa: a cadaveric shoulder study with computed tomographic analysis. Arthroscopy. 2015 Feb;31(2):209–14. Epub 2014 Sep 30.

18. Davidson PA, Tibone JE. Anterior-inferior (5 o'clock) portal for shoulder arthroscopy. Arthroscopy. 1995 Oct;11(5):519–25.

19. Pearsall AW 4th, Holovacs TF, Speer KP. The low anterior five-o'clock portal during arthroscopic shoulder surgery performed in the beach-chair position. Am J Sports Med. 1999 Sep-Oct;27(5):571–4.

20. Oh JH, Kim SH, Lee HK, Jo KH, Bae KJ. Trans-rotator cuff portal is safe for arthroscopic superior labral anterior and posterior lesion repair: clinical and radiological analysis of 58 SLAP lesions. Am J Sports Med. 2008 Oct;36(10):1913–21. Epub 2008 May 21.

21. Neviaser TJ. Arthroscopy of the shoulder. Orthop Clin North Am. 1987 Jul;18(3):361–72.

22. Lafosse L, Tomasi A, Corbett S, Baier G, Willems K, Gobezie R. Arthroscopic release of suprascapular nerve entrapment at the suprascapular notch: technique and preliminary results. Arthroscopy. 2007 Jan;23(1):34–42.

23. Hanypsiak BT, DeLong JM, Simmons L, Lowe W, Burkhart S. Knot strength varies widely among expert arthroscopists. Am J Sports Med. 2014 Aug;42(8):1978–84. Epub 2014 Jun 12.

24. Lo IK, Ochoa E Jr, Burkhart SS. A comparison of knot security and loop security in arthroscopic knots tied with newer high-strength suture materials. Arthroscopy. 2010 Sep;26(9 Suppl):S120–6. Epub 2010 May 31.

25. Riboh JC, Heckman DS, Glisson RR, Moorman CT 3rd. Shortcuts in arthroscopic knot tying: do they

affect knot and loop security? Am J Sports Med. 2012 Jul;40(7):1572–7. Epub 2012 May 10.

26. Moen TC, Rudolph GH, Caswell K, Espinoza C, Burkhead WZ Jr, Krishnan SG. Complications of shoulder arthroscopy. J Am Acad Orthop Surg. 2014 Jul;22(7):410–9.

27. Lo IK, Lind CC, Burkhart SS. Glenohumeral arthroscopy portals established using an outside-in technique: neurovascular anatomy at risk. Arthroscopy. 2004 Jul;20(6):596–602.

28. Meyer M, Graveleau N, Hardy P, Landreau P. Anatomic risks of shoulder arthroscopy portals: anatomic cadaveric study of 12 portals. Arthroscopy. 2007 May;23(5):529–36.

29. Nottage WM. Arthroscopic portals: anatomy at risk. Orthop Clin North Am. 1993 Jan;24(1):19–26.

30. Zmistowski B, Austin L, Ciccotti M, Ricchetti E, Williams G Jr. Fatal venous air embolism during shoulder arthroscopy: a case report. J Bone Joint Surg Am. 2010 Sep 1;92(11):2125–7.

3 Surgical Exposures

Adequate exposure is critical for any of the open surgical procedures that are described in the remaining chapters of this book. Although exposures may need to be modified, the same approaches generally are used for various procedures. There are also small variations on exposures that are based on surgeons' preferences.

All shoulder exposures are somewhat complicated by 3 particular issues related to the anatomy of the shoulder region. First, the deltoid is a large muscle that wraps around the front, side, and back of the shoulder; deep exposure oftentimes requires either mobilizing the deltoid or splitting the deltoid fibers in a controlled fashion. Second, the rotator cuff, so important for shoulder function, oftentimes needs to be divided and repaired; subscapularis tenotomy (or any of its alternatives) is commonly required for open treatment of anterior instability or arthroplasty. Finally, a number of neurovascular structures are very close to the shoulder joint and at risk for injury, including the cephalic vein in the deltopectoral interval, the brachial plexus and subclavian vessels medial to the coracoid and conjoined tendon, the axillary nerve inferior to the glenoid and around the proximal aspect of the humeral neck, the musculocutaneous nerve in close proximity to the conjoined tendon, and the radial nerve more distally.

In this chapter, we review the most commonly used exposures for open shoulder surgery (Table 3.1), although I will not cover every single exposure described. Exposures for the scapula and periscapular muscles will be covered in chapters 6, The Rotator Cuff and Biceps Tendon, and 10, The Scapula. Some aspects of patient positioning and anesthesia, already discussed in chapter 2 on arthroscopy, also apply to open shoulder surgery, although there is less need for hypotensive anesthesia in open surgery. As detailed later, the posterior approach to the shoulder joint can be

Table 3.1 • Common Surgical Exposures in Open Shoulder Surgery
Deltopectoral approach
Standard deltopectoral approach
Long deltopectoral approach
Inferior deltopectoral approach
Anteromedial approach
Posterior approach to the glenohumeral joint
Direct posterior approach
Subdeltoid
Deltoid split
Deltoid detachment
Deltoid splitting approaches
Superior (or anterosuperior) approach
Mini-open deltoid split
Extended lateral deltoid split
Posterior deltoid split

performed with the patient prone or in the lateral decubitus position.

A Few Words About Skin Preparation

Before I dive into details on various surgical exposures, it is important to emphasize the need for proper skin preparation prior to shoulder surgery and other efforts that may be needed in order to decrease the chances of a deep surgical site infection. These concepts apply to both open and arthroscopic shoulder surgery, so please take them into account when you plan to perform arthroscopic shoulder procedures (see chapter 2, Arthroscopic Shoulder Surgery).

Infection is a devastating complication after any orthopedic surgical procedure, particularly when implants are

Table 3.2 • Considerations Related to Shoulder Surgery and *Cutibacterium* (*Propionibacterium*) spp Infection

Propionibacterium spp are slow-growing, gram-positive rods that behave as facultative anaerobes and colonize the pilosebaceous glands of the dermis

The axillary region harbors a higher concentration of *Staphylococcus* spp and other bacteria compared with the rest of the shoulder skin; the concentration of *Propionibacterium* spp is actually higher in the chest and back areas contiguous to the shoulder than in the axilla itself

Preparation of the skin for shoulder surgery with topical antiseptics helps decrease the chance of infection with non-*Propionibacterium* spp microorganisms, but probably does little to prevent *Propionibacterium* spp infection

Deep infections with *Propionibacterium* spp manifest as low grade infections
No classic signs of infection
Inflammatory markers (i.e., complete blood count, sedimentation rate, C-reactive protein) may be normal
Cultures from aspirated fluid may not grow; cell count often is normal
Intraoperative pathology does not show acute inflammation; it may show chronic inflammation
Isolation in culture may require surgical biopsies obtained through an open or arthroscopic approach, and longer culture times (e.g., 2–3 weeks)

Prevention of infection with *Propionibacterium* spp
Avoid operating on patients with active skin acne without treatment
Proper intravenous antibiotic prophylaxis
Change the knife blade after the skin is incised
Avoid contact between dermis and implants as much as possible
Consider bathing percutaneous implants in an antiseptic solution just prior to implantation
Consider bathing the surgical site at the end of the procedure with antiseptic solutions for a few minutes
Consider placing vancomycin powder at the surgical site at the end of the procedure prior to closure
Consider perioperative skin treatment with topical benzoyl peroxide and/or clindamycin

used. The shoulder region is somewhat vulnerable to a very specific group of microorganisms, *Propionibacterium* spp (recently renamed *Cutibaterium acnes*). These microorganisms were thought for the longest time to be only commensal bacteria not responsible for true infections. However, we now know that *Propionibacterium* spp are responsible for some opportunistic deep infections around the shoulder (Table 3.2) (1).

The axillary region is perceived to have a higher content of bacteria, which is true for *Staphylococci* and other species but not for *Propionibacterium* spp. When the shoulder is ready for skin preparation, it is wise to apply a topical antiseptic to the surgical site, ending with the axilla last to avoid dragging bacteria from the axillary region into the front or back of the shoulder. When draping, the axilla is also isolated first with adhesive film. However, these standard precautions will not address the *Propionibacterium* spp residing in the dermal sebaceous glands, and further actions are needed, as summarized at the end of Table 3.2.

Deltopectoral Approach

Exposure of the glenohumeral joint and adjacent structures through the natural anterior interval between the pectoralis major medially and the deltoid laterally is the most common approach used in open shoulder surgery (🔘 Video 3.1) (2). There are some variations in terms of the location of the skin incision, the proximal to distal portion of the interval used, and extending the approach if needed by controlled partial release of the deltoid origin or insertion.

Terminology

The standard deltopectoral approach utilizes most of the extent of the deltopectoral interval from proximal to distal. The term *long deltopectoral approach* (or extended deltopectoral approach) was introduced to emphasize the more ample exposure that is obtained when the deltopectoral interval is developed proximally all the way to the clavicle and distally all the way to the humeral shaft. As detailed later, my preference is to use a relatively lateral skin incision (Figure 3.1 line A), but others prefer to place the skin incision directly over the deltopectoral interval (Figure 3.1 line B). Shoulder hemiarthroplasty and simple proximal humerus fractures may be exposed through a shorter portion of the deltopectoral interval, but glenoid exposure in total shoulder arthroplasty and management of the more complex proximal humerus fractures benefit from a truly long deltopectoral approach.

Access to the anterior glenoid rim for management of anterior glenoid fractures and anterior instability (e.g., open Bankart repair and capsular shift, coracoid transfer procedures [see chapter 7, Shoulder Instability and the Labrum]) is best achieved using a more limited medial skin incision and developing the lower part of the deltopectoral approach; this represents the so-called inferior deltopectoral approach (or limited deltopectoral approach) (Figure 3.1, line C).

Occasionally, the long deltopectoral approach needs to be extended. Distal extension can be achieved by partially releasing the distal insertion of the deltoid. Proximal extension is only required for more complex procedures such as glenohumeral arthrodesis or extremely complex arthroplasty; proximal extension is achieved through the anteromedial approach (see later).

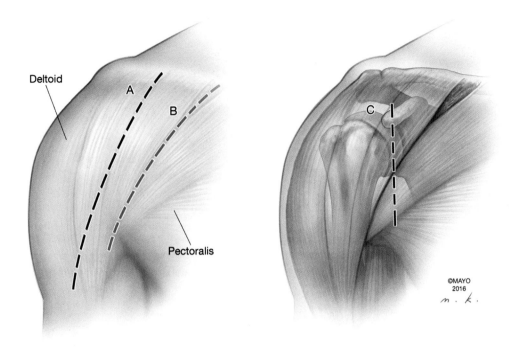

Figure 3.1 *Line* **A**, *Preferred skin incision for a long deltopectoral approach (note: other surgeons prefer a more medial oblique incision over the interval itself, as shown in Line* **B**; *see Table 3.3). Line* **C**, *Skin incision for the inferior deltopectoral approach.*

Long Deltopectoral Approach

This approach is typically performed in the beach chair position. Figure 3.2 summarizes this approach step by step. As mentioned before, my preference is to place the skin incision relatively lateral (Figure 3.1, line B; Figure 3.2, line A). In my opinion, placing the skin incision laterally (approximately 2 cm lateral to the tip of the coracoid) has a number of benefits (Table 3.3).

The deltopectoral interval is easiest to find proximally. The deltoid and the pectoralis are separated by a triangular space of adipose tissue (Mohrenheim fossa) (3). For a long deltopectoral approach, my preference is to preserve the cephalic vein and mobilize it medially with the pectoralis. This requires coagulation of the multiple feeding vein branches from the deltoid. Some surgeons prefer to ligate the vein or mobilize it laterally with the deltoid. Preservation of the cephalic vein theoretically decreases the chances of hand swelling. In addition, the vein can be left superficial to the deltopectoral interval at the time of closure, serving as a very useful landmark if revision surgery becomes necessary. As discussed later, for an inferior deltopectoral approach I typically mobilize the vein laterally with the deltoid.

The transverse branches (artery and veins) of the thoracoacromial arch cross the upper third of the deltopectoral interval just deep to the cephalic vein (Figure 3.3). It is wise to identify and coagulate or ligate these vessels before further developing the deltopectoral interval bluntly because, when these vessels are iatrogenically injured during exposure, they retract and bleed throughout the procedure and make visualization more difficult.

Mobilization of the deltoid is required for most procedures and is especially necessary for shoulder arthroplasty and plate fixation of the proximal humerus. Two pointed levering retractors (such as Hohmann retractors) are placed over the coracoid proximally and around the humeral shaft distally, just proximal to the deltoid insertion, where a natural subdeltoid space is very easy to identify and develop bluntly. My preference is to release the subdeltoid adhesions with the arm in abduction, typically by resting the arm and forearm on a Mayo stand at this point of the procedure. Placing the arm in abduction relaxes the deltoid muscle fibers, making it easier to develop the subdeltoid plane with less risk of injury to the axillary nerve or underlying rotator cuff. Deltoid retraction is best accomplished with a large, wide Browne retractor.

Selective release of the upper portion of the pectoralis tendon can aid exposure in large or muscular patients. Most of the time, no more than 1 or 2 cm are released. Most surgeons do not formally repair this partial pectoralis release at the time of closure.

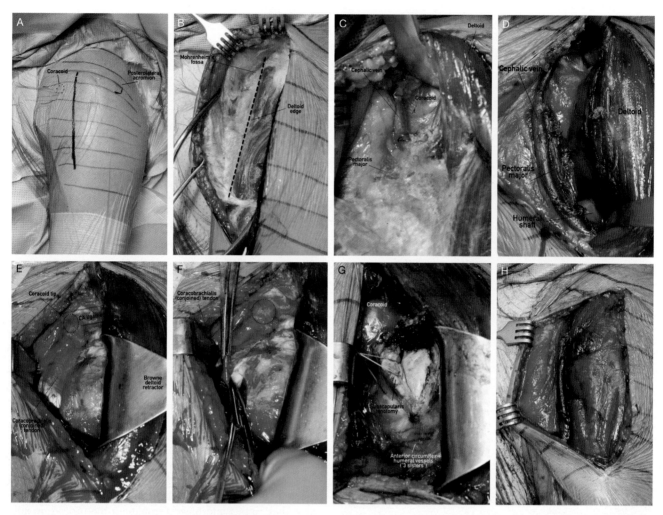

Figure 3.2 *The long deltopectoral approach step by step (left shoulder).* **A,** *Skin incision,* **B,** *Identification of the medial margin of the deltoid.* **C,** *Proximal development of the deltopectoral interval.* **D,** *Interval developed, cephalic vein preserved and mobilized medially.* **E and F,** *Identification and mobilization of the conjoined tendon.* **G,** *Subscapularis tenotomy.* **H,** *Closure.*

When needed, further exposure may also be gained by partial release of the distal insertion of the deltoid off the humeral shaft. This is particularly useful for plate fixation of proximal humerus fractures (chapter 4, Proximal Humerus Fractures) and revision shoulder arthroplasty (chapter 9,

---

Table 3.3 • Benefits of a Lateral Skin Incision for the Long Deltopectoral Approach Over Others

Better centered over the glenoid: facilitates glenoid exposure in shoulder arthroplasty

Better centered over the anterolateral aspect of the humeral shaft: facilitates plate fixation for proximal humerus fractures

Further away from the axillary region: may help decrease the potential for bacteria from the axilla to contaminate the surgical field

More cosmetic healing: it lies on top of the deltoid muscle as opposed to the interval, healing with less indentation

---

Shoulder Arthritis and Arthroplasty). The distal insertion of the deltoid measures between 5 and 7 cm in length and approximately 2 cm in width; in addition, the distal deltoid fibers continue partially into the fascia of the arm and intermuscular septum (4). Subperiosteal detachment of the distal deltoid is safe to some extent.

The next step of the exposure is to develop the plane between the conjoined tendon (which is superficial) and the subscapularis (which is deep). The coracobrachialis and the short head of the biceps are identified as a single structure. Oftentimes the most medial aspect of this conjoined tendon is fleshy (i.e., muscular) and not tendinous. Pulling up on the medial edge of the conjoined tendon clearly identifies the plane of dissection, which is more evident distally than proximally. The clavipectoral fascia can then be released all the way up to the coracoid tip and coracoacromial ligament. The axillary nerve can be felt by hooking a finger inferiorly in the space between the conjoined tendon and the subscapularis.

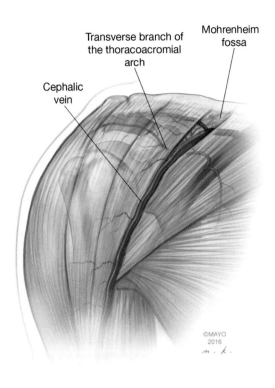

Cephalic vein

Transverse branch of the thoracoacromial arch

Mohrenheim fossa

©MAYO 2016
m. k.

Figure 3.3 Relationship between the cephalic vein and the transverse branch of the thoracoacromial arch.

Remember that the brachial plexus and the axillary vessels are close, deep, and medial to the conjoined tendon and the coracoid. Some have termed the coracoid process "the lighthouse of the shoulder," since it alerts the proximity of neurovascular structures in danger if dissection continues medially. When further medial exposure is required (i.e., locked anterior dislocations, removal of an anteriorly dislocated, fractured humeral head, exploration of the brachial plexus), the conjoined tendon can be detached from the coracoid for additional exposure, and repaired at the end of the case. Alternatively, the coracoid may be osteotomized and fixed at the end of the procedure.

The rest of the exposure depends on the nature of the procedure. When deeper articular exposure is gained through the subscapularis, care must be taken to ligate or coagulate the anterior humeral circumflex vessels (the so-called "three sisters") at the inferior edge of the subscapularis. When further exposure is required, the deltopectoral approach may be converted to an anteromedial approach (see later).

Inferior Deltopectoral Approach

The inferior, low, or limited deltopectoral approach was developed mainly for open procedures to manage recurrent anterior instability (open Bankart repair and capsular shift, coracoid transfer procedures, see chapter 7, Shoulder

Table 3.4 • Low (Inferior) Deltopectoral Approach: Tips and Tricks

Modified beach chair position
Patient is not seated as high as in the typical beach chair position
A folded towel under the medial border of the scapula *opens* the anteroinferior shoulder

Skin incision more medial and inferior (from tip of the coracoid to axilla)

The cephalic vein is mobilized medially

Change the position of the arm as needed
Lateral structures are exposed with the arm in abduction
Medial structures are exposed with the arm in adduction

Instability and the Labrum) or fractures of the anterior glenoid (⬤ Video 3.2).

Exposure of the anteroinferior aspect of the glenohumeral joint is facilitated by placing the patient in a modified beach chair position, not too high, and with a folded towel underneath the medial aspect of the scapula posteriorly (Table 3.4). Since the anteroinferior aspect of the glenohumeral joint is low and medial, the skin incision is typically different than for a long deltopectoral approach (Figure 3.1, line C). My preferred skin incision is centered over the tip of the coracoid and extends distally toward the axillary crease (Figure 3.4). Some authors have described use of an incision in the axilla for either open soft-tissue procedures for instability or for biceps tenodesis. The benefit of an axillary incision is improved cosmesis, but it may be more difficult to extend if needed and may increase the chance of bacterial contamination.

The inferior deltopectoral approach uses the inferior two thirds of the deltopectoral interval, and the cephalic vein is best mobilized laterally with the deltoid. Deep exposure is gained by mobilizing the deltoid laterally and developing the plane between the conjoined tendon and the subscapularis, as described earlier. Self-retaining retractors with interchangeable blades (such as the Kölbel retractor) are particularly useful for the low deltopectoral approach. If the medial blade is placed under the conjoined tendon, care must be taken to avoid a compression injury to the musculocutaneous nerve.

Since the exposure is more limited than when the whole deltopectoral approach is developed, remember to change the position of the arm to facilitate exposure in different portions of the procedure. Exposure of lateral structures (biceps, subscapularis tendon) is facilitated by placing the arm in abduction to relax the deltoid. Exposure of medial structures such as the conjoined tendon and pectoralis minor is facilitated by placing the arm in adduction. External rotation of the shoulder exposes the subscapularis muscle-tendon unit but also tends to lead to anterior subluxation, which may make medial exposure more difficult.

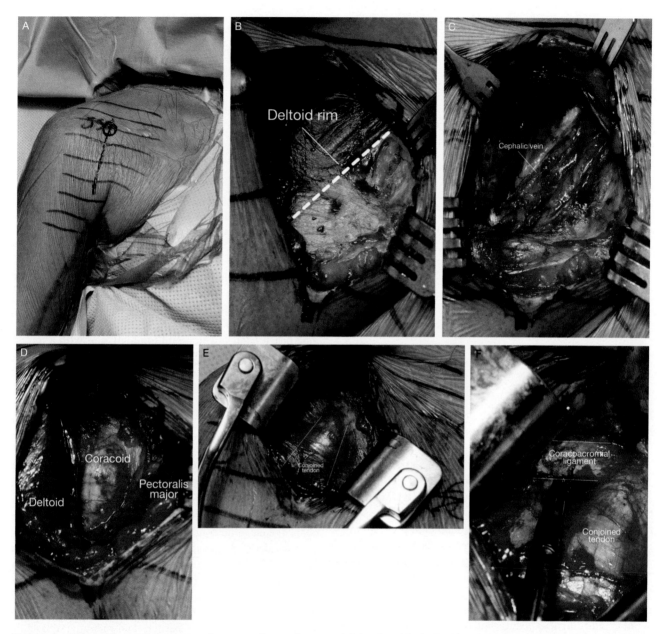

Figure 3.4 *The inferior deltopectoral approach step by step (right shoulder).* **A,** *Skin incision.* **B,** *Identification of the medial edge of the deltoid.* **C and D,** *Developing the deltopectoral interval.* **E,** *Self-retaining retractor and identification of the conjoined tendon.* **F,** *Detail of the location of the coracoacromial ligament.*

Exposure of the anteroinferior aspect of the glenoid and glenohumeral joint can be obtained by detaching or splitting the subscapularis (see chapter 7, Shoulder Instability and the Labrum). A subscapularis tenotomy is more commonly used when capsular shifting is considered, since adequate dissection of the plane between the subscapularis and capsule is best achieved that way. Horizontal splitting of the subscapularis along the line of its fibers is favored for glenoid bone grafting and internal fixation. In the Latarjet procedure, the coracoid is osteotomized and transferred to the anteroinferior glenoid (see chapter 7, Shoulder Instability

and the Labrum). Osteotomizing the coracoid and mobilizing the conjoined tendon first facilitates deep exposure of the glenoid. As mentioned before, taking down the conjoined tendon or osteotomizing the coracoid is a very useful step to improve medial exposure for other procedures when needed.

Anteromedial Approach

The anteromedial approach is used to describe extending the deltopectoral approach by progressive detachment of the origin of the deltoid from the clavicle, acromion, and

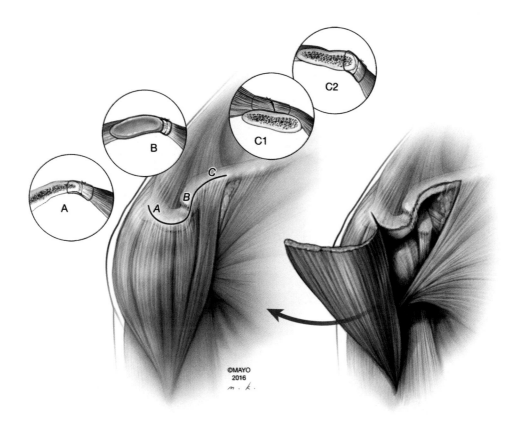

Figure 3.5 The anteromedial approach. **A,** *Transosseus deltoid repair to the acromion.* **B,** *Repair to the capsule at the acromioclavicular joint level.* **C,** *Repair of the deltoid to the trapezius;* **C1,** *standard repair;* **C2,** *alternative repair through clavicular bone.*

spine of the scapula, allowing complete mobilization of the deltoid laterally (Figure 3.5) (5,6). This approach was described and utilized more commonly decades ago but was largely replaced by the long deltopectoral approach. However, I currently use this approach for shoulder arthrodesis (see chapter 11, Salvage Procedures) and, rarely, for complex reconstructive shoulder surgery in patients with marked deformity or stiffness and in those with a severely scarred anterior deltoid that could tear in an uncontrolled way unless detached (Table 3.5, ◐ Video 3.3).

The long deltopectoral approach is first completed as detailed earlier. The deltoid origin is then carefully

---

Table 3.5 • Current Indications for the Anteromedial Approach

Glenohumeral arthrodesis

Complex reconstructive surgery in the presence of
Severe scarring of the anterior deltoid
Severe osteopenia and stiffness with risk of humeral shaft
    fracture
Need for more ample glenoid exposure

---

detached (Figures 3.5 and 3.6) starting medially over the clavicle and proceeding laterally over the acromioclavicular joint, anterior acromion, lateral acromion and, if needed, spine of the scapula (5–7). The key for a successful repair is to detach the deltoid subperiosteally with all its fascial tissue. In some cases all that is needed is to detach the anterior deltoid to protect it from uncontrolled tearing, whereas the detachment can continue posteriorly as needed depending on the extent of exposure required. Three medium-size Kocher clamps may be placed on the edge of the incised deltoid origin and allowed to fall laterally and posteriorly, keeping the detached deltoid out of the surgical field.

A strong repair is needed at the end of the procedure. Most surgeons use nonabsorbable sutures; however, our preference at Mayo Clinic is to use absorbable sutures. Sutures are placed through bone (at the acromion and clavicle) as well as through the capsule of the acromioclavicular joint. When the exposure has been extended posteriorly over the spine of the scapula, that portion of the repair can be reinforced with sutures between the deltoid and trapezius. Healing of the deltoid origin is facilitated by use of a sling or immobilizer for 6 weeks, avoiding active shoulder motion for the same period of time. When exposure, repair,

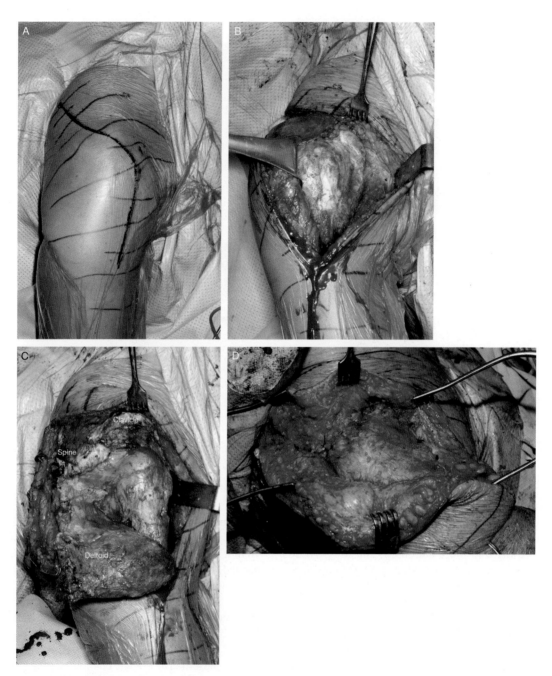

Figure 3.6 *The anteromedial approach step by step (right shoulder).* **A,** *Skin incision.* **B,** *Deltopectoral approach.* **C,** *Deltoid origin detached off bone.* **D,** *Closure.*

and protection are all performed carefully, the deltoid origin heals predictably (5,6).

Posterior Approach to the Glenohumeral Joint

Most shoulder surgeons are less familiar with open exposure of the posterior aspect of the glenohumeral joint. Advances in shoulder arthroscopy provide a very useful alternative for procedures performed through an open approach in the past, particularly open repair of the posterior labrum and capsule, now largely abandoned. However, approaching the posterior aspect of the glenohumeral joint and the posterior aspect of the scapular body may be indicated for certain fractures of the posterior glenoid cavity, fractures of the scapular body, bone block augmentation procedures for posterior shoulder instability, certain tendon transfers, axillary nerve repair or reconstruction, glenoid osteotomy, and resection of tumors.

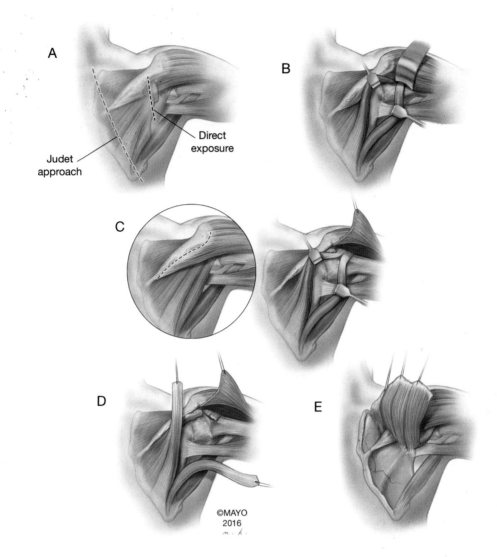

Figure 3.7 Posterior surgical exposures. **A,** *Skin incisions for the direct posterior approach and the Judet approach.* **B,** *Posterior approach without deltoid detachment.* **C,** *Posterior approach with deltoid detachment.* **D,** *Posterior approach with deltoid detachment and infraspinatus/teres minor tenotomy.* **E,** *Posterior approach with deltoid detachment and elevation of the supraspinatus and/or infraspinatus from medial to lateral (classic Judet approach).*

Many surgeons use the term *Judet approach* to refer to an extensile exposure to the posterior aspect of the scapula, initially described for fracture fixation (8) (Figure 3.7). This approach involves detachment of the posterior deltoid off the scapular spine and subperiosteal elevation of the supraspinatus and/or infraspinatus from medial to lateral. Although this approach provides great exposure, it is associated with substantial morbidity and carries the risk of supraspinatus and infraspinatus atrophy (9–12). Currently, most surgeons favor trying to achieve good exposure through the interval between the teres minor and the supraspinatus (2,9,11). In addition, the deltoid origin is preserved intact whenever possible (10,13) and detached selectively only if additional exposure is required.

Careful patient positioning is important. The patient may be placed prone or in the lateral decubitus position. When placed prone, the affected upper extremity is draped so that it is free and may then be supported in a Mayo stand throughout the procedure; this allows easy adjustment of the position of the upper extremity for various portions of the procedure. When the patient is placed in the lateral decubitus position, use of an articulated arm holder is extremely useful.

Direct Posterior Approach

For procedures that require access to the posterior aspect of the glenohumeral joint without extension toward the scapular body, the exposure can be performed using a

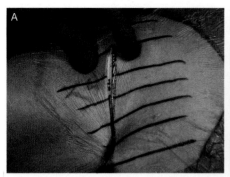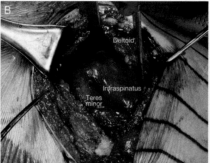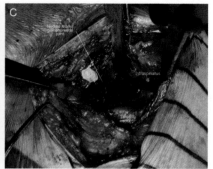

Figure 3.8 *Direct posterior approach.* **A**, *Skin incision.* **B**, *Identification of the interval between teres minor and infraspinatus.* **C**, *Deep exposure.*

straight vertical incision centered over the glenohumeral joint, slightly medial to the posterior corner of the acromion (Figure 3.8, ⬤ Video 3.4) (13). The posteroinferior rim of the deltoid is identified and the plane between the deltoid and the underlying cuff muscles is developed bluntly. Placing the arm in abduction will facilitate this step by bringing the deltoid edge superior and relaxing the deltoid fibers.

Once the deltoid is retracted superiorly, the raphe between the infraspinatus and teres minor is identified and developed from medial to lateral. Separation of these 2 muscle bellies allows exposure of the posterior aspect of the scapular body and glenoid. Dissection may be carried further laterally to the capsule of the glenohumeral joint. A needle may be used to identify the glenohumeral joint line posteriorly. Depending on the procedure to be performed, the joint may be opened. If further proximal exposure is required, an infraspinatus tenotomy and later repair may be performed, although this last step is seldom needed.

When exposure is difficult secondary to a very bulky deltoid that cannot be retracted enough out of the way, consideration may be given to partly releasing the most medial aspect of the origin of the posterior deltoid from the spine of the scapula (13). Sometimes, releasing 2 to 3 cm is all that is required to improve exposure. Deltoid reattachment should be performed through bone at the end of the procedure. Alternatively, a longitudinal split of the posterior deltoid has also been described for a direct posterior approach to the glenohumeral joint (14). However, distal exposure may be limited when splitting the posterior deltoid due to the location of the axillary nerve (15).

Extensile Posterior Approach

When more ample exposure is required, typically in the setting of fractures involving the body of the scapula, many surgeons favor a curvilinear incision placed horizontally along the spine of the scapula from medial to lateral, that then curves inferiorly at the posterior corner of the acromion (Figure 3.7). In the classic description of the extensile posterior approach, the deltoid origin is detached from the spine of the scapula from medial to lateral and retracted laterally, and the origin of the supraspinatus, the infraspinatus, or both is elevated subperiosteally from the respective fossae. Care must be taken to avoid injury to the suprascapular nerve or its branches as the dissection progresses medially and superiorly (8,9). Currently, most surgeons try to gain exposure of the scapular body by working in the interval between the teres minor and the infraspinatus as described earlier (9,10).

Deltoid Splitting Exposures

Exposure of the rotator cuff and greater tuberosity (by splitting the deltoid in line with its fibers) represents another classic shoulder exposure; it was universally used by most surgeons for open cuff surgery (see chapter 6, The Rotator Cuff and Biceps Tendon). With the development of arthroscopic techniques for cuff repair, this exposure is less commonly used for that particular indication, but at the same time interest has grown in using a superior approach for reverse shoulder arthroplasty (16) (see chapter 9, Shoulder Arthritis and Arthroplasty) and a more distal deltoid split for proximal humerus fracture plate fixation (2,17–19). As mentioned before, splitting the posterior deltoid has also been described to perform a direct posterior approach to the glenohumeral joint (14) (Table 3.6).

Deltoid splitting exposures are somewhat limited by the location of the axillary nerve. Since the axillary nerve runs somewhat horizontally and perpendicular to the deltoid fibers, uncontrolled distal deltoid split may result in iatrogenic damage to the axillary nerve or its branches. The distance between the acromion and the location of the axillary nerve is proportional to the length of the arm (i.e., size of the patient) and varies from anterior to posterior and with arm positioning (15,20). A detailed study reported an average distance of 6 cm (range, 5–7 cm) between the anterior acromion and the axillary nerve, whereas the posterior distance was 5 cm (range, 4–6 cm) (15). However, the distance seems

Table 3.6 • Deltoid Splitting Exposures

Superior (anterosuperior) approach
Open cuff repair
Fractures of the greater tuberosity
Reverse shoulder arthroplasty

Mini-open deltoid split
Mini-open rotator cuff repair
Intramedullary nailing for proximal humerus/humeral shaft
    fractures

Lateral deltoid split
Plate fixation for proximal humerus fractures

Posterior deltoid split
Direct posterior approach

to decrease with arm abduction (20). Figure 3.9 represents the safe deltoid zone for a lateral split of the deltoid. In general, most surgeons agree on not splitting the deltoid more than 5 cm from the lateral acromion (2,16).

Superior (Anterosuperior) Approach

This exposure involves detachment of part of the deltoid from the acromion and splitting of the deltoid; it is used most commonly for open cuff repair, fixation of greater tuberosity fractures, and sometimes for implantation of a reverse shoulder arthroplasty (Video 3.5). Several variations have been described in terms of both skin incisions and deltoid detachment (Table 3.7).

Most surgeons favor use of a lateral skin incision starting over the anterior aspect of the acromioclavicular joint and extended laterally over the anterior acromion and lateral deltoid. The deltoid is split along the raphe between its anterior and middle portions, and the anterior deltoid is detached subperiosteally from the anterior acromion and lateral clavicle. The raphe between the anterior and the middle deltoid represents a watershed intervascular zone, since the posterior and middle deltoid are vascularized by branches of the posterior circumflex vessels, whereas the anterior deltoid is vascularized by branches of the thoracoacromial arch or the anterior circumflex vessels (21). The deltoid is repaired through bone to the acromion and side to side for the split portion (2,11,16).

As discussed in chapter 6, The Rotator Cuff and Biceps Tendon, when the anterosuperior approach is used for open rotator cuff repair surgery, I prefer a variation of the approach just described (Figure 3.10). The skin incision is oblique (*saber cut*), and the deltoid is detached from the anterior acromion and lateral acromion; the deltoid split is more anterior, in line with the acromioclavicular joint, and the deltoid flap thus created is retracted laterally, as a *piece of a pie* or a *number 7*. This modification of the anterosuperior approach provides a number of benefits for cuff repair surgery (Table 3.8).

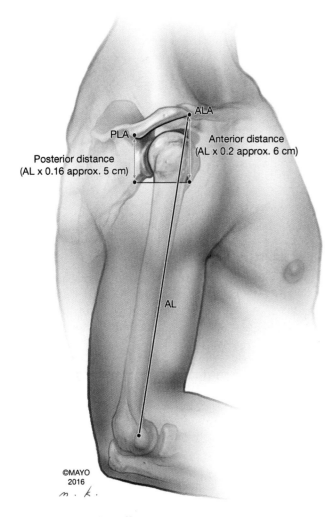

©MAYO
2016
m. k.

Figure 3.9 Safe axillary nerve zone.

Table 3.7 • Variations in the Superior (Anterosuperior) Splitting Approach

Skin incision
Lateral (in line with the anterior acromion)
Oblique (saber-cut)
Transverse (along Langer lines)
U-shaped

Deltoid detachment
From the anterior acromion, acromioclavicular joint and
    clavicle only
        Continues into a lateral split
From the anterior and lateral acromion
        Continues as an anterior split

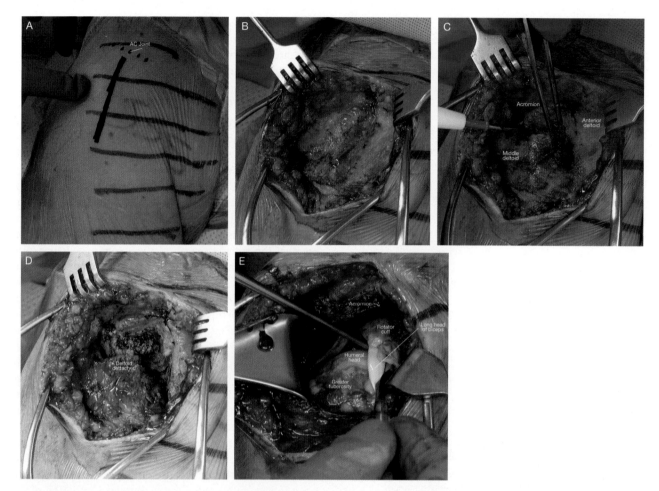

Figure 3.10 *Anterosuperior approach with anterior deltoid splitting (right shoulder).* **A,** *Skin incision.* **B,** *Mobilizing skin flaps.* **C and D,** *Deltoid detachment.* **E,** *Deep exposure.*

Table 3.8 • Benefits of the Anterosuperior Deltoid Splitting Approach for Open Cuff Repair
Can be extended distally and medially into the deltopectoral interval
Can be extended proximally and posteriorly into the anteromedial approach
If the axillary branches are inadvertently damaged, less deltoid is denervated

The anterosuperior approach has a number of potential issues. It seems to be more painful than the deltopectoral approach. As mentioned before, care must be taken to avoid damage to the axillary nerve. In addition, if the deltoid origin does not heal, late repair or reconstruction is unpredictable and functional losses are typically substantial (22). Luckily, healing seems to happen reliably in the absence of infection, provided the exposure, repair, and postoperative protection are adequate (23). However, late deltoid detachment has been reported when reverse arthroplasty

is performed through a deltopectoral approach in patients with a previous superior approach (24).

Mini-Open Deltoid Split

A limited split of the deltoid fibers without detachment of the deltoid origin from bone has been used for so-called "mini-open" rotator cuff repairs as well as for intramedullary nailing of fractures of the proximal humerus and humeral shaft.

As arthroscopic techniques for cuff repair continued to evolve, surgeons started to perform bursectomy, acromioplasty, associated intra-articular procedures, and cuff releases arthroscopically; however, difficulties with skills and instrumentation would make it difficult to complete the repair arthroscopically. In these circumstances, after all the arthroscopic work is completed, the surgeon splits the deltoid just lateral to the acromion to complete the repair. This has largely been abandoned now that arthroscopic cuff procedures are more streamlined, but it is important to keep in the armamentarium of the shoulder surgeon in case difficulties with arthroscopic cuff repair arise.

Intramedullary nailing for fractures of the proximal humerus or humeral shaft is also commonly performed through a limited deltoid split. The deltoid is split in line with the anterolateral acromion to gain access to the entry point for the humeral nail. Some nails are designed to be introduced through the greater tuberosity and some are inserted through the most lateral portion of the articular cartilage of the humeral head. In any event, the supraspinatus tendon needs to be split or detached in order to access the entry point. Both the supraspinatus and the deltoid are repaired at the end of the procedure.

Extended Lateral Deltoid Split

This approach was developed for plate fixation of proximal humerus fractures. Although a long deltopectoral approach offers (in my opinion) great exposure for proximal humerus plate fixation, some surgeons have reported difficulties in getting the plate positioned laterally enough (which typically requires releasing some of the distal deltoid from the humeral shaft) and gaining control of the greater tuberosity. Splitting the deltoid laterally from the acromion and past the location of the axillary nerve facilitates lateral plate placement and control of the greater tuberosity (2,17–19). However, it requires dissecting the axillary nerve and working through 2 separate proximal and distal windows.

The proximal window of the extended lateral deltoid approach corresponds to a classic superior approach: the deltoid is split through the raphe between the anterior and the middle deltoid for a distance of approximately 4 to 5 cm. The deltoid can be partially detached off the anterior acromion if needed. Once the proximal window has been fully developed, the surgeon palpates through the split distally and posteriorly to identify the location of the axillary nerve. The nerve is dissected and protected with a vessel loop, and more deltoid is split distal to the location of the nerve, creating the distal window (2,17,18). The plate used for fracture fixation can then be slid under the axillary nerve from the proximal and into the distal window. Studies reported on the use of this approach for fracture fixation have not reported axillary nerve dysfunction postoperatively (17,18).

KEY POINTS

✓ Surgical exposures for open shoulder surgery are complicated by the need to mobilize, split, or detach the deltoid muscle, divide or split the rotator cuff, and protect various neurovascular structures, in particular the axillary nerve.

✓ The deltopectoral interval is most commonly used for open shoulder surgery. The long deltopectoral approach provides great exposure for proximal humerus fracture fixation and arthroplasty, whereas a more limited inferior deltopectoral approach is ideal for access to the anteroinferior glenoid rim.

✓ Extension of the deltopectoral approach by a limited release of the distal insertion of the deltoid is easy to perform and well tolerated. The long deltopectoral approach can also be extended into the anteromedial approach (i.e., controlled detachment of the deltoid origin) for shoulder arthrodesis and complex reconstructive shoulder surgery.

✓ A direct posterior approach with deltoid preservation and development of the interval between teres minor and infraspinatus provides adequate exposure to the posterior aspect of the glenohumeral joint.

✓ A more extensile posterior approach can be achieved by detaching the deltoid origin off the spine of the scapula and occasionally elevating the posterior cuff muscles off their respective fossae.

✓ The superior deltoid splitting approach, formerly often used for open cuff repair surgery, is now used mostly for reverse joint replacement and fixation of proximal humerus fractures involving the greater tuberosity.

✓ A limited split of the anterolateral deltoid may also be used to access the entry point for nails used for fixation of proximal humerus or humeral shaft fractures.

✓ The extended lateral deltoid split approach, developed for plate fixation of proximal humerus fractures, requires use of 2 windows separated by the axillary nerve, which needs to be dissected and protected. It allows direct lateral plate fixation and great exposure of the greater tuberosity. Although axillary nerve dysfunction seems to be uncommon, it remains a potential concern.

REFERENCES

1. Hsu JE, Bumgarner RE, Matsen FA 3rd. Propionibacterium in shoulder arthroplasty: what we think we know today. J Bone Joint Surg Am. 2016 Apr 6;98(7):597–606.
2. Chalmers PN, Van Thiel GS, Trenhaile SW. Surgical exposures of the shoulder. J Am Acad Orthop Surg. 2016 Apr;24(4):250–8.
3. Gadea F, Bouju Y, Berhouet J, Bacle G, Favard L. Deltopectoral approach for shoulder arthroplasty: anatomic basis. Int Orthop. 2015 Feb;39(2):215–25. Epub 2015 Jan 16.
4. Rispoli DM, Athwal GS, Sperling JW, Cofield RH. The anatomy of the deltoid insertion. J Shoulder Elbow Surg. 2009 May-Jun;18(3):386–90. Epub 2009 Jan 30.
5. Foruria AM, Oh LS, Sperling JW, Cofield RH. Anteromedial approach for shoulder arthroplasty: current indications, complications, and results. J Shoulder Elbow Surg. 2010 Jul;19(5):734–8. Epub 2010 Feb 10.
6. Gill DR, Cofield RH, Rowland C. The anteromedial approach for shoulder arthroplasty: the importance of the anterior deltoid. J Shoulder Elbow Surg. 2004 Sep-Oct;13(5):532–7.
7. Kumar VP, Satku K, Liu J, Shen Y. The anatomy of the anterior origin of the deltoid. J Bone Joint Surg Br. 1997 Jul;79(4):680–3.

8. Judet R. [Surgical treatment of scapular fractures]. Acta Orthop Belg. 1964;30:673–8. French.

9. Harmer LS, Phelps KD, Crickard CV, Sample KM, Andrews EB, Hamid N, et al. A comparison of exposure between the classic and modified judet approaches to the scapula. J Orthop Trauma. 2016 May;30(5):235–9.

10. Salassa TE, Hill BW, Cole PA. Quantitative comparison of exposure for the posterior Judet approach to the scapula with and without deltoid takedown. J Shoulder Elbow Surg. 2014 Nov;23(11):1747–52. Epub 2014 May 24.

11. Hoyen H, Papendrea R. Exposures of the shoulder and upper humerus. Hand Clin. 2014 Nov;30(4):391–9. Epub 2014 Oct 23.

12. Jones CB, Cornelius JP, Sietsema DL, Ringler JR, Endres TJ. Modified Judet approach and minifragment fixation of scapular body and glenoid neck fractures. J Orthop Trauma. 2009 Sep;23(8):558–64.

13. Brodsky JW, Tullos HS, Gartsman GM. Simplified posterior approach to the shoulder joint: a technical note. J Bone Joint Surg Am. 1987 Jun;69(5):773–4.

14. Wirth MA, Butters KP, Rockwood CA Jr. The posterior deltoid-splitting approach to the shoulder. Clin Orthop Relat Res. 1993 Nov;(296):92–8.

15. Cetik O, Uslu M, Acar HI, Comert A, Tekdemir I, Cift H. Is there a safe area for the axillary nerve in the deltoid muscle? A cadaveric study. J Bone Joint Surg Am. 2006 Nov;88(11):2395–9.

16. Mole D, Wein F, Dezaly C, Valenti P, Sirveaux F. Surgical technique: the anterosuperior approach for reverse shoulder arthroplasty. Clin Orthop Relat Res. 2011 Sep;469(9):2461–8.

17. Robinson CM, Murray IR. The extended deltoid-splitting approach to the proximal humerus: variations and extensions. J Bone Joint Surg Br. 2011 Mar;93(3):387–92.

18. Gardner MJ, Boraiah S, Helfet DL, Lorich DG. The anterolateral acromial approach for fractures of the proximal humerus. J Orthop Trauma. 2008 Feb;22(2):132–7.

19. Robinson CM, Khan L, Akhtar A, Whittaker R. The extended deltoid-splitting approach to the proximal humerus. J Orthop Trauma. 2007 Oct;21(9):657–62.

20. Burkhead WZ Jr, Scheinberg RR, Box G. Surgical anatomy of the axillary nerve. J Shoulder Elbow Surg. 1992 Jan;1(1):31–6. Epub 2009 Feb 2.

21. Hue E, Gagey O, Mestdagh H, Fontaine C, Drizenko A, Maynou C. The blood supply of the deltoid muscle: application to the deltoid flap technique. Surg Radiol Anat. 1998;20(3):161–5.

22. Groh GI, Simoni M, Rolla P, Rockwood CA. Loss of the deltoid after shoulder operations: an operative disaster. J Shoulder Elbow Surg. 1994 Jul;3(4):243–53. Epub 2009 Feb 13.

23. Cofield RH, Parvizi J, Hoffmeyer PJ, Lanzer WL, Ilstrup DM, Rowland CM. Surgical repair of chronic rotator cuff tears: a prospective long-term study. J Bone Joint Surg Am. 2001 Jan;83-A(1):71–7.

24. Whatley AN, Fowler RL, Warner JJ, Higgins LD. Postoperative rupture of the anterolateral deltoid muscle following reverse total shoulder arthroplasty in patients who have undergone open rotator cuff repair. J Shoulder Elbow Surg. 2011 Jan;20(1):114–22. Epub 2010 Aug 30.

4 Proximal Humerus Fractures

Fractures of the proximal humerus are common. A relatively large number of these injuries will heal with nonoperative treatment without major residual pain or functional loss. However, internal fixation or arthroplasty leads to a much better outcome for selected fractures.

The orthopedic surgeon dealing with these injuries is faced with 3 challenges. First, it is difficult to understand these fractures based on imaging studies and to select those patients that will do better with surgery. Second, internal fixation and arthroplasty for proximal humerus fractures are difficult procedures fraught with technical complications. And third, complications often require challenging salvage procedures. Fracture personality and patient age and comorbidities all play a role in treatment selection.

Epidemiology

Proximal humerus fractures are the third-most-common nonvertebral osteoporotic fracture in patients over age 65 (following hip fractures and distal radius fractures) (1–3). Over the past few years, the annual incidence of proximal humerus fractures has been reported to be 61/100,000 men and 125/100,000 women. The frequency of proximal humerus fractures is increasing; in the United States, the number of patients presenting with a proximal humerus fracture is expected to reach 275,000 by 2030. Proximal humerus fractures often occur in the fit, independent, elderly patient who is still a contributing member of society but might well become socially dependent after a fracture.

History and Physical Examination

The key pieces of information to be obtained in every patient with a proximal humerus fracture are summarized in Table 4.1. The management strategy will be completely

Table 4.1 • Important Factors for Patients With a Proximal Humerus Fracture

Shoulder status prior to this injury (completely normal, cuff, arthritis)

Age, comorbidities, anticipated functional demands, lower extremities, support systems

Fragility/fracture history (Do I need to worry about osteopenia/osteoporosis?)

Associated injuries: clavicle, elbow, forearm, wrist, hand, head, others

Status of the axillary nerve, the brachial plexus, other nerve injuries

Pulse

different for a young patient with a previously normal shoulder and interest in return to sports versus an elderly patient who needs to use a walker on a regular basis and had already complained of pain and loss of motion prior to the fracture.

Patients with prior shoulder complaints may be best served by surgery either acutely or once the fracture has healed, depending on the nature of the previous pathology. Elderly debilitated patients may be best served by avoidance of surgery, even for fractures with substantial displacement. However, some elderly patients who enjoy an independent life may suddenly be rendered dependent by the poor outcome of a proximal humerus fracture. Fractures of the proximal humerus are a classic example of fragility fractures; evaluation and prevention strategies (e.g., bone mineral density evaluation, calcium, vitamin D, bisphosphonates, PTH-analogues) should be considered when appropriate.

Assessments of active range of motion or cuff strength through physical examination are pointless in the acute fracture setting. The examination should be directed to identifying associated injuries. Carefully palpate the clavicle and assess the elbow, forearm, wrist, and hand. Arterial injuries are uncommon but must be ruled out. Axillary nerve injuries are relatively common; check for sensory changes in the lateral aspect of the deltoid region and assess contraction of the posterior deltoid muscle. A complete neurologic evaluation should be directed to identifying associated brachial plexus injuries.

During the first days to weeks after a proximal humerus fracture, ecchymosis will develop in the medial aspect of the arm and lateral aspect of the chest wall. Patients should be educated about this anticipated hematoma so that they do not become alarmed by extensive bruising.

Imaging and Other Complementary Studies

Radiographs

Plain radiographs are essential for the evaluation of proximal humerus fractures (Table 4.2). The anteroposterior projection must be performed in the scapular plane (trunk angled approximately 30° with the noninjured side forward); commonly referred to as the Grashey view, this position will avoid projection overlapping of the humeral head and the glenoid (Figure 4.1). The Grashey view is performed best in some external rotation to optimize evaluation of the greater tuberosity to head relationship. The axillary view may be obtained by abduction of the arm

---

Table 4.2 • Pitfalls for Imaging Studies in Proximal Humerus Fractures

- Do not accept suboptimal radiograph projections; it is important to obtain optimal views (i.e., Grashey, Neer, Axillary, or Velpeau Axillary)

- Do not miss dislocation of the head posteriorly or anteriorly

- Arm rotation will influence projection of the head-shaft varus/valgus angulation

- Axillary radiographs will overestimate shaft angulation; check the Y view

- Identify any possible associated glenoid rim fractures

- Identify pre-existing pathology (e.g., arthritis) and associated injuries (e.g., clavicle fracture)

- Spin the 3D renderings of the CT scan first, then evaluate the 2D cuts

- Assess greater tuberosity comminution and size

- Use CT scan to assess the cuff status (atrophy, fatty infiltration)

- Use CT scan to assess bone quality and pre-existing arthritis

Abbreviations: CT, computed tomography; 2D, 2-dimensional; 3D, 3-dimensional.

(Figure 4.1D) or by keeping the arm in an immobilizer (Velpeau axillary projection, Figure 4.1C). The scapular lateral, or Y (i.e., Neer), projection is obtained with the patient facing the cassette, the torso rotated 60°, and the source located posteriorly (Figure 4.1B) (2).

Fracture lines are quite consistent (4). When the greater tuberosity is fractured, the fracture plane starts lateral to the bicipital groove and exits posteriorly, sometimes including a small portion of the articular cartilage. When the lesser tuberosity is fractured, the fragment includes not only the lesser tuberosity but also the bicipital groove. The head segment may be fractured off the shaft flush with the articular cartilage rim or more distally along the calcar region.

Fracture-dislocations typically will not do well without surgery; interestingly, the dislocation component of the injury is not uncommonly missed. Start by assessing the head–glenoid relationship in all 3 views. Posterior dislocation of the head segment is best identified by outlining the contour of the subchondral bone on the axillary radiograph and determining its relationship to the glenoid articular surface (Figure 4.2). With posterior head dislocation, the head will be overlapping the glenoid in a true Grashey view. Anterior dislocation of the head segment is easier to identify in the anteroposterior radiograph and also is visualized well in axillary projections (Figure 4.3).

Displacement of the greater tuberosity needs to be assessed in both the anteroposterior (is the profile of the greater tuberosity higher than the head?) and axillary (is the greater tuberosity displaced posteriorly enough to impinge with the posterior glenoid rim?) projections. Displacement of the greater tuberosity is best assessed in the axillary radiograph (Figure 4.4). Head–shaft relationships are assessed in terms of translation, angulation, and varus-valgus malalignment. Translation and angulation are best assessed in the anteroposterior and Y views; the axillary view will show various degrees of angulation, depending on how the arm is positioned by the radiology technician at the time. Translation and angulation are surrogates for instability and lack of contact and may lead to malunion or nonunion. Varus-valgus malalignment is best assessed in the anteroposterior view. Take into account that when the shoulder is in internal rotation, the head projects as varus (articular cartilage pointing up); thus, varus malalignment is oftentimes overestimated.

Computed Tomography

Computed tomography (CT) with 3-dimensional reconstruction is extremely useful for both evaluation and surgical planning (Figure 4.5). In my opinion, CT should not be used routinely; however, it should be obtained in every fracture scheduled for the operating room and in every instance when the evaluating orthopedic surgeon is unclear about the choice between nonoperative and operative treatment.

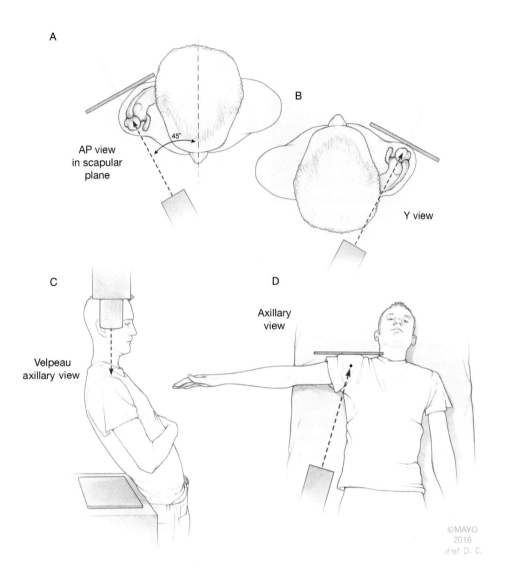

Figure 4.1 *Patient positioning for radiographs commonly used in the evaluation of proximal humerus fractures.* **A,** *Grashey (anteroposterior [AP]) view;* **B,** *Neer (lateral [Y]) view;* **C,** *Velpeau axillary view;* **D,** *Axillary view.*

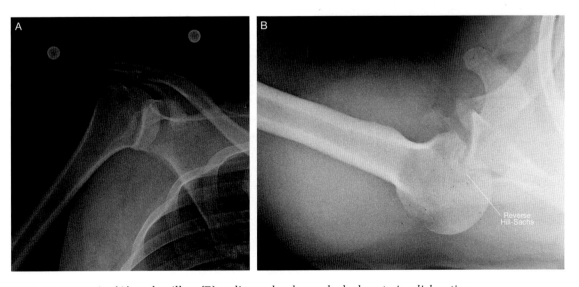

Figure 4.2 *Anteroposterior* **(A)** *and axillary* **(B)** *radiographs show a locked posterior dislocation.*

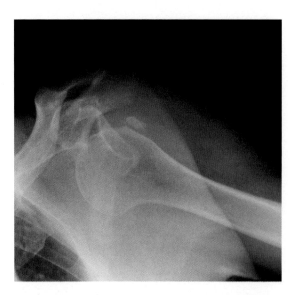

Figure 4.3 Anterior dislocation with a small greater tuberosity fracture.

In my experience, it is best to look at the 3-dimensional reconstruction first. Rotation of the images builds a mental representation of the fracture in the mind of the evaluating physician. Once the fracture personality is understood, the 2-dimensional images (and plain radiographs) can then be assessed for details and measurements (i.e., millimeters of greater tuberosity displacement, length of calcar attachment to the head segment).

CT provides added value in terms of assessing pre-existing pathology such as cuff atrophy or fatty infiltration (indicative of cuff pathology), as well as identifying associated glenoid rim fractures that may be extremely difficult to visualize in plain radiographs.

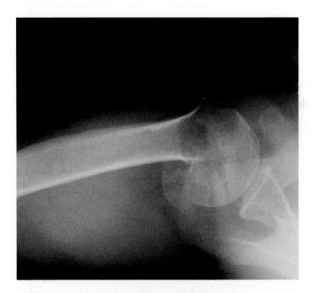

Figure 4.4 Greater tuberosity displacement is sometimes best appreciated on the axillary radiograph.

Other Studies

Magnetic resonance has limited value in patients with proximal humerus fractures except for occult fractures of the greater tuberosity or surgical neck. *Vascular studies* (i.e., angiography or magnetic resonance angiogram) may need to be considered when an associated injury to the axillary vessels is suspected or in chronic anterior fracture-dislocations where the head segment may be scarred to blood vessel walls. *Nerve conduction studies* should be considered in patients with associated nerve injuries, but do not provide much useful information until week 4 (see chapter 1, Evaluation of the Shoulder).

Classification versus Understanding: The Decision-Making Process

You have confirmed that your patient has a proximal humerus fracture. You need to decide if surgery is best and, in that case, what type of surgery. *How do you do that?* Great minds in shoulder surgery have proposed various classification systems, but the reality is that, when using various classifications, intraobserver and interobsever agreement have been suboptimal. However, trying to apply one classification system (or several) does help the surgeon understand fracture patterns and appreciate displacement.

Neer concepts on fracture displacement and classification continue to be used as a frame of reference (Table 4.3) (5). A proximal humerus part (e.g., head, tuberosities, or shaft) is considered displaced when there is more than 1 cm of distance or more than 45° of angulation. It is important to emphasize that these criteria for displacement were not based on data analysis; they were set arbitrarily. Identification of displacement was not meant to set the indication for surgery or dictate the type of procedure to be used. Intuitively, displaced fractures should do worse than nondisplaced fractures when allowed to heal in their displaced position; however, the correlation between fracture pattern and displacement and outcome has been difficult to establish.

Fracture Patterns and Displacement

The proximal humerus may fracture in many different ways. However, a few patterns are seen much more commonly than others (6–8). Figure 4.6 does not include every single possible fracture subtype, but it does present a useful algorithmic way to understand common fracture patterns.

Fractures through the articular surface of the humeral head are not very common but need to be identified when present. **Head-depression fractures** typically are the result of a dislocation, with the glenoid rim impacting and depressing a portion of the articular surface (similar to the imprint

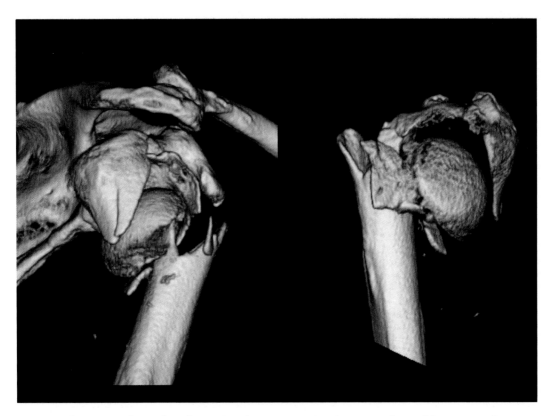

Figure 4.5 *Computed tomography with 3-dimensional reconstruction is extremely useful to assess fracture pattern and displacement.*

Table 4.3 • Neer Concepts on Displacement and Classification for Proximal Humerus Fractures

Displacement of a given part or segment
Distance >1 cm
Angulation >45°
Fracture types
Nondisplaced fracture
Head-splitting fracture
Head-depression fracture
Displaced fracture (1, 2, 3, or 4-part with or without dislocation)

Issues
Displacement criteria were set arbitrarily
The specifics on how to measure displacement were not precisely detailed
Displacement did not imply "always requires surgery" or dictate the type of surgery
Few studies have tried to correlate displacement or fracture pattern with outcome
Agreement is suboptimal, probably due to difficulty in reading imaging studies

---

left by a thumb pressing on a ping-pong ball) (Figure 4.7). Anterior dislocations lead to an impaction fracture of the posterosuperior aspect of the humeral head (Hill-Sachs lesion), whereas posterior dislocations lead to an impaction

of the anterior aspect of the humeral head (reverse Hill-Sachs lesion). In posterior fracture-dislocations, the glenoid rim may remain impacted in the head-depression fracture; this results in the head becoming locked in the dislocated position (locked posterior dislocation, or fracture dislocation).

A second fracture pattern splits the humeral head into 2 or more pieces. Radiographs and CT show a double-contour head (2 or more overlapping subchondral lines at different levels). The tuberosities and shaft also may be fractured, but (in terms of prognosis and treatment options) the presence of a **head-splitting fracture** is more important than other elements of the fracture (Figure 4.8).

Fractures of only 1 tuberosity may occur as well. **Isolated fractures of the greater tuberosity** are seen almost always in the context of an anterior dislocation (Figure 4.3); as the head dislocates anteriorly (with the lesser tuberosity and the shaft), the greater tuberosity remains posterior (held by the posterosuperior cuff). Residual tuberosity displacement must be evaluated after closed reduction. **Isolated fractures of the lesser tuberosity** are rare; they may be associated with a posterior dislocation.

Surgical neck fractures are very common (Figure 4.9). The fracture line separates the shaft from the head and tuberosities. Most commonly, the proximal aspect of the shaft is displaced medially secondary to the pull of the

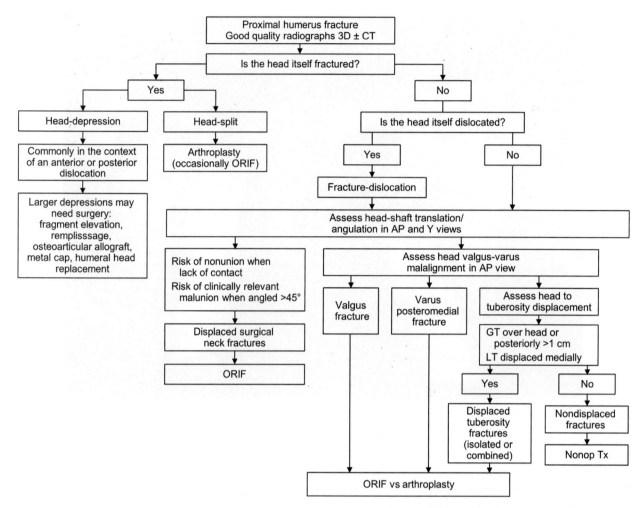

Figure 4.6 *Algorithmic approach for the evaluation and management of proximal humerus fractures. AP indicates anteroposterior; CT, computed tomography; GT, greater tuberosity; LT, lesser tuberosity; ORIF, open reduction internal fixation; 3D, 3-dimensional; Tx, treatment; Y, lateral Y view.*

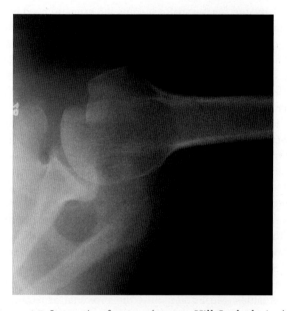

Figure 4.7 *Impaction fracture (reverse Hill-Sachs lesion).*

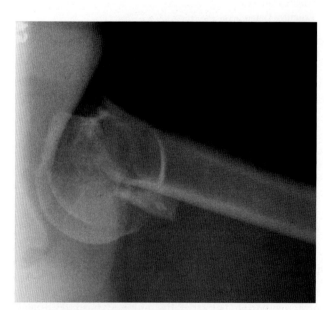

Figure 4.8 *Head-splitting fracture.*

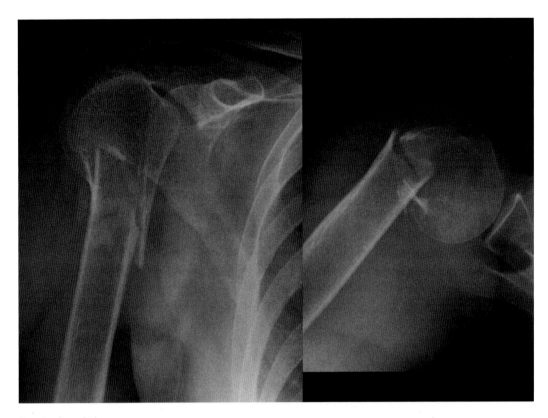

Figure 4.9 Surgical neck fracture.

pectoralis major. The head remains in normal valgus-varus and rotational alignment.

Varus posteromedial fractures are very common as well (Figure 4.10). The fracture line at the head-shaft level results in posteromedial comminution and malalignment in 3 planes: varus, internal rotation, and flexion. Most of the time (but not always), there is a fracture of the greater tuberosity (3-part varus posteromedial fracture); more rarely, there is a fracture of both tuberosities (4-part varus posteromedial fracture).

In **valgus-impacted fractures,** the head-shaft deformity occurs in the opposite direction: the head rotates laterally, almost straight into valgus, with comminution of the cancellous bone on the lateral aspect of the humeral head (Figure 4.11). The greater tuberosity is fractured (3-part, valgus-impacted fracture) most of the time; the lesser tuberosity may be fractured as well (4-part, valgus-impacted fracture).

The term *fracture-dislocation* is added when the humeral head is completely dislocated from the glenoid in combination with a head split, head depression, tuberosity fracture, varus posteromedial fracture, or valgus-impacted fracture in 2, 3, or 4 parts.

When to Operate: Sometimes It Is Pretty Clear, Sometimes It Is Not

Although hard to believe, deciding on when to recommend surgical treatment for a proximal humerus fracture remains extremely difficult in many cases. Patient factors may tip the balance in favor of nonoperative treatment for fractures that otherwise should be treated surgically. These factors include age, comorbidities, mental status, compliance, preexisting shoulder pathology, bone quality, and anticipated physical demands.

The lack of strong evidence to support a better outcome with surgical treatment for displaced fractures is one of the reasons why I still have difficulty in deciding when to operate and what operation to recommend (9–11). This lack of evidence likely is due to the fact that different researchers have classified fractures differently, making comparisons difficult. Also, hemiarthroplasty for proximal humerus fractures has been associated in the past with a relatively high failure rate secondary to tuberosity nonunion (12). Likewise, internal fixation has been associated with a high rate of complications initially due to poor fixation systems and, more recently, to a lack of understanding about how to reduce the fracture, how to best manage the tuberosities, and progressive fracture settling during healing (9,13,14). The general guidelines presented in Table 4.4 apply to patients without risk factors for an adverse outcome with surgery and need to be understood as guidelines rather than strict indications.

Head-Splitting Fractures

Most head-splitting fractures should be treated surgically. Otherwise, intra-articular incongruity will lead to poor

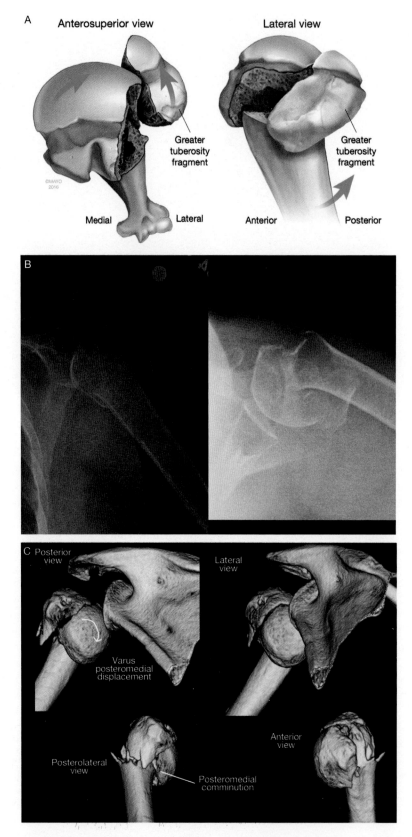

Figure 4.10 *Varus posteromedial fracture (in this example, the greater tuberosity is fractured).* **A,** *Schematic.* **B,** *Radiographs.* **C,** *3-dimensional computed tomography.*

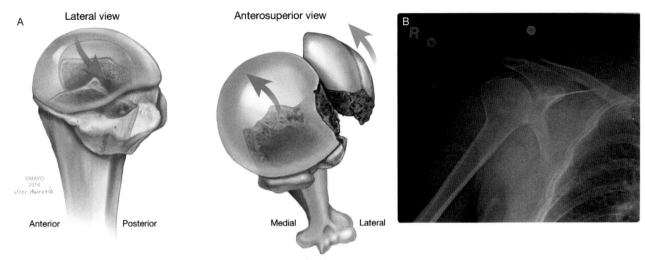

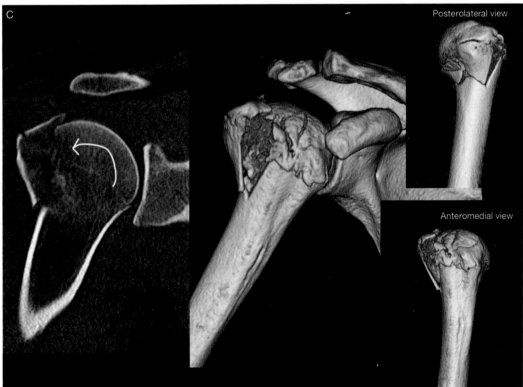

Figure 4.11 *Valgus impacted fracture (in this example, the greater tuberosity is fractured).* **A,** *Schematic.* **B,** *Radiograph.* **C,** *3-Dimensional computed tomography.*

function and progressive osteoarthritis. Head splitting is a classic indication for arthroplasty; however, internal fixation of the fracture can be considered in younger patients, provided anatomical reduction of the articular surface can be achieved.

Head-Depression Fractures

Posterosuperior Hill-Sachs fractures are typically evaluated in the context of shoulder instability; their treatment is discussed in chapter 7, Shoulder Instability and the Labrum. Anterior reverse Hill-Sachs fractures need to be evaluated in the context of a locked posterior fracture-dislocation (see later).

Surgical Neck Fractures

The main complication of this fracture pattern is nonunion (15). Surgical neck nonunions are much more difficult to address surgically than acute surgical neck fractures. It is thus important not to miss the opportunity to intervene acutely for those fractures with a high risk of nonunion.

Table 4.4 • Characteristics That Support Surgical Treatment

Head splitting

Large head depression (take into account shoulder instability)

Surgical neck fractures if
Gross instability
Complete translation
Angulation >45°

Varus posteromedial fractures if
Tuberosity displacement dictates surgery
Varus malalignment over 30°–45°
Angulation over 30°–45°

Valgus impacted fractures if
Tuberosity displacement dictates surgery
Humeral head pointing straight up or laterally

Isolated tuberosity fractures displaced >1 cm
Greater tuberosity
Lesser tuberosity

Fracture-dislocations

However, most surgical neck fractures heal with a good functional outcome with nonoperative treatment. When surgery is recommended acutely, internal fixation is the treatment of choice. I consider internal fixation for fractures with marked clinical instability (gross motion at the fracture site with gentle stress), complete translation (absolutely no contact between the fractured fragments), and angulation greater than 45° with the arm resting by the side (ignore the axillary radiograph for this particular displacement).

Valgus-Impacted Fractures

When the greater or lesser tuberosity is displaced more than 1 cm in any direction, surgery probably should be considered. In this fracture pattern, the typical location of the greater tuberosity is occupied by the displaced head, so the humeral head needs to be elevated out of valgus for the greater tuberosity to be reduced. Currently, it is not completely clear how much valgus malalignment can be tolerated clinically. Most surgeons would agree on recommending surgery when the subchondral bone outline of the humeral head is pointing straight up or laterally; however, remember that valgus displacement of the humeral head is overestimated when radiographs are obtained with the arm in internal rotation.

Varus Posteromedial Fractures

As with valgus impacted fractures, tuberosity displacement per se is oftentimes the main deciding factor in recommending surgery, since tuberosity nonunion or malunion can lead to poor outcomes. Varus posteromedial displacement of the humeral head in reference to the shaft correlates with decreased elevation and can contribute to limited internal rotation as well. Most surgeons would agree on recommending surgery when the head-shaft malalignment is greater than 30° to 45° of varus, depending on patient expectations.

Isolated Greater Tuberosity Fractures

These fractures may occur in conjunction with an anterior dislocation or be truly isolated. When they occur in the setting of an anterior dislocation, residual displacement should be assessed after closed reduction of the dislocation; once the humeral head is relocated, the residual displacement is oftentimes minimal. Most surgeons agree about operative treatment of these fractures if there is residual displacement greater than 1 cm; in patients with high physical demands, displacement greater than 0.5 cm may lead to incomplete restoration of the desired function without surgery.

Isolated Lesser Tuberosity Fractures

These are rare fractures. When isolated and displaced more than 1 cm, they are best treated surgically, since they are the equivalent of an acute subscapularis tear (see chapter 6, Rotator Cuff and Biceps Tendon). When associated with a posterior dislocation, they oftentimes have minimal residual displacement after closed reduction and may be amenable to conservative treatment.

Fracture-Dislocations with Head-Shaft Displacement

In those injury patterns when the humeral head is dislocated and fractured off the shaft, surgical treatment is almost always universally recommended. Internal fixation may be attempted if either or both tuberosities are not fractured, providing some vascularity to the head segment. For the true 4-part fracture dislocation, arthroplasty is oftentimes the treatment of choice.

Risk of Avascular Necrosis (and Nonunion)

Avascular necrosis (AVN) is considered a classic complication of certain proximal humerus fractures that disrupt the vascularity to the humeral head. As detailed in Table 4.5, the topic of posttraumatic AVN after proximal humerus fractures is somewhat confusing and controversial (2).

Symptomatic AVN is likely when the humeral head is completely disconnected from the tuberosities and shaft (isolated fractures of the anatomical neck or, more commonly, true Neer 4-part fracture and fracture dislocations); these patterns are best treated with arthroplasty in most cases. Other fracture patterns are associated with decreased humeral head perfusion that does not always lead to symptomatic AVN, and to base treatment decisions (i.e., whether to operate or not and whether to

Table 4.5 • **Current Thoughts on AVN After Proximal Humerus Fractures**

When AVN is confirmed on radiographs or a CT scan, does it create any clinical issues?

Classic teaching is that small areas of AVN after nonoperative treatment of proximal humerus fractures are well tolerated

However, there are patients who clearly develop symptoms secondary to AVN and eventually require shoulder arthroplasty

In patients with symptomatic AVN, it is sometimes difficult to determine how much of the pain and dysfunction is due to necrosis vs. commonly associated malunion/nonunion

AVN is really problematic after internal fixation with hardware in the humeral head: humeral head collapse leaves protruding hardware that may damage the glenoid (Figure 4.12)

Which vessels are involved in the genesis of AVN after proximal humerus fractures?

The anterolateral ascending branch of the anterior circumflex humeral artery penetrates the head as the arcuate artery; it is classically considered the main source of blood supply for the humeral head and it is the most common branch interrupted in proximal humerus fractures

Branches from the posterior circumflex humeral artery penetrating the posteromedial humeral metaphysis are less commonly injured and may provide enough blood supply in certain fracture patterns and patients

Which fracture patterns are the most prone to decreased humeral head perfusion and/or AVN?

Fractures through the anatomical neck

Disruption of the medial periosteal hinge

Distal metaphyseal extension of the head fragment <8 mm

Complete disconnection and displacement of the humeral head from the tuberosities and shaft

    True Neer 4-part fractures

    Neer 4-part fracture-dislocations

Abbreviations: AVN, avascular necrosis; CT, computed tomography.

replace or not) on the risk of AVN becomes a challenge. Internal fixation should probably be avoided in fractures with some risk of AVN since the worse clinical scenario represents the patient with prominent hardware after head collapse and secondary destruction of the glenoid (Figure 4.12) (13). If the risk of AVN is high and the fracture is considered surgical, arthroplasty is a better option.

Most likely, the same risk factors listed for AVN also increase the risk of nonunion, since fracture union requires vascularity. In addition, fractures with severe displacement

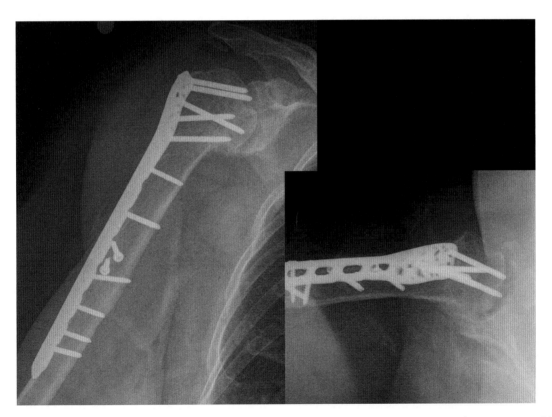

Figure 4.12 *Avascular necrosis after locking-plate fixation becomes extremely problematic secondary to potential hardware penetration and glenoid damage.*

and/or instability are prone to nonunion as well; these would include markedly displaced 2-part fractures at the surgical neck level.

Internal Fixation, Hemiarthroplasty, or Reverse Arthroplasty?

A little bit of history is very useful in understanding current views regarding surgical treatment of proximal humerus fractures. In general terms, when surgery is recommended, the alternatives are to either fix the fracture or proceed with joint replacement.

Internal Fixation

Internal fixation devices and techniques have been refined over time. In the early years of orthopedic surgery, fracture fixation often involved partial fragment resection, suture, or pin fixation. Blade-plate fixation and old-style nails have given way to 2 main methods of fixation: locking plates and modern intramedullary nails (some surgeons still favor percutaneous pinning for some fractures). A central concept when fixing proximal humerus fractures is that secure tuberosity fixation is as important or more important than head-shaft fixation.

When locking plates were introduced for proximal humerus fractures, they were perceived as the ultimate improvement in the management of these injuries. Locking-plate technology does provide improved head-to-shaft support and fixation compared with older techniques. However, the reported outcomes of locking-plate fixation for proximal humerus fractures have been plagued with complications, namely those caused by poor head-to-shaft reduction, poor tuberosity management, and/or late screw penetration with secondary glenoid damage (13,16–18). Internal fixation of proximal humerus fracture using a locking compression plate is a great procedure, but it is technically demanding and should be performed with meticulous attention to both fracture-reduction and fixation techniques (9,17).

The problems observed with using locking compression plates, poor tuberosity management, and glenoid destruction have led to a resurgence in use of modern nails that rely on tuberosity fixation and indirect head support to provide adequate fracture fixation.

Arthroplasty

Dr. Neer introduced the concept of replacing the humeral head with a metal implant and fixing the tuberosities to each other and the shaft for those fractures deemed "unfixable" with the techniques available in the later part of the last century. His overall rate of excellent and satisfactory results was pretty good, but it was seldom reproduced by other surgeons. The orthopedic community now recognizes that the outcome of shoulder hemiarthroplasty (humeral head replacement) for proximal humerus fractures is largely dependent on anatomical union of the greater tuberosity (12).

Table 4.6 • **Risk Factors for Nonunion or Malunion of the Greater Tuberosity in Shoulder Hemiarthroplasty or Reverse Arthroplasty**

Poor intraoperative tuberosity reduction
Poor intraoperative tuberosity fixation
Excessive humeral component retroversion
Humeral component inserted too high or too low
Female sex
Advanced age
Immobilization in internal rotation
Too aggressive early motion exercises
Systemic factors compromising bone healing (i.e., smoking)

Any factor that compromises anatomical greater tuberosity fixation (Table 4.6) leads to poor motion and overall outcome, although pain is not severe in the absence of marked superior subluxation (19). On the other hand, humeral head replacement can restore shoulder function to almost normal with proper tuberosity healing.

Reverse arthroplasty was introduced as "the solution" for those fractures that needed arthroplasty but were not doing quite well with a hemiarthroplasty secondary to tuberosity problems. Since reverse arthroplasty compensates to some extent for rotator cuff function, reverse arthroplasty should be ideal for proximal humerus fractures. In fact, in the early experience with reverse arthroplasty for proximal humerus fractures, some surgeons advocated resecting or ignoring the tuberosities. It was soon realized that a reverse arthroplasty without a greater tuberosity does not lead to a great outcome; there is little pain and good active elevation but poor active external rotation and an increased risk of dislocation.

Surgeons' Current Thoughts

Complications (reported with locking-plate fixation) and poor functional outcomes obtained in a large number of patients after hemiarthroplasty have led many surgeons to reconsider the role of nonoperative treatment, develop improved surgical techniques for locking-plate fixation, explore alternative nail-fixation techniques, and favor reverse arthroplasty over hemiarthroplasty. However, internal fixation continues to provide the best solution for fixable fractures when properly indicated and executed. Likewise, the best hemiarthroplasty for fracture is better than the best reverse for fracture; having said that, reverse arthroplasty is more reliable for a number of fracture patterns in the hands of most surgeons.

In our practice, patient factors play a major role in the decision-making process. At one extreme, patients with major comorbidities, limited anticipated shoulder demands, and major risks for surgery are treated nonoperatively even for severely displaced fractures. At the other extreme, younger patients with anticipated high functional demands may benefit from surgery even if the fracture displacement is borderline.

Currently, arthroplasty is typically recommended for fracture-dislocations with head-shaft displacement, head-splitting fractures (although internal fixation may be considered in the ultra-young patient), head-depression fractures affecting over 40% to 45% of the humeral head articular cartilage (unless the depression can be elevated acutely), true Neer 4-part fractures (more so in the varus posteromedial variety), and fractures perceived to have a high risk of AVN or nonunion. All other displaced fractures are typically first addressed with attempted internal fixation. However, when successful fixation is perceived as the best possible option but concerns about bone quality or comminution exist, patients should give consent for both procedures, with the final choice dependent on intraoperative findings.

Once internal fixation is selected, the fixation technique may vary. In our practice, locking plates are the "workhorse" for most proximal humerus fractures treated with internal fixation (20). However, intramedullary nailing is a very attractive option for displaced surgical neck fractures. Percutaneous pinning is another very good alternative for selected fractures in patients with good bone quality.

When arthroplasty is recommended, reverse arthroplasty is more forgiving and reliable, but complications can be catastrophic. The long-term outcome for reverse arthroplasty remains unknown, and internal rotation is not restored in many patients (21,22). Hemiarthroplasty is selected most often for younger patients with large greater tuberosity fragments and no major risk factors for union. Reverse arthroplasty is selected for older patients, fractures with severe greater tuberosity comminution and/or osteopenia, and for those at an increased risk of nonunion (e.g., active smokers or those receiving chemotherapy) (23,24).

Nonoperative Treatment

As much as we like to operate, orthopedic surgeons also need to know how to obtain the best outcome when nonoperative treatment is selected. In my opinion, there are a couple of misconceptions and some simple guidelines to be considered that will lead to the best possible outcome for proximal humerus fractures treated nonoperatively (Table 4.7).

The Myth and Reality of Early Motion

Early motion has likely been overemphasized for nonoperative treatment of proximal humerus fractures. Whereas it is true that prolonged immobilization may lead to stiffness and stable fractures can be moved safely early in treatment, many patients who complain of stiffness after nonoperative treatment of proximal humerus fractures

---

Table 4.7 • Nonoperative Treatment of Proximal Humerus Fractures

Misconceptions
Early range of motion is always safe and necessary
The shoulder is best immobilized in internal rotation

Program
Immobilize until motion exercises are safe (timing must be tailored)
Immobilize in external rotation
Close follow-up (physical examination and radiographs)
Once motion is safe, work on motion, then strength—do not forget the scapula (see Chapter 12, Rehabilitation and Injections)
Assess and treat for fragility fracture
Follow for long-term adverse events (e.g., AVN, nonunion, posttraumatic OA)

Abbreviations: AVN, avascular necrosis; OA, osteoarthritis.

---

actually have limited motion secondary to malunion, not stiffness. In addition, nonunion and malunion secondary to aggressive motion are much more difficult to correct surgically than stiffness around a minimally deformed, well-healed, proximal humerus where an arthroscopic release has little morbidity and a good outcome.

Immobilize in Some External Rotation

Most patients across the world are advised to use a conventional sling or immobilizer after fracture. If you think about it, resting the forearm and hand on the belly during fracture healing may lead to healing of the shaft in internal rotation in relation to the head segment and poor greater tuberosity-to-head relationship.

If the greater tuberosity is fractured, it is brought closer to the humeral head when the arm is immobilized in some external rotation. In addition, when the humeral shaft is fractured from the head segment, the best rotational alignment is probably achieved with the wrist and hand pointing almost straight forward.

A Program of Nonoperative Treatment for Proximal Humerus Fractures

If the recommendation is to proceed with nonoperative treatment, provide the patient with an immobilizer that will keep the limb in some external rotation and schedule a follow-up appointment in approximately 2 weeks. In addition to analgesics, patients often find that they cannot sleep or rest when lying completely flat but can in a somewhat upright position. (Typically, they sleep in a reclining armchair.) Most patients develop a pretty substantial subcutaneous ecchymosis in the lateral aspect of the chest and the inside of the arm several days after injury, and they should be advised to expect it so that they do not become alarmed. Skin care is important to avoid moisture accumulation and blisters, especially in the axillary region.

The ideal time to start range-of-motion exercises should be tailored to each patient and fracture. Compliant patients with stable fractures may start gentle range-of-motion exercises at week 2. Typically, fracture stability is assessed clinically as the examiner uses one hand at the elbow to rotate the humerus while the other hand is placed around the humeral head to detect if the whole bone moves as a unit; when in doubt, stability can be assessed with fluoroscopy. Patients with questionable fracture stability or poor compliance may need to be immobilized for 6 weeks or longer. Once motion is started, patients are advised to complete a program of passive, rather than active, motion followed by stretching and strengthening, as outlined in chapter 12, Rehabilitation and Injections.

Surgical Exposures for Internal Fixation and Arthroplasty

The **deltopectoral approach** is most commonly used for both plate fixation and arthroplasty after proximal humerus fractures, similar to other procedures around the shoulder (see chapter 3, Surgical Exposures). However, some surgeons prefer alternate approaches for some procedures or fracture types.

The **superior approach** has become popular for 2 procedures: intramedullary nailing and reverse arthroplasty for fracture. Intramedullary nailing for displaced surgical neck fractures can be performed elegantly through a minimally invasive, almost percutaneous approach splitting the deltoid. A more formal, superior, deltoid-splitting approach is attractive because it provides excellent exposure of the greater tuberosity and the humeral canal for either nailing or humeral prosthetic stem insertion; it also provides good glenoid access for reverse arthroplasty after removal of the fractured head. This approach, however, is not ideal for plate fixation.

Plate fixation can be performed well through a deltopectoral approach. However, without complete mobilization and partial elevation of the deltoid insertion distally, it may be difficult to place the plate lateral enough or control the greater tuberosity. **Splitting the deltoid** along its nearly entire length has become popular among surgeons with training and background in traumatology (15,25). Fracture exposure is excellent, but formal identification, dissection, and protection of the axillary nerve is required. Surgeons with a background in arthroplasty tend to prefer a deltopectoral approach for both arthroplasty and plate fixation.

Internal Fixation

Locking-Plate Fixation

Periarticular, precontoured locking plates have become a blessing and a curse for internal fixation of proximal

Table 4.8 ∘ Benefits and Dangers of Locking-Plate Fixation for Proximal Humerus Fractures, Including Clinical Pearls

Benefits
Locked screws provide better head support and shaft fixation
Precontouring provides low-profile, anatomical fixation

Dangers
Shaft-head centered systems: may lead to poor tuberosity management
Plate placement too proximal, anterior, or oblique may facilitate
    Plate impingement superiorly or anteriorly
    Poor reduction or suboptimal fixation
Screw penetration/prominent hardware

Pearls
Place your plate lateral and inferior enough
Fracture reduction and tuberosity management are key
Screws placed in the humeral head
    Avoid hardware penetration/prominence
    Inferior screws vs. superior screws
    Intentional incomplete drilling
    Excessive screw length (avoid)
    Blunt-tipped screws/pegs
    Inferior screws for calcar support are important in varus posteromedial fractures
Hybrid fixation
    Fix (anchor) the tuberosities using sutures through the rotator cuff and the plate
Selective void filling/support with bone graft or substitutes

humerus fractures. They are very useful devices to provide head support and head-to-shaft fixation, and their precontoured nature reduces impingement and facilitates placement. However, they do not compensate for poor fracture reduction, they do not emphasize tuberosity fixation, and can result in screw penetration into the glenohumeral joint. In our practice, precountoured proximal humerus locking plates currently represent the most common treatment modality when internal fixation is selected (◉ Video 4.1). Table 4.8 summarizes the benefits, pitfalls, and pearls of proximal humerus fracture fixation using periarticular plates.

Reduction Maneuvers

Different fracture patterns require different reduction maneuvers (Figure 4.13). Traction, rotation, and translation are all useful in controlling the shaft. The tuberosities are best controlled using traction sutures through the rotator cuff; if 1 or both tuberosities are in continuity with the head segment, these sutures through the cuff can also help with head reduction.

In varus posteromedial fracture patterns the head needs to be derotated out of varus, flexion, and internal rotation; this can be accomplished with a periosteal elevator to lever on the head through the fracture site or by inserting 1 or more wires into the head at a steep angle and using them as a joystick. In valgus patterns, the head needs to be

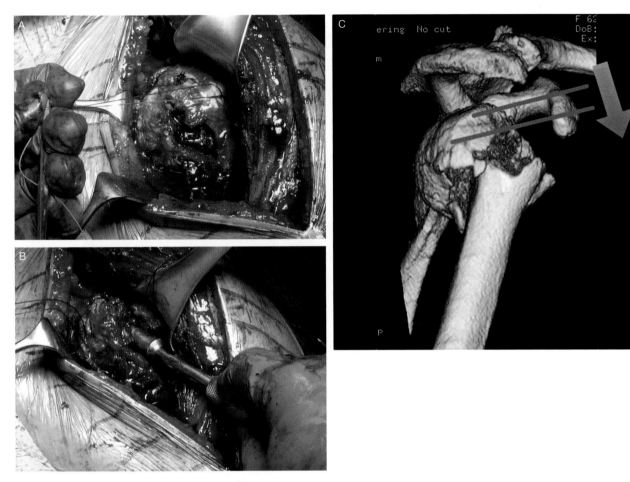

Figure 4.13 *Reduction techniques for proximal humerus fractures.* **A,** *Sutures through the rotator cuff.* **B,** *Elevator.* **C,** *K-wires as a joystick.*

elevated out of valgus, and this can be accomplished with an impactor or a lamina spreader. Care must be taken not to excessively displace the medial side of the fracture, which could make the fracture more unstable or disrupt the medial osteoperiosteal hinge.

When the head is dislocated posteriorly, use of a bone hook on the shaft to laterally provide traction may result in better space for head reduction. When the head is dislocated anteriorly, careful dissection behind and medial to the conjoined tendon should help free up the head and avoid injury to the brachial plexus or adjacent vessels. The conjoined tendon may be detatched for exposure if needed and repaired at the end of the procedure.

Fixation Strategy

The relative position of the head and shaft may be maintained provisionally with 1 or more wires inserted so that they will not interfere with plate placement. The plate can then be fixed to the shaft provisionally with a non-locking screw through 1 oblong hole, and the proximal-to-distal plate position may be adjusted under fluoroscopic control. Shaft fixation can be completed with additional

screws, and the head is supported with multiple locking screws. In order to avoid intra-articular screw penetration, care must be taken to avoid drilling all the way through the bone (I typically only drill the lateral cortex) and to use screws long enough to support the head but not reach all the way to the subchondral bone. Screws aimed toward the calcar region are considered to be extremely important by some in preventing loss of reduction in varus posteromedial patterns. Plate-and-screw fixation is augmented with multiple sutures placed though the cuff and through small holes present in most modern plates (Figure 4.14).

Bone Augmentation

Some fractures present with a high grade of comminution, leaving a large void after reduction. Filling this void with bone graft or substitutes helps prevent loss of reduction. In valgus fractures oftentimes the defect can be successfully addressed with particulate allograft or substitutes. In varus posteromedial fractures requiring bone graft, structural support may be needed. In these circumstances, use of a structural allograft (typically fibula) has gained popularity;

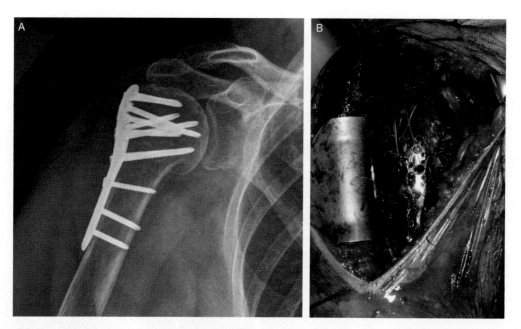

Figure 4.14 *Hybrid internal fixation: plate fixation augmented with sutures through the rotator cuff.* **A,** *Postoperative radiograph;* **B,** *Intraoperative photo.*

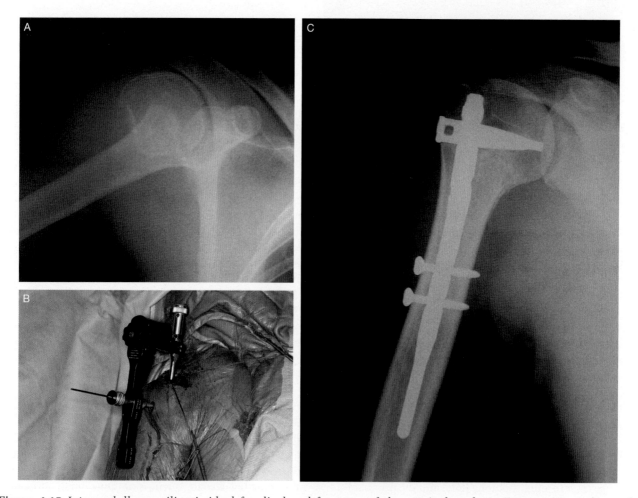

Figure 4.15 *Intramedullary nailing is ideal for displaced fractures of the surgical neck.* **A,** *Preoperative radiograph.* **B,** *Percutaneous intramedullary nailing.* **C,** *Radiograph at 2 months shows fracture healing.*

it supports the head segment and provides additional cortices for screw purchase distally. However, when healed inside the canal, allograft may make revision to an arthroplasty difficult. Alternatively, the structural graft can be placed extramedullary along the medial cortex of the humeral shaft to support the calcar region.

Intramedullary Nailing

Dedicated nails for proximal humerus fractures provide intramedullary stability and various interlocking options (26). In our practice, a displaced surgical neck fracture is the ideal indication for this technique since the fixation may be performed almost percutaneously through a superior approach and the tuberosities are not fractured from the head (Figure 4.15). This option is also attractive for a 3-part greater tuberosity fracture with minimal displacement of the head and severe tuberosity displacement; through a superior approach, the head and shaft are stabilized with the nail and the greater tuberosity can be controlled and reduced very well.

Percutaneous Pinning and Screws

Some recommend percutaneous pinning for fractures without major head-shaft instability in patients with good bone quality (Figure 4.16). Terminally threaded pins are ideal. The reduction is achieved under fluoroscopy with closed manipulation and selective percutaneous use of elevators. Distal-to-proximal, shaft-to-head fixation is achieved with pins. Greater tuberosity fragments may be pinned from proximal to distal, or these pins may be replaced with cannulated screws. Shoulder immobilization for 6 weeks is

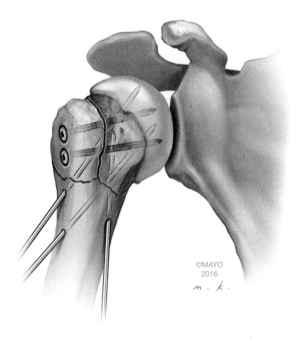

Figure 4.16 Percutaneous pinning.

recommended. The pins are left buried under the skin and removed at 6 to 8 weeks after surgery.

Arthroplasty

As mentioned before, those fractures considered for shoulder replacement may be treated with hemiarthroplasty or reverse arthroplasty (23,24) (Figure 4.17). While the relative indications for these 2 techniques keep evolving, both procedures have the need for adequate tuberosity management and healing in common in order to obtain the best possible outcome.

Hemiarthroplasty for Fracture

The 2 goals of hemiarthroplasty for fracture are anatomical restoration of the height and version of the humeral head and adequate reduction and fixation of the tuberosities (Table 4.9). Although there is interest in the development of reliable cementless components for fracture, cemented fixation is considered the gold standard since it does not rely on the support provided by the metaphysis in nonfracture applications and it allows setting the height and version of the humeral head prior to tuberosity fixation (Figure 4.18).

Once exposure is obtained, my first step is to identify the long head of the biceps tendon and follow it proximally to identify the space between the fractured greater and lesser tuberosities, typically just posterior to the bicipital groove. The biceps is tenodesed in situ. The fractured lesser tuberosity is then mobilized medially, and the head is removed and saved for bone graft prior to mobilizing the greater tuberosity because the removal of the humeral head creates a workspace that facilitates access to the cuff–greater tuberosity interface.

Multiple methods and reference points (e.g., bicipital groove and pectoralis tendon) have been proposed to guide placement of the humeral component in the right height and version. I favor 20° to 25° of retroversion for most patients, since slight anteversion of the component leaves more room posteriorly for the greater tuberosity. For height, I prefer that the trial humeral head is perfectly centered on the glenoid once the shoulder is relocated. It is important to use a system that allows accurate trials and replication of humeral component position; most commonly, this is achieved with jigs and laser marks on the trials and final components.

Greater tuberosity malreduction is not uncommon. It is important to advance the greater tuberosity over the shoulder of the prosthesis; this is facilitated by placing the shoulder in abduction to relax the deltoid and using traction sutures or atraumatic clamps. External rotation of the humerus will also facilitate reduction of the greater tuberosity. Most surgeons recommend a combination of horizontal cerclage fixation (e.g., tuberosity to tuberosity and tuberosities to prosthesis) and vertical fixation of each tuberosity

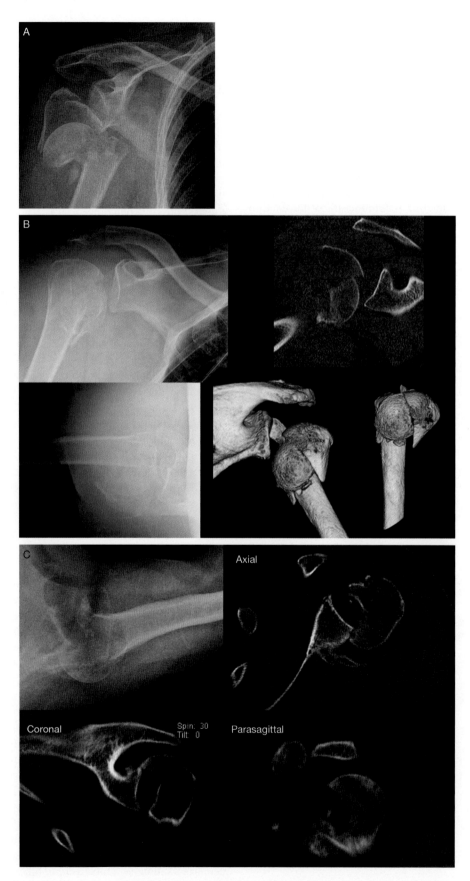

Figure 4.17 *Classic indications for arthroplasty in proximal humerus fractures.* **A,** *True 4-part fracture.* **B,** *Head split.* **C,** *Impaction over 40%.*

Table 4.9 • Hemiarthroplasty and Reverse Arthroplasty for Fracture

Surgical steps
Follow biceps to fracture site and tenodese
Mobilize the lesser tuberosity medially
Extract the head and save for bone graft
Get control of the greater tuberosity
Implant sizing and positioning
  Hemiarthroplasty
    Head diameter same size or one size smaller than fractured
      humeral head
    20°–25° retroversion
    Trial faces the glenoid at the perfect height with the
      shoulder reduced
  Reverse arthroplasty
    Place glenoid component first
    Trial reduction with thinnest bearing, apply traction,
      mark height
    Soft-tissue tension may need to be increased with thicker
      bearings
Tuberosity reduction and fixation, bone grafting

Factors that may help with tuberosity healing
Stem
  Use a fracture-friendly or fracture-specific stem
    Small, non-bulky body
    Ingrowth or ongrowth surface treatment
  Aim for relative anteversion (retroversion 20°–25°)
  Do not position the stem too high or too low (use jigs, marks,
    references)
Tuberosity management
  Adequate reduction
  Horizontal and vertical stable fixation
  Bone grafting
Immobilization
  Immobilize in relative external rotation
  Delay range of motion exercises

to the shaft using heavy nonabsorbable sutures. Cancellous bone chips from the fractured head are packed underneath the tuberosities to promote healing (Figure 4.19).

Reverse Arthroplasty for Fracture

Many of the technical pearls described for hemiarthroplasty also apply to reverse arthroplasty for fracture (● Video 4.2). The humeral component is most commonly fixed with cement, version is set between 20° and 25°, and tuberosity management is very similar (horizontal and vertical suture fixation and bone grafting; Figure 4.20). When reverse arthroplasty is used for fractures, the ideal height for the stem is largely unknown. On one hand, the humerus needs to be somewhat lengthened to avoid postoperative dislocation; on the other hand, excessive lengthening may compromise tuberosity to shaft contact and thus tuberosity healing. I typically place the glenoid component first and then relocate the humeral component trial with the thinnest humeral bearing; moderate traction is applied to the arm and the height of the trial is marked or noted. Alternatively, some trialing systems allow reduction at a given height to confirm adequate tuberosity reduction. Once the final component is implanted, soft-tissue tension may be increased further if needed by using thicker bearings (Figure 4.21).

Complications

Proximal humerus fractures may be associated with various complications, including infection, injuries to the brachial plexus or axillary nerve, vascular injuries, stiffness, chronic regional pain syndrome, nonunion, malunion,

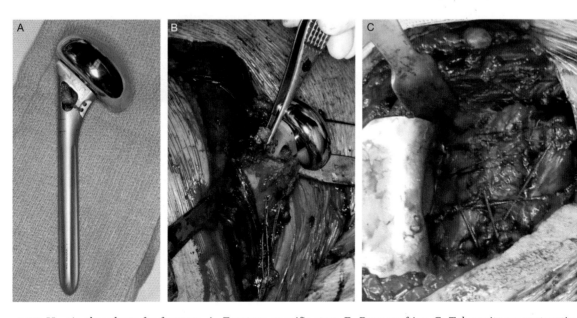

Figure 4.18 *Hemiarthroplasty for fracture.* **A,** *Fracture-specific stem.* **B,** *Bone grafting.* **C,** *Tuberosity reconstruction.*

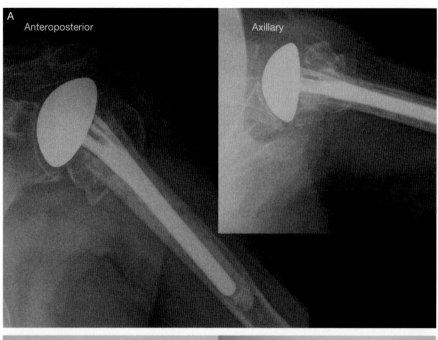

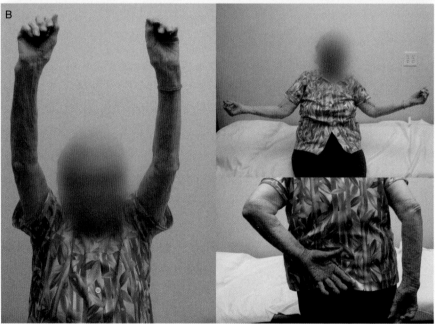

Figure 4.19 **A,** *Hemiarthroplasty performed for a proximal humerus fracture led to successful healing of both tuberosities.* **B,** *Patient range of motion at follow-up.*

AVN, and posttraumatic osteoarthritis; I will briefly discuss the last 4 (2).

Nonunion

Nonunion is particularly common at the head-shaft junction, especially for unstable surgical neck fractures with or without fractures of the tuberosity. The humeral head loses bone stock very quickly, and osteopenia, joint contracture, and varus malalignment are not uncommon. Internal fixation with bone grafting is considered for younger patients with relatively well-preserved bone stock in the head segment. Arthroplasty is considered for salvage for those nonunions not amenable to internal fixation. Although hemiarthroplasty may be considered, reverse arthroplasty is generally preferred due to patient age, compromised bone stock, or compromised tuberosities.

Malunion

Some patients tolerate certain degrees of malunion and adapt to their functional limitations. Rarely, osteotomies

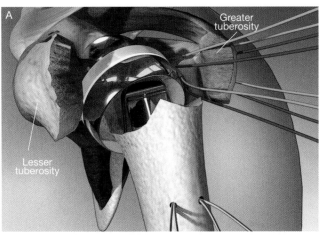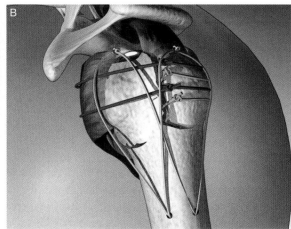

Figure 4.20 *Tuberosity reconstruction around reverse arthroplasty for fracture. The technique used is similar for hemiarthroplasty and reverse shoulder arthroplasty.*

are considered for patients with severe malunions and no posttraumatic arthrosis. Greater tuberosity malunions can oftentimes be addressed by tuberosity remodeling with or without rotator cuff detachment and repair (sometimes combined with acromioplasty). Arthroplasty may be considered for the salvage of severe malunions. Hemiarthroplasty is successful when the tuberosities are united in good position; otherwise, if the tuberosities are malunited or nonunited, reverse arthroplasty is preferred.

Avascular Necrosis

AVN in fractures treated nonoperatively or with limited fixation (i.e., percutaneous pinning) is oftentimes well tolerated and requires no treatment. Otherwise,

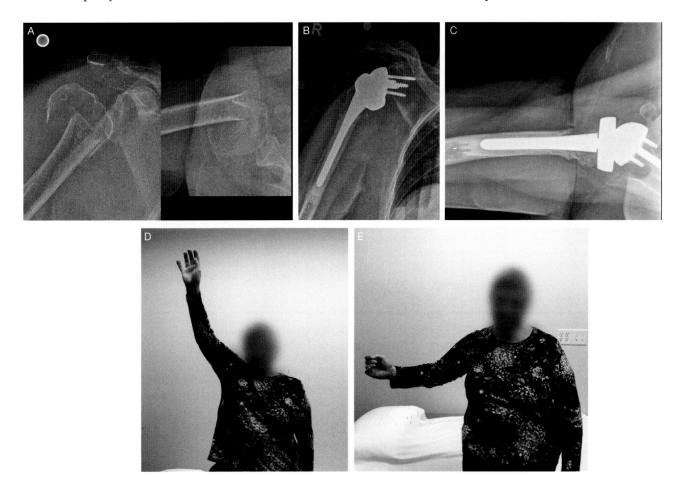

Figure 4.21 **A,** *Comminuted proximal humerus fracture in a 73-year-old patient treated with a reverse arthroplasty.* **B and C,** *Successful tuberosity healing led to good range of motion.*

hemiarthroplasty or reverse arthroplasty is considered, depending on the status of the tuberosities. As mentioned before, care must be taken to avoid delayed arthroplasty in patients with AVN and hardware penetration, since severe glenoid damage may compromise arthroplasty alternatives.

Posttraumatic Osteoarthritis

Some patients will develop secondary degenerative changes after a proximal humerus fracture. This may happen after a fracture heals in relatively good position with no additional complications or it may be associated with malunion, nonunion, or AVN. Anatomical total shoulder arthroplasty is selected in uncomplicated cases, whereas reverse arthroplasty is favored for patients with severe malunion or nonunion.

KEY POINTS

✓ Proximal humerus fractures are common and have the potential to decrease independence in otherwise highly functional elderly patients.

✓ High-quality imaging studies (plain radiographs ± CT scan) need to be carefully analyzed to understand fracture pattern and displacement.

✓ Although there are multiple fracture patterns considered in comprehensive classifications, a few patters are especially common: surgical neck fractures, greater tuberosity fractures, varus posteromedial fractures, valgus impacted fractures, fracture-dislocations, head splits, and head depressions.

✓ The decision of whether or not to operate is based on fracture factors (e.g., pattern, displacement) and patient factors.

✓ Fractures treated nonoperatively should be immobilized in some external rotation; early motion is beneficial only if it does not lead to fracture displacement.

✓ Internal fixation using periarticular plates, intramedullary nails, or percutaneous pins or screws is the treatment of choice for most fractures requiring surgery. Poor results are typically related to incomplete reduction, poor tuberosity management, or hardware penetration.

✓ Hemiarthroplasty and reverse arthroplasty are considered for fractures with severe head destruction or marked comminution. Satisfactory stem placement in the right height and version can be difficult. Tuberosity reduction, fixation, and healing are paramount for the success of hemiarthroplasty and important for reverse arthroplasty as well, although reverse arthroplasty is more forgiving.

REFERENCES

1. Launonen AP, Lepola V, Saranko A, Flinkkila T, Laitinen M, Mattila VM. Epidemiology of proximal humerus fractures. Arch Osteoporos. 2015;10:209. Epub 2015 Feb 13.

2. Streubel PN, Sanchez-Sotelo J, Steinmann SP. Proximal humeral fractures. In: Court-Brown CM, Heckman JD, McQueen MM, Ricci WM, Tornetta P, editors. Rockwood and Green's fractures in adults. 8th ed. Vol. 1. Philadelphia (PA): Wolters Kluwer Health; c2015. p. 1341–425.

3. Khatib O, Onyekwelu I, Zuckerman JD. The incidence of proximal humeral fractures in New York State from 1990 through 2010 with an emphasis on operative management in patients aged 65 years or older. J Shoulder Elbow Surg. 2014 Sep;23(9):1356–62. Epub 2014 Apr 13.

4. Sanchez-Sotelo J. Proximal humerus fractures. Clin Anat. 2006 Oct;19(7):588–98.

5. Neer CS 2nd. Four-segment classification of proximal humeral fractures: purpose and reliable use. J Shoulder Elbow Surg. 2002 Jul-Aug;11(4):389–400.

6. Foruria AM, de Gracia MM, Larson DR, Munuera L, Sanchez-Sotelo J. The pattern of the fracture and displacement of the fragments predict the outcome in proximal humeral fractures. J Bone Joint Surg Br. 2011 Mar;93(3):378–86.

7. Robinson BC, Athwal GS, Sanchez-Sotelo J, Rispoli DM. Classification and imaging of proximal humerus fractures. Orthop Clin North Am. 2008 Oct;39(4):393–403.

8. Shrader MW, Sanchez-Sotelo J, Sperling JW, Rowland CM, Cofield RH. Understanding proximal humerus fractures: image analysis, classification, and treatment. J Shoulder Elbow Surg. 2005 Sep-Oct;14(5):497–505.

9. Gupta AK, Harris JD, Erickson BJ, Abrams GD, Bruce B, McCormick F, et al. Surgical management of complex proximal humerus fractures-a systematic review of 92 studies including 4500 patients. J Orthop Trauma. 2015 Jan;29(1):54–9.

10. Launonen AP, Lepola V, Flinkkila T, Laitinen M, Paavola M, Malmivaara A. Treatment of proximal humerus fractures in the elderly: a systemic review of 409 patients. Acta Orthop. 2015 Jun;86(3):280–5. Epub 2015 Jan 9.

11. Rangan A, Handoll H, Brealey S, Jefferson L, Keding A, Martin BC, et al; PROFHER Trial Collaborators. Surgical vs nonsurgical treatment of adults with displaced fractures of the proximal humerus: the PROFHER randomized clinical trial. JAMA. 2015 Mar 10;313(10):1037–47.

12. Antuna SA, Sperling JW, Cofield RH. Shoulder hemiarthroplasty for acute fractures of the proximal humerus: a minimum five-year follow-up. J Shoulder Elbow Surg. 2008 Mar-Apr;17(2):202–9. Epub 2008 Jan 11.

13. Jost B, Spross C, Grehn H, Gerber C. Locking plate fixation of fractures of the proximal humerus: analysis of complications, revision strategies and outcome. J Shoulder Elbow Surg. 2013 Apr;22(4):542–9. Epub 2012 Sep 6.

14. Sudkamp N, Bayer J, Hepp P, Voigt C, Oestern H, Kaab M, et al. Open reduction and internal fixation of proximal humeral fractures with use of the locking proximal humerus plate. Results of a prospective, multicenter, observational study. J Bone Joint Surg Am. 2009 Jun;91(6):1320–8.

15. Murray IR, Amin AK, White TO, Robinson CM. Proximal humeral fractures: current concepts in

classification, treatment and outcomes. J Bone Joint Surg Br. 2011 Jan;93(1):1–11.

16. Petrigliano FA, Bezrukov N, Gamradt SC, SooHoo NF. Factors predicting complication and reoperation rates following surgical fixation of proximal humeral fractures. J Bone Joint Surg Am. 2014 Sep 17;96(18):1544–51.

17. Ockert B, Siebenburger G, Kettler M, Braunstein V, Mutschler W. Long-term functional outcomes (median 10 years) after locked plating for displaced fractures of the proximal humerus. J Shoulder Elbow Surg. 2014 Aug;23(8):1223–31. Epub 2014 Feb 16.

18. Sproul RC, Iyengar JJ, Devcic Z, Feeley BT. A systematic review of locking plate fixation of proximal humerus fractures. Injury. 2011 Apr;42(4):408–13. Epub 2010 Dec 19.

19. Boileau P, Winter M, Cikes A, Han Y, Carles M, Walch G, et al. Can surgeons predict what makes a good hemiarthroplasty for fracture? J Shoulder Elbow Surg. 2013 Nov;22(11):1495–506. Epub 2013 Jul 5.

20. Barlow JD, Sanchez-Sotelo J, Torchia M. Proximal humerus fractures in the elderly can be reliably fixed with a "hybrid" locked-plating technique. Clin Orthop Relat Res. 2011 Dec;469(12):3281–91.

21. Bonnevialle N, Tournier C, Clavert P, Ohl X, Sirveaux F, Saragaglia D; la Société française de chirurgie orthopédique et traumatologique. Hemiarthroplasty versus reverse shoulder arthroplasty in 4-part displaced fractures of the proximal humerus: multicenter retrospective study. Orthop Traumatol Surg Res. 2016 Sep;102(5):569–73. Epub 2016 Apr 23.

22. Grubhofer F, Wieser K, Meyer DC, Catanzaro S, Beeler S, Riede U, et al. Reverse total shoulder arthroplasty for acute head-splitting, 3- and 4-part fractures of the proximal humerus in the elderly. J Shoulder Elbow Surg. 2016 Oct;25(10):1690–8. Epub 2016 Apr 15.

23. Ferrel JR, Trinh TQ, Fischer RA. Reverse total shoulder arthroplasty versus hemiarthroplasty for proximal humeral fractures: a systematic review. J Orthop Trauma. 2015 Jan;29(1):60–8.

24. Namdari S, Horneff JG, Baldwin K. Comparison of hemiarthroplasty and reverse arthroplasty for treatment of proximal humeral fractures: a systematic review. J Bone Joint Surg Am. 2013 Sep 18;95(18):1701–8.

25. Gavaskar AS, Chowdary N, Abraham S. Complex proximal humerus fractures treated with locked plating utilizing an extended deltoid split approach with a shoulder strap incision. J Orthop Trauma. 2013 Feb;27(2):73–6.

26. Dilisio MF, Nowinski RJ, Hatzidakis AM, Fehringer EV. Intramedullary nailing of the proximal humerus: evolution, technique, and results. J Shoulder Elbow Surg. 2016 May;25(5):e130–8. Epub 2016 Feb 16.

5 The Clavicle, the Acromioclavicular Joint, and the Sternoclavicular Joint

The management of traumatic injuries to the clavicle and its 2 joints, acromioclavicular and sternoclavicular, has evolved substantially over the last few years.

Regarding clavicle fractures, we now realize that nonoperative treatment of certain fracture patterns does lead to poor outcomes more frequently than previously thought; precontoured plates and modern intramedullary devices facilitate fixation techniques.

Regarding the acromioclavicular joint, techniques have been developed for the management of both injuries and arthritis, while augmentation techniques using allograft or synthetic devices are being used with increasing frequency. More emphasis is placed on anatomical reconstruction of all ligamentous structures, and there is substantial interest in arthroscopically assisted techniques.

Fear of a major vascular complication when dealing with sternoclavicular joint pathology still lingers, but more and more surgeons feel they can manage this particular area of the shoulder region with reliable reconstructive techniques.

Anatomical and Functional Considerations

The clavicle functions as a suspensory stabilizing strut connecting the whole upper extremity to the trunk. Some find it useful to think of the sternum and the 2 clavicles as the body (sternum) and wings (clavicle) of a plane. The sternoclavicular joints are the sturdy take-off points of these wings, and the weight of each upper extremity is suspended off the lateral end of the clavicles through the acromioclavicular joint, other connections between the clavicle and the scapula, as well as the scapulothoracic joint (Figure 5.1).

Pathology involving the clavicle or its joints can result in symptomatic functional alterations of the scapula and

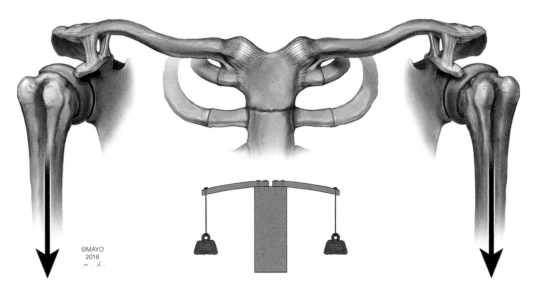

Figure 5.1 *The suspensory mechanism of the upper extremity is formed by the clavicle, the scapula, stabilizing structures between the 2, and the scapulothoracic area.*

periscapular muscles. This is extremely important to realize, since a number of patients with clavicle malunion or chronic acromioclavicular joint injuries will present in the office complaining mostly of periscapular pain (see chapter 10, The Scapula).

Clavicle

The clavicle has an interesting lazy-S shape with a fair amount of variation among individuals. The lateral clavicle shaft is concave anteriorly, whereas the medial shaft is anteriorly convex. The average straight length of the clavicle in adults is 15 cm (range, 11 to 17 cm). Something that I always find somewhat noteworthy at the time of surgery is how wide the lateral end of the clavicle is from anterior to posterior. Other interesting facts regarding the clavicle are its embryonic development, and how close it is to both the skin and a number of neurovascular structures (Table 5.1).

The fact that the clavicles undergo a process of endomembranous ossification during development has been proposed to explain the relatively high union rates of clavicle fractures even when displaced, and maybe influenced how strongly nonoperative treatment was recommended for most clavicle fractures in the past.

Other anatomic details that have direct orthopedic implications are the fact that the clavicle is so subcutaneous, as well as its proximity to a number of important neurovascular structures (Figure 5.2). The clavicle is essentially under the skin, which results in real risk of skin compromise by fractured fragments, as well as easily visible cosmetic and sometimes bothersome consequences secondary to callus formation, malunion, and hardware placed on the clavicle.

Multiple cutaneous branches from the cervical brachial plexus descend in the anterior aspect of the clavicle region. Skin incisions in this area may result in areas of hypoesthesia or painful neuroma formation. The brachial plexus and subclavian vessels lie just under the clavicle; care must be taken not to injure these structures iatrogenically when mobilizing fragments (especially in nonunions) or with hardware placement (special drills and screw tips).

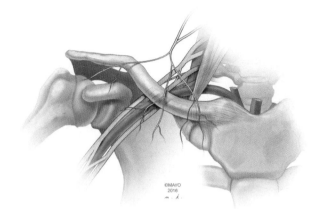

Figure 5.2 *Clavicle shape and relationships between the clavicle and superficial and deep neurovascular structures.*

Acromioclavicular Joint

As mentioned before, the scapula and the rest of the upper extremity hang off the lateral end of the clavicle (with additional support from the scapulothoracic musculature). The acromioclavicular joint complex (Figure 5.3) serves as the main interconnecting area between the clavicle and the scapula.

The lateral end of the clavicle is covered by articular cartilage and articulates with the articular surface of the acromion. The capsule of the joint is particularly thick superiorly and inferiorly, and the terms *superior* and *inferior acromioclavicular ligaments* are commonly used to refer to these thicker capsular areas.

In addition, 2 distinct ligamentous structures attach the superior aspect of the coracoid to the inferior cortex of the clavicle: these coracoacromial ligaments are named

---

Table 5.1 • Clavicle Facts

Endomembranous ossification during embryonic development

Lazy S shape, anteriorly concave laterally, anteriorly convex medially

Average adult length 15 cm

The lateral end is really wide from anterior to posterior

Subcutaneous location

Proximity to cutaneous branches of the superficial cervical plexus

Proximity to the brachial plexus and subclavius vessels

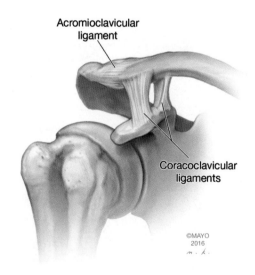

Figure 5.3 *The acromioclavicular joint complex.*

Table 5.2 • **Coracoacromial Ligaments: Dimensions and Attachment Sites**

	Clavicle Attachment	Coracoid Attachment	Width, cm	Length, cm
Trapezoid (lateral)	25 mm from the lateral end	Broad, lateral upper side	0.8–2.5	0.8–2.5
Conoid (medial)	50 mm from the lateral end	Smaller, medial posterior	0.4–0.95	0.7–2.5

conoid and trapezoid. The dimensions and attachment sites of these 2 ligaments have been carefully studied in an effort to design reconstructive techniques that replicate anatomy as much as possible (Table 5.2). As detailed in the section on injuries to the acromioclavicular joint (see "Traumatic Injuries"), without section or injury of both coracoacromial ligaments, major instability in the vertical plane does not seem to occur.

The trapezius and the deltoid muscles also contribute some to the stability of the acromioclavicular joint. Interestingly, cross-sectional histologic studies demonstrate that no muscular or tendinous fibers cross over the top of the acromioclavicular joint capsule. However, as detailed later, advancing the trapezius anteriorly and the deltoid posteriorly at the time of surgery helps cushion this subcutaneous area superiorly and may provide added joint stability.

Sternoclavicular Joint

The medial end of the clavicle is strongly connected to the sternum and first rib, providing a very stable take-off point for the clavicular strut in its function to provide support to the whole shoulder girdle (Figure 5.4). The sternal ossification center of the clavicle gets ossified and fuses late in life; ossification occurs between the ages of 12 and 19 years, whereas fusion to the rest of the clavicle occurs at the age of 22 to 25, which explains why some sternoclavicular joint dislocations are actually epiphyseal fractures of the medial clavicle.

The medial end of the clavicle is covered by articular cartilage and articulates with the clavicular facet of the sternum. This joint contains a meniscus or intra-articular disk. The lower aspect of the medial clavicle also has an articular facet for the first rib inferiorly.

The bone architecture of this joint makes it inherently unstable. However, it is made remarkably stable by a

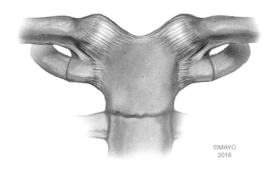
©MAYO 2016

Figure 5.4 The sternoclavicular joint complex.

number of capsular and ligamentous structures. Classically, 4 ligaments are considered to contribute to sternoclavicular joint stability. The posterior sternoclavicular ligament appears as a diffuse thickening of the posterior joint capsule. The anterior sternoclavicular joint ligament is identified as an oblique capsular thickening running from inferomedial to superolateral. The interclavicular ligament is commonly identified as a discrete ligament connecting the medial ends of both clavicles superiorly across the top of the sternum. Finally, the costoclavicular ligament (also known as rhomboid ligament) is short, robust, and has the largest footprint of all these ligaments.

Controversy remains regarding the relative contribution of all these ligaments to sternoclavicular joint stability. Some studies seem to indicate that the anterior and posterior sternoclavicular ligaments are most important (1,2), whereas others suggest that the costoclavicular ligament is most important (3). In any event, when the ligamentous support of this joint is disrupted, it becomes unstable easily. Since the costoclavicular ligament seems to attach to the inferior clavicle 10 mm lateral to the inferior sternoclavicular articular margin, in the management of sternoclavicular joint arthritis, resection of no more than 10 mm of medial clavicle should be considered whenever possible in order to preserve the origin of this ligament.

Biomechanically, the majority of clavicle motion during scapulothoracic motion occurs at the sternoclavicular joint. The medial clavicle translates with shoulder elevation, and also with scapular protraction and retraction; commonly, these combined motions require as much as 50° of rotation at the sternoclavicular joint (4). For these reasons, stiffness of the sternoclavicular joint compromises overall shoulder motion, and arthrodesis of this joint is never a great option.

Fractures of the Clavicle

Epidemiology and Mechanisms of Injury

Clavicle fractures are the fourth most common upper extremity fracture (after fractures of the distal radius, phalangeal and metacarpal fractures, and proximal humerus fractures). They comprise between 2% and 4% of all fractures in adults (5,6). Some studies have reported an incidence of 5.8 per 10,000 people (7). Interestingly, clavicle fractures are relatively common at birth. They also tend to affect infants, children, and young adults; their incidence is highest in the second and third decades of life (5).

The overall incidence of clavicle fractures in neonates has been reported to vary between 0.5 and 7.2 per 1,000 births (8).

Table 5.3 • Clavicle Fractures at Birth

Epidemiology and risk factors
Between 0.5 and 7.2 per 1,000 births
Large newborn
Older maternal age
Breech presentation
Delivery by less experienced health care providers

Evaluation
Painful pseudoparalysis
Deformity and crepitus
Rule out associated brachial plexus injury

Treatment
Short period of immobilization (shirt pinning)

Risk factors for neonatal clavicle fractures include large size of the newborn, older maternal age, breech presentation, and delivery by less experienced health care providers.

Details regarding the evaluation and management of clavicle birth fractures exceed the scope of this book (Table 5.3). Most neonates with a fractured clavicle avoid moving the affected upper extremity secondary to pain. Painful pseudoparalysis (which can occur as a consequence of a fracture of the clavicle, a proximal humerus fracture, or septic arthritis of the shoulder) must be distinguished from a neonatal brachial plexus injury (presenting as painless paralysis). Neonatal clavicle fractures and neonatal brachial plexus injuries can coexist. Most neonatal clavicle fractures heal uneventfully, and management is limited to a short period of immobilization of the affected upper extremity for comfort.

Most fractures in infants, children, and adolescents occur as a result of falls from a height or accidents while playing sports. Bicycle and motorcycle accidents are particularly common. Older patients can also sustain fractures as a result of a car accident. Stress fractures of the clavicle have occasionally been reported in gymnastics and other sports such as rowing, basketball, and cheerleading (9). Spontaneous fractures of the clavicle can also occur in the setting of radical neck dissection or malignancy.

Evaluation

History and Physical Examination
Clavicle fractures present with a number of classic features. Most patients experience acute onset of pain at the time of injury and avoid motion of the affected upper extremity. Deformity is typically obvious due to the subcutaneous location of the clavicle. Inspection may show areas of bruising, erosion or tenting of the skin, and occasionally patients will present with an open clavicle fracture. The clinical length of the fractured clavicle can be measured with tape and compared with the opposite side to provide an estimation of shortening. Displaced fractures of the distal end of the clavicle may resemble acromioclavicular joint dislocations.

After inspection, the clavicle can be gently palpated when in doubt in order to identify areas of tenderness and

deformity. Special attention should be paid to the identification of associated injuries (distal radius fractures, elbow injuries, neurovascular injuries, and, in cases of severe trauma, scapulothoracic disassociation). Range of motion of the shoulder in rotation may be evaluated to assess the integrity of the glenohumeral joint, but elevation is seldom tested—to avoid unnecessary pain. When pain allows, dynamic evaluation of the scapula should also be performed, since scapular dyskinesia seems to be associated with worse clinical outcomes after conservative management of displaced midshaft clavicle fractures (10).

Radiographs
Plain radiographs typically provide enough information for proper evaluation and decision making when managing clavicle fractures. Standard views include an anteroposterior view and a 30° cephalic tilt view with the patient standing at a 45° angle in reference to the beam. Use of these 2 views improves fracture classification agreement (11).

As detailed later, clavicle shortening through the fracture is a major decision-making point regarding treatment; comparative radiographs of the contralateral clavicle are helpful in that regard. In addition, radiographs obtained with the patient lying supine underestimate vertical displacement; in one study, complete lack of contact was identified in more than 40% of radiographs obtained in the upright position, and was not seen in any radiographs obtained in the supine position (on average, radiographs obtained in the supine position underestimated vertical displacement by almost 9 mm or 90%) (12).

Clavicle fractures are typically classified according to their anatomical location as midshaft fractures (fractures of the middle third), fractures of the medial clavicle, and lateral clavicle fractures (Figure 5.5; Table 5.4). Fractures involving each of these anatomical locations are further subclassified as follows.

Fractures of the Medial End of the Clavicle (Type 1)
These fractures are classified as undisplaced (A) or displaced (B), and then as extra-articular (1A1 and 1B1) or intra-articular (1A2 or 1B2).

Midshaft Clavicle Fractures (Type 2)
These fractures are subclassified as type 2A if they maintain some cortical contact (less than 100% of displacement—2A1 are nondisplaced and 2A2 are angulated). Types 2B have no cortical contact (displacement over 100%) and are further classified into 2B1 if they have no comminution or at the most a simple wedge fragment, or 2B2 if they are segmental or have marked comminution.

Fractures of the Lateral End of the Clavicle (Type 3)
These fractures are further subclassified by depending on the location of the fracture relative to the coracoacromial ligaments and the presence or absence of intra-articular extension (see later).

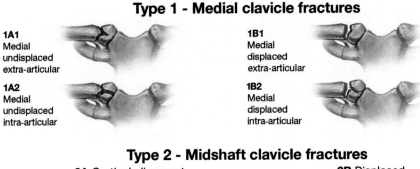

Type 1 - Medial clavicle fractures

1A1
Medial
undisplaced
extra-articular

1A2
Medial
undisplaced
intra-articular

1B1
Medial
displaced
extra-articular

1B2
Medial
displaced
intra-articular

Type 2 - Midshaft clavicle fractures

2A Cortical alignment

2B Displaced

2A1
Undisplaced

2A2
Angulated

2B1
Simple

or

Single
butterfly

2B1
Segmented

or

Comminuted

Type 3 - Distal clavicle fractures

3A Distal third undisplaced

3B Distal third displaced

3A1
Undisplaced
extra-articular
(Neer I)

3A2
Undisplaced
intra-articular
(Neer III)

3B1
Displaced
extra-articular
(Neer II)

3B2
Displaced
intra-articular

Figure 5.5 *Clavicle fracture classification.*
(Adapted from Robinson [56]. Used with permission.)

Table 5.4 • Classifications Commonly Used for Clavicle Fractures

Fractures of the middle third (mid-shaft clavicle fractures)—Altman/Robinson

Fractures of the lateral third—Neer/Robinson

Fractures of the medial third—Craig/Robinson

Advanced Imaging Studies

Additional imaging studies are seldom necessary in patients with fractures of the clavicle. However, computed tomography (CT) may be of help when good quality radiographs sitting or standing cannot be obtained (i.e., polytrauma patient) or when evaluating the medial end of the clavicle, which may be difficult to assess secondary to the overlap of the sternum, ribs, clavicle, and spine. CT helps determine if medial clavicle injuries resulted in an intra-articular fracture, a physeal injury, or an isolated dislocation. CT is also very helpful to assess union in patients with persistent symptoms after management of a clavicle fracture: plain radiographs do not reliably distinguish nonunions and malunions (13). Vascular studies and electromyography with nerve conduction studies may be necessary when an associated vascular or nerve injury is suspected.

Midshaft Fractures of the Clavicle

Decision-Making: When Should Surgery Be Considered?

Traditionally, nonoperative management was the treatment of choice for the majority of patients presenting with midshaft clavicle fractures. These injuries were expected to unite with little functional consequences even in the presence of marked displacement and residual malunion. Surgery used to be considered only for open fractures, fractures with associated vascular injuries, severe tenting of the skin, or the need to return to activities as soon as possible (e.g., professional motorcycle riders). However, a number of relatively recent studies seem to indicate that certain displaced fractures are associated with a substantial rate of nonunion, malunion, and dysfunction in adults, and internal fixation provides a better outcome for select displaced fractures. When treating clavicle fractures, the information provided by some landmark studies needs to be taken into consideration.

For decades, nonoperative treatment was preferred over surgical treatment based on studies by Rowe and Neer reporting very low rates of nonunion with conservative treatment, and a three-fold increase in nonunion using the internal fixation techniques available back then. In 1997, Hill et al. (14) published the first modern study describing a high rate of dissatisfaction with nonoperative treatment of clavicle fractures. Since then, a number of studies have analyzed in detail the rates of malunion and nonunion after nonoperative management of clavicle fractures, and have also compared nonoperative treatment and internal fixation. Some authors have reported an approximately 25% incidence of poor functional outcomes with conservative management of displaced clavicle fractures (15).

Age is a major risk factor for nonunion after conservative management (15); fractures occurring under the age of 18 years have been reported to have a nonunion rate close to zero (16,17). Children and adolescents seem to do quite well with nonoperative treatment of displaced fractures (18). This is partly due to their remodeling potential. Even in children with established clavicle malunions, little to no functional deficits can be identified (17).

Displacement is a second risk factor for nonunion and malunion, with very low rates for nondisplaced fractures. The rate of nonunion increases to approximately 15% for displaced fractures (those with no cortical contact), and in this group of injuries the main risk factors for nonunion include smoking (odds ratio, ≈4), comminution (odds ratio, ≈2), and fracture displacement (odds ratio, 1.17). Controversy remains about the relative contribution of shortening and vertical displacement (15).

Prospective, randomized studies have compared the outcome of nonoperative management and plate fixation for *displaced* clavicle fractures. The Canadian Orthopaedic Trauma Society (19) reported lower rates of nonunion, shorter times to union, and better functional outcomes in the operative group, although the operative group had a complication rate of 37% and a reoperation rate of 18%. Robinson et al. (13) reported nonunion rates of 15% and 1%, respectively, for nonoperative treatment versus plate fixation. Interestingly, when patients with non-united fractures were excluded, the functional outcomes were identical between the 2 groups, although plate fixation led to faster recovery and nonoperative treatment was associated with an additional 10% delayed union rate (union after 6 months). The rates of reoperation for nonunion, malunion, or a new clavicle fracture were 5% in the surgical group and 12% in the nonoperative group, but this difference did not reach statistical significance. The rate of plate removal was 10%. Other recent studies have confirmed faster recovery and lower nonunion rates with plate fixation, but at the expense of a higher complication rate (20,21).

Data from all these studies seem to indicate that even though surgery provides faster recovery and a lower nonunion rate, many displaced clavicle fractures can be treated successfully without surgery. Robinson et al. (13) estimated that it would be necessary to operate on 6.2 fractures surgically in order to prevent 1 nonunion. On the other hand, financial analysis seems to indicate decreased costs with internal fixation of displaced clavicle fractures (22). Thus, despite the great quality of several recent studies reported, refined prognostic criteria to predict nonunion and malunion are still required.

Some studies have tried to determine if bridges are burned when patients are treated nonoperatively, they develop a nonunion, and eventually require plate fixation. In other words, how do patients who undergo internal fixation of an acute clavicle fracture recover compared with those who fail to heal and eventually develop a nonunion requiring internal fixation? Patients treated with late plate fixation seem to have less endurance than patients treated acutely, even though healing and good restoration of function is achieved in both groups of patients (23).

Based on the study by Murray et al. (16), displacement over 2.5 cm increases the nonunion rate to over 15% in nonsmokers, so that severity of displacement seems to break even with the overall results of nonoperative treatment. In a separate study, the nonunion rate increased with vertical displacement over 100% (15). A poor DASH (Disabilities of the Arm, Shoulder, and Hand) score at 6 weeks has also been found to be predictive of nonunion (24). Based on the data available to date and summarized earlier, we currently recommend internal fixation for midshaft clavicle fractures in the circumstances summarized in Table 5.5.

Table 5.5 • Current Indications for Surgical Management of Midshaft Clavicle Fractures

Displaced fractures (no cortical contact—displacement over 100%)
Overall displacement more than 25 mm
Tenting of the skin

Need to operate for other reasons
Open fracture
Associated vascular injury requiring surgical repair
Associated nerve injury requiring surgical repair

Scapulothoracic disassociation (floating shoulder)

True need to return to activities as soon as possible

Severe associated scapular dyskinesia

Poor DASH score at 6 weeks (relative)

Abbreviation: DASH, Disabilities of the Arm, Shoulder, and Hand.

Nonoperative Management

Nonoperative management of clavicle fractures consists of immobilization of the affected upper extremity until some healing has occurred, followed by physical therapy for patients with residual periscapular pain. Classically, displaced midshaft clavicle fractures were immobilized with a figure-of-8 bandage to facilitate fracture healing in a better position of fractured fragments (Figure 5.6). However, figure-of-8 bandages have not been demonstrated to decrease the rate of malunion or nonunion (25,26). Figure-of-8 bandages are also uncomfortable: not uncommonly, patients feel that

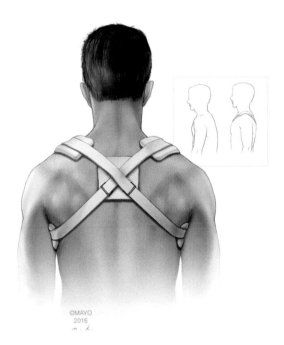

Figure 5.6 Figure-of-8 bandage for conservative management of clavicle fractures.

their hands go to sleep, and sleeping at night can be close to impossible without placing a folded towel or pillow in the thoracic spine area, so that the shoulders will rest on the mattress with the spine properly supported. For these reasons, most surgeons currently favor immobilization with a sling.

The length of immobilization varies depending on the age of the patient and the severity of the fracture. Clavicle fractures in young children heal very rapidly, and in some children within a couple of weeks no motion can be identified by stressing the fracture site. On the other hand, elderly individuals may be best served by immobilization for 6 to 8 weeks. Most patients do well with 4 to 6 weeks of immobilization, recognizing that radiographic fracture healing lags behind clinical healing.

Once the fracture is healed, most patients experience little difficulty regaining motion. However, depending on the amount of residual displacement at the time of healing, some patients may complain of periscapular pain secondary to mild scapular dyskinesis. Physical therapy is specifically aimed at strengthening and rebalancing the periscapular musculature (see chapter 12, Rehabilitation and Injections). Contact sports may be resumed in 4 to 6 months, or earlier in younger patients (6).

Plate Fixation

Open reduction and internal fixation using a plate and screws is the most common treatment modality when surgical treatment is performed. The main area of controversy remains placement of the plate superiorly or anteriorly.

Plate Selection
When surgery is indicated for a midshaft clavicle fracture (Table 5.5), internal fixation using a plate and screws is most commonly used. Plate fixation of midshaft clavicle fractures has evolved substantially over time. Traditional stainless-steel straight plates were problematic: these relatively thick plates are quite prominent for such a subcutaneous bone, and also difficult to adapt to the very particular shape of the clavicle. In an effort to use lower profile plates that could be contoured more easily, surgeons turned to other alternatives, such as reconstruction plates; however, fatigue led to either plate angulation resulting in malunion, or plate breakage and nonunion. Luckily, improvements in implant design have led to modern precontoured plates with a number of extremely useful features (Table 5.6). The need for hardware removal has decreased with the use of these lower profile precontoured plates (27).

Plate length is extremely important as well, and many failures of fixation are secondary to inadequate plate length. As a minimum, 3 bicortical screws should be placed on each side of the fracture past the areas of comminution. Most of the time this can only be achieved using a 7- or 8-hole plate; longer plates are used in patients with poor bone quality, severe comminution, or risk factors for delayed union or nonunion.

Table 5.6 • Modern Clavicle Plate Features

Precontoured (accommodate multiple clavicle shapes)

Strong (resist fatigue failure)

Low profile (less prominence and discomfort, possibly lowering removal rates)

Multiple screw options (locking, variable-angle locking and nonlocking, large and small, clustered at the ends)

Dedicated holes for suture augmentation (particularly useful for severe comminution or when temporary elastic fixation to the coracoid is considered beneficial)

Table 5.7 • Superior versus Anteroinferior Plating

Superior	Anteroinferior
Biomechanically stronger (placed on the tension side of the bone)	Deformation mode similar to intact clavicle
Most precontoured plates fit better the shape of the clavicle when placed superiorly	Less subcutaneous prominence
More risk of neurovascular injury with drills and screws directed from superior to inferior	

Plate Position

One of the main current controversies regarding clavicle plate fixation is the ideal positioning of the plate (Figure 5.7). Traditionally, plates have been placed on the superior cortex of the clavicle; more recently, plate placement on the anteroinferior aspect of the clavicle has been advocated mostly to decrease plate prominence and hopefully decrease the need for reoperation. The relative advantages and disadvantages of these 2 plate locations are summarized in Table 5.7 (28–30). Clinical studies have not clearly shown lower rates of either subjective discomfort secondary to plate irritation or plate removal, although when only patients with retained plates are compared, the rate of soft-tissue irritation seems to be less with anteroinferior plates (30). In my practice, I favor superior plating, especially when there is comminution; however, anteroinferior plating is considered for very thin patients with more simple fracture patterns, as well as when the skin covering the superior aspect of the clavicle is compromised.

Patient Position

There are a number of additional technical details that may facilitate plate fixation of the clavicle and hopefully lead to better outcomes. Patient positioning in the operating room is critical, especially for superior plating. I prefer to position the patients in a standard table and raise the head of the table 30° to 40°, and secure the head and neck of the patient rotated toward the opposite shoulder; otherwise, it is difficult to use drills and screws in the correct trajectory on the medial side of the plate (Figure 5.8). The arm is draped free, since motion of the upper extremity will aid with fracture reduction.

Exposure

My preference is to place a transverse skin incision along the anteroinferior aspect of the clavicle and divide the platysma colli directly onto bone without raising skin flaps. At the time of closure, the skin incision does not rest directly over a superiorly placed plate. The fracture is then exposed subperiosteally, trying to preserve vascularity as much as possible.

One potential issue related to surgical exposure for plate fixation of the clavicle has to do with the sensory branches of the cervical plexus. A number of these sensory nerves cross the surgical field from proximal to distal. Some surgeons advocate dissecting and preserving these branches, mobilizing them sideways for fracture reduction and plate placement. Others ignore these branches and blindly divide them during exposure. Dysfunction of these nerves leads to numbness in the anterior chest wall. The reported rate of numbness has varied depending on how carefully patients are questioned about it. Even with nerve preservation, the rate of anterior chest wall numbness is over 80% at 2 weeks,

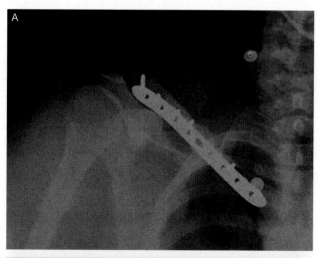

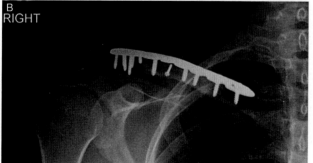

Figure 5.7 *Radiographs showing* **A,** *Superior plating and* **B,** *Anteroinferior plating.*

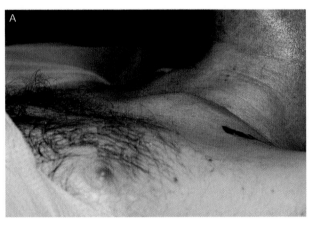
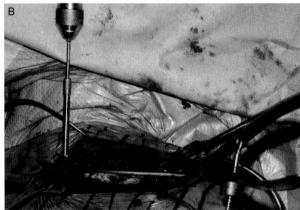

Figure 5.8 **A,** *Patient positioning for plate fixation of a clavicle fracture.* **B,** *Adequate insertion of medial screws may be difficult if the head and neck are not rotated to the opposite shoulder.*

decreasing to under 50% at 1 year (31). Interestingly, the presence of numbness does not lead to worse overall patient reported outcomes or dissatisfaction.

Since numbness seems to be very common even with nerve preservation, in my practice I do not make an effort to identify and protect these nerve branches. However, prior to surgery it is important to let patients know that they have a very high chance of anterior chest wall numbness and that the area of numbness will decrease in size over time but may never get back to normal.

Plate Application

All basic principles of diaphyseal fracture plate fixation should be applied. Interfragmentary screw fixation of smaller comminuted cortical fragments is followed by compression plating whenever possible. Occasionally, the fracture pattern does not allow compression plating, and the plate is applied as a neutralizing or bridging device. My preference is to use 1 nonlocking screw on each side of the plate to compress the fracture and intimately apply the plate to the cortex; locking screws are used in the remaining holes, especially when variable angle locking screws are available. Very small fragments can be secured with sutures through or around the plate. Wires are avoided due to their risk of migration (Figure 5.9).

Care must be taken when drilling and placing screws to avoid inadvertent damage of the underlying neurovascular structures. Accurate measurement of screw length is critical, since bicortical purchase is extremely beneficial, but prominent screws can impinge on neurovascular structures or, for lateral screws, invade the subacromial space. I favor cancellous fully threaded screws for holes positioned directly over the acromion or the very medial end of the clavicle.

Postoperative Management

Provided adequate fixation is achieved, a sling is used for comfort the first 1 or 2 weeks, and shoulder range of motion

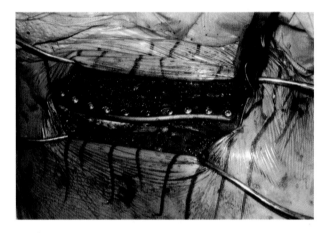

Figure 5.9 *Open reduction and plate fixation of a clavicle fracture.*

exercises and scapular isometrics are initiated at week 3 or 4. Most patients can be allowed to return to heavier use of their upper extremity by 2 to 3 months and to initiate contact sports by 4 to 6 months.

Reported Outcomes

Plate fixation of displaced clavicle fractures has been reported to provide good clinical outcomes and very high union rates in the majority of modern published studies (13,20,27,30,32–34). Most patients recover complete motion of the upper extremity and have no pain and no functional restrictions. However, complications such as deep infection, nonunion, and malunion can happen. In addition, as mentioned before, many patients experience numbness in the anterior chest wall (31).

The rate of reoperation for any reason has been reported to vary between 15% and 40% (27,32,34). The most common reason for reoperation is hardware-related discomfort secondary to plate prominence. Plate removal is more commonly performed in smaller patients and females, and is less common with precontoured plates (27,34).

The rate of serious complications has ranged between 7% and 15%, with equal rates of infection and nonunion, and slightly lower rates of malunion. Risk factors for these complications include diabetes mellitus, alcohol and drug abuse, multiple comorbidities, female sex, and older age. Other uncommon but serious complications reported include pneumothorax, and injury to the axillary vessels or branches of the brachial plexus (34).

Intramedullary Nailing

Intramedullary nailing of the clavicle was developed to avoid some of the disadvantages of plate fixation, including long skin incisions, anterior chest wall numbness, and plate prominence. However, the particular shape of the clavicle does not lend itself to easy nailing, and there are some concerns regarding the relative stability of plate versus nail fixation (especially in fractures with comminution) as well as the potential for nail migration (Figure 5.10). Biomechanically, plate fixation seems to be superior to intramedullary nailing against rotational stress (35). Some authors have reported relatively higher rates of nonunion than those reported with plate fixation (36). However, a few comparative and prospective randomized studies have reported equal results with both fixation modalities (37–39).

Modern flexible nails designed for clavicle fracture fixation are made of titanium. The patient is typically placed supine on a radiolucent line, and the procedure is performed under fluoroscopic control. The nail is introduced from the medial end of the clavicle through a perforation in the anterior cortex. If the fracture can be aligned properly, the nail is advanced across the fracture site to the lateral end of the clavicle. If the fracture cannot be reduced closed, a limited horizontal or vertical skin

incision is used to align the fragments. Once the nail is fully advanced, it is cut flush at the entrance.

As mentioned before, two prospective randomized studies have demonstrated no major differences when plate and nail fixation have been compared (38,39). One study reported on 59 fractures randomized to either a reconstruction plate or a nail (38). Plate bending during healing occurred in a number of shoulders; reconstruction plates have largely been abandoned for this reason. Nails were associated with skin irritation more commonly, and the only nonunion occurred in a fracture stabilized with a nail (38). In a separate prospective randomized study (39), 120 fractures were randomized to plate or nail fixation; again, there were no differences in final outcome. Plate fixation led to a faster recovery (39).

Management of Complications
Nonunion
As mentioned, clavicle nonunion seems to occur in approximately 15% of clavicle fractures in the adult treated nonoperatively (16,19); nonunion can also occur in fractures treated surgically with either plate or intramedullary fixation (20,32). Risk factors for nonunion were discussed previously. Some patients adapt to their established nonunion and do not seek additional treatment. Others complain of various degrees of pain and dysfunction and elect to undergo surgery.

Evaluation Table 5.8 summarizes the key elements to be learned from patients with an established clavicle nonunion. It is extremely important to identify known risk factors for nonunion, since those that are modifiable (e.g., smoking) should be addressed prior to surgical treatment. Clinical measurement of the length of both clavicles, as mentioned in the section on evaluation of acute fractures (see "Evaluation"), is even more important in nonunions (Figure 5.11). Severe shortening may prompt the need for

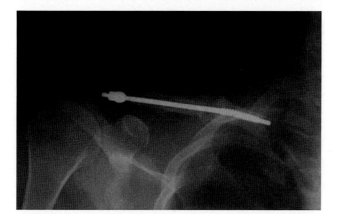

Figure 5.10 Clavicle fracture stabilized with an intramedullary nail.

Table 5.8 • Key Elements When Evaluating Patients With an Established Clavicle Nonunion
Mechanism of initial injury
Time elapsed
Risk factors for nonunion Open fracture Smoking Other
Clinical shortening compared with opposite side
Secondary scapular dyskinesis
Neurovascular symptoms
Prior surgical treatments, if any

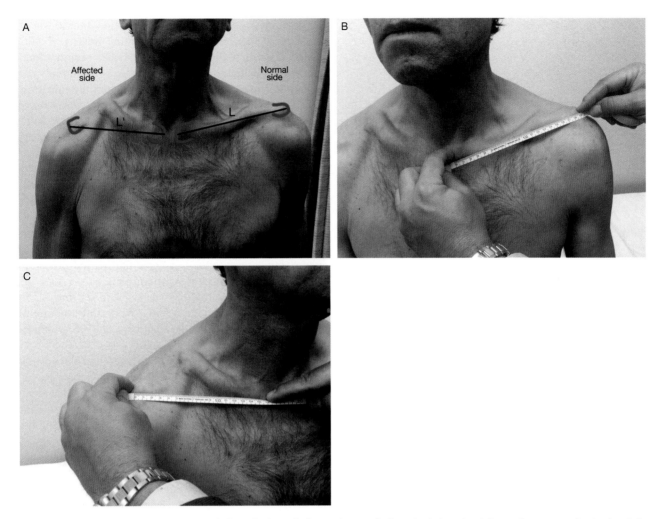

Figure 5.11 *Clinical measurement of clavicle length from the medial end of the clavicle to the sternoclavicular joint. L indicates normal length; L', length on affected, shortened side.*

special bone augmentation techniques. In addition, restoration of adequate length can be confirmed intraoperatively by comparison with the opposite side. Patients should also be assessed for secondary scapular dyskinesis, since a dedicated program of scapular exercises may be needed after surgery, and patients should be counseled about the fact that secondary scapular dyskinesis may be extremely difficult to overcome even after satisfactory clavicle union. Patients with previous failed surgery need to be assessed further regarding the location of previous skin incisions, the condition of the soft tissues, details on the procedures performed before, and the possibility of deep infection.

Most nonunions are easily identified in plain radiographs (Figure 5.12). However, the radiographic aspect may occasionally suggest *mal*union rather than *non*union, and vice versa. Radiographs should be assessed for bone quality. Retained hardware, if any, should be noted (Figure 5.13). In addition, the amount of shortening and missing bone

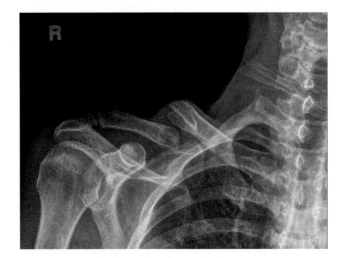

Figure 5.12 *Plain radiograph of a clavicle nonunion complicating nonoperative treatment.*

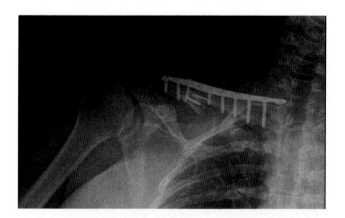

Figure 5.13 *Failed plate fixation with ensuing nonunion.*

should be estimated; most of the time, the amount of shortening overestimates missing bone, since there may be some fragment overlapping. Contralateral radiographs are used for comparison of length.

CT is particularly useful when union is questionable, especially for nonunions complicating surgical treatment (Figure 5.14). It can also be used to more accurately measure the size of the fragments, and hence estimate bone loss. Finally, CT with 3-dimensional reconstruction can be used for 3-dimensional printing. The opposite side can be mirrored and printed in a mold that can be taken to the operating room to replicate as close as desired the length and shape of the clavicle.

Occasionally, clavicle nonunions may be associated with neurologic or vascular changes that merit evaluation using electromyography with nerve conduction studies

or vascular studies. Ruling out infection should also be considered in nonunions complicating internal fixation, especially when the history or physical examination is suggestive. Laboratory studies can also be selectively used to monitor nicotine levels in smokers and the nutritional status of malnourished individuals. My preference is to not offer surgical treatment for patients with risk factors for nonunion (particularly smokers) until these risk factors are corrected.

Surgical Management Established nonunions are considered for surgical management in individuals affected by the condition. As mentioned, efforts are made to correct any risk factors for nonunion prior to embarking on a surgical intervention. Open reduction and internal fixation with plates and screws is the most commonly used procedure. Hypertrophic nonunions with minimal bone loss may not require bone grafting. However, bone grafting is commonly required to promote union, and more importantly add length if needed. Infected nonunions are oftentimes addressed in a staged fashion.

The surgical technique for plate fixation of clavicle nonunions follows the same principles described for acute fractures. However, internal fixation of nonunions is typically more complicated due to the need to remove interposed fibrous tissue, mobilize the fragments, and understand how to achieve the best possible reduction.

Regarding bone grafting, iliac crest bone grafting is the most commonly used source. Sometimes, a tricortical graft needs to be harvested and interposed at the nonunion site to gain enough length. However, not uncommonly adequate length can be re-established with proper reduction

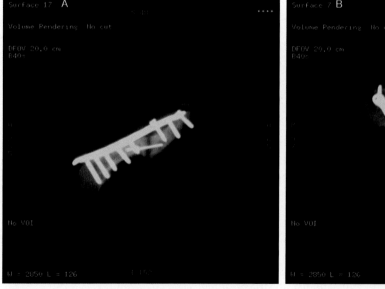
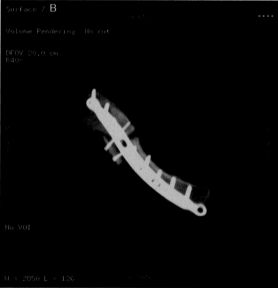

Figure 5.14 **A and B,** *Computed tomography with 3-dimensional reconstruction can be particularly useful for the evaluation of clavicle nonunions after failed internal fixation.*

of the fragments, but only with a small contact area. In those circumstances, my preference is to fashion a small unicortical bone plate with a cancellous back and fix the plate across the nonunion site anteriorly with small screws, packing cancellous chips all around it. This anterior bone plate does not migrate away from the nonunion site postoperatively and may also provide some additional stability (Figure 5.15).

When more than 3 to 4 centimeters of intercalary graft are required to restore adequate length, the rate of union using iliac crest is suboptimal, and consideration should be given to a vascularized fibular autograft (40). Vascularized fibular autografting is also considered for patients presenting after multiple failed procedures (Figure 5.16). Obviously, this procedure is associated with increased complexity and morbidity. For patients with compromised healing potential but no major segmental bone deficiency, we have been very successful in our practice using a vascularized graft from the medial femoral

condyle. A thin layer of bone and periosteum is harvested with its vascularity and ends up being flexible enough to be rolled around the clavicle (41).

Outcome A number of studies have reported on the outcome of internal fixation with or without various bone grafting techniques for clavicle nonunions. Most publications from the 1980s and 1990s reported very high union rates and satisfactory clinical outcomes when compression plating was associated with autologous bone grafting (42–47). Later, some studies reported good outcomes using compression plating without bone grafting (48,49). Reported union rates have exceeded 90% in most of these studies. Fewer studies have reported on the outcome of internal fixation and bone grafting using a free vascularized fibular autograft or a free vascularized corticoperiosteal bone graft, but the results have been uniformly satisfactory in terms of both healing rates and restoration of function (40,41).

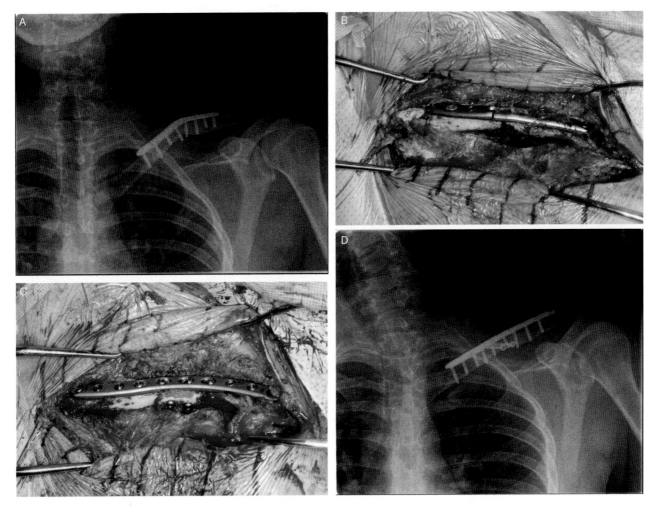

Figure 5.15 *Clavicle nonunion treated with plate fixation and structural iliac crest bone grafting using an anterior unicortical bone plate fixed in place with small screws.* **A,** *Preoperative radiograph.* **B,** *Intraoperative photograph shows broken plate.* **C,** *Internal fixation with a superior plate and anterior iliac crest bone graft.* **D,** *Postoperative radiograph.*

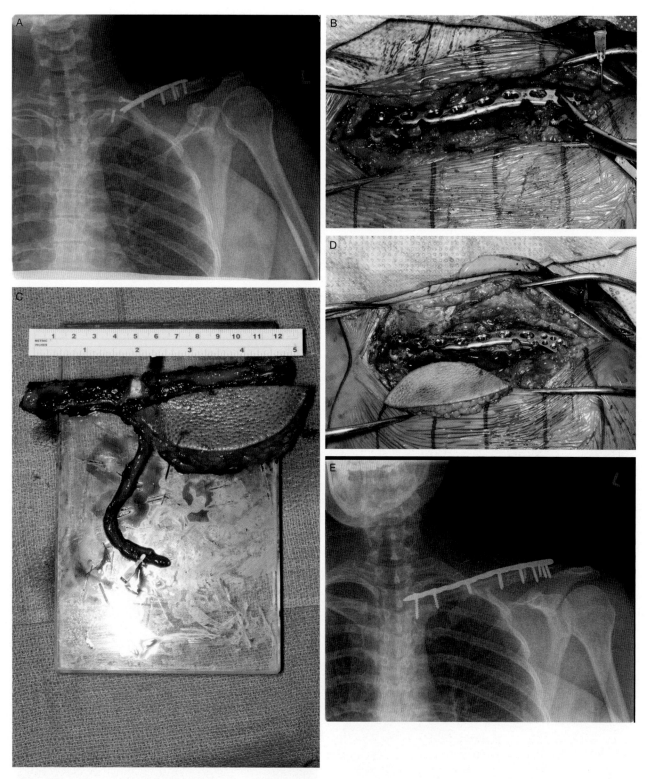

Figure 5.16 *Vascularized fibular autograft reconstruction.* **A,** *Preoperative radiograph.* **B,** *Preliminary fracture fixation to determine the length of deficiency after restoration of length.* **C,** *Harvested vascularized fibula autograft with skin island to monitor healing.* **D,** *Autograft fibula in place.* **E,** *Postoperative radiograph.*

Table 5.9 • **Possible Clinical Manifestations of Symptomatic Clavicle Malunions**

Local pain and deformity

Various degrees of scapular dyskinesis and periscapular pain

Compression of underlying neurovascular structures

Weakness and loss of endurance

Difficulty with certain activities, such as carrying a backpack or wearing clothing with straps

---

Malunion

Many individuals tolerate certain severity of clavicle malunion without major symptoms or functional deficits. However, severe clavicle malunion may lead to substantial issues (Table 5.9) (50). Occasionally, patients may complain of neurovascular symptoms secondary to compression of the brachial plexus or subclavian vessels. More commonly, patients with symptomatic malunions complain of periscapular pain, loss of endurance, and difficulty with certain activities. Women can be upset by difficulties with clothing, as straps in bras, swimming suits, tank tops, and t-shirts may fall off on the affected side.

Physical examination of the shoulder typically shows an obvious deformity of the clavicle as well as shortening of the shoulder girdle with protraction and drooping of the scapula. Patients may have periscapular pain with various degrees of objective scapular dyskinesia. A careful neurovascular examination is warranted to detect sensory or even motor changes in various components of the brachial plexus, as well as changes in the radial pulse. The clinical length of both clavicles may be measured, as mentioned before, for acute fractures. The malunion site may be stressed manually to detect abnormal motion that might indicate occult nonunion.

Plain radiographs of both clavicles may be enough to assess the severity of the malunion. CT is oftentimes considered to rule out an associated nonunion. As mentioned before, 3-dimensional reconstructions and printing based on CT may facilitate surgical planning. In patients with associated neurovascular symptoms, consideration should be given to electromyography with nerve conduction studies and vascular studies. If vascular studies show intimate proximity of the subclavian vessels to the malunion site, dissection in surgery must proceed very cautiously, and consideration should be given to partnering with a vascular surgeon.

When to recommend surgery in patients with symptomatic clavicle malunions is oftentimes a difficult decision to make, and it must be individualized. Although the reported results of clavicle osteotomy for malunion have been pretty good, there are instances of osteotomy nonunion, and plate removal is occasionally required later (51). When periscapular pain and dyskinesia are the only complaints, a well-structured program of physical therapy focused on scapular stabilizing exercises may provide enough improvement.

For patients severely affected by a clavicle malunion, osteotomy of the clavicle may be considered (Figure 5.17). As mentioned before, most studies on the topic have reported high healing rates and good functional results (23,51–53). However, patients need to be counseled about the rare possibility of nonunion, and possible issues related to plate prominence and the cosmetic consequence of the scar.

Although intramedullary nailing has been reported for fixation of clavicle osteotomies (53), my preference is to use plate fixation. All considerations reviewed for plate fixation of acute fractures (exposure, plate selection, plate location) apply to malunions as well. The location and orientation of the osteotomy should be planned carefully based on clinical measurements of clavicle length and preoperative imaging studies, including 3-dimensional printing for more complex cases. Most of the time, an oblique osteotomy allows restoration of clavicle length without the need for a structural or intercalary graft, but consent should be obtained from patients to add bone-grafting techniques if they are deemed necessary at the time of surgery. Before performing the osteotomy, the clavicle should be examined carefully to identify the occasional patient with an occult nonunion, since the correction would then be performed through the nonunion site.

A few studies have reported on the outcome of clavicle osteotomy for malunion. Bosch et al. (52) reported satisfactory outcomes in all 4 extension osteotomies with bone grafting included in their study. McKee et al. (51) reported very good results as well in 15 shoulders treated with clavicle osteotomy; however, there was 1 nonunion, and 2 patients requested plate removal.

Deep Infection

Deep infection is an uncommon but devastating complication of surgical management for clavicle fractures. Some studies have reported infection rates between 2% and 3% (34), but in most the reported infection rate has been less than 1% (20,27,39,54). The most commonly identified risk factors for infection include active smoking and diabetes mellitus. A major problem with infection after internal fixation of a clavicle fracture is that the soft-tissue envelope is frail, since the clavicle is almost subcutaneous.

Superficial infections may be treated with antibiotic therapy and, if needed, irrigation and débridement. Deep infection may contribute to nonunion. If the fracture is healing, most surgeons would favor managing the infection with antibiotics and débridement, maintaining the internal fixation hardware in place until fracture union, at which time all hardware can be removed. On the other hand, if the patient develops an infected nonunion, most of the time staged surgery is warranted. In the first procedure, all hardware is removed, a thorough débridement is

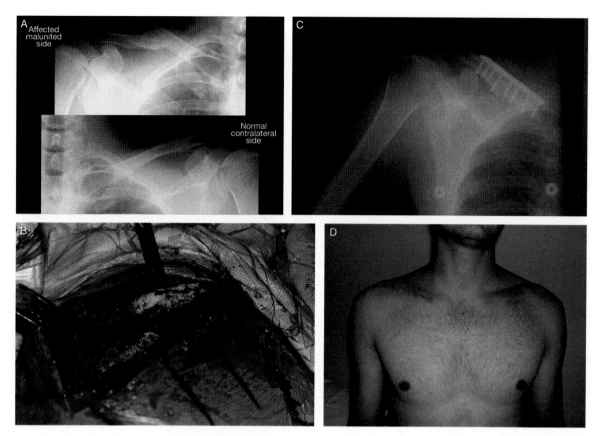

Figure 5.17 *Clavicle malunion.* **A,** *Radiographs at presentation,* **B,** *Osteotomy.* **C,** *Postoperative radiograph.* **D,** *Postoperative clinical aspect with normal restoration of length and shape.*

performed, and consideration is given to soft-tissue coverage techniques. After a course of intravenous antibiotics (typically 6 weeks), and once the infection is resolved, the second procedure almost always involves revision internal fixation and bone grafting. Unfortunately, union is not consistently achieved (55).

Fractures of the Distal Third of the Clavicle

Fractures of the lateral or distal end of the clavicle receive particular attention because they have the potential to compromise stability between the clavicle and the scapula when the fracture line is just medial to the coracoclavicular ligaments. In these more unstable fracture patterns, the weight of the arm can lead to substantial displacement and facilitate nonunion. If surgical management is attempted, the small size of the lateral fragment may make stable internal fixation very difficult to achieve.

Classification

These fractures were originally classified in 5 separate types. Later on, a simpler classification with better observer agreement was proposed (see Figure 5.5) (56,57). In nondisplaced fractures (with cortical alignment), one or both coracoclavicular ligaments are still

attached to the medial fragment, whereas in displaced fractures (with no cortical alignment) the medial clavicle is completely disconnected from the coracoclavicular ligaments (Figure 5.18). Either fracture type may or may not extend into the acromioclavicular joint.

Evaluation

The general principles of evaluation outlined previously for all clavicle fractures apply to fractures of the distal third. Most commonly, these fractures are the result of a medially directed impact on the shoulder or a fall on the outstretched hand (56,58). Nondisplaced fractures may be associated with some swelling and ecchymosis but minimal deformity, whereas displaced fractures usually present with substantial deformity and may even tent the skin; their clinical aspect is similar to that of acromioclavicular joint dislocations. Gentle strength testing of the rotator cuff should be part of the evaluation, since associated injuries to the suprascapular nerve have been described (59). Plain radiographs are oftentimes sufficient to evaluate these injuries. CT may be useful in patients with questionable union after nonoperative treatment. Magnetic resonance imaging may be considered for the evaluation of physeal injuries.

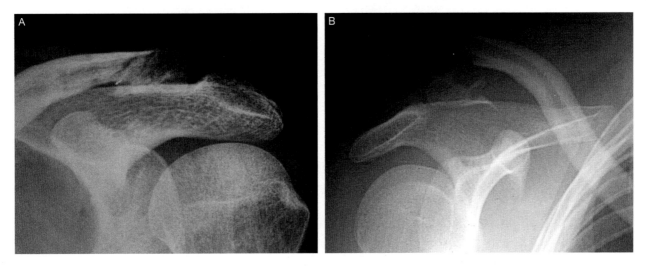

Figure 5.18 Radiographic examples of nondisplaced (A) and displaced (B) fractures of the distal clavicle.

Management

Nondisplaced Fractures

Fractures with cortical alignment and no disruption of the ligamentous attachments between the medial fragment and the coracoclavicular ligaments are treated with a short period of immobilization for comfort. Fractures with intra-articular extension are theorized to predispose to symptomatic acromioclavicular joint arthritis, but the frequency of late symptoms at the acromioclavicular joint requiring management is unclear (58).

Displaced Fractures

Lack of radiographically visible fracture union at 1 year is very common after nonoperative treatment of displaced fractures of the distal clavicle. However, nonunion is not always bothersome enough to justify further treatment. Age and displacement are the main risk factors for nonunion of a displaced distal clavicle fracture (56). The reported rates of nonunion have ranged between 30% and 50%, although isolated studies have reported rates as high as 75% (58,60). This information is shared with patients at the time of evaluation. If the patient is interested in avoiding the possibility of a nonunion, surgery is recommended. If the patient is willing to wait and see if the fracture will unite without surgery, surgery can be initially avoided and considered only if the patient develops a symptomatic nonunion.

Multiple procedures have been described for the surgical management of displaced fractures of the distal end of the clavicle (Figure 5.19). Early on, transacromial wire fixation was the most commonly recommended procedure; however, wire migration around the shoulder region is known to be a potentially disastrous problem. Currently, when addressing these fractures surgically, 2 options are considered: resection of smaller fragments (combined with primary repair or reconstruction of the coracoclavicular ligaments) or internal fixation. The same strategies may be considered for management of established symptomatic nonunions, with addition of grafting procedures if needed.

Fragment resection combined with coracoclavicular ligament repair or reconstruction is attractive when fragment size, comminution, or osteopenia makes stable internal fixation unlikely to be achieved. However, it may result in substantial shortening of the clavicle, with some loss of the strut function. The details of repair or reconstruction of the coracoclavicular ligaments are discussed in the section on traumatic injuries of the acromioclavicular joint.

Internal fixation techniques are facilitated by use of precontoured, periarticular plates specifically designed for the lateral end of the clavicle. Modern plates are shaped to fit the clavicle; provide a number of clustered lateral holes for use of multiple, relatively small locking screws; and may occasionally provide the opportunity to augment fixation by anchoring on the coracoid using either high tensile sutures or a screw (Figure 5.20). Sutures may be placed around the coracoid or fixed with suture anchors or a button. Another alternative to improve fracture stability is to extend the fixation over the acromioclavicular joint and into the acromion, either using a hook plate or a traditional plate fixed to the acromion as well. A second operation for hardware removal is typically necessary when a screw is placed into the coracoid, as well as to remove hook plates or plates across the acromioclavicular joint. If the fragment is very small, it can be fixed with heavy nonabsorbable suture in a tension band configuration, typically combined with suture augmentation into or around the coracoid. Suture augmentation to the coracoid may be performed with arthroscopically assisted techniques (61). Multiple small studies have reported successful outcomes with all these techniques (58,62–64).

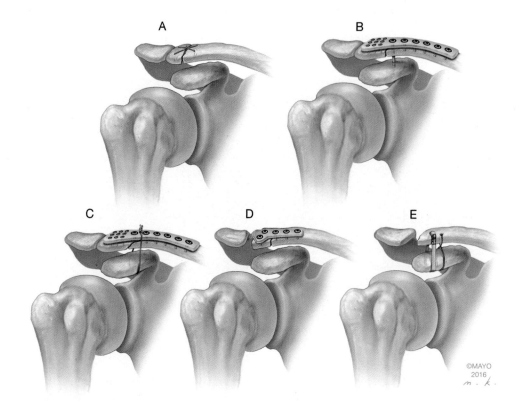

Figure 5.19 *Surgical management of displaced fractures of the distal end of the clavicle.* **A,** *Suture fixation.* **B,** *Plate fixation with screw into the coracoid.* **C,** *Plate fixation with suture around the coracoid.* **D,** *Hook plate.* **E,** *Fragment resection and primary coracoclavicular ligament repair or reconstruction.*

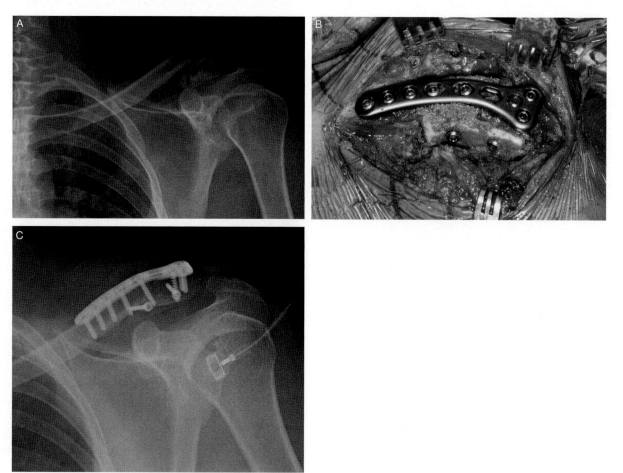

Figure 5.20 **A,** *Radiograph of left distal clavicle nonunion.* **B,** *Internal fixation with a dedicated lateral clavicle plate.* **C,** *Postoperative radiograph.*

Fractures of the Medial End of the Clavicle

Fractures of the medial end of the clavicle are rare, representing only 2% to 5% of all clavicle fractures (5,6). In children and adolescents, they occur through the physis and can be difficult to distinguish from sternoclavicular joint dislocations. In adults, they are almost always the result of high-energy injuries (motor vehicle accidents) and may be associated with chest injuries or a floating shoulder. They are classified as displaced or undisplaced with or without intra-articular extension (see Figure 5.5).

These fractures are oftentimes treated nonoperatively with temporary immobilization for comfort. Traditionally, surgery is reserved for fractures with posterior displacement and the potential to compromise mediastinal structures, as well as for open fractures. However, some studies on the nonoperative management of displaced fractures of the medial clavicle have reported persistent symptoms in approximately 50% of the patients (65). Internal fixation is performed with high-tensile suture fixation for physeal injuries and for smaller fractures in the adult; precontoured, periarticular locking plates are preferred for most fractures in adults. Reported union rates and functional results have been satisfactory (54). As with fractures of the lateral end of the clavicle, it is occasionally better to remove small fracture fragments and reconstruct the sternoclavicular ligaments (see "The Sternal Docking Technique").

Acromioclavicular Joint Conditions

Degenerative and Inflammatory Conditions

The acromioclavicular joint can become a source of pain and dysfunction secondary to joint degeneration, synovitis in chronic inflammatory diseases such as rheumatoid arthritis, and rarely septic arthritis. Acromioclavicular degenerative joint disease is very commonly seen on radiographs or MRI of patients being evaluated for either cuff disease or glenohumeral arthritis (Figure 5.21). The clinical evaluation and management of the acromioclavicular joint in patients being treated for rotator cuff problems is discussed in detail in chapter 6, The Rotator Cuff and Biceps Tendon. Most commonly, isolated pain-related acromioclavicular joint degeneration is due to primary osteoarthritis, typically in older patients. Traumatic injuries to the acromioclavicular joint and distal clavicle fractures with extension into the joint may also lead to posttraumatic joint degeneration.

Atraumatic distal clavicle osteolysis is another condition that may affect the acromioclavicular joint, typically in younger patients (Figure 5.22). In this condition a spontaneous stress fracture develops on the articular surface of the distal clavicle, resulting in various degrees of fragmentation. Patients with distal clavicle osteolysis are almost always heavy laborers or involved in sports that require weight training; the combination of throwing sports

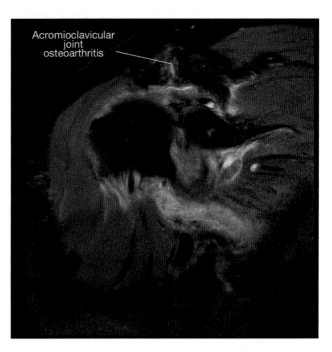

Figure 5.21 *Magnetic resonance imaging of a patient with primary osteoarthritis of the acromioclavicular joint.*

(e.g., volleyball, basketball, tennis, or even swimming) and supplemental weight training is not uncommon in adolescents with distal clavicle osteolysis.

Clinically, these patients develop tenderness over the acromioclavicular joint that can be reproduced with direct pressure, cross-body adduction, and all other maneuvers described in chapter 1, Evaluation of the Shoulder, for evaluation of this joint. Radiographs can be essentially negative or may show subchondral sclerosis and fragmentation on the articular surface of the clavicle; in advanced

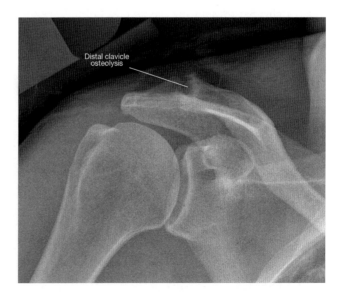

Figure 5.22 *Atraumatic distal clavicle osteolysis.*

cases, the acromioclavicular joint space may look widened. Magnetic resonance imaging shows increased signal changes in the distal clavicle and occasionally the acromion, with various degrees of articular cartilage damage, thickening of the capsule, and sometimes periosteal stress reactions (66,67).

The management of all these conditions is similar, except for septic arthritis. Due to the very high frequency of asymptomatic osteoarthritis of the acromioclavicular joint, it is important to confirm through history and physical examination that the acromioclavicular joint contributes to the patient's symptoms. If that is the case, some patients may respond to nonoperative treatment; surgery is considered for the rest.

Nonoperative management of acromioclavicular joint conditions includes activity modifications, nonsteroidal anti-inflammatory drugs, and the occasional use of intra-articular corticosteroid injections (see chapter 12, Rehabilitation and Injections). Overhead lifting and forceful pushing should be avoided. In patients with atraumatic distal clavicle osteolysis, the inciting activity should be temporarily discontinued. Patients not responding to conservative management are considered for surgical resection of the distal end of the clavicle; some surgeons associate resection of the acromial articular surface as well. This can be done through an open or arthroscopic approach.

Open Resection of the Distal End of the Clavicle
This is a relatively straightforward procedure that requires attention to a few details in order for it to be successful. The amount of clavicle resected needs to be just right: very small resections may not adequately alleviate symptoms, but large resections may lead to instability. Care must be taken to preserve the ligamentous and capsular attachments of the joint inferiorly, anteriorly, and posteriorly. Finally, the lateral end of the clavicle needs to be adequately covered by suturing the deltoid to the trapezius over the gap.

My preference is to perform the procedure through a superior 3-cm skin incision placed in the coronal plane over the distal clavicle (Figure 5.23). Subperiosteal exposure of the lateral end of the clavicle and division of the superior aspect of the capsule are followed by bone resection using a microsagittal saw. We typically remove less than 1 cm of bone. Care must be taken to avoid piercing the inferior capsule with the saw blade, and to create an even resection from anterior to posterior. Prominent osteophytes from the acromial side of the joint may be removed as well, and some surgeons favor removing a thin sliver of bone off the acromion. Once the resection has been completed, I imbricate securely the deltoid and the trapezius over the area so that the distal end of the clavicle does not end being subcutaneous, as the defect may be otherwise quite visible and sometimes bothersome. After surgery, patients are recommended use of a sling for comfort and resume activities of daily living with no restrictions within 2 weeks.

Arthroscopic Resection of the Distal End of the Clavicle
The distal end of the clavicle can also be resected arthroscopically. Some surgeons prefer to visualize with the arthroscopic camera in a standard posterior subacromial position (indirect approach), whereas others prefer insertion of the camera directly into the joint (direct approach), either from the beginning or in the later portions of the procedure. An arthroscopic bur is used to remove bone from the distal clavicle; some surgeons also remove bone from the acromial side of the joint. The most common error in performing this procedure is incomplete removal of bone, especially posteriorly. Benefits of arthroscopic distal clavicle resection include better preservation of the capsule and ligaments of the joint, more cosmetic incisions, and the potential of treating other associated pathology arthroscopically. However, for patients needing just a resection of the distal end of the clavicle, open resection is faster, cheaper, and easier. Selection of one or the

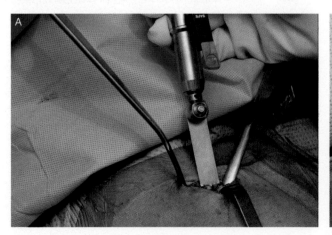
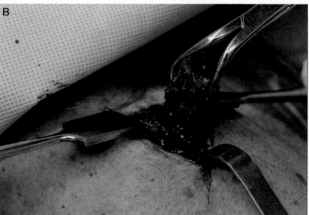

Figure 5.23 Mini open distal clavicle resection. **A,** *Resection using a microsagittal saw.* **B,** *Resected distal clavicle end.*

other should be solely based on surgeon and patient preferences, since both approaches seem to be equally effective. The postoperative management is similar as well.

Traumatic Injuries

Injury to the ligaments stabilizing the distal clavicle and scapula (acromion and coracoid) results in sprains and various degrees of separation or dislocation of the acromioclavicular joint. The indications for surgical management of the more severe grades of injury continue to be debated, and the techniques for reconstruction have continued to evolve over time.

Classification

Most surgeons use the classification system proposed by Rockwood and Williams (Table 5.10; Figure 5.24) (68). In types I and II, the coracoclavicular ligaments are intact or at the most sprained, deformity is absent or minimal, the stability of the suspensory complex of the shoulder is not completely disrupted, and most heal uneventfully without treatment. In types III and V, disruption of the coracoclavicular ligaments (and the trapezius and deltoid in type V) creates the classic deformity seen in acromioclavicular joint separations, with an abnormally low position of the acromion and rest of the shoulder region compared with the lateral end of the clavicle. Types IV (posterior, with the clavicle piercing the trapezius) and VI (inferior) are very uncommon.

Evaluation

Acromioclavicular joint injuries are the result of an inferiorly directed force on the superior aspect of the shoulder.

They most commonly occur in falls, particularly biking accidents. The rare type VI injury is typically the result of a much more severe injury, such as a car accident. In acute injuries, bruising or skin erosions may be seen over the acromial region.

In type I, there is no deformity, only pain at the acromioclavicular joint, and radiographs are completely negative. In type II, there may be no or mild deformity, the clavicle and acromion cannot be displaced in the vertical plane, but the fingers of the examiner can displace the clavicle some in the horizontal plane anteriorly and posteriorly; radiographs may be normal or may show widening of the joint line and at the most less than 25% of vertical displacement (widening of the space between the coracoid and clavicle).

Types III and V have similar findings: there is obvious deformity where the clavicle seems to be sticking up under the skin, although in reality the deformity is created by inferior displacement of the scapula and rest of the arm (Figure 5.25). In type III, the deformity can be fully reduced by supporting the arm of the patient by the elbow and pushing the arm up, whereas in type V the distal clavicle is felt literally under the skin, and the deformity cannot be fully corrected passively. Radiographically, both injuries show vertical separation of the joint; the space between the coracoid and the clavicle is increased up to double in type III and more than double in type V.

In type IV injuries, the clavicle is quite posterior compared with the acromion, and this is best appreciated by looking at the patient from a superior view (Figure 5.26). The posterior displacement is also best appreciated in the axillary radiograph. In type VI the acromion is actually

---

Table 5.10 • Classification of Acromioclavicular Joint Injuries

Type	AC Joint	AC Ligaments	CC Ligaments	Deltoid and Trapezius	Radiographic Findings	Treatment
I	Intact	Sprained	Intact	Intact	Normal	Conservative
II	Mild displacement	Torn	Intact or sprained	Intact	Mild displacement	Conservative
III				Intact	Marked displacement (CC spaced increased 25%–100%)	Conservative vs surgical— controversial
IV	Marked vertical displacement			Torn	The clavicle is displaced posteriorly (axillary view)	Surgical
V			Torn (maybe intact in VI subacromial)	Torn	Severe displacement (CC spaced increased over 100%)	Surgical
VI	Clavicle under the acromion or coracoid			Torn	Clavicle under the acromion or coracoid	Surgical

Abbreviations: AC, acromioclavicular; CC, coracoclavicular.

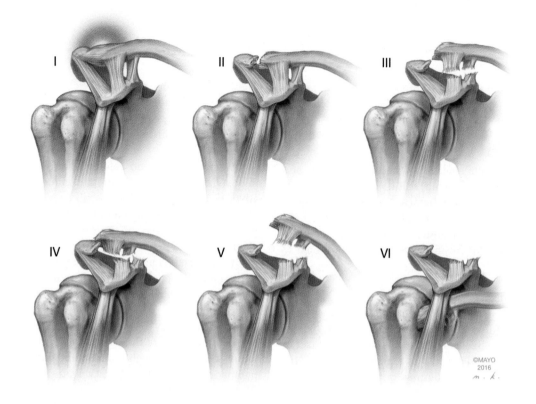

Figure 5.24 *Rockwood and Williams classification of acromioclavicular joint dislocations.*

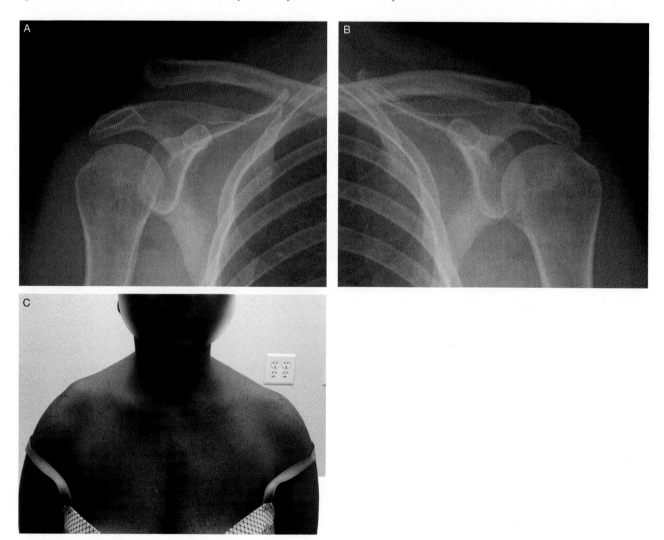

Figure 5.25 *Type III acromioclavicular joint injury.* **A,** *Injured side.* **B,** *Normal side.* **C,** *Clinical aspect.*

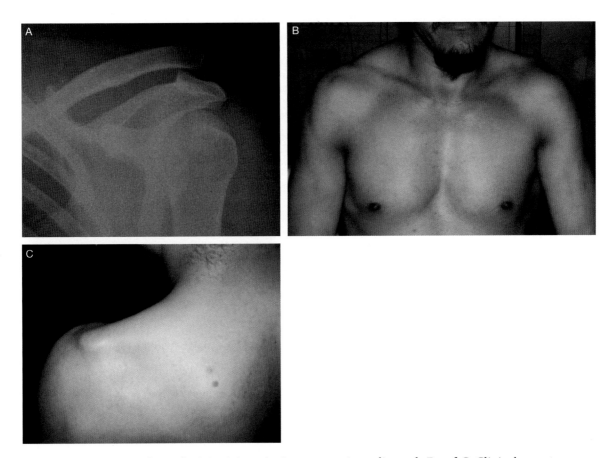

Figure 5.26 *Type IV acromioclavicular joint injury.* **A,** *Anteroposterior radiograph.* **B and C,** *Clinical aspect.*

higher than the clavicle, and there commonly are other severe associated injuries.

Substantial agreement has been proven when classifying acromioclavicular joint injuries based on radiographs only (69). A panoramic anteroposterior radiograph that includes both clavicles and both acromioclavicular joint is useful to detect subtle changes in type II. Axillary radiographs are particularly useful in type IV. In the past, anteroposterior views of both shoulders were obtained with weights suspended from the wrists, but these stress-weighted views have fallen out of favor (70). CT is only useful to evaluate associated injuries to the coracoid and other structures.

When to Consider Surgery

Most orthopedic surgeons agree on treating type I and II injuries conservatively and treating types IV, V and VI surgically. However, controversy persists about conservative versus surgical treatment of the very common type III injury (71–74).

Nonoperative management consists of use of a sling for comfort for a few days in type I and up to 2–3 weeks in a type II. Ice and nonsteroidal anti-inflammatory drugs can be added initially. Most patients recover back to normal, and the occasional patient with persistent discomfort a few months after sustaining a type II injury can be offered an

intra-articular injection with corticosteroids. If conservative treatment is selected for a patient with a type III, rehabilitation needs to be more involved: prevention of contracture and shortening of the pectoralis minor, and to less extent the pectoralis major, is important, and a program of periscapular stabilization needs to be instituted early on.

Regarding surgical treatment for types IV, V, VI, and those patients with a type III in whom surgery is considered indicated, the principles of surgery involve reducing the dislocation and re-establishing the ligamentous stability of the suspensory complex. However, as detailed later, there are some controversies regarding the ideal technique to achieve these goals.

So why do surgeons still not know how to best treat type III injuries? Because most studies that have compared the outcome of nonoperative versus surgical treatment for type III acromioclavicular joint injuries have found no differences (75). However, a fair number of patients treated nonoperatively do return to the orthopedic surgeon because they do want their injury fixed. In a recent study 30% of all patients treated conservatively eventually requested surgical reconstruction (71). Unfortunately, no study has identified great predictive factors to understand who will not do well without surgery. Anecdotally, we have observed some risk factors

---

Table 5.11 • Possible Risk Factors for Eventual Surgery in Type III Acromioclavicular Injuries

Functional scapular dyskinesis at presentation

Evidence of associated pathology
Labral tears
Cuff tears
Other

Use of upper extremity to bear load (e.g., bicycle—motorcycle riders)

Use of upper extremity overhead for prolonged periods of time (e.g., painters)

Thin patients with a very obvious cosmetic deformity

---

that seem to lead patients with grade III injuries to end up having surgery (Table 5.11).

Advocates of treating all type III injuries conservatively in the acute phase argue that the complexity and outcome of surgery in the acute and chronic phase are identical, and furthermore subjective satisfaction may be higher with surgery in the chronic phase, since the patient will compare how things are after surgery with a chronically dislocated state versus a normal state. Advocates of treating some type III injuries surgically in the acute phase argue that the torn coracoclavicular ligaments are given an opportunity to heal, and patients are not wasting time waiting to see if they will be able to cope or not with the functional status of their shoulder with conservative treatment. However, surgery is more expensive, seems to be associated with longer medical leave of absence, and carries the risk of surgical complications (75).

So how do I deal with it in my practice? As mentioned in chapter 6, The Rotator Cuff and Biceps Tendon, when dealing with chronic cuff tears, there is a difference between recommending and offering surgery. The type III acromioclavicular joint dislocation is one example of pathology when I believe the patient needs to be informed of the pluses and minuses of one option versus the other. Surgery can be offered to any patient interested but it cannot be strongly recommended, since more than two thirds of patients will choose to never have surgery, and if they do, the outcome in the chronic phase seems to be similar. Patients interested in surgery only for cosmetic reasons need to know that they will trade their current deformity for a scar in a visible area and that surgery does not always restore the aspect of the joint back to normal, even when successful otherwise. Surgery is definitely offered, although not strongly recommended, to patients with any of the features summarized in Table 5.11.

Surgical Techniques for Acromioclavicular Joint Reconstruction

Once the decision to operate is made in a patient with a grade III–VI injury, a number of additional questions

---

Table 5.12 • Techniques for the Surgical Treatment of Acromioclavicular Joint Injuries

Repair
Direct suture coracoclavicular ligaments ± temporary fixation clavicle to acromion and/or clavicle to coracoid
Hook plate (temporary)

Reconstruction
Transfer of the coracoid tip to the clavicle (largely abandoned)
Transfer of the acromial end of the coracoacromial ligament to the acromion (Weaver-Dunn procedure)
Clavicle to coracoid fixation with synthetic material (i.e., TightRope, Lockdown)
Tendon graft reconstruction of the coracoclavicular ligaments
  Autograft vs allograft
  ± Acromioclavicular stabilization as well
Temporary protection of the reconstruction
Nonabsorbable sutures (around the coracoid, anchor, button)
Screw fixation from clavicle to coracoid

---

arise (Table 5.12): In the acute setting, do the coracoclavicular ligaments heal if sutured or approximated with a hook plate? What is the ideal method to restore the function of the coracoclavicular ligaments? Does the reconstruction need to be augmented temporarily? Is it necessary to resect a little bit of the distal clavicle? How important is it to reconstruct the acromioclavicular ligaments for additional horizontal stability? Is it best to perform these procedures with open or arthroscopic techniques?

Probably, primary repair works only in acute injuries. In the past, direct suture of the coracoclavicular ligaments was combined with wire fixation across the acromioclavicular joint, but this has largely been abandoned due to concerns with wire migration and poor stability. Primary healing is also the goal of temporary neutralization of the acromioclavicular joint with a hook plate; however, this implant requires routine removal after the first 3 months, and a number of complications, mostly related to acromion bone loss or even fracture, have been reported. Consequently, the popularity of this device has decreased recently.

The most commonly performed classic reconstruction involves detaching the coracoacromial ligament from the acromion and transferring it to the end of the clavicle (Weaver-Dunn procedure, Figure 5.27A). Concerns with the variability of this ligament transfer in terms of length and quality, combined with interest in reconstructing also the horizontal stability of the acromioclavicular joint has led to the development of reconstructive techniques using tendon graft (76). In addition, there is interest in solely using synthetic materials to re-establish the stability of the suspensory complex (77–79). It is important to realize that even though most patients seem to do well clinically with surgical reconstruction, complications can happen, the most devastating

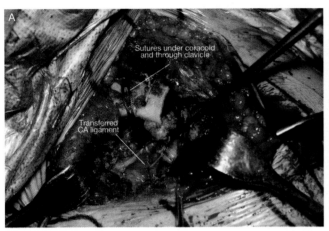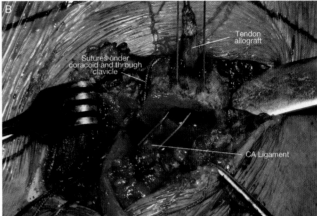

Figure 5.27 A, *Classic Weaver-Dunn reconstruction.* **B,** *Reconstruction using coracoacromial (CA) ligament transfer combined with allograft tendon reconstruction of the coracoclavicular and acromioclavicular ligaments, unloading the reconstruction with heavy, nonabsorbable suture.*

being fractures of the clavicle or coracoid through fixation sites. A wide range of loss of reduction has been reported with various techniques, ranging from 5% to 80% (80).

My preference is to combine transfer of the coracoacromial ligament to the distal clavicle with allograft reconstruction of the coracoclavicular and acromioclavicular ligaments, unloading the reconstruction with heavy nonabsorbable suture though the clavicle and under the coracoid (Figure 5.27B; ⊙ Video 5.1). This technique relies partly on autograft (the transferred ligament) and partly on allograft, is relatively inexpensive (no anchoring devices such as screws, buttons, or anchors are used), and does not require a second operation to remove temporary coracoclavicular fixation.

After surgery, it is extremely important to prevent stretching of the reconstruction by keeping the arm supported for approximately 6 weeks. Scapular isometrics may be initiated as soon as pain subsides. Stiffness is uncommon after this procedure, so once patients come out of their immobilizer, therapy continues to be centered in scapular stabilizing exercises.

Sternoclavicular Joint Conditions

The sternoclavicular joint may become symptomatic secondary to traumatic injuries, degenerative or inflammatory arthritis, as well as infectious arthritis and osteomyelitis. Surgery on the sternoclavicular joint is always somewhat intimidating secondary to the very close proximity of neurovascular and other mediastinal structures (81). In general, patients presenting with symptoms related to the sternoclavicular joint fall into one of three categories (Table 5.13): traumatic injuries, atraumatic instability secondary to excessive laxity, and

Table 5.13 • Sternoclavicular Joint Conditions

Traumatic
Anterior or posterior dislocation
Physeal fracture of the medial clavicle
Fracture of the medial clavicle with intra-articular extension

Atraumatic instability
Collagen disorders (e.g., Ehlers-Danlos, Marfan syndrome)
Idiopathic dynamic instability

Degenerative and inflammatory conditions
Primary osteoarthritis
Inflammatory arthritis (i.e., rheumatoid arthritis)
Septic arthritis and osteomyelitis
Malignancy/metastasis
Sternoclavicular hyperostosis syndrome

degenerative or inflammatory conditions. Fractures of the medial end of the clavicle and physeal injuries were described earlier.

Sternoclavicular Joint Instability

Evaluation
Instability of the sternoclavicular joint can be secondary to trauma or develop spontaneously in patients with collagen disorders or idiopathic hyperlaxity. It is classified as anterior or posterior, depending on the position of the clavicle relative to the sternum.

Traumatic Instability
Dislocation of the sternoclavicular joint requires substantial energy. Most posterior dislocations are the result of blunt trauma to the central aspect of the chest wall, although they may also be the result of lateral compression of the shoulder with the arm flexed. Anterior dislocations

are most commonly the result of a fall on the outstretched hand or the side of the shoulder, resulting in medial compression and extension of the clavicle.

The clinical presentation of posterior dislocations may be subtle or more dramatic. Patients report pain centered over the sternoclavicular joint region, but associated injuries may demand more attention, and the posterior sternoclavicular joint dislocation may be missed. Typically, patients hold the upper extremity with the scapula protracted, and the shoulder girdle may look shortened or asymmetrical. Close inspection reveals the lack of fullness normally present at the medial aspect of the clavicle. Occasionally, patients may complain of dysphagia, stridor, cough, a feeling of choking, shortness of breath, venous congestion of the face or upper extremity, or distal peripheral nerve abnormalities; these signs and symptoms are consistent with compression of the esophagus, trachea, subclavian vein, or brachial plexus. Compression of these mediastinal structures has been estimated to occur in approximately 30% of these injuries (82). Although shortness of breath may be secondary to airway compression by the dislocated clavicle only, a chest radiograph should be obtained to exclude an associated pneumothorax or other chest injuries.

Anterior dislocations present as abnormal anterior prominence of the medial end of the clavicle compared with the sternum and the opposite side (Figure 5.28A). The medial clavicle may be in the dislocated position all the time, or patients may experience dynamic dislocation, where the clavicle is reduced with the arm in the resting position, but dislocates with every episode of active elevation. When evaluated right after their injury, these patients typically complain of pain over the dislocated joint, whereas in chronic dislocations pain may be minimal. Anterior dislocations can mimic fractures of the medial end of the clavicle, where the lateral fragment typically protrudes medially and anterior close to the skin and can be felt as more irregular.

Dislocations of the sternoclavicular joint may be difficult to visualize with standard radiographs of the shoulder and clavicle, but these should be obtained anyway to rule out associated injuries. Better visualization of the sternoclavicular joints may be obtained with the radiography beam centered over the sternoclavicular area and angled 40° from superior to inferior (this projection has been termed by some the *serendipity view*) (82). In a posterior dislocation, the medial clavicle would appear inferior, whereas in an anterior dislocation it would appear superior (4). The *Heinig view* (patient supine and radiography beam perpendicular to the joint line, ie oblique to the patient) can also be useful.

CT with 3-dimensional reconstruction is extremely useful in the evaluation of these patients (Figure 5.28B). It will demonstrate the presence and direction of instability, as well as any bone fragments that may be present after fracture-dislocations or physeal injuries. In patients with a longstanding chronic posterior dislocation, vascular studies should be obtained. Computed angiotomography allows assessment of both the articular/bony injuries and the location and proximity of adjacent blood vessels. Not uncommonly, the wall of the subclavian vessels is scarred to the dislocated clavicle, and thus at risk when surgery is performed. Magnetic resonance with or without intravascular contrast can also be considered, especially when compression of the esophagus or airway is suspected.

Atraumatic Instability
Patients with abnormal collagen disorders (e.g., Ehlers-Danlos) or excessive laxity may develop instability of the sternoclavicular joint without major trauma, although some report a minor injury (4). Patients with atraumatic instability should be assessed for abnormal collagen disorders if they have not been fully evaluated (see Table 7.12 for Beighton criteria).

Most commonly, the pattern of instability is dynamic anterior: in certain positions of the shoulder (typically extension in various degrees of elevation), the clavicle

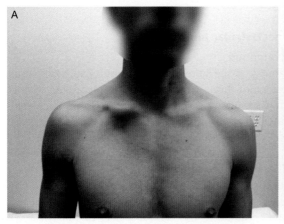
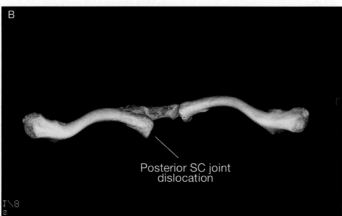

Posterior SC joint dislocation

Figure 5.28 A, *Clinical aspect of a patient with an anterior sternoclavicular (SC) joint dislocation.* **B,** *Computed tomography of a patient with a posterior SC joint dislocation.*

subluxes or dislocates anteriorly, but in the resting position no subluxation or dislocation is appreciated. Some patients may have global instability (the clavicle displaces excessively both anteriorly and posteriorly), and the instability may also be bilateral in some. The instability may also be static (the joint is dislocated all the time). Some individuals are bothered by the sense of instability but do not complain of pain, whereas others develop pain over time. Scapular dyskinesia is common in patients with hyperlaxity, partly due to loss of the strut function of the clavicle and partly due to associated dysfunction of the periscapular musculature. Multidirectional atraumatic glenohumeral instability may also be present in some patients.

As mentioned before, assessment of the sternoclavicular joint on plain radiographs is not easy. CT is oftentimes necessary to confirm the diagnosis. However, in patients with dynamic instability, CT does not always show the joint in the dislocated position, or it may show subtle subluxation.

Management

Instability of the sternoclavicular joint is managed differently depending on the direction, timing, and symptoms. Figure 5.29 summarizes the management of these injuries.

Acute Posterior Dislocation

Reduction of posterior dislocations is the treatment of choice, especially in patients with evidence of compression of mediastinal structures. Closed reduction under general anesthesia is attempted first, and if unsuccessful it should be followed by open reduction. It is wise to have a thoracic or vascular surgeon available in case injury to the mediastinal structures occurs during reduction.

For closed reduction of a posterior dislocation, the patient is placed supine with a pad between the scapulae to retract the shoulders. The surgeon applies longitudinal traction to the limb with the shoulder in abduction, and the shoulder is slowly brought into extension. If reduction does not happen, a towel clip can be used to grab the medial end of the clavicle percutaneously and translate the medial end of the clavicle anteriorly into the reduced position. Most of the time, the sternoclavicular joint is stable after closed reduction of an acute posterior dislocation. Patients are recommended immobilization of the shoulder for 6 weeks to allow for ligament healing. Figure-of-8 immobilization may be considered to maintain the scapulae retracted. Contact sports can be initiated in 3 to 4 months.

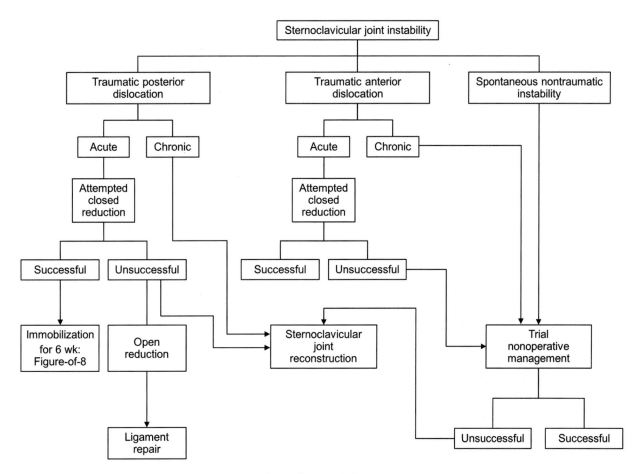

Figure 5.29 *Algorithm for management of sternoclavicular instability.*

If closed reduction cannot be performed, or the reduction is lost and the clavicle dislocates posteriorly as soon as the arm is placed in the neutral position, open reduction can be performed through an anterior approach. Care must be taken to identify and address interposed soft tissues, and to very gently lever the clavicle anteriorly, with close attention paid to the possibility of abrupt bleeding that might indicate a vascular injury requiring repair. Direct repair of the ligaments may be enough to maintain stability after a successful open reduction. Some authors have reported internal fixation using a plate and screws over the superior aspect across the sternoclavicular joint (83). Alternatively, any of the reconstructive techniques described later for chronic instability may be utilized.

Acute Anterior Instability

Traumatic anterior sternoclavicular joint dislocations have a high rate of recurrent instability after closed reduction. Some surgeons do offer the patient the option of a closed reduction, where others prefer to treat the patient symptomatically and offer surgery in the chronic phase only to those patients unable to cope with their permanent anterior dislocation.

Closed reduction is again best performed under general anesthesia to avoid painful manipulation and muscle

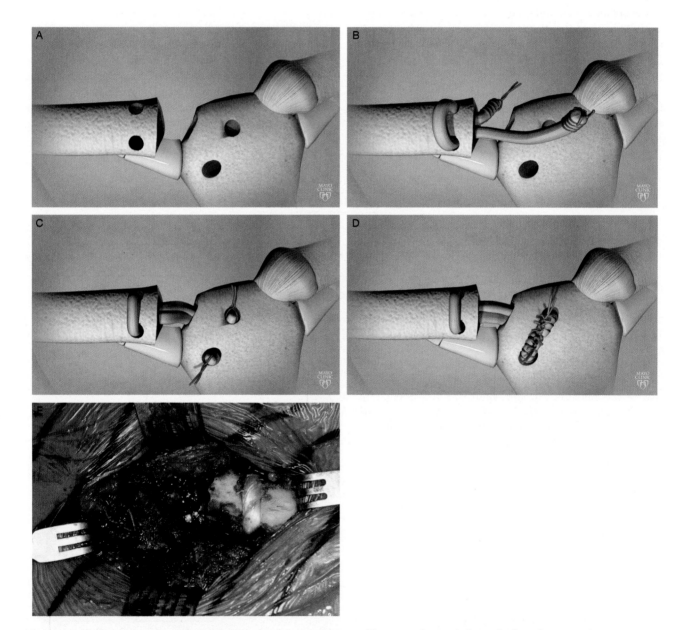

Figure 5.30 *The sternal docking technique, step by step.* **A,** *Tunnel location.* **B,** *Graft through clavicle.* **C,** *Graft into sternum. Final reconstruction shown in illustration (***D***) and operative photo (***E***).*

spasms that may make the reduction more difficult. The patient is also positioned supine with a pad between the scapulae. Longitudinal traction of the limb and shoulder flexion are combined with direct posterior pressure on the dislocated medial end of the clavicle. If the reduction is successful, patients are immobilized in a sling for 6 weeks and counseled to avoid scapular retraction and shoulder extension.

Unfortunately, some authors have estimated than more than 50% of patients undergoing closed reduction of an anterior dislocation experience recurrent instability soon after the reduction, sometimes even while the patient is still under anesthesia (4,82). Although open reduction can be considered in these circumstances, most surgeons favor treating the patient's symptoms. As mentioned before, surgery would be considered only for those patients unable to adjust to their new situation due to pain or poor function.

Chronic Instability

Closed reduction is not recommended for patients with chronic posttraumatic instability, since the rate of success is very low and it could actually be dangerous in patients with posterior dislocations. In general, surgery is recommended for patients with a chronic posterior dislocation, especially if they have symptoms, but even in the absence of symptoms to avoid erosion into mediastinal structures (Figure 5.30). In contrast, surgery for chronic posttraumatic anterior instability and for patients with atraumatic spontaneous instability is considered only if symptoms are bothersome enough after a failed trial of nonoperative treatment.

Most patients come to the orthopedic surgeon to explore the possibility of surgical correction because they are bothered by their subjective feeling of instability. Some patients also complain of pain over the sternoclavicular joint area or the periscapular region. Occasionally, patients will also describe 1 or more symptoms indicative of mediastinal compression (hoarseness, shortness of breath, difficulty swallowing, choking sensation, and so on). Nonoperative treatment for patients with chronic anterior or atraumatic instability concentrates on pain management modalities and scapular stabilizing exercises. When nonoperative treatment fails, surgery is considered.

Surgical Procedures for Reconstruction of the Sternoclavicular Joint

Multiple procedures have been described for surgical reconstruction of the sternoclavicular joint (Table 5.14, 🔘 Video 5.2). Temporary internal fixation with wires or pins has been abandoned due to risks associated with hardware migration in this particular location. Several small series have reported good outcomes with most other techniques. One biomechanical study suggested that reconstruction with a tendon graft results in a stronger construct (1). For these reasons, this technique has been more widely

Table 5.14 • Surgical Techniques for Reconstruction of the Sternoclavicular Joint

Imbrication of the anterior ligaments and capsule

Intramedullary ligament reconstruction

Reconstruction with a local musculotendinous structure
Subclavius
Sternocleidomastoid

Allograft tendon reconstruction
Figure-of-8
Docking technique

Synthetic materials
Artificial ligament
Enveloping mesh

Temporary internal fixation
Kirschner wires or Steinmann pins
Screws
Plate fixation

adopted lately. However, there are no comparative studies to understand the superiority of one technique over the rest. As mentioned before, it is wise to have a thoracic or vascular surgeon available in case complications arise.

Over the past decade, most surgeons have favored routing the tendon graft in a figure-of-8 fashion (Figure 5.31A). I have used this technique in my practice in the past. Although effective in restoring stability, we noted that at the end of the procedure, as the graft is tied in the front, it displaces the clavicle anteriorly; in addition, passing the graft behind the clavicle and the sternum can be difficult and potentially dangerous, and the bulk of the graft knot

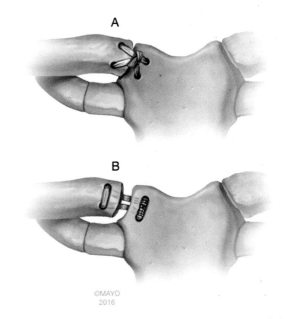

Figure 5.31 **A,** *Figure-of-8 reconstruction.* **B,** *Sternal docking technique.*

can be felt by patients once the surgical swelling subsides. In order to benefit from the biomechanical properties of tendon graft reconstruction, but improve some of the features of the figure-of-8 technique, I developed the sternal docking technique (Figure 5.31B), which has become my procedure of choice for most patients.

The Sternal Docking Technique

The sternal docking technique (⊙ Video 5.2) involves the graft entering the medial clavicle, exiting inferiorly through a cortical perforation, and re-entering the canal superiorly through a second cortical perforation. The 2 ends of the graft are then introduced into the sternal facet of the joint and retrieved through perforations on the anterior cortex of the sternum. This graft configuration facilitates graft passage and keeps the graft centralized without any anterior translation or prominence (see Figure 5.30).

Surgery is performed under general anesthesia with the patient supine and the head of the table raised approximately 30° from horizontal. The affected upper extremity is draped free, and both sternoclavicular joints are included in the surgical field. Exposure is performed through an anterior skin incision centered across the inferior aspect of the affected sternoclavicular joint.

Once the joint is exposed, the intra-articular disk is resected and the medial 5- to 10-mm portion of the clavicle is also resected with a microsagittal saw. In cases of posterior instability, the joint may need to be reduced before bone resection can be safely performed. The goal is to remove just enough bone to enter the medullary canal, but in some patients removal of more bone is needed in order to eliminate osteophytes or allow reduction. Sequels of physeal injuries or intra-articular fracture-dislocations require separate removal of the fractured fragments. Care is taken to remove all these fragments subperiosteally without undue traction, in order to prevent injury to the structures posterior to the joint.

Two holes are then created on the anteroinferior and anterosuperior aspects of the medial clavicle exiting into the medullary canal using a high-speed 4.0-mm bur. A curette may be used to remove cancellous bone between the canal and the clavicle perforations. Using the same bur, an oblong hole is created on the sternal facet of the sternoclavicular joint; 2 additional holes are created on the anterior cortex of the sternum superiorly and inferiorly, and a curette is used to communicate these 2 holes with the 1 oblong hole created on the sternal articular facet.

I favor use of a semitendinous allograft. The allograft can be split in half for smaller patients, whereas the whole diameter of the graft is used in larger patients. The length of the graft may be measured with a suture passed along the planned graft trajectory, or it can be determined in situ after the graft has been placed. A heavy, nonabsorbable suture is placed in a running locking configuration on each end of the graft.

The graft is then passed in a sternal docking fashion. One end of the graft enters the medullary canal of the clavicle, exits through the inferior hole and re-enters through the superior hole. This leaves 2 ends of the graft exiting the clavicle medullary canal. Both ends are then fed into the oblong hole at the sternal facet of the joint, and separately retrieved though the anterosuperior and anteroinferior holes in the anterior cortex of the clavicle. Traction applied to both ends of the graft keeps the clavicle stable and centralized on the sternum. The sutures placed on the ends of the graft are tied together, and the reconstruction is reinforced further if needed with multiple interrupted sutures connecting the 2 limbs of the graft. The remainder of the closure is routine.

After surgery, patients are placed in a shoulder immobilizer for 6 weeks. Active range of motion exercises of the elbow, wrist, and hand are encouraged, but shoulder motion is discouraged. At 6 weeks, the shoulder immobilizer is discontinued, and patients are started on a program of active assisted range of motion exercises with stretching. Strengthening of the deltoid, rotator cuff, and periscapular muscles is started at week 8 to 10, and strengthening with elastic bands is started at week 10 to 12. Patients are allowed unrestricted use of the affected shoulder 6 months after surgery.

Outcome of Surgical Reconstruction of the Sternoclavicular Joint

As mentioned before, since surgical reconstruction for sternoclavicular joint instability is relatively uncommon, most studies have included a small number of patients. Bak and Fogh (84) reported 32 reconstructions using autograft tendon; mean Western Ontario Shoulder Instability scores statistically improved from 44% to 75%, and there were only 2 failures (7.4%), although persistent discomfort was reported by 40% of the patients and almost 70% complained of donor site morbidity. Sabatini et al. (85) reported 10 reconstructions using allograft in a figure-of-8 fashion; pain improved from a Visual Analog Score (VAS) of 7 preoperatively to 1.15 postoperatively, with improvement in American Shoulder and Elbow Surgeons scores as well. Other authors have reported similar results (85–88).

I recently reviewed my outcomes using the sternal docking technique in 19 consecutive reconstructions. The indications for surgery included instability (16—anterior in 13, posterior in 3) or medial clavicle resection for osteoarthritis (3). During the follow-up period, 2 reconstructions (10.5%) underwent revision surgery for recurrent instability, 1 additional patient had occasional subjective instability, and the remaining 16 reconstructions (84%) were considered stable. Sternoclavicular joint reconstruction was associated with improved pain and restoration of normal motion. The cosmetic appearance of the shoulder as it relates to the position of the medial end of the clavicle compared with the opposite side was satisfactory in 16 reconstructions (84%), with a median of 10 points on the VAS for overall satisfaction.

Degenerative and Inflammatory Arthritis of the Sternoclavicular Joint

Evaluation

The sternoclavicular joint may be affected by osteoarthritis, inflammatory arthritis, or infection. Some patients with osteoarthritis may recall a previous injury to the sternoclavicular joint, but most report no history of trauma. Pain and swelling are the most common complaints for patients with degenerative or inflammatory arthritis; patients with infection may also present warmth and erythema.

Physical examination shows prominence of the sternoclavicular joint secondary to inflammation and bone changes. Pain is reproduced with palpation over the sternoclavicular joint, shoulder motion, and cross-body adduction. Plain radiographs and CT are the imaging modalities of choice. Magnetic resonance is particularly useful when infection is suspected (89,90); the joint may be aspirated as well, and *Staphylococcus* spp is most commonly isolated. Patients with inflammatory arthritis should be managed in conjunction with a rheumatologist. Patients with septic arthritis should be assessed for immunosuppressive conditions, particularly human immunodeficiency virus infection.

The sternocostoclavicular hyperostosis syndrome was first described in middle-aged Japanese men. It is characterized by ossification of the manubrium, sternum, clavicles, upper ribs, and periarticular ligaments. In 60% of patients, palmoplantar pustulosis occurs and many consider the condition to be related to diffuse idiopathic skeletal hyperostosis and ankylosing spondylitis (4). Diagnosis is mainly by exclusion. Laboratory tests exclude metabolic bone disease; histologic studies reveal chronic inflammation and microbiologic studies should be negative, although *Propionibacterium acnes* has been isolated in a few patients.

Management

Most patients with symptomatic osteoarthritis or inflammatory arthritis of the sternoclavicular joint are initially treated symptomatically (4,82). Optimization of medical management needs to be assessed in patients with inflammatory conditions. Intra-articular injections with corticosteroids may be considered, and they are best performed under ultrasonographic guidance (91). Patients with confirmed septic arthritis may be started on a course of intravenous antibiotics. The natural history of sternocostoclavicular hyperostosis syndrome is uncertain, and treatment is mainly symptomatic, but oral antibiotics seem to reduce pain and pustulosis, and a short course should be used during a flare-up.

Surgical management is considered for patients with septic arthritis as well as those with degenerative and inflammatory conditions not responding to nonoperative treatment modalities. Joint débridement with removal of the intra-articular disk and any bone prominences is the treatment of choice. This procedure can be performed through open or arthroscopic techniques (82,92,93). As mentioned in the section on instability, care must be taken during open or arthroscopic procedures on the sternoclavicular joint to avoid iatrogenic damage to vital mediastinal structures. If the débridement procedure allows preservation of major ligamentous stabilizing structures, no additional reconstruction is required. Otherwise, tendon graft reconstruction of the sternoclavicular joint using the techniques mentioned earlier should be associated to resection of the medial end of the clavicle to avoid symptomatic instability, with the exception of patients with an active infection.

KEY POINTS

✓ The clavicle and its connections with the sternum and scapula function as a suspensory stabilizing strut connecting the whole upper extremity to the trunk.

✓ Fractures of the clavicle are extremely common and associated with a relatively high union rate. However, older age, fracture displacement, fracture comminution, and certain comorbidities (e.g., smoking) increase the risk of symptomatic nonunion or malunion.

✓ Evaluation of displacement is best performed in radiographs obtained with the patient in the upright position, since radiographs obtained supine underestimate displacement.

✓ Indications for surgical management of midshaft clavicle fractures include severe displacement, need to operate for other reasons, and scapulothoracic dissociation. Relative indications include need to return to activities very quickly, scapular dyskinesia, or a DASH score under 60 at 6 weeks.

✓ Plate fixation and intramedullary nailing may be considered for internal fixation of clavicle fractures. Plate fixation is more commonly utilized. Precontoured plates facilitate the procedure, and they can be placed superiorly or anteroinferiorly.

✓ Displaced fractures of the lateral end of the clavicle oftentimes lead to lack of radiographic union, although well tolerated by many. Internal fixation with plates or sutures in the acute phase seems to be quite reliable.

✓ Degenerative arthritis of the acromioclavicular joint is very common and not always symptomatic. Open or arthroscopic distal clavicle resection is extremely effective when patients need surgery.

✓ Injuries of the acromioclavicular joint are classified in 6 types. Nonoperative treatment is of choice for types I and II, whereas surgery is recommended for types IV–VI. The treatment of type III is controversial.

✓ Surgical reconstruction of the acromioclavicular joint is commonly performed with tendon graft reconstruction.

✓ Posterior sternoclavicular joint dislocations should be treated acutely with close or open reduction with a vascular or thoracic surgeon on standby. The risk of injury to vital mediastinal structures is real.

✓ Anterior sternoclavicular joint instability is tolerated well by many and may be the consequence of trauma or collagen abnormalities. Patients not responding to nonoperative treatment may be considered for reconstruction using a tendon graft.

✓ The sternoclavicular joint can also be affected by primary osteoarthritis, inflammatory conditions, septic arthritis, or idiopathic hyperostosis.

REFERENCES

1. Spencer EE Jr, Kuhn JE. Biomechanical analysis of reconstructions for sternoclavicular joint instability. J Bone Joint Surg Am. 2004 Jan;86-A(1):98–105.
2. Renfree KJ, Wright TW. Anatomy and biomechanics of the acromioclavicular and sternoclavicular joints. Clin Sports Med. 2003 Apr;22(2):219–37.
3. Lee JT, Campbell KJ, Michalski MP, Wilson KJ, Spiegl UJ, Wijdicks CA, et al. Surgical anatomy of the sternoclavicular joint: a qualitative and quantitative anatomical study. J Bone Joint Surg Am. 2014 Oct 1;96(19):e166.
4. Sewell MD, Al-Hadithy N, Le Leu A, Lambert SM. Instability of the sternoclavicular joint: current concepts in classification, treatment and outcomes. Bone Joint J. 2013 Jun;95-B(6):721–31.
5. Donnelly TD, Macfarlane RJ, Nagy MT, Ralte P, Waseem M. Fractures of the clavicle: an overview. Open Orthop J. 2013 Sep 6;7:329–33. Epub 2013.
6. van der Meijden OA, Gaskill TR, Millett PJ. Treatment of clavicle fractures: current concepts review. J Shoulder Elbow Surg. 2012 Mar;21(3):423–9. Epub 2011 Nov 6. Review.
7. Karl JW, Olson PR, Rosenwasser MP. The epidemiology of upper extremity fractures in the United States, 2009. J Orthop Trauma. 2015 Aug;29(8):e242–4.
8. Beall MH, Ross MG. Clavicle fracture in labor: risk factors and associated morbidities. J Perinatol. 2001 Dec;21(8):513–5.
9. Fallon KE, Fricker PA. Stress fracture of the clavicle in a young female gymnast. Br J Sports Med. 2001 Dec;35(6):448–9.
10. Shields E, Behrend C, Beiswenger T, Strong B, English C, Maloney M, et al. Scapular dyskinesis following displaced fractures of the middle clavicle. J Shoulder Elbow Surg. 2015 Dec;24(12):e331–6. Epub 2015 Jul 10.
11. Stegeman SA, Fernandes NC, Krijnen P, Schipper IB. Reliability of the Robinson classification for displaced comminuted midshaft clavicular fractures. Clin Imaging. 2015 Mar-Apr;39(2):293–6. Epub 2014 Aug 7.
12. Backus JD, Merriman DJ, McAndrew CM, Gardner MJ, Ricci WM. Upright versus supine radiographs of clavicle fractures: does positioning matter? J Orthop Trauma. 2014 Nov;28(11):636–41.
13. Robinson CM, Goudie EB, Murray IR, Jenkins PJ, Ahktar MA, Read EO, et al. Open reduction and plate fixation versus nonoperative treatment for displaced midshaft clavicular fractures: a multicenter, randomized, controlled trial. J Bone Joint Surg Am. 2013 Sep 4;95(17):1576–84.
14. Hill JM, McGuire MH, Crosby LA. Closed treatment of displaced middle-third fractures of the clavicle gives poor results. J Bone Joint Surg Br. 1997 Jul;79(4):537–9.
15. Fuglesang HF, Flugsrud GB, Randsborg PH, Stavem K, Utvag SE. Radiological and functional outcomes 2.7 years following conservatively treated completely displaced midshaft clavicle fractures. Arch Orthop Trauma Surg. 2016 Jan;136(1):17–25. Epub 2015 Nov 4.
16. Murray IR, Foster CJ, Eros A, Robinson CM. Risk factors for nonunion after nonoperative treatment of displaced midshaft fractures of the clavicle. J Bone Joint Surg Am. 2013 Jul 3;95(13):1153–8.
17. Bae DS, Shah AS, Kalish LA, Kwon JY, Waters PM. Shoulder motion, strength, and functional outcomes in children with established malunion of the clavicle. J Pediatr Orthop. 2013 Jul-Aug;33(5):544–50.
18. Parry JA, Van Straaten M, Luo TD, Simon AL, Ashraf A, Kaufman K, et al. Is there a deficit after nonoperative versus operative treatment of shortened midshaft clavicular fractures in adolescents? J Pediatr Orthop. 2017 Jun;37(4):227–233. Epub 2015 Aug 28t
19. Canadian Orthopaedic Trauma Society. Nonoperative treatment compared with plate fixation of displaced midshaft clavicular fractures: a multicenter, randomized clinical trial. J Bone Joint Surg Am. 2007 Jan;89(1):1–10.
20. van der Ven Denise JC, Timmers TK, Flikweert PE, Van Ijseldijk AL, van Olden GD. Plate fixation versus conservative treatment of displaced midshaft clavicle fractures: functional outcome and patients' satisfaction during a mean follow-up of 5 years. Injury. 2015 Nov;46(11):2223–9. Epub 2015 Aug 10.
21. Virtanen KJ, Remes V, Pajarinen J, Savolainen V, Bjorkenheim JM, Paavola M. Sling compared with plate osteosynthesis for treatment of displaced midshaft clavicular fractures: a randomized clinical trial. J Bone Joint Surg Am. 2012 Sep 5;94(17):1546–53.
22. Althausen PL, Shannon S, Lu M, O'Mara TJ, Bray TJ. Clinical and financial comparison of operative and nonoperative treatment of displaced clavicle fractures. J Shoulder Elbow Surg. 2013 May;22(5):608–11. Epub 2012 Sep 7.
23. Potter JM, Jones C, Wild LM, Schemitsch EH, McKee MD. Does delay matter? The restoration of objectively measured shoulder strength and patient-oriented outcome after immediate fixation versus delayed reconstruction of displaced midshaft fractures of the clavicle. J Shoulder Elbow Surg. 2007 Sep-Oct;16(5):514–8. Epub 2007 Jul 12.
24. Clement ND, Goudie EB, Brooksbank AJ, Chesser TJ, Robinson CM. Smoking status and the disabilities of the arm shoulder and hand score are early predictors of symptomatic nonunion of displaced midshaft fractures of the clavicle. Bone Joint J. 2016 Jan;98-B(1):125–30.
25. Lenza M, Belloti JC, Andriolo RB, Faloppa F. Conservative interventions for treating middle third clavicle fractures in adolescents and adults. Cochrane Database Syst Rev. 2014 May 30;(5):CD007121.
26. Ersen A, Atalar AC, Birisik F, Saglam Y, Demirhan M. Comparison of simple arm sling and figure of eight

clavicular bandage for midshaft clavicular fractures: a randomised controlled study. Bone Joint J. 2015 Nov;97-B(11):1562–5.

27. Schemitsch LA, Schemitsch EH, Kuzyk P, McKee MD. Prognostic factors for reoperation after plate fixation of the midshaft clavicle. J Orthop Trauma. 2015 Dec;29(12):533–7.

28. Iannotti MR, Crosby LA, Stafford P, Grayson G, Goulet R. Effects of plate location and selection on the stability of midshaft clavicle osteotomies: a biomechanical study. J Shoulder Elbow Surg. 2002 Sep-Oct;11(5):457–62.

29. Favre P, Kloen P, Helfet DL, Werner CM. Superior versus anteroinferior plating of the clavicle: a finite element study. J Orthop Trauma. 2011 Nov;25(11):661–5.

30. Hulsmans MH, van Heijl M, Houwert RM, Timmers TK, van Olden G, Verleisdonk EJ. Anteroinferior versus superior plating of clavicular fractures. J Shoulder Elbow Surg. 2016 Mar;25(3):448–54. Epub 2015 Dec 6.

31. Christensen TJ, Horwitz DS, Kubiak EN. Natural history of anterior chest wall numbness after plating of clavicle fractures: educating patients. J Orthop Trauma. 2014 Nov;28(11):642–7.

32. Naimark M, Dufka FL, Han R, Sing DC, Toogood P, Ma CB, et al. Plate fixation of midshaft clavicular fractures: patient-reported outcomes and hardware-related complications. J Shoulder Elbow Surg. 2016 May;25(5):739–46. Epub 2015 Dec 15.

33. Rehn CH, Kirkegaard M, Viberg B, Larsen MS. Operative versus nonoperative treatment of displaced midshaft clavicle fractures in adults: a systematic review. Eur J Orthop Surg Traumatol. 2014 Oct;24(7):1047–53. Epub 2013 Dec 10.

34. Leroux T, Wasserstein D, Henry P, Khoshbin A, Dwyer T, Ogilvie-Harris D, et al. Rate of and risk factors for reoperations after open reduction and internal fixation of midshaft clavicle fractures: a population-based study in Ontario, Canada. J Bone Joint Surg Am. 2014 Jul 2;96(13):1119–25. [Epub ahead of print]

35. Wilson DJ, Scully WF, Min KS, Harmon TA, Eichinger JK, Arrington ED. Biomechanical analysis of intramedullary vs. superior plate fixation of transverse midshaft clavicle fractures. J Shoulder Elbow Surg. 2016 Jun;25(6):949–53. Epub 2016 Jan 14.

36. Millett PJ, Hurst JM, Horan MP, Hawkins RJ. Complications of clavicle fractures treated with intramedullary fixation. J Shoulder Elbow Surg. 2011 Jan;20(1):86–91. Epub 2010 Nov 3.

37. Kleweno CP, Jawa A, Wells JH, O'Brien TG, Higgins LD, Harris MB, et al. Midshaft clavicular fractures: comparison of intramedullary pin and plate fixation. J Shoulder Elbow Surg. 2011 Oct;20(7):1114–7. Epub 2011 Jul 1.

38. Andrade-Silva FB, Kojima KE, Joeris A, Santos Silva J, Mattar R Jr. Single, superiorly placed reconstruction plate compared with flexible intramedullary nailing for midshaft clavicular fractures: a prospective, randomized controlled trial. J Bone Joint Surg Am. 2015 Apr 15;97(8):620–6.

39. van der Meijden OA, Houwert RM, Hulsmans M, Wijdicks FJ, Dijkgraaf MG, Meylaerts SA, et al. Operative treatment of dislocated midshaft clavicular fractures: plate or intramedullary nail fixation? A randomized controlled trial. J Bone Joint Surg Am. 2015 Apr 15;97(8):613–9.

40. Momberger NG, Smith J, Coleman DA. Vascularized fibular grafts for salvage reconstruction of clavicle nonunion. J Shoulder Elbow Surg. 2000 Sep-Oct;9(5):389–94.

41. Fuchs B, Steinmann SP, Bishop AT. Free vascularized corticoperiosteal bone graft for the treatment of persistent nonunion of the clavicle. J Shoulder Elbow Surg. 2005 May-Jun;14(3):264–8.

42. Manske DJ, Szabo RM. The operative treatment of mid-shaft clavicular non-unions. J Bone Joint Surg Am. 1985 Dec;67(9):1367–71.

43. Olsen BS, Vaesel MT, Sojbjerg JO. Treatment of mid-shaft clavicular nonunion with plate fixation and autologous bone grafting. J Shoulder Elbow Surg. 1995 Sep-Oct;4(5):337–44.

44. Bradbury N, Hutchinson J, Hahn D, Colton CL. Clavicular nonunion. 31/32 healed after plate fixation and bone grafting. Acta Orthop Scand. 1996 Aug;67(4):367–70.

45. Ebraheim NA, Mekhail AO, Darwich M. Open reduction and internal fixation with bone grafting of clavicular nonunion. J Trauma. 1997 Apr;42(4):701–4.

46. Ballmer FT, Lambert SM, Hertel R. Decortication and plate osteosynthesis for nonunion of the clavicle. J Shoulder Elbow Surg. 1998 Nov-Dec;7(6):581–5.

47. Laursen MB, Dossing KV. Clavicular nonunions treated with compression plate fixation and cancellous bone grafting: the functional outcome. J Shoulder Elbow Surg. 1999 Sep-Oct;8(5):410–3.

48. Endrizzi DP, White RR, Babikian GM, Old AB. Nonunion of the clavicle treated with plate fixation: a review of forty-seven consecutive cases. J Shoulder Elbow Surg. 2008 Nov-Dec;17(6):951–3. Epub 2008 Sep 20.

49. Baker JF, Mullett H. Clavicle non-union: autologous bone graft is not a necessary augment to internal fixation. Acta Orthop Belg. 2010 Dec;76(6):725–9.

50. McKee MD, Pedersen EM, Jones C, Stephen DJ, Kreder HJ, Schemitsch EH, et al. Deficits following nonoperative treatment of displaced midshaft clavicular fractures. J Bone Joint Surg Am. 2006 Jan;88(1):35–40.

51. McKee MD, Wild LM, Schemitsch EH. Midshaft malunions of the clavicle. J Bone Joint Surg Am. 2003 May;85-A(5):790–7.

52. Bosch U, Skutek M, Peters G, Tscherne H. Extension osteotomy in malunited clavicular fractures. J Shoulder Elbow Surg. 1998 Jul-Aug;7(4):402–5.

53. Smekal V, Deml C, Kamelger F, Dallapozza C, Krappinger D. Corrective osteotomy in symptomatic midshaft clavicular malunion using elastic stable intramedullary nails. Arch Orthop Trauma Surg. 2010 May;130(5):681–5. Epub 2009 Nov 3.

54. Sidhu VS, Hermans D, Duckworth DG. The operative outcomes of displaced medial-end clavicle fractures. J Shoulder Elbow Surg. 2015 Nov;24(11):1728–34. Epub 2015 Jul 2.

55. Duncan SF, Sperling JW, Steinmann S. Infection after clavicle fractures. Clin Orthop Relat Res. 2005 Oct;439:74–8.

56. Robinson CM. Fractures of the clavicle in the adult: epidemiology and classification. J Bone Joint Surg Br. 1998 May;80(3):476–84.

57. Bishop JY, Jones GL, Lewis B, Pedroza A; MOON Shoulder Group. Intra- and interobserver agreement in the classification and treatment of distal third clavicle fractures. Am J Sports Med. 2015 Apr;43(4):979–84. Epub 2015 Jan 13.

58. Banerjee R, Waterman B, Padalecki J, Robertson W. Management of distal clavicle fractures. J Am Acad Orthop Surg. 2011 Jul;19(7):392–401.

59. Huang KC, Tu YK, Huang TJ, Hsu RW. Suprascapular neuropathy complicating a Neer type I distal clavicular fracture: a case report. J Orthop Trauma. 2005 May-Jun;19(5):343–5.

60. Edwards DJ, Kavanagh TG, Flannery MC. Fractures of the distal clavicle: a case for fixation. Injury. 1992;23(1):44–6.

61. Cisneros LN, Reiriz JS. Arthroscopic-assisted management of unstable distal-third clavicle fractures: conoid ligament reconstruction and fracture cerclage with sutures. Arthrosc Tech. 2015 Nov 9;4(6):e655–61. Epub 2015 Dec.

62. Shin SJ, Ko YW, Lee J, Park MG. Use of plate fixation without coracoclavicular ligament augmentation for unstable distal clavicle fractures. J Shoulder Elbow Surg. 2016 Jun;25(6):942–8. Epub 2015 Dec 23.

63. Fleming MA, Dachs R, Maqungo S, du Plessis JP, Vrettos BC, Roche SJ. Angular stable fixation of displaced distal-third clavicle fractures with superior precontoured locking plates. J Shoulder Elbow Surg. 2015 May;24(5):700–4. Epub 2014 Oct 29.

64. Duralde XA, Pennington SD, Murray DH. Interfragmentary suture fixation for displaced acute type II distal clavicle fractures. J Orthop Trauma. 2014 Nov;28(11):653–8.

65. Throckmorton T, Kuhn JE. Fractures of the medial end of the clavicle. J Shoulder Elbow Surg. 2007 Jan-Feb;16(1):49–54. Epub 2006 Dec 12.

66. Roedl JB, Nevalainen M, Gonzalez FM, Dodson CC, Morrison WB, Zoga AC. Frequency, imaging findings, risk factors, and long-term sequelae of distal clavicular osteolysis in young patients. Skeletal Radiol. 2015 May;44(5):659–66. Epub 2015 Jan 7.

67. de la Puente R, Boutin RD, Theodorou DJ, Hooper A, Schweitzer M, Resnick D. Post-traumatic and stress-induced osteolysis of the distal clavicle: MR imaging findings in 17 patients. Skeletal Radiol. 1999 Apr;28(4):202–8.

68. Rockwood CA Jr, Williams GR Jr, Young DC. Disorders of the acromioclavicular joint. In: Rockwood CAJr, Matsen FAIII, editors. The shoulder. 2nd ed. Vol. 1. Philadelphia (PA): W. B. Saunders Company; c1998. p. 483–553.

69. Schneider MM, Balke M, Koenen P, Frohlich M, Wafaisade A, Bouillon B, et al. Inter- and intraobserver reliability of the Rockwood classification in acute acromioclavicular joint dislocations. Knee Surg Sports Traumatol Arthrosc. 2016 Jul;24(7):2192–6. Epub 2014 Nov 16.

70. Yap JJ, Curl LA, Kvitne RS, McFarland EG. The value of weighted views of the acromioclavicular joint: results of a survey. Am J Sports Med. 1999 Nov-Dec;27(6):806–9.

71. Petri M, Warth RJ, Greenspoon JA, Horan MP, Abrams RF, Kokmeyer D, et al. Clinical results after conservative management for grade III acromioclavicular joint injuries: does eventual surgery affect overall outcomes? Arthroscopy. 2016 May;32(5):740–6. Epub 2016 Feb 4.

72. Stucken C, Cohen SB. Management of acromioclavicular joint injuries. Orthop Clin North Am. 2015 Jan;46(1):57–66. Epub 2014 Oct 11.

73. Brand JC, Lubowitz JH, Provencher MT, Rossi MJ. Acromioclavicular joint reconstruction: complications and innovations. Arthroscopy. 2015 May;31(5):795–7.

74. Barth J, Duparc F, Baverel L, Bahurel J, Toussaint B, Bertiaux S, et al; Société Française d'Arthroscopie. Prognostic factors to succeed in surgical treatment of chronic acromioclavicular dislocations. Orthop Traumatol Surg Res. 2015 Dec;101(8 Suppl):S305–11. Epub 2015 Oct 23.

75. Smith TO, Chester R, Pearse EO, Hing CB. Operative versus non-operative management following Rockwood grade III acromioclavicular separation: a meta-analysis of the current evidence base. J Orthop Traumatol. 2011 Mar;12(1):19–27. Epub 2011 Feb 23.

76. Tauber M, Valler D, Lichtenberg S, Magosch P, Moroder P, Habermeyer P. Arthroscopic stabilization of chronic acromioclavicular joint dislocations: triple- versus single-bundle reconstruction. Am J Sports Med. 2016 Feb;44(2):482–9. Epub 2015 Dec 9.

77. Vascellari A, Schiavetti S, Battistella G, Rebuzzi E, Coletti N. Clinical and radiological results after coracoclavicular ligament reconstruction for type III acromioclavicular joint dislocation using three different techniques: a retrospective study. Joints. 2015 Nov;3(2):54–61. Epub 2015 Apr-Jun.

78. Taranu R, Rushton PR, Serrano-Pedraza I, Holder L, Wallace WA, Candal-Couto JJ. Acromioclavicular joint reconstruction using the LockDown synthetic implant: a study with cadavers. Bone Joint J. 2015 Dec;97-B(12):1657–61.

79. Struhl S, Wolfson TS. Continuous loop double endobutton reconstruction for acromioclavicular joint dislocation. Am J Sports Med. 2015 Oct;43(10):2437–44. Epub 2015 Aug 10.

80. Woodmass JM, Esposito JG, Ono Y, Nelson AA, Boorman RS, Thornton GM, et al. Complications following arthroscopic fixation of acromioclavicular separations: a systematic review of the literature. Open Access J Sports Med. 2015 Apr 10;6:97–107. Epub 2015.

81. Ponce BA, Kundukulam JA, Pflugner R, McGwin G, Meyer R, Carroll W, et al. Sternoclavicular joint surgery: how far does danger lurk below? J Shoulder Elbow Surg. 2013 Jul;22(7):993–9. Epub 2013 Jan 16.

82. Martetschlager F, Warth RJ, Millett PJ. Instability and degenerative arthritis of the sternoclavicular joint: a current concepts review. Am J Sports Med. 2014 Apr;42(4):999–1007. Epub 2013 Aug 16.

83. Quispe JC, Herbert B, Chadayammuri VP, Kim JW, Hao J, Hake M, et al. Transarticular plating for acute posterior sternoclavicular joint dislocations: a valid treatment option? Int Orthop. 2016 Jul;40(7):1503–8. Epub 2015 Aug 11.

84. Bak K, Fogh K. Reconstruction of the chronic anterior unstable sternoclavicular joint using a tendon autograft: medium-term to long-term follow-up results. J Shoulder Elbow Surg. 2014 Feb;23(2):245–50. Epub 2013 Jul 10.

85. Sabatini JB, Shung JR, Clay TB, Oladeji LO, Minnich DJ, Ponce BA. Outcomes of augmented allograft figure-of-eight sternoclavicular joint reconstruction. J Shoulder Elbow Surg. 2015 Jun;24(6):902–7. Epub 2014 Dec 3.

86. Kusnezov N, Dunn JC, DeLong JM, Waterman BR. Sternoclavicular reconstruction in the young active patient: risk factor analysis and clinical outcomes at short-term follow-up. J Orthop Trauma. 2016 Apr;30(4): e111–7.

87. Uri O, Barmpagiannis K, Higgs D, Falworth M, Alexander S, Lambert SM. Clinical outcome after reconstruction for sternoclavicular joint instability using a sternocleidomastoid tendon graft. J Bone Joint Surg Am. 2014 Mar 5;96(5):417–22.

88. Quayle JM, Arnander MW, Pennington RG, Rosell LP. Artificial ligament reconstruction of sternoclavicular joint instability: report of a novel surgical technique with early results. Tech Hand Up Extrem Surg. 2014 Mar;18(1):31–5.

89. Bodker T, Tottrup M, Petersen KK, Jurik AG. Diagnostics of septic arthritis in the sternoclavicular region: 10 consecutive patients and literature review. Acta Radiol. 2013 Feb 1;54(1):67–74. Epub 2012 Oct 26.

90. Higginbotham TO, Kuhn JE. Atraumatic disorders of the sternoclavicular joint. J Am Acad Orthop Surg. 2005 Mar-Apr;13(2):138–45.

91. Pourcho AM, Sellon JL, Smith J. Sonographically guided sternoclavicular joint injection: description of technique and validation. J Ultrasound Med. 2015 Feb;34(2):325–31.

92. Tytherleigh-Strong G, Griffith D. Arthroscopic excision of the sternoclavicular joint for the treatment of sternoclavicular osteoarthritis. Arthroscopy. 2013 Sep;29(9):1487–91. Epub 2013 Jul 30.

93. Tytherleigh-Strong GM, Getgood AJ, Griffiths DE. Arthroscopic intra-articular disk excision of the sternoclavicular joint. Am J Sports Med. 2012 May;40(5):1172–5. Epub 2012 Mar 28.

6 The Rotator Cuff and Biceps Tendon

Rotator cuff disease is the most common condition responsible for shoulder pain worldwide (1,2). The understanding and treatment of rotator cuff disease has advanced tremendously over the past few years, mostly due to both technological advances (magnetic resonance, ultrasonography, arthroscopic surgery, and reverse arthroplasty) and a better understanding of the biology of healing and of muscle changes over time.

Not uncommonly, the long head of the biceps tendon presents structural pathology in patients with cuff disease; however, determining the contribution of biceps pathology to patients' symptoms is not always straightforward. Since the long head of the biceps tendon is anatomically in continuity with the labrum, I debated whether to discuss biceps pathology in this chapter, or in chapter 7, Shoulder Instability and the Labrum, but in my practice treatment of the biceps is much more common in the setting of cuff disease, so I kept it in this chapter.

Anatomy and Function

Rotator Cuff

The rotator cuff is a group of muscles that surrounds the glenohumeral joint anteriorly, superiorly, and posteriorly (Figure 6.1A). It includes the subscapularis, supraspinatus, infraspinatus, and teres minor (Table 6.1). The supraspinatus, infraspinatus, and teres minor tendons attach to the greater tuberosity as a continuous tissue sheath, whereas the subscapularis is separated from the supraspinatus at the so-called interval region, where the biceps tendon is located along with the superior glenohumeral ligament (deep) and the coracohumeral ligament (superficial).

The rotator cuff tendons insert in specific areas of the proximal humerus (Figure 6.1B) (3,4). The subscapularis inserts into the lesser tuberosity, and its area of attachment or footprint lies directly adjacent to the rim of the humeral head articular cartilage. The greater tuberosity has 3 insertional facets. The footprint of the supraspinatus on the

greater tuberosity is also directly adjacent to the articular cartilage, whereas the infraspinatus attaches a few millimeters lateral to the articular cartilage, leaving a bare area. The teres minor attachment is the most inferior. Multiple investigators have reported various dimensions for these footprint areas (Table 6.1).

The tendons of the rotator cuff are particularly prone to tendinopathy and degenerative rupture with aging. Rotator cuff dysfunction can also be secondary to traumatic rupture at the tendon-bone or, less commonly, muscle-tendon junction. Compression of the suprascapular nerve by cysts, repetitive traction, or thickening of the transverse superior scapular ligament may also lead to cuff dysfunction. Finally, some patients may have poor control or imbalance of the rotator cuff. The clinical expression of these different conditions varies.

The rotator cuff functions to provide motion to the glenohumeral joint, but also contributes to joint stability. A rotator cuff tear may present with only pain, but most commonly it leads to weakness in internal rotation, abduction, and/or external rotation, depending on the tendons involved.

Contraction of the rotator cuff muscles also contributes to keeping the humeral head centered on the glenoid during motion. As discussed in chapter 7, Shoulder Instability and the Labrum, the humeral head translates on the glenoid as it rotates. The behavior of the glenohumeral joint with poor control of the rotator cuff could be compared with trying to run using loose shoes with the laces untied: the foot would move all over the place in the shoe, making it difficult to run. With poor control of the rotator cuff, the humeral head glides excessively all over the glenoid and makes it difficult for the prime movers (deltoid, pectoralis, etc.) to provide effective function secondary to this dynamic instability.

Tendon of the Long Head of the Biceps

The biceps brachii muscle consists of a short portion originating from the coracoid process and a long

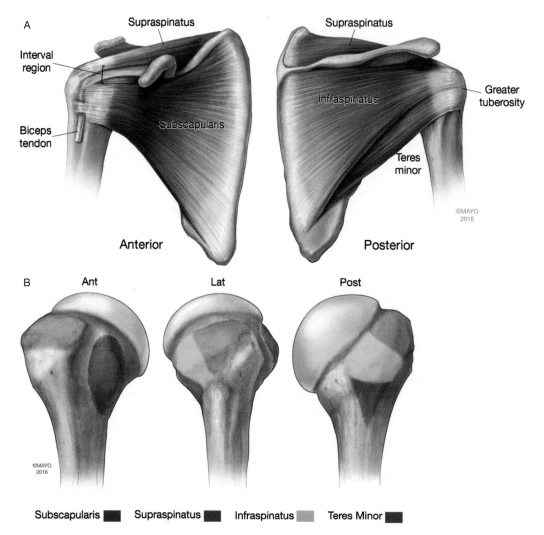

Figure 6.1 **A,** *The rotator cuff and the biceps tendon (gross anatomy).* **B,** *Attachment footprints for the rotator cuff tendons. Ant indicates anterior; Lat, lateral; Post, posterior.*

portion, the long head of the biceps (Figure 6.2). The tendon of the long head of the biceps typically originates from the labrum and the supraglenoid tubercle. Its intra-articular portion passes over the anterior aspect of the humeral head in the interval between the subscapularis and the supraspinatus before exiting the glenohumeral joint through the bicipital groove, in between the lesser and the greater tuberosity. The tendon of the long head of the biceps is approximately 5 mm in diameter and 10 cm in length. It is important to realize that multiple anatomical variants have been described for this tendon (5,6).

Table 6.1 • The Rotator Cuff

	Origin	Insertion	Footprint Area	Innervation	Action
Subscapularis	Anterior aspect scapular body	Lesser tuberosity	Sup-Inf – 40 mm ML – 20 mm	Subscapularis nerves	Internal rotation
Supraspinatus	Supraspinous fossa	Greater tuberosity	AP – 1.5–2.5 cm ML – 7–30 mm	Suprascapular nerve	Abduction
Infraspinatus	Infraspinous fossa	Greater tuberosity	AP – 1.5–3.0 cm ML – 10–30 mm	Suprascapular nerve	External rotation
Teres minor	Middle part of the lateral border of the scapula	Greater tuberosity	AP – 30 mm ML – 20 mm	Axillary nerve	External rotation

Abbreviations: AP, anterior to posterior; ML, medial to lateral; Sup-Inf, superior to inferior.

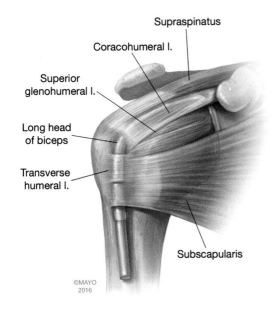

©MAYO 2016

Figure 6.2 *Tendon of the long head of the biceps, bicipital pulley, and interval region structures. l indicates ligament.*

A soft-tissue sling stabilizes the tendon of the long head of the biceps as it enters the bicipital groove—the bicipital pulley, formed by the coalescence of fibers from the cora-cohumeral ligament, the superior glenohumeral ligament, and portions of the subscapularis tendon. In the groove, the long head of the biceps tendon is covered by the transverse humeral ligament (formed by fibers from the subscapularis tendon) and then by an expansion of the pectoralis major tendon.

The specific function of the tendon of the long head of the biceps has been difficult to determine (5–8). Cadaveric studies seem to suggest that the biceps tendon contributes to glenohumeral stability, especially against an anterosuperiorly directed force. However, in vivo studies using electromyography (EMG) or imaging have provided inconsistent results regarding the function of the long head of the biceps. As discussed at the end of the chapter, when the long head of the biceps is divided (biceps tenotomy or rupture), patients do not seem to lose much strength in the shoulder, but they can experience a 20% decrease of strength in elbow flexion or forearm supination.

Basic Science

The Muscle-Tendon-Bone Unit and Rotator Cuff Tears

The transition zones between muscle and tendon, and between tendon and bone are fascinating. The myotendinous junction is particularly prone to injury with a sudden eccentric load; myotendinous cuff injuries have been reported to affect mostly the infraspinatus tendon (9). However, most rotator cuff tears affect the tendon to bone transition zone.

The rotator cuff tendon to bone attachment consists of 4 zones: tendon, uncalcified fibrocartilage, calcified fibrocartilage, and bone (Figure 6.3) (10–13). In histology preparations, a dense line called tidemark separates calcified from uncalcified fibrocartilage, and it continues with the tidemark that separates the calcified and uncalcified layers of the articular cartilage. Collagen fibers from the tendon

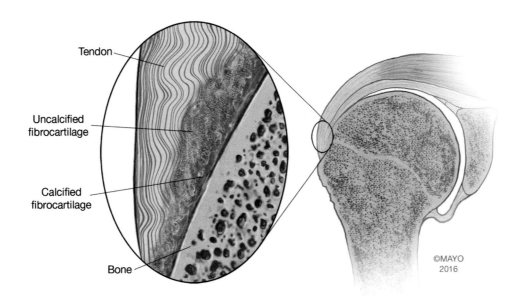

©MAYO 2016

Figure 6.3 *Ultrastructure of direct tendon to bone attachment.*

approach the tidemark perpendicularly. Tendon fiber rupture forms the basis of rotator cuff disease.

Initiation of fiber rupture happens when applied loads exceed fiber strength. The most common reason for progressive decrease of fiber strength is aging. However, many other factors may contribute as well: some individuals are likely genetically predisposed to decreased fiber strength at a younger age; inflammatory joint conditions, chronic exposure to corticosteroids, and microvascular insufficiency secondary to diabetes, smoking, and other conditions are associated with tendinopathy; and repetitive overload may also lead to fiber failure.

A sudden traumatic event will disrupt fibers at a specific location depending on the direction of the energy applied. For example, an anterior dislocation of the shoulder may create a tear of the subscapularis tendon fibers. However, most commonly, rotator cuff tears

occur slowly over time, and in those circumstances the first fibers disrupted are typically the deep fibers of the supraspinatus approximately 1 centimeter posterior to the anterior edge of the tendon (2,14,15). Fiber disruption may affect part of the thickness of the tendon (partial-thickness tears) or the whole thickness of the tendon (full-thickness tears).

Once some fibers are disrupted, the stage for progression is set (Figure 6.4): adjacent fibers are overloaded; blood vessels are distorted with progressive local ischemia; the area of fiber rupture is exposed to articular fluid that may abolish the healing response (both by washing out the hematoma and by biochemical actions of enzymes and other molecules); and fewer muscle fibers are connected to bone, so that less force can be delivered by the affected muscle-tendon unit. As tear size increases, the humeral head tends to migrate proximally, partly due to

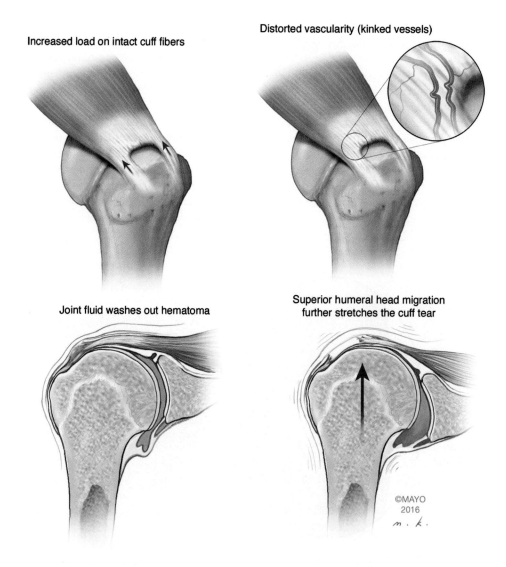

Increased load on intact cuff fibers

Distorted vascularity (kinked vessels)

Joint fluid washes out hematoma

Superior humeral head migration further stretches the cuff tear

©MAYO
2016
m. k.

Figure 6.4 *Tendon fiber disruption leads to tear progression through several mechanisms.*

the lack of a cushioning tendon superiorly and partly due to the loss of the stabilizing function of the cuff.

The contributions of primary tendon degeneration and mechanical compression of the rotator cuff on fiber tearing continue to be argued. Since a thick acromion with an anteroinferior spur is commonly observed in patients with cuff disease, some authors have proposed that the resultant narrowing of the subacromial space leads to repetitive impingement and compression, with resultant secondary tendon degeneration. Others interpret that subacromial spurs are traction osteophytes that develop as a response to abnormal loads on the coracoacromial ligament as the humeral head migrates superiorly once the cuff is torn. As discussed later, the role of enlarging the subacromial space at the time of surgery by removing bone from the undersurface of the anterior acromion (acromioplasty) continues to be debated (16).

Rotator Cuff Tears and Symptoms

The lack of correlation between rotator cuff tears and symptoms continues to puzzle me daily. Since chronic nontraumatic tears are related to aging, the existence of asymptomatic tears should not come as a surprise; as detailed later, this has been noticed both in cadaver dissections and in imaging studies on asymptomatic patients. To add to the picture, some patients with a relatively small tear complain of severe pain and poor motion, whereas other patients with large tears have little pain. Finally, attempted surgical repair will oftentimes lead to improvements in pain and function even if tendon healing does not occur (2,14,15,17–19).

The pathways through which rotator cuff tearing generates pain are not fully understood. Possible mechanisms include altered joint mechanics, local accumulation of pain mediators, and an inflammatory response in adjacent structures, like the capsule, synovium, and bursa.

The mechanics of the rotator cuff have been analyzed extensively to understand why some patients with cuff tears maintain good arcs of active motion (Figure 6.5). The terms *force couple* (20) and *rotator cable* (21) are commonly used in this context. Theoretically, the force vectors of the subscapularis anteriorly, and the infraspinatus and teres minor posteriorly, can be so well balanced that the patient can actively elevate the shoulder in the presence of a relatively large rotator cuff tear (balanced force couple) (20). In addition, disrupted tendon fibers may still be able to transmit force to bone through adjacent intact fibers, since the posterior and the anterior portions of the cuff are connected by bundles of fibers perpendicular to the direction of the tendons (rotator cable) (21).

Tendon-to-Bone Healing

When the torn rotator cuff is surgically repaired, the dream of the orthopedic surgeon would be to ensure that the

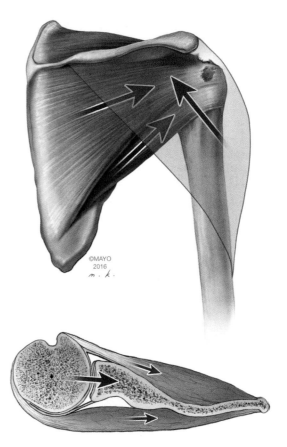

Figure 6.5 *Force couples concept.*

native attachment at the tendon-to-bone transition area is re-established in all individuals. Unfortunately, as detailed later, healing fails to occur in 1 of every 4 patients who undergo surgical repair; and even when tendon-to-bone continuity is re-established, it does not replicate the zonal configuration just described, with interposed fibrocartilage and firm direct attachment to bone. Tendon-to-bone healing is characterized by the formation of connective tissue with vastly inferior biomechanical properties in comparison with normal, uninjured tendon (22). Luckily, pain relief and improved function are experienced by most patients, sometimes even those without restoration of tendon to bone continuity.

In simple terms, tendon-to-bone healing after surgery requires 2 conditions: adequate mechanical tendon-to-bone fixation and a good biologic healing response. Ways to obtain adequate fixation are discussed later under Treatment. Enhancement of the biologic healing response can theoretically be attempted on the bone side, the tendon side, and/or the healing environment. Cell therapy and/ or growth factors have been investigated without a major breakthrough so far. Regarding rehabilitation, basic science studies have shown that early mobilization seems to be detrimental for tendon-to-bone healing (22). However, complete removal of load from the healing insertion site (simulated with botulinum toxin injections) is also detrimental.

Muscle and Nerve Changes After Rupture

Chronic absence of tendon-to-bone continuity leads to muscular changes that seem to be directly correlated with the outcome of treatment (23,24). Contraction of muscle fibers no longer connected to bone leads to retraction. In addition, muscle bulk may decrease (atrophy), and the relative content of adipose tissue within the epimysium and perimysium may increase (fatty infiltration). These changes may become partly irreversible even if healing occurs after cuff repair, compromising the clinical outcome.

Moderate to severe degrees of muscle retraction have been theorized by some to kink the neurovascular pedicles of the posterosuperior cuff (25,26). Scarring associated with chronic retraction may lead to permanent compression or stretching of the suprascapular nerve, which could again compromise the clinical outcome of an otherwise successful repair. Some studies have found evidence of suprascapular neuropathy in patients with rotator cuff tears, whereas others have failed to do so.

Rotator Cuff Tears

Epidemiology

The epidemiology of rotator cuff disease has been investigated in patients with and without symptoms. The burden of symptomatic rotator cuff disease is difficult to analyze. The incidence of symptomatic cuff pathology has been reported to be at least 90 per 100,000 person-years (1,27). Some studies have reported an even higher rate of rotator cuff repair, up to 130 per 100,000 person-years (28). Smoking, hypercholesterolemia, and a positive family history have been shown to predispose individuals to rotator cuff tearing (2).

Cadaver and imaging studies have shown an overall rate of full-thickness rotator cuff tears in approximately 15% to 20% of the individuals over the age of 60 and 50% to 80% of the individuals over the age of 80 (2). Magnetic resonance imaging (MRI) evaluation of asymptomatic persons has shown a 15% rate of full-thickness tears and a 20% rate of partial thickness tears (19). Asymptomatic full-thickness rotator cuff tears are present in approximately 50% of patients over the age of 65 with a contralateral symptomatic full-thickness tear (2). Approximately 15% of the patients with a symptomatic tear will develop a new tear in the contralateral shoulder (15).

Natural History

A key question in counseling patients presenting in the office with a rotator cuff tear relates to the likelihood of progression of both symptoms and tear size. Approximately 50% of the individuals with asymptomatic full-thickness tears develop symptoms within 2 or 3 years (2). Larger tears are more likely to lead to symptoms over time, and 50% of the patients developing symptoms will also experience an increase in tear size. Tear enlargement has been reported in approximately 60% of asymptomatic full-thickness tears and 44% of asymptomatic partial-thickness tears (15). Regarding symptomatic full-thickness tears, 50% increase in size at an average of 2 years. Small tears (under 1.5 cm) have a lower rate of size progression (25% at 2 years). Tear size progression is correlated with increased symptoms and also with muscle degeneration (15).

Evaluation

History and Physical Examination

Shoulder pain, weakness, and motion loss may all be present to some extent in patients with impingement, cuff tendinopathy, partial or full-thickness rotator cuff tears, or secondary articular degenerative changes. Table 6.2 summarizes the goals of the evaluation. History and physical examination findings will help identify all potential sources of pain or other symptoms (chapter 1, Evaluation of the Shoulder). The history should also attempt to identify prognostic factors for tendon healing (Table 6.3) and help understand the anticipated demands and expectations of the patient.

Most patients complain of pain centered over the deltoid region, felt as a dull ache in a relatively wide lateral area of the shoulder. For many patients, pain is especially bothersome at night, interfering with the ability to sleep. Pain is typically worse with attempted overhead activities or when trying to lift objects. The acromioclavicular joint, biceps tendon, and articular cartilage loss should be specifically assessed to identify associated pathology.

Table 6.2 • Goals of Patient Evaluation

Identify all sources of symptoms
Rotator cuff tendinopathy or tear
Impingement
Biceps tendon and labral pathology
Acromioclavicular osteoarthritis
Cartilage loss

Grade severity of disease
Physical examination
Radiographs
Advanced imaging studies (MRI, ultrasonography, CT)
Previous trauma (acute tear vs chronic extension)

Understand patient's demands and expectations

Identify risk factors for poor tendon healing (see Table 6.3)

Abbreviations: CT, computed tomography; MRI, magnetic resonance imaging.

Table 6.3 • Factors Associated With Poor Tendon Healing

Structural pathology
Tear size
Tendon quality (multiple corticosteroid injections)
Muscle atrophy and fatty infiltration
Bone quality

Poor healing response
Smoking
Diabetes
Hyperlipidemia
Advanced age
Chemotherapy
Inflammatory arthritis (i.e., rheumatoid arthritis)
Individual predisposition (host variation)

Surgical factors
Incomplete repair
Poor construct
  Tear pattern poorly understood
  Subscapularis tears not repaired
  Unstable repair construct
  Lack of tendon to bone contact and compression (?)

It is important to carefully question patients about previous injuries and to distinguish acute rotator cuff tears from traumatic extension of a chronic tear. Patients with a truly acute rotator cuff tear deny any shoulder symptoms prior to a specific injury; most of these patients know that something bad has happened to their shoulder with their injury, complaining of various degrees of pain and loss of active motion. In a few days to weeks, pain and motion may improve, but rarely to normal. Tendon retraction may be identified in imaging studies, but there is absence of muscular atrophy and fatty infiltration (see later).

The term *acute extension of a chronic tear* refers to those circumstances in which a patient had developed a degenerative chronic tear over time and experiences rupture of additional tendon fibers as a consequence of an injury. The hallmark is the presence of atrophy and fatty infiltration on imaging studies. Some patients may not have known that they had a previous asymptomatic rotator cuff tear, but every patient should be carefully questioned about symptoms prior to the injury. Radiographs oftentimes reveal findings consistent with chronicity (sclerosis, osteopenia or cysts at the greater tuberosity, as well as acromial spurring).

Physical examination of the shoulder should be aimed at identifying all locations of pain, recording active and passive range of motion, and assessing strength and cuff integrity (chapter 1, Evaluation of the Shoulder). Patients with impingement and cuff disease may present with a painful arc and a drop arm sign. Patients with full-thickness tears may have limited active motion with relatively good passive motion, but there is a subset of patients who present with stiffness secondary to longstanding cuff disease; in these patients, the associated stiffness must be addressed in order to obtain a good outcome with any type of intervention for

cuff disease. The supraspinatus, infraspinatus, teres minor, and subscapularis should be individually examined using the maneuvers described in chapter 1, Evaluation of the Shoulder. The examination is completed with maneuvers to assess the acromioclavicular joint, biceps tendon, and glenohumeral articular surface (articular shear test), and to identify any associated scapular dyskinesis.

Radiographs
Plain radiographs should be obtained in every patient evaluated for cuff disease. Radiographic changes will vary depending on the stage of cuff disease and the presence of associated pathology. Radiographs are extremely useful in identifying calcific tendinopathy that could otherwise be misdiagnosed (see later). In patients with tendinopathy, partial thickness tears, and small full-thickness tears, plain radiographs may be completely normal. Radiographic changes thought to be related to rotator cuff disease are discussed in the following sections.

Acromial Changes
There is some controversy regarding the role of acromial morphology in the genesis of rotator cuff disease. The shape of the acromion is different from individual to individual. In the parasagittal plane, the inclination of the anterior acromion is classified into types I, II, and III (Figure 6.6); some believe that type II and especially type III acromions contribute to cuff impingement and tearing (29). In the coronal plane, a wider acromion is believed by some to also contribute to cuff disease (an increase in the so-called critical shoulder angle). Regardless of the individual shape of the acromion, in a number of patients a subacromial spur develops over time. It is hypothesized to represent a traction enthesophyte off the origin of the coracoacromial ligament. All these changes theoretically contribute to cuff impingement by narrowing the supraspinatus outlet.

Another change possibly related to cuff pathology is the presence of an os acromiale. This term refers to lack of complete fusion of the ossifying centers of the acromion (Figure 6.7). The most common subtype is the meso os acromiale. The synchondrosis between the 2 portions of the acromion allows inferior tipping of the anterior portion with deltoid contraction. This is believed to contribute to dynamic impingement in some patients. The os acromiale is best identified in the axillary radiograph (as well as the axial cuts of an MRI or a computed tomography [CT] scan).

Proximal Humeral Head Migration
Larger rotator cuff tears lead to progressive proximal migration of the humeral head in reference to the glenoid. The amount of migration may be assessed by measuring the acromiohumeral distance; a distance of less than 6 to 8 mm seems to be associated with the presence of a full-thickness cuff tear (Figure 6.8). In severe cases, the humeral head migrates until it is in contact with the acromion, which

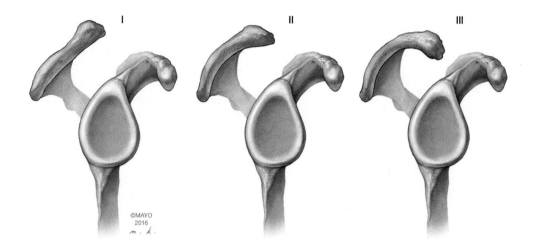

Figure 6.6 Acromion types.

may eventually become eroded and even develop a stress fracture (Figure 6.9).

Tuberosity Changes

Cuff disease may be reflected by tuberosity changes, most commonly in the greater tuberosity. There may be sclerosis, osteopenia, spurring, or cysts. Beware of large cysts or marked osteopenia, as they may compromise tendon to bone fixation at the time of surgery. Larger tuberosity spurs may give the false impression of a very narrow acromiohumeral distance.

Acromioclavicular Joint Degeneration

Radiographic changes consistent with osteoarthritis of the acromioclavicular joint (narrowing, sclerosis, and osteophytes) are extremely common even in completely asymptomatic patients. It is extremely important to correlate these changes with symptoms by using the examination maneuvers described in chapter 1, Evaluation of the Shoulder. Inferior osteophytes may contribute to cuff impingement in some patients.

Secondary Glenohumeral Joint Degeneration (Cuff-Tear Arthropathy)

Longstanding full-thickness cuff tears may lead to progressive articular cartilage damage, and eventually various degrees of bone loss (Figure 6.9). The term *cuff-tear arthropathy* was coined to describe this situation (30); in the initial description, it was required for the humeral head to have collapsed in order for the term to be applied (Figure 6.9B). Joint degeneration likely results from a combination of abnormal joint biomechanics, leading to areas of excessive joint contact pressure as well as biochemical changes due to chronic escape of articular fluid through the cuff defect. Interestingly, like in other areas of orthopedics, there is not a perfect correlation between radiographic changes and symptoms; some individuals with end-stage cuff-tear arthropathy complain of little pain and have good elevation, whereas many present with severe pain and/or various degrees of motion loss, including pseudoparalysis.

Advanced Imaging Studies

Magnetic Resonance Imaging

Currently, magnetic resonance is the advanced imaging modality of choice across the world to assess patients with rotator cuff disease (31). It is mostly used to assess tendon fiber disruption and muscle changes, but it is also useful to assess changes in the articular cartilage, biceps, labrum, and bone. It is important to be systematic when assessing a patient's MRI so that abnormalities are not missed and at the same time realize that many individuals will present with abnormal findings that are completely asymptomatic.

Tendinopathy and Partial Thickness Tears Disruption of some of the tendon fibers is seen as a bright signal in T2-weighted images. The term *tendinopathy* is commonly used when the bursal and articular sides of the tendon are intact (seen as continuity of dark fibers all the way to the footprint), but there are areas of intratendinous bright signal (intratendinous tear). Partial-thickness tears may extend into the articular or the bursal surface of the tendon. Tendinopathy and partial thickness tears most commonly affect the supraspinatus tendon. It may be extremely difficult to establish the relationship between partial-thickness tears and symptoms.

Full-Thickness Tears Discontinuity of the complete tendon thickness is best identified as a bright gap in T2-weighted images in between the dark torn tendon edge and the bone footprint (Figure 6.10). Understanding tear size and pattern is important to establish prognosis and treatment

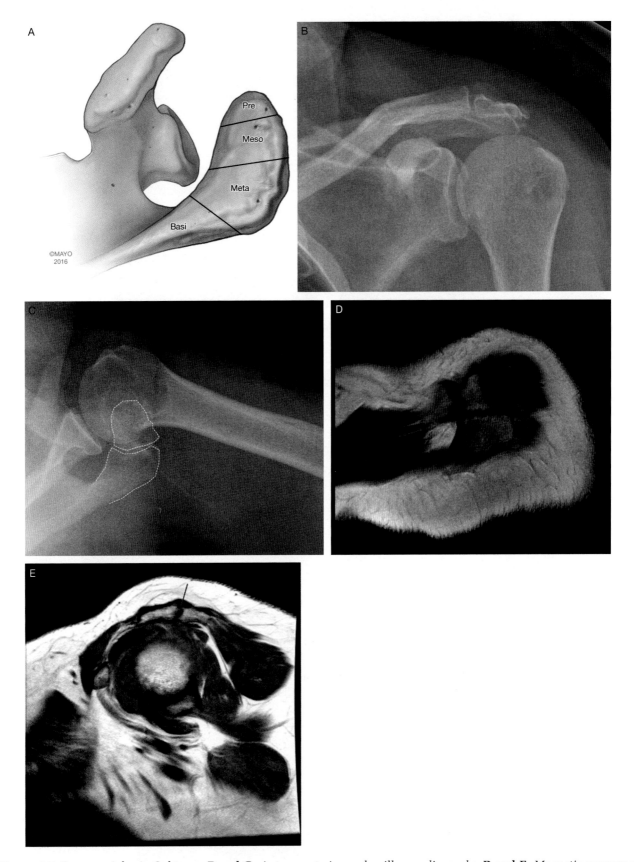

Figure 6.7 *Os acromiale.* **A,** *Subtypes.* **B and C,** *Anteroposterior and axillary radiographs.* **D and E,** *Magnetic resonance imaging. Red line indicates the location of synchondrosis.*

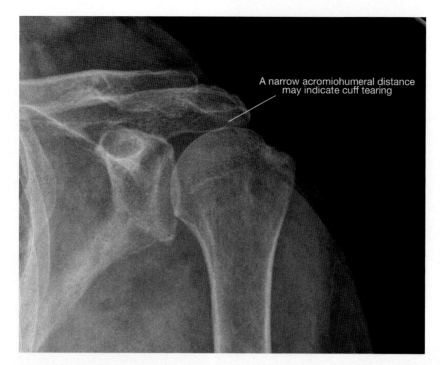

Figure 6.8 *Plain radiograph shows proximal migration, subacromial spur, tuberosity changes, and acromioclavicular joint degeneration.*

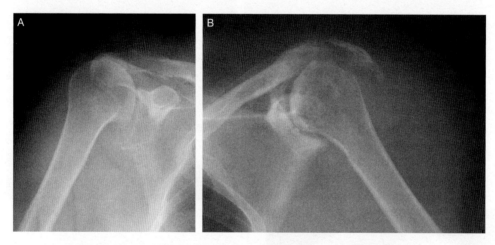

Figure 6.9 *Radiographs showing cuff tear arthropathy.* **A,** *Precollapse.* **B,** *After collapse.*

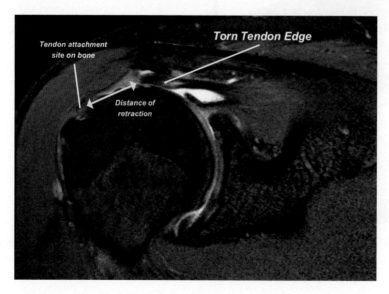

Figure 6.10 *Magnetic resonance imaging of a full-thickness tear.*

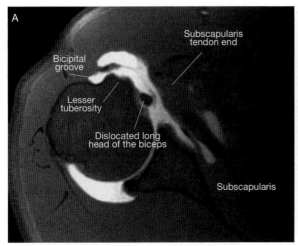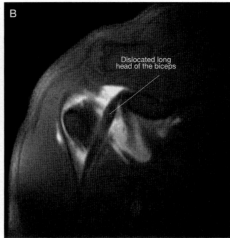

Figure 6.11 *Magnetic resonance imaging of a subscapularis tear.* **A,** *Axial cut.* **B,** *Coronal cut. Note dislocation of the tendon of the long head of the biceps.*

recommendations, as well as planning when surgery is considered.

Supraspinatus tears are best identified in coronal cuts. Tears of the subscapularis, infraspinatus, and teres minor are best identified in axial cuts. Full-thickness tears of the subscapularis tendon are commonly associated with dislocation of the long head of the biceps tendon off the bicipital groove (Figure 6.11). The subscapularis tendon may tear in continuity; MRI will show an excessively long tendon. Parasagittal cuts are useful to understand the true extent of the tear from anterior to posterior: a U-shaped tear may seem extremely retracted and unfixable in the coronal cut though the apex of the U, but will look more amenable to repair by margin convergence when analyzed in the parasagittal plane (Figure 6.12). Rarely, rotator cuff tendon tears occur at the muscle-tendon junction. The infraspinatus seems to be particularly prone to this tear pattern, which can be easily missed (9). It is best identified as a bright gap at the muscle-tendon junction posteriorly in the axial and parasagittal cuts (Figure 6.13).

Muscle Bulk, Fatty Infiltration, and Atrophy As discussed previously, chronic tendon ruptures lead to secondary

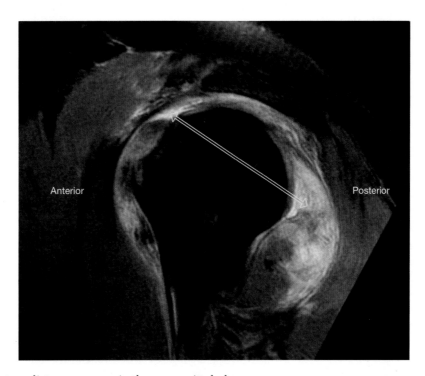

Figure 6.12 *Cuff rupture distance as seen in the parasagittal plane.*

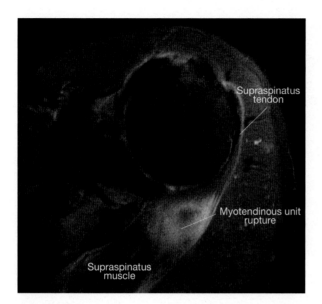

Figure 6.13 *Tear of the infraspinatus at the muscle-tendon junction.*

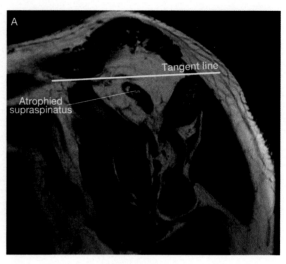

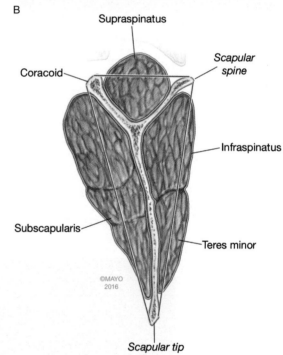

Figure 6.14 *Muscle retraction and atrophy, tangent line.* **A,** *Magnetic resonance imaging.* **B,** *Anatomical tangent lines.*

changes in the muscle (32). There is some confusion about terminology. Since muscles are fusiform, muscle retraction after tendon rupture will lead to a narrower cross-section in the parasaggital plane (Figure 6.14). Thus, muscle atrophy is oftentimes overestimated. When the bulk of muscle seen on MRI is decreased secondary to either retraction or atrophy, the empty portions of the fossae are seen as filled with fatty and connective tissue; this is not what we call fatty infiltration. Fatty infiltration is an increase in the relative content of fat *inside the muscle body*, seen as streaks of brighter signal (Figure 6.15) (33). Most of the assessments described later are performed on the most parasagittal image where the scapular spine is in contact with the scapular body.

The importance of fatty infiltration was first recognized using CT (Goutallier system) (24), but is now more commonly assessed on MRI (Fuchs-Gerber system) (23) (Table 6.4). On the other hand, rotator cuff atrophy can be quantified with the occupation ratio, defined as the ratio of the surface area of the muscle over the surface area of the corresponding fossa (33). A ratio of 1.0 to 0.6 is normal or slight atrophy, 0.4 to 0.6 moderate, and under 0.4 severe atrophy. Decreased supraspinatus muscle bulk may be assessed using the so-called tangent lines (33,34) (Figure 6.14B): if the muscle bulk is under lines tangent to specific scapular landmarks, it indicates moderate to severe atrophy. These lines are drawn from the edge of the coracoid to the scapular spine for the supraspinatus, from the edge of the coracoid to the inferior scapular tip for the subscapularis, and from the scapular spine to the inferior scapular tip for the infraspinatus and teres minor. Normal muscles are convex above these lines, in mild atrophy the muscle contour is at the lines, in moderate atrophy it is

under the lines, and in severe atrophy there is barely any muscle visible.

Ultrasonography

Ultrasonographic evaluation of the rotator cuff has become the standard of care in many practices (Table 6.5) (31,33). Some orthopedic surgeons have learned to use ultrasonography evaluation in the office. The goals of the evaluation are similar to those of MRI, mainly, identify the presence of partial-thickness and full-thickness tears and associated pathology. Ultrasonography offers a dynamic evaluation and allows comparison with the contralateral side, as well

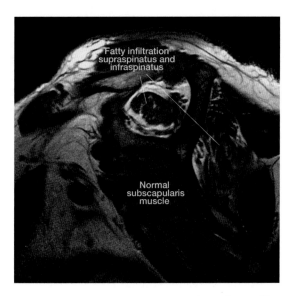

Figure 6.15 Magnetic resonance imaging shows fatty infiltration.

as relatively easy assessment of the shoulder at multiple time points.

Computed Tomography
When MRI is contraindicated (i.e., patients with certain implanted metallic objects) and ultrasonography is not available, CT can be used to assess the rotator cuff for both tears and atrophy. Intra-articular injection of iodine contrast (CT arthrogram) provides better images for evaluation of the rotator cuff.

Arthrogram
Prior to the generalized use of CT, MRI, or ultrasonography, arthrograms were commonly used. They provide only a yes/no answer: if contrast injected under radiographic or fluoroscopic control into the glenohumeral joint leaks into the subacromial space, the diagnosis of a full-thickness rotator cuff tear is established. Capsular contracture and synovitis can also be identified as a joint space with

Table 6.5 • Advantages and Disadvantages of Ultrasonography in the Evaluation of the Rotator Cuff

Advantages
Less expensive
No radiation
Allows dynamic assessment
Allows easy comparison with contralateral side
Facilitates diagnostic injections

Disadvantages
Extremely operator dependent
Difficult to interpret by a secondary observer from static images
Less useful for evaluation of muscle, bone, and cartilage

very small capacity or irregular outline of the intra-articular contrast, respectively.

Concise Alphanumeric Coding
Once the anticipated structural pathology is known, it can be summarized using the concise alphanumeric code proposed by Lafosse et al. (35) (Table 6.6). For example, the code D- AC 3 BP 320 would mean that when the patient was evaluated, there was acromioclavicular joint osteoarthritis, a tear of the upper two-thirds of the subscapularis, a pathologic biceps, and a tear of the supraspinatus to the level of the glenoid and the infraspinatus to the level of the humeral head. The code D ACr 0 BT 100 would mean that surgery included resection of the acromioclavicular joint, biceps tenodesis, and a complete repair of the subscapularis and infraspinatus but an incomplete repair of the supraspinatus with minimal retraction.

Other
The evaluation of patients with rotator cuff disease may need to be completed using diagnostic injections or EMG/nerve conduction studies. Diagnostic injections are discussed in chapter 12, Rehabilitation and Injections. Nerve compression syndromes involving the rotator cuff are discussed later.

Table 6.4 • Classification of Fatty Infiltration in Rotator Cuff Disease

Goutallier Classification[a]		Fuchs-Gerber Classification[b]	
Grade 0	Normal muscle	Normal	No fat to minimal intramuscular fat
Grade 1	Some fatty streaks		
Grade 2	Less than 50% fatty muscle infiltration	Moderate	Less fat than muscle
Grade 3	50% fatty muscle infiltration	Advanced	Equal amounts of fat and muscle or more fat than muscle
Grade 4	More than 50% fatty muscle infiltration		

[a] Based on computed tomography scan.
[b] The magnetic resonance imaging assessment is based on the most lateral parasagittal image where the scapular spine is in contact with the scapular body.
Data from Fuchs et al. (23) and Goutallier et al. (24).

Table 6.6 • Alphanumeric Coding for Patients With Rotator Cuff Pathology

Side	R – Right
	L – Left
Date	D- Consultation
	D Surgery date, observed pathology
	D+ Surgery performed
	+xW – weeks postop
	+xY – years postop
Acromioclavicular joint	AC – Osteoarthritis
	ACr – Surgical resection
Subscapularis	0 – Normal
	1 – Upper third partial
	2 – Upper third full thickness
	3 – Upper two-thirds
	4 – Complete tear, fatty infiltration 1–3
	5 – Complete tear, fatty infiltration >3, eccentric
Long head of the biceps	BN – Biceps normal
	BP – Biceps pathologic
	BA – Biceps absent or tenotomized
	BT – Biceps tenodesis
	BY – Biceps "tenodesis" in Y
Supraspinatus	0 – Normal
Infraspinatus	1 – Nonretracted
Teres minor	2 – Retracted to mid head level
	3 – Retracted to glenoid

Treatment

Rotator cuff disease may present at so many different stages that the treating orthopedic surgeon must be ready to consider multiple treatment options (Figure 6.16). Treatment recommendations are quite different for partial versus full-thickness tears, as well as for acute versus chronic tears.

Symptomatic partial thickness tears merit a program of nonoperative treatment almost universally; surgery can always be considered if a good program of nonoperative treatment fails (36). It is important to exclude and treat other possible associated problems and to follow patients over time not to miss "silent" extension of a high-grade partial thickness tear to a full-thickness tear.

Treatment of acute, traumatic, full-thickness tears is straightforward; most patients benefit from an attempted tendon repair as soon as possible (37). Healing is quite predictable in the acute setting even if the tendon tear is large and retracted. The key is to make sure that the patient presents a truly acute tear as opposed to an acute extension of a chronic tear (were there symptoms before the index injury? Is there atrophy and fatty infiltration?) (38).

Chronic full-thickness tears are most common, and decision-making is much more complicated. In fact, evidence-based treatment algorithms seem to guide toward avoiding surgery more often than not (39). In my practice, this is the central question I try to answer for patients with a chronic full-thickness tear: *What are the chances that I can*

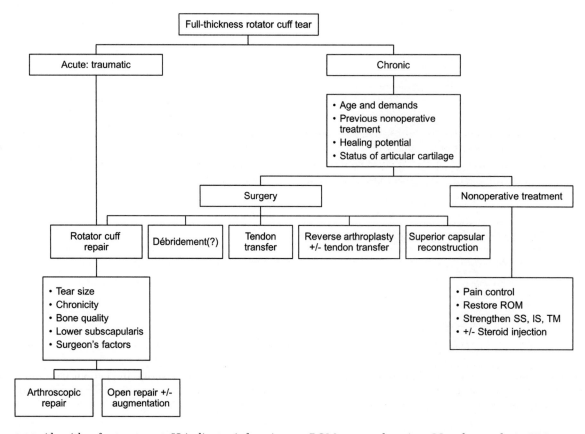

Figure 6.16 *Algorithm for treatment. IS indicates infraspinatus; ROM, range of motion; SS, subscapularis; TM, teres minor.*

repair the tear with some degree of confidence that the tendon will heal?

That is such a hard question to answer! A full-thickness tear affecting only the supraspinatus in a younger patient with no risk factors for incomplete healing is easy: surgical repair will likely work. A full-thickness tear affecting the whole supraspinatus and infraspinatus with substantial fatty infiltration in a 75-year-old smoker is also easy: tendon repair should probably be avoided. The problem is that most patients fall into a "grey area" where many factors must be considered by the surgeon before establishing a treatment plan.

If the answer to my initial question is "yes," I tend to offer surgical repair. It is important to emphasize that offering surgery in these circumstances without a trial of nonoperative treatment is not widely accepted. There is an important distinction between *offering* and *recommending* surgery. Surgery is strongly recommended for patients with an acute traumatic tear. Surgery is offered as a good option for patients with a chronic fixable tear provided they understand 4 important factors outlined below.

Tendon healing does not seem to occur in 20% to 25% of the patients undergoing surgery. Recovery time is slow. A trial of 3 months of nonoperative treatment is unlikely to change the chances of success much for a given patient if surgery is eventually undertaken. Advanced imaging studies should be repeated in a few months to a year to avoid missing "silent" extension of the cuff tear if nonoperative treatment is selected.

If the answer to my question is "no" (in my hands, the tendon tear is unlikely to be fixable, or there are substantial negative factors for tendon healing), conservative treatment is again warranted prior to considering salvage procedures, which range from débridement to tendon transfers or reverse shoulder arthroplasty. The exception may be the patient with a massive irreparable rotator cuff tear and pseudoparalysis, as well as the patient with end-stage cuff-tear arthropathy; in these circumstances, conservative treatment is unlikely to be successful, and reverse shoulder arthroplasty may be offered without a trial of nonoperative treatment.

Nonoperative Treatment

Not uncommonly, I see individuals with rotator cuff disease who should respond to nonoperative treatment and do not respond: the patient states that physical therapy made the shoulder worse. The importance of using an adequate program of physical therapy cannot be overemphasized, as for many of these patients the program used was not ideal. The goals of nonoperative treatment include alleviating pain; treating associated stiffness; strengthening the subscapularis, infraspinatus, and teres minor; and addressing associated scapular dyskinesia (when present) (40–42).

Pain

Use of acetaminophen and/or nonsteroidal anti-inflamatory drugs represents the first line of pain relief for patients with cuff disease. Use of narcotic pain medications is not recommended. Local injection of corticosteroids in the subacromial space can be very effective in alleviating pain, at least on a temporary basis (see chapter 12, Rehabilitation and Injections). Empirically, it is recommended to consider 1 to 3 subacromial corticosteroid injections; multiple injections have the potential to weaken tendon fibers further. Injection of a soluble nonsteroidal drug may be considered as well, although it is perceived to be less effective.

Stiffness

A subset of patients with a chronic rotator cuff tear develops secondary stiffness. Physical examination in the office reveals restriction not only of active but also of passive motion, most commonly elevation. Stretching exercises, once pain is somewhat controlled, are the next step of the physical therapy program.

Strengthening

Chronic rotator cuff tears commonly involve the supraspinatus tendon. As the patient tries to elevate the arm, the vector of the deltoid muscle would tend to shear the humeral head on the glenoid superiorly and cause it to migrate toward the supraspinatus defect. In addition, the capacity of the rotator cuff to keep the head centered is compromised by the tear. In these circumstances, strengthening of elevation would make the deltoid relatively stronger than the remaining rotator cuff and worsen symptoms. For these reasons, selective strengthening of the inferior cuff seems to be more beneficial, as the vectors of the subscapularis and external rotators opposes superior translation of the humeral head.

A good way to block deltoid activation during strengthening is to have the patient actively adduct the shoulder by keeping a magazine or folded towel under the armpit (Figure 6.17). With the shoulders in this position, the inferior cuff is strengthened with isometrics in internal and external rotation followed by elastic band training, again in internal and external rotation. In addition, scapular stabilizing exercises are added if needed (see chapter 12, Rehabilitation and Injections).

Acromioplasty/Débridement

Although removal of subacromial spurs and bone and cuff débridement were described as open procedures, currently these procedures are performed arthroscopically almost universally. This procedure is considered on 2 ends of the spectrum of injury severity: the patient with impingement and tendinopathy or a partial-thickness tear, and selected patients with an irreparable tear.

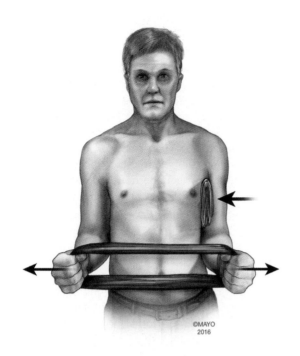

Figure 6.17 Performing exercises with a magazine under the armpit.

Acromioplasty for Impingement

Arthroscopic acromioplasty is considered for patients with well-defined chronic subacromial impingement and either tendinopathy or a partial thickness tear involving, at most, 50% to 60% of the tendon thickness (if the partial tear involves 70% to 90% of the thickness, a tendon repair is probably best). Patients should be carefully selected for this procedure only after failure of a good program of nonoperative treatment (43). The 3 most common reasons for poor outcome after arthroscopic subacromial decompression are performing an acromioplasty for the wrong diagnosis (e.g., labral and biceps pathology, acromioclavicular joint osteoarthritis, mild glenohumeral osteoarthritis), failure to address associated pathology (i.e., a high-grade, partial-thickness rotator cuff tear), and incomplete bone removal. I tend not to offer an acromioplasty to patients who have not experienced improvement of most of their pain with a subacromial corticosteroid injection for at least a few days.

The procedure starts with an arthroscopic evaluation of the glenohumeral joint in order to identify associated pathology at the labrum, biceps, articular cartilage, capsule, and articular side of the rotator cuff and, the pathology is treated accordingly. When a partial thickness tear is identified, an arthroscopic shaver is used to remove torn, loose fibers; if arthroscopic assessment reveals that the tear might involve more than half the thickness of the tendon, the location of the area of tendon damage is marked with sutures (typically #1 PDS) for identification of the same area

from the subacromial space. After the intra-articular portion of the procedure is completed, the arthroscopic camera is redirected to the subacromial space from a posterior portal, and a subtotal bursectomy is followed by removal of bone from the anteriorinferior acromion with an arthroscopic bur (Figure 6.18). Portals may be switched to visualize from the lateral portal and work from the posterior portal, confirming that the slope of the spine of the scapula continues anteriorly without any residual prominent inferior bone. The cuff is then assessed for treatment of partial thickness tearing with débridement or repair if needed. If no cuff repair is necessary, I typically will inject the subacromial space with steroids prior to closure. After surgery, patients use a sling for comfort for 1 or 2 weeks and most recover motion without dedicated physical therapy.

Débridement for Irreparable Cuff Tears

Patients with large tears that are deemed not repairable are commonly considered for either repair with augmentation, tendon transfers, or a reverse shoulder arthroplasty. However, in selected elderly, low-demand patients who complain mostly of pain and have good active motion, tendon débridement with bursectomy and acromioplasty may be considered (44). Patients must understand that the procedure is unpredictable, although much less involved than the alternatives. The procedure seems to be especially helpful in patients who present with an irreparable cuff but an intact biceps; performing a biceps tenotomy or tenodesis in these patients helps with pain relief (see Biceps Tendon Pathology later). If the rotator cuff tear is found to have irregular flaps, they are regularized at the time of surgery as well.

Tendon Repair

Rotator cuff repair is one of the most commonly performed procedures in orthopedic surgery and can be performed with open or arthroscopic techniques. In selected patients, the procedure is associated with surgery on the biceps tendon, acromioclavicular joint, suprascapular nerve, or an associated os acromiale. Tendon augmentation with allograft or synthetic materials may be considered to cover residual gaps in incomplete repairs.

Cuff repair should always start with assessment of passive glenohumeral motion under anesthesia. As mentioned previously, a subset of patients with chronic tears will develop stiffness. Failure to restore a complete arc of motion at the time of surgery may lead to an unsuccessful outcome, despite complete tendon healing. If the patient is noted to be stiff in the office and stiffness is confirmed under anesthesia, options include closed manipulation of the shoulder prior to starting the cuff repair, or an arthroscopic capsular release (see chapter 8, Adhesive Capsulitis) (45). For patients with severe stiffness and a cuff tear, some surgeons prefer to stage the procedures, performing surgery to restore motion first, and delaying the cuff repair until motion has

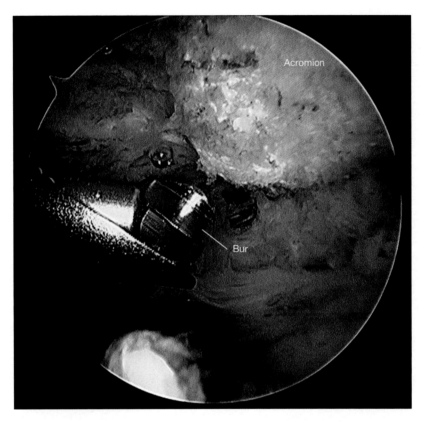

Figure 6.18 *Arthroscopic acromioplasty.*

been restored. This is due to the fact that therapy programs after contracture release and tendon repair are opposite, and also to the fact that the healing response, which is desired to occur after cuff repair, may end up contributing to recurrent loss of motion.

Open Repair

The 3 goals of open cuff repair are preparation of the bone surfaces (of the cuff footprint on the tuberosities) to enhance healing, cuff mobilization to restore normal excursion, and secure anchoring of tendon to bone (46). There is some variation among surgeons in terms of exposure and cuff repair techniques (⊙ Video 6.1).

Skin Incision My preference is to use a so-called *cup de sabre* (saber cut) incision starting just lateral to the acromioclavicular joint and extending laterally and distally about 5 to 6 cm (see Superior Approach in chapter 3, Shoulder Exposures). This incision can easily be extended distally into the deltopectoral interval if needed (Figure 6.19A). Others prefer an incision along Langer lines more parallel to the parasagittal plane.

Deltoid Management Meticulous deltoid detachment and repair is paramount for the outcome of rotator cuff repair: iatrogenic deltoid damage or postoperative deltoid dehiscence will lead to a poor outcome, is difficult

to repair, and might compromise the option of a reverse arthroplasty later. My preference is to detach the deltoid from the anterior and lateral margins of the acromion and split through the muscle fibers of the anterior portion of the deltoid (Figure 6.19B); this allows easy exposure posteriorly by detaching more and more deltoid from the lateral acromion and the spine of the scapula (if needed), as well as anteriorly by merging into the deltopectoral interval. Other surgeons prefer to detach the deltoid only off of the anterior acromion and continue splitting at the raphe between the anterior and middle deltoid. Care must be taken not to extend this lateral split beyond 5 cm approximately in order to avoid injury to the axillary nerve, which would result in denervation of the anterior deltoid. Regardless of the detachment technique, a secure reattachment through bone is extremely important at the end of the case.

Tendon Repair The areas of bone where the tendon end will be reattached are cleaned of fibrous tissue. A rongeur or bur is then used to create a bleeding surface without weakening the bone. Cysts encountered in these locations may be curetted and bone grafted. The cuff is then mobilized with use of traction sutures by dividing adhesions on the bursal side and occasionally on the articular side. The pattern of tear is then analyzed. Some tears are best repaired only to bone (small to medium U tears), whereas

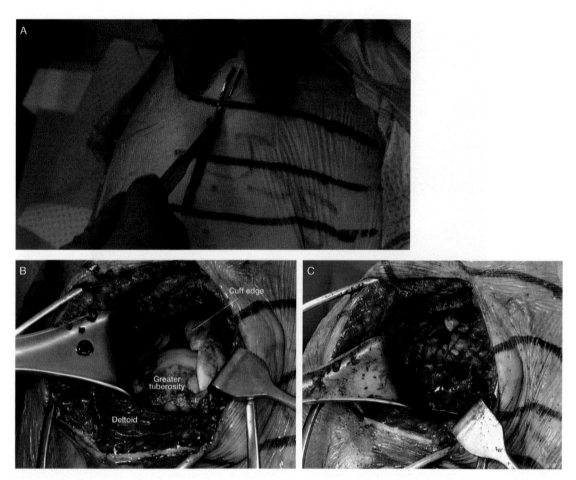

Figure 6.19 *Open cuff repair.* **A,** *Skin incision.* **B,** *Deltoid detachment.* **C,** *Repaired cuff.*

L-shaped tears and larger U tears benefit from use of so-called margin convergence sutures prior to reattachment to bone.

For tendon to bone fixation, my preference is to use simple transosseous sutures that start at the articular margin and exit laterally (Figure 6.19C). This suture configuration uses large bone tunnels and really compresses the tendon to bone. Other surgeons prefer to use a Mason-Allen suture configuration, with the 2 limbs of the suture exiting laterally; this technique provides better tendon grasp but leaves smaller bone tunnels that could fracture and does not compress tendon to bone as much. Alternatively, suture anchors may be used through an open approach as described in the following text for arthroscopic repairs, but I find it difficult to justify the extra cost of using suture anchors in open surgery.

Arthroscopic Repair

Major improvements in arthroscopic instrumentation and implants have translated into the possibility of achieving excellent outcomes when cuff repair is performed arthroscopically (◯ Video 6.2) (47–53). Arthroscopic repair of larger tendon tears is still a difficult procedure,

though, and conversion to an open procedure may be necessary when difficulties are encountered. Many surgeons feel frustrated when they need to abandon the arthroscopic attempt and expose the cuff using open techniques, but it is better to convert to an open procedure than to let the patient leave the operating room with a poor repair. A surgical technique cannot violate a surgical principle. Thus, the principles of arthroscopic cuff repair are the same as those of open cuff repair: prepare the bone surface, mobilize the cuff, and securely anchor the cuff to bone.

The procedure starts in the glenohumeral joint. The articular cartilage, biceps, and labrum are assessed and addressed, if needed. If the patient has stiffness, a contracture release may be performed. The extent of cuff tearing is then assessed. Sutures inserted percutaneously with use of a needle across the subacromial space may be placed in order to mark the location of the tear; this is extremely important for high-grade, partial thickness tears treated with completion of the detachment and repair of the tendon (Figure 6.20).

For the repair itself, my preference is to establish a posterolateral subacromial portal for visualization and a lateral subacromial portal to start the bursectomy. Extensive

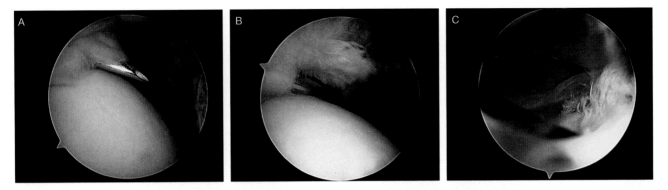

Figure 6.20 *Suture marking of partial thickness tears.* **A,** *Needle marking.* **B,** *Suture marking from the joint.* **C,** *Identifying sutures at the subacromial space.*

removal of bursal tissue is very important for arthroscopic repair. It aids not only with tendon mobilization but also with adequate visualization. Once this step is completed, cuff excursion and tendon tear pattern are assessed. It is useful to assess the tear not only from the posterior view but also from the lateral view, by switching portals. Most repairs require tendon to bone fixation; in many shoulders, tendon-to-tendon sutures are also necessary (margin-convergence sutures). The value of changing the position of the shoulder for various portions of the repair cannot be overemphasized.

Tendon to bone fixation may be performed using transosseous sutures or suture anchors. There are 3 broad categories of arthroscopic tendon to bone cuff repair: single-row repair, double-row repair, and transosseous sutures (Figure 6.21) (48,49). In single-row repairs, anchors are typically placed centered in the tuberosity from lateral to medial, and the cuff is attached in a relatively narrow area of bone. In double-row repairs, anchors are placed in 2 locations: medial anchors are placed close to the articular cartilage, and sutures or tapes passed through tendon are anchored in a second row of lateral anchors, leading to a wider area of tendon to bone attachment. The third alternative is to use transosseous sutures instead of anchors (54). Biomechanically, double-row and transosseous repairs provide a stronger construct and, in addition, compress the tendon across a larger area of bone. Most studies have not been able to demonstrate differences in clinical outcomes when compared with single-row repairs (48,49). My preference is to perform a double-row repair, except for those patients with a very retracted tear that will not have enough excursion to reach the whole tuberosity area (Figure 6.22).

Arthroscopic repair of tears involving the subscapularis can be more difficult (51,55) (● Video 6.3). Adequate visualization of the lesser tuberosity and subscapularis identification and mobilization can be challenging. In addition, the lower third of the subscapularis is muscular and may provide less suture-holding power. Planning for arthroscopic repair of a subscapularis tear includes identification of the superolateral corner of the subscapularis (so-called "comma tissue," since it looks like a comma sign when seen from

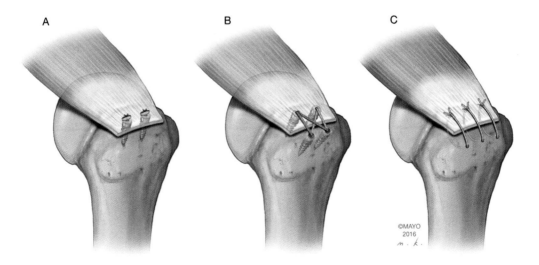

Figure 6.21 *Tendon-to-bone cuff repair.* **A,** *Single row.* **B,** *Double row.* **C,** *Transosseous.*

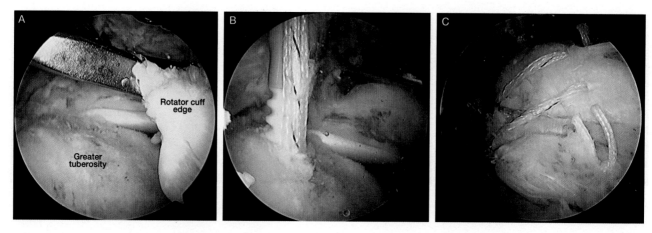

Figure 6.22 *Arthroscopic photographs of a double-row repair.* **A,** *Cuff mobilization.* **B,** *Anchor placement.* **C,** *Completed repair.*

a posterior intra-articular portal); preparation of the lesser tuberosity and anchor placement visualized from the gle-nohumeral joint; posterior displacement of the proximal humerus by an assistant, use of a 70° arthroscope; and use of anterior subacromial portals. Most surgeons repair tears of the upper one-third of the subscapularis looking through the intra-articular portal and tears of the upper two-thirds or entire subscapularis looking through an anterior subacromial portal.

Associated Procedures
Acromioplasty When open cuff repair techniques were developed, bone removal from the anteroinferior acromion was performed almost universally. As open and arthroscopic techniques evolved, some questioned the added value of performing an acromioplasty, and most comparative studies have failed to show a difference (16). Benefits of acromioplasty include removal of impinging bone, a larger space to work during the repair, and the potential from a bleeding bone surface to provide a local postoperative hematoma that might carry beneficial cells and growth factors. Disadvantages of acromioplasty include longer operating time and increased bony bleeding, which might impair visualization during arthroscopic surgery. My preference is to perform an acromioplasty in almost all patients undergoing cuff repair, the exception being acute traumatic tears involving only the subscapularis.

Biceps As discussed previously, the biceps and labrum may contribute to pain in some patients with a full-thickness rotator cuff (6). The rate of associated procedures on the biceps has increased over time. This is partly due to the fact that the biceps tendon can be assessed more carefully (and, many times, looks worse than expected) with arthroscopic techniques, and also to the fact that in some anterosuperior tears, removing the biceps facilitates arthroscopic cuff repair. Most substantial subscapularis tears are

associated with biceps tendon subluxation or dislocation. My indications for addressing the biceps surgically at the time of cuff repair include clear biceps symptoms during preoperative physical examination; a partially torn, subluxed, or dislocated biceps; and repair of tears involving the subscapularis. The roles of tenotomy versus tenodesis when addressing the tendon of the long head of the biceps are discussed later.

Acromioclavicular Joint As mentioned previously, acromioclavicular joint arthritis is very commonly seen on radiographs of patients with cuff pathology. When symptomatic, the acromioclavicular joint is addressed by resecting the distal end of the clavicle (56,57). My impression is that the rate of distal clavicle resections performed in the setting of cuff repair is excessive, since many patients do not have symptoms when this particular joint is examined. Resection of the distal end of the clavicle is discussed further in chapter 5, The Clavicle, the Acromioclavicular Joint, and the Sternoclavicular Joint.

Suprascapular Nerve As discussed at the beginning of this chapter, some believe that retracted posterosuperior tears lead to secondary suprascapular neuropathy and advocate release of the suprascapular ligament in some patients (25,26). In my practice, I consider electromyographic evaluation of the cuff and nerve conduction studies when the amount of weakness and atrophy are disproportionate to the size and chronicity of the tear, and consider adding an arthroscopic decompression of the suprascapular nerve if these tests confirm neurologic abnormalities. The details of suprascapular nerve decompression are discussed later.

Augmentation
Addition of structural material to augment the rotator cuff tissue has been considered by some, especially when a repair is attempted and either the tissue quality is poor

or a complete repair cannot be accomplished. Various authors have reported use of synthetic materials or allograft (58). Some animal-derived synthetic materials have been associated with an unacceptable rate of adverse effects and poor outcomes. The outcome of augmentation is likely very different when the structural material is used to thicken a complete repair versus bridging an incomplete repair. In my practice, I do use Achilles tendon allograft augmentation for chronic subscapularis tears, and also to extend tendon length at the time of a transfer if needed (see later). I also consider using it when I attempt a repair of a posterosuperior tear and it is not possible to seal the joint otherwise. The published outcome of cuff augmentation has been very variable, and its use has decreased with improved tendon transfers and reverse arthroplasty.

Os Acromiale Management

Indications Management of the os acromiale at the time of cuff repair is very controversial. Some surgeons completely ignore it on every single occasion. I consider acting surgically on the os acromiale if I suspect it contributes to the patient's symptoms, or if it is found to dynamically impinge on the cuff at the time of surgery (59). Ideally, I want to confirm that the patient has pain with direct inferior pressure over the ununited anterior acromion. Diagnostic injections with local anesthesia into the synchondrosis may be considered. Ultimately, os mobility and dynamic impingement are assessed intraoperatively.

Techniques Resection of the united fragment and primary reattachment of the deltoid origin to the remaining acromion is considered only for small fragments (pre os acromiale); resection of a larger portion of acromion may lead to substantial deltoid weakness and facilitate anterosuperior escape if the cuff repair were to fail. Internal fixation is preferred for larger fragments (meso os acromiale). Fixation may be attempted with wires or screws with or without additional tension band wiring. A final alternative is to perform an acromioplasty and ignore the os acromiale; this is difficult if the os is very mobile (59–62).

When an open cuff repair is performed and the os acromiale is planned to be fixed, my preference is to take down the synchondrosis as part of the exposure (treating the os acromiale as if it were an acromion osteotomy). When the cuff is repaired arthroscopically, fixation of the os acromiale can be attempted percutaneously under arthroscopic visualization, or it can be performed through a dedicated superior exposure (Figure 6.23). Percutaneous fixation is more attractive, but it makes it more difficult to remove fibrous tissue and cartilage at the synchondrosis or to add bone grafting, and it does not allow adding tension band wiring. My current preference is to use percutaneous cannulated screws without tension band wiring at the time of arthroscopic repair; tension band wiring is added if the acromion is too thin for screw fixation (wire fixation does probably

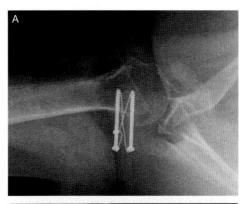

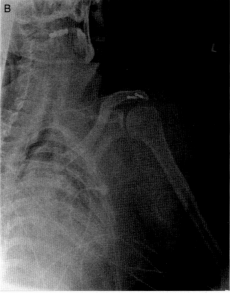

Figure 6.23 *Open reduction and internal fixation (ORIF) of os acromiale.* **A,** *Tension band.* **B,** *Percutaneous screws.*

require additional tension band wiring) or if the cuff repair is performed open. Suture fixation of the bone fragments in a tension band configuration without supplemental wire or screw fixation can also be considered.

Outcomes The added value of fixing or resecting an os acromiale at the time of cuff repair is difficult to tease out, since the overall outcome is also determined by the success or failure of cuff repair. The few studies that have analyzed this topic report that satisfactory outcomes can be achieved in most patients, solid union is not universally achieved, and some patients experience adverse effects related to the hardware used for fixation (e.g., wires can actually migrate and require removal, especially in the absence of an associated tension band) (59–62).

Postoperative Management

A dedicated program of physical therapy is very important for the success of rotator cuff repair (63,64). During the early postoperative phase, protection takes precedence over motion. The program should be individualized to each patient based on the appearance of the repair at the end of the procedure, as well as tendon and bone quality and compliance. Safe ranges of motion during the first few weeks after surgery are determined intraoperatively by recording the extent of motion in each direction that does not seem to compromise the repair. Motion is limited in different directions depending on the tear pattern: tears involving the subscapularis require limiting external rotation and elevation, whereas tears involving the infraspinatus and teres minor require limiting internal rotation.

Although the physical therapy program must be individualized, my general protocol of physical therapy either starts with no motion or passive shoulder motion for the first 6 weeks after the procedure. At that time point, provided there are no surprises during physical examination, patients start active assisted range-of-motion exercises with stretching, adding isometrics at week 10 and elastic bands at week 12. Active use of the elbow, wrist, and hand is encouraged early on, although active elbow flexion may need to be limited in patients with an associated biceps tenodesis. Avoidance of motion is particularly common after arthroscopic cuff repair, but differences in outcome based on when to initiate passive motion have been difficult to prove. I do avoid shoulder motion for the first 6 weeks after repair of a very large tear and in patients with poor bone quality. Individual exercises are covered in more detail in chapter 12, Rehabilitation and Injections.

Results

The results of rotator cuff repair are difficult to interpret (47–49,65–69). This is due partly to changes in technique over time (especially after the introduction of arthroscopic techniques), the wide range of pathology (tear pattern, size, chronicity, associated pathology, patient-related factors), and the striking lack of correlation in some studies between rates of confirmed tendon healing and clinical outcomes. A complete summary of the outcomes of tendon repair exceeds the scope of this book, but I will summarize some useful information.

Clinical Results With the information currently available, it is fair to say that rotator cuff repair leads to improved patient-reported outcomes in approximately 85% of the patients. Interestingly, some patients will experience improved clinical outcomes in the absence of tendon healing. The mean improvement in scores is approximately 75% of normal. Age does not seem to correlate with clinical outcomes.

Tendon Healing Rates Approximately 20% to 25% of rotator cuff repairs do not heal, as evidenced by areas of tendon discontinuity on advanced imaging studies. Tendon healing does not correlate with most patient-reported outcomes, but leads to worse strength. Lack of tendon healing correlates with age, tear size, and fatty infiltration, and (as

noted before) there seem to be a few additional risk factors that decrease the chances of tendon healing (Table 6.3).

Tendon Tear Size and Clinical Outcome Even though it has been difficult to demonstrate a correlation between clinical results and tendon healing, there is a clear correlation between tendon tear size and clinical outcome. Patients with smaller tendon tears have a higher risk of stiffness. With open surgery, clinical outcomes clearly correlate with tendon tear size: repair of a small, medium, large, and massive tear was associated with a successful clinical outcome in 95%, 85%, 70%, and 30% of the shoulders, respectively; the exception is the acute tear.

A word of caution is required regarding patients with a large or massive cuff tear, severe pain, and good motion: an attempt to repair the rotator cuff in these circumstances is successful in improving pain in most patients, but some may end up losing motion, likely as a result of a change in force-couple balance with incomplete tendon healing.

Biologic Enhancement of Healing Since the rates of tendon healing have not improved over time despite the development of better repair techniques, it is felt that further improvement in the management of patients with a rotator cuff tear will require biologic techniques to enhance healing. Unfortunately, most attempts to date have not clearly demonstrated improved clinical outcomes or healing rates (12,70–72). Different researchers have used local administration of individual growth factors, a blood clot, platelet-rich plasma, stem cells, and other strategies. At this point, the best practical way to enhance healing seems to be avoidance of known modifiable risk factors for healing, such as smoking.

Insertion of a resorbable spacer in the subacromial space represents another interesting thought to promote tendon healing, although there are very limited data to support its use. An inflatable balloon can be inserted arthroscopically in the subacromial space and expanded with saline. The material of the balloon is absorbable, so that theoretically it completely disappears in a few months. Although some surgeons use it in isolation, it makes more sense to me to use it as a complement to cuff repair in patients with preoperative proximal humeral head migration. The expanded balloon will help keep the humeral head centered and resist proximal humeral head migration while the cuff is healing. In addition, theoretically the balloon provides additional compression of the cuff to the footprint, which could also enhance healing.

Tendon Transfers

Transfer of a healthy muscle-tendon unit to compensate for the irreparable rotator cuff has been considered for a number of years. The field of tendon transfers for cuff disease has changed substantially over the past few years. On one hand, the availability and success of reverse shoulder arthroplasty (RSA) has made RSA the procedure of choice for a number of patients who were previously considered for tendon transfer. On the other hand, transfer of specific tendons has been successful in the hands of some surgeons and unsuccessful in the hands of others, creating the need to explore new alternatives.

Tendon transfers are considered for patients with an irreparable posterosuperior tear (supraspinatus and infraspinatus with or without extension into the teres minor) or an irreparable anterosuperior tear (a chronic subscapularis tear with various degrees of extension into the supraspinatus). Options for posterosuperior tears include transfer of the latissimus dorsi with or without the teres major, and transfer of the lower portion of the trapezius. Options for anterosuperior tears include transfer of the pectoralis major or anterior transfer of the latissimus dorsi. Some authors have considered transferring a portion of the deltoid. Comparative studies would be required in order to understand which of these transfers is best for each indication.

A prolonged period of protection and a tailored physical therapy program are paramount for the success of any of these transfers. For posterosuperior tears, the shoulder is immobilized in a fair amount of external rotation and some abduction using an external rotation brace. For anterosuperior tears, the shoulder is immobilized in internal rotation. Immobilization is maintained for 6 to 8 weeks, with either no motion or passive motion only to safe ranges as determined intraoperatively.

Latissimus Dorsi Transfer (or Latissimus Dorsi/Teres Major Transfer)

This tendon transfer was originally developed for posterosuperior tears (73), but currently there is some interest in using it for irreparable subscapularis tears (74).

Posterosuperior Tears There are some variations in terms of exposure, tendons transferred, and attachment location. The tendinous attachment of the latissimus dorsi and teres major on the humeral shaft is contiguous from proximal to distal; in some individuals it is difficult to separate the 2 tendons. Some authors transfer only the latissimus dorsi and some prefer to transfer both.

In terms of exposure, there are 2 options. The patient may be placed in the lateral position, so that the latissimus dorsi and teres major are harvested and mobilized using a posterior approach, tunneled under the deltoid and retrieved though a classic superior open rotator cuff deltoid splitting exposure (Figure 6.24) (73). Currently, there is interest in arthroscopically assisted techniques for latissimus dorsi transfer. For posterosuperior tears, the latissimus dorsi harvest is performed in the beach chair position through an axillary approach, and fixation is completed arthroscopically. Alternatively, the tendons can be harvested through a deltopectoral approach by dividing and later repairing the pectoralis major tendon; the tendons are then transferred around the humeral shaft and under the deltoid, as initially described for brachial plexus injuries

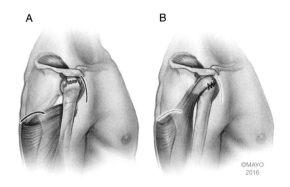

Figure 6.24 *Latissimus dorsi transfer through 2 incisions.*

(modified Sever-L'Episcopo procedure) (Figure 6.25) (75). This modality of tendon transfer is occasionally combined with a reverse arthroplasty in selected patients (see chapter 9, Shoulder Arthritis and Arthroplasty).

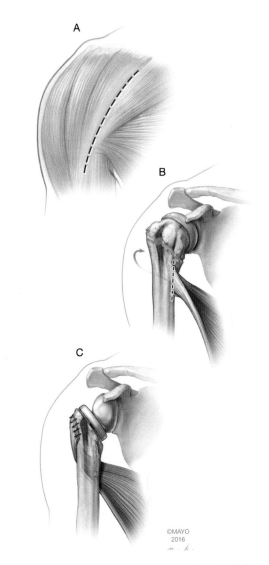

Figure 6.25 *Latissimus dorsi transfer through deltopectoral for posterior cuff in combination with a reverse prosthesis.*

Most descriptions of this tendon transfer for postero-superior tears recommend reattachment of the transferred tendons to the greater tuberosity using anchors or bone tunnels. The transferred tendons are also sutured to any intact subscapularis and any remaining posterosuperior cuff. In some patients, the tendon excursion does not allow reaching the tuberosity, and some have augmented the transfer with Achilles tendon allograft. Alternatively, the transferred tendons can be attached more distally on the lower part of the tuberosity and the humeral shaft, as initially described for the L'Episcopo procedure.

Results published using this procedure have been mixed. Some authors have reported satisfactory results even after 10 years of follow-up, whereas others have reported poor results and abandoned this procedure (73,75). A theoretical challenge with this transfer is that the latissimus dorsi and teres major are native internal rotators; EMG studies have failed to show that patients learn how to use them as external rotators after the transfer, and some argue that these tendons function more as a tenodesis or a vascularized graft providing healthy tissue as opposed to a dynamically active muscle-tendon unit. Results are worse for patients with no subscapularis and those with less than 90° of active elevation preoperatively. More distal transfers to the upper humeral shaft are expected to provide more gains in external rotation, whereas more proximal transfers close to the tuberosity are expected to improve both elevation and external rotation. Dedicated physical therapy and biofeedback training are very important for the success of this technique.

Subscapularis Tears Since the latissimus dorsi is an internal rotator and its line of action and location are so close to the subscapularis, recently some have explored the possibility of transferring the latissimus dorsi to compensate for an irreparable subscapularis (74). Using a deltopectoral approach, the latissimus dorsi can be harvested just distal to the lesser tuberosity and transferred superiorly. The line of pull of the transferred tendon should provide more power in internal rotation and also resist proximal humeral head migration (Figure 6.26). This transfer also can be completed with arthroscopically assisted techniques.

Lower Trapezius Transfer

The line of action of the lower portion of the trapezius is very close to the orientation of the infraspinatus and teres minor. Transfer of the lower trapezius has emerged as a very good alternative to transfer of the latissimus dorsi for posteriosuperior tears (76–78). This is especially useful for the uncommon isolated tear of the infraspinatus at the muscle-tendon junction, but can be successfully used for the salvage of chronic irreparable posterosuperior cuff tears.

The procedure may be performed with or without arthroscopic assistance. The open procedure is currently performed through 2 separate incisions (Figure 6.27). A more medial incision is used to harvest the lower trapezius by detaching it from the scapula; care must be taken to protect the neurovascular bundle, and removal of some bone from the medial aspect of the spine of the scapula may be necessary in order to avoid compression of the pedicle.

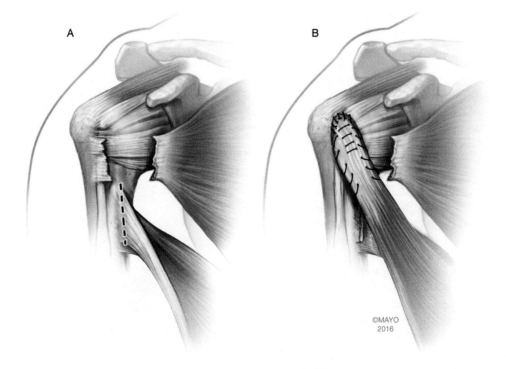

©MAYO
2016

Figure 6.26 Latissimus dorsi transfer through deltopectoral for subscapularis deficiency.

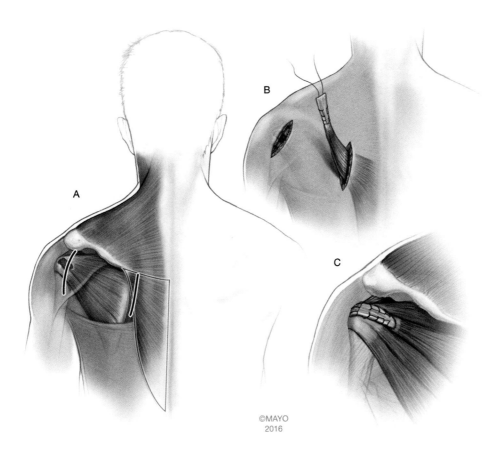

©MAYO
2016

Figure 6.27 *Lower trapezius transfer.*

The tendon is then tunneled under the skin and attached to the posterior aspect of the greater tuberosity or any remaining tendon still attached to the tuberosity in myotendinous tears. As with the latissimus dorsi, sometimes the tendon is not long enough and can be extended using an Achilles tendon allograft. Alternatively, the attachment of the Achilles tendon to the greater tuberosity may be performed arthroscopically (arthroscopically assisted lower trapezius transfer) (⊙ Video 6.4).

Some authors have expressed concerns about violating the lower trapezius due to the fact that trapezius dysfunction is associated with scapular dyskinesia (see chapters 1, Evaluation of the Shoulder and 10, The Scapula). However, published results so far using this transfer for irreparable cuff tears have been promising in terms of pain relief and restoration of function without scapular dyskinesia.

Pectoralis Major Transfer
Transfer of the pectoralis major tendon from the humeral shaft to the lesser tuberosity can be considered for patients with an irreparable subscapularis tear (79). The transfer may be performed superficial or deep to the conjoined tendon (Figure 6.28). The former is easier to perform but leads to a worse line of pull than the latter. However, transfer deep to the conjoined tendon puts the musculocutaneous nerve at risk, and oftentimes only part of the pectoralis tendon fits in the space between the musculocutaneous nerve and the coracoid. This procedure has been reported to provide mixed results, and has been especially unsuccessful when attempted in the setting of anterior instability after arthroplasty (79).

Shoulder Arthroplasty
Reverse shoulder arthroplasty has emerged as a very appealing alternative for patients with massive irreparable rotator cuff tears (Figure 6.29). It is considered by most the treatment of choice for cuff tear arthropathy. It is also commonly considered for older patients with irreparable cuff tears involving the anterior and posterosuperior cuff even in the absence of arthritis, especially in the presence of pseudoparalysis (80–82). Hemiarthroplasty was the procedure of choice for cuff tear arthropathy prior to the introduction of reverse shoulder arthroplasty; it continues to represent a useful alternative for selected patients, especially in the setting of severe glenoid bone loss. The role of shoulder arthroplasty in patients with rotator cuff disease

A

B

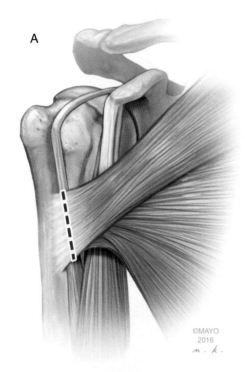
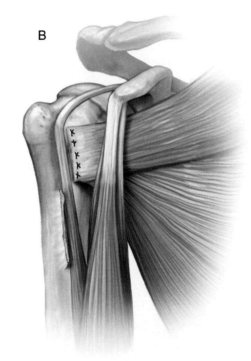

©MAYO
2016
m. k.

Figure 6.28 Pectoralis transfer under conjoined tendon.

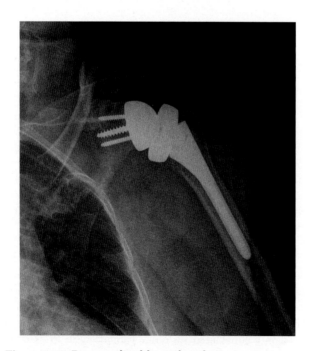

Figure 6.29 Reverse shoulder arthroplasty.

is discussed further in chapter 9, Shoulder Arthritis and Arthroplasty.

Superior Capsular Reconstruction

This procedure is becoming increasingly popular despite the fact that good mid-term and long-term outcome data

are lacking. It involves implantation of a structural patch fixed to the superior aspect of the glenoid neck and the greater tuberosity (Figure 6.30, ● Video 6.5) (83,84). This static restraint between the humeral head and the glenoid keeps the head better centered on the glenoid, avoids painful contact between the superior aspect of the humeral head and the coracoacromioal arch, and results in a better fulcrum that allows active elevation of the arm in the absence of a posterosuperior cuff (85,86).

The patch most commonly used currently is fabricated with human dermis and measures approximately 3.5 mm in thickness (83). It is fashioned intraoperatively into a trapezoid narrower medially and wider laterally. Implantation is performed arthroscopically using anchors into the glenoid and the greater tuberosity. Any remaining posterior cuff is anchored to the patch as well.

Although some authors have reported impressive early results in terms of pain relief and active elevation (84), there are a number of unanswered questions: Will the dermal patch be eroded in time, leading to high failure rates in the mid and long term? How common are fixation failures at the glenoid or greater tuberosity? Will some patients experience adverse allergic reaction to the patch? Is the outcome the same in patients who receive only the patch versus those who have the cuff partially repaired to the patch? Can the patch in these latter cases function as a way to indirectly transmit forces to the tuberosity? Only time and good quality research will tell!

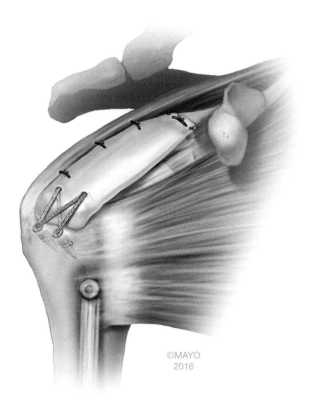

Figure 6.30 Schematic representation of reconstruction of the superior capsule of the glenohumeral joint.

Failed Rotator Cuff Repair

Management of patients presenting with persistent symptoms and evidence of persistent cuff tearing after repair is challenging (87,88). There are 2 key questions: (1) Why did the attempted repair fail to achieve healing and symptomatic relief? and (2) Can another repair be considered, or is it best to proceed with a tendon transfer or a reverse arthroplasty? The goals of the evaluation of a patient presenting with a failed rotator cuff repair are summarized in Table 6.7. Special attention needs to be paid to risk factors for healing, the condition of the deltoid, and the possibility of a low-grade, deep infection.

Revision rotator cuff repair has been associated with a relatively high rate of failure. However, some patients do benefit from a second attempt to repair their rotator cuff primarily (87–89). This is especially the case for the younger patient with a fixable tear, particularly if the prior attempt was suboptimal or if risk factors for failure (smoking, diabetes, poor compliance) can be modified. Otherwise, it may be best to avoid surgery altogether or to consider salvage procedures. Severe deltoid damage as a result of the first surgery may make all salvage options unreliable.

Table 6.7 • Evaluation of the Patient With a Failed Rotator Cuff Repair

Identify factors associated with poor healing potential (see Table 6.3)

Review surgical report and progress notes
Was the index repair performed properly?
Was the postoperative program appropriate?
Was the patient compliant?

Assess current pathology
Tear size
Muscle quality
Tendon quality
Bone quality
Glenohumeral joint cartilage
Deltoid status

Consider the possibility of an infected cuff repair
Was there drainage or prolonged redness after the index procedure?
Was the patient placed on a course of antibiotics?
If high index of suspicion, consider aspiration

Calcifying Tendinitis

This is a common disorder of unknown etiology in which calcium crystals are deposited in the substance of a rotator cuff tendon. The calcific deposit is typically located a few millimeters away from the tendon to bone junction, most commonly in the supraspinatus followed by the infraspinatus; calcific deposits can rarely be identified in the teres minor or subscapularis (90).

Not all individuals with calcific deposits have symptoms; cuff calcifications have been reported in approximately 5% to 10% of individuals without symptoms (91). Approximately 5% of the patients evaluated in the office for shoulder pain present with a calcific deposit; this rate increases to 20% if we consider only patients under the age of 40 and to 40% if we include only patients with subacromial syndrome (91). Symptomatic calcific tendinitis is more common in women. Calcifying tendinitis seems to be a self-resolving condition in many patients: calcium deposits are slowly laid down over time and eventually fragment and disappear.

Clinical Presentation

Pain is the cardinal symptom of calcifying tendinitis. Patients may present with either a chronic dull ache or an episode of exquisite, acute shoulder pain. Some believe that while calcium is being deposited, patients experience either no symptoms or mild to moderate pain, whereas episodes of severe acute pain occur with resorption of deposits and release of crystals that irritate the subacromial space. Not everyone shares this view.

Patients presenting with an acute episode of excruciating pain cannot sleep at night and can barely move their shoulder. Pain is centered over the deltoid region but can radiate toward the upper arm or the neck. Patients with chronic dull ache can typically move their shoulder with some discomfort and may experience occasional catching. Weakness is secondary only to pain; strength testing is otherwise normal. Calcifying tendinitis can lead to secondary frozen shoulder in some individuals (see chapter 8, Adhesive Capsulitis).

Imaging Studies

Radiographs

Depending on the amount of calcium deposited and the stage of the disease, the calcification may be easily noticed on plain radiographs or barely visible. As mentioned before, the deposits of calcium are localized inside the tendon and do not extend into bone (Figure 6.31). Supraspinatus calcifications are easily identified in anteroposterior views in neutral or external rotation; infraspinatus calcifications are projected behind the humeral head on external rotation views, and are best seen in anteroposterior views in internal rotation. Subscapularis calcifications are best seen on axillary views.

Advanced Imaging Studies

Most patients with classic calcifying tendinitis do not benefit from additional imaging. However, when the calcifications are very faint and difficult to visualize on plain radiographs, ultrasonography, MRI, or CT can be helpful. Some patients may be referred to the orthopedic surgeon with an MRI already performed. Calcific deposits are hypointense in both T1- and T2-weighted sequences, although hyperintensity may be seen surrounding the deposit in T2-weighted sequences.

Management

Acute Presentation

Patients presenting with excruciating acute pain secondary to calcifying tendinitis are best helped with either an injection in the subacromial space or percutaneous decompression of the calcification with partial removal using a needle. The relative efficacy of these 2 interventions for the acute episode is unclear.

One option is to inject the subacromial space with a combination of a local anesthetic and a corticosteroid. Patients typically experience pain relief soon after the injection, but symptoms may recur. There is no evidence to suggest that corticosteroids per se accelerate resorption of the calcification.

Another option is to try to pierce the surface of the involved tendon with a needle percutaneously in an effort to decrease intratendinous pressure and hopefully evacuate part or most of the calcific deposit. Ultrasonography

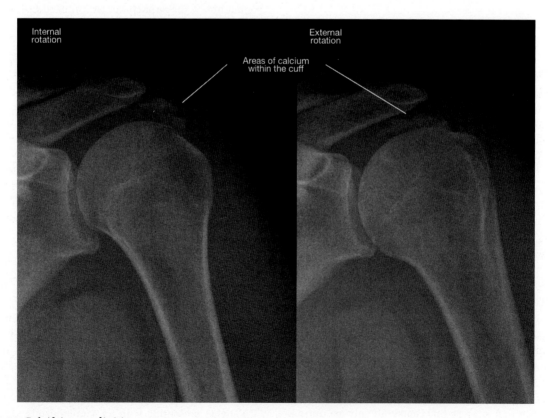

Figure 6.31 Calcifying tendinitis.

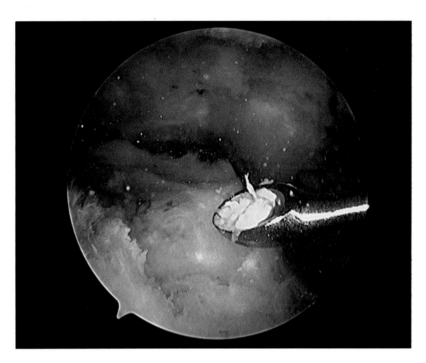

Figure 6.32 *Arthroscopic removal of calcific deposits.*

guidance is extremely helpful. Aspiration, lavage, and injection of corticosteroids can be added as well.

Chronic Presentation
Nonoperative Treatment
Patients presenting with dull achiness can initially be treated nonoperatively with activity modifications, a short course of nonsteroidal anti-inflamatory drugs, and occasionally a corticosteroid injection in the subacromial space. If symptoms persist and are bothersome enough to consider additional treatment, removal of the calcific deposit can be attempted with a percutaneous needle under ultrasonography, as described earlier. Some authors have proposed the use of extracorporeal shock wave therapy or radiation, but I have no personal experience. Physical therapy may be added to any of these treatment modalities in order to maintain motion and strength.

Arthroscopic Surgery
When patients do not respond to nonoperative treatment, surgery is a very good alternative. The main goal of surgery is removal of the calcific deposit (◯ Video 6.6). Prior to surgery, it is important to discuss with the patient the possibility of persistent calcium deposits on postoperative radiographs. Rarely, this is due to the fact that the calcification cannot be identified in surgery; more commonly, it is not possible to remove absolutely every particle of calcium without compromising the rotator cuff. Removal of most of the deposit seems to be enough to provide relief.

Currently, most perform this procedure arthroscopically (Figure 6.32) (92,93). After evaluation of the glenohumeral joint to identify possible associated pathology, the subacromial space is carefully assessed to identify the area of calcification. Location of the calcific deposit can be a challenge. Occasionally, a zone of hyperemia, seen as a reddish spot during arthroscopy, can be present over the area of calcification. Most of the time the calcification needs to be identified by probing with a blunt instrument or a needle. Once the calcification is located, the tendon fibers over the calcification are divided and the calcific deposit is removed with arthroscopic graspers, a curette, or a shaver. Care must be taken to avoid inadvertent damage to the adjacent intact rotator cuff.

Once no more particles of calcium can be removed, the subacromial space is thoroughly lavaged with arthroscopic fluid. Some authors add an acromioplasty routinely and others never do; in my practice, I add an acromioplasty selectively for patients with evidence of impingement. I also inject subacromial corticosteroids at the end of the procedure. After surgery, patients are provided with a sling for comfort and start a gentle program of physical therapy to regain motion and strength. Most patients respond to surgery, and recurrence is rare.

Neuropathies and the Rotator Cuff

In certain patients, rotator cuff dysfunction is due primarily to nerve compression or stretching of the suprascapular nerve, the axillary nerve, or branches of the axillary nerve to the teres minor. As mentioned before, some believe that large retracted posterosuperior cuff tears lead to secondary dysfunction of the suprascapular nerve (25,26).

Suprascapular Nerve

Anatomy

The suprascapular nerve originates from the C5 and C6 roots at the junction of the upper trunk and its divisions (Figure 6.33). It enters the scapular region through the suprascapular notch, bridged by the superior transverse scapular ligament. After exiting the suprascapular notch, it gives branches to innervate the supraspinatus as well as sensory branches to the glenohumeral joint. It continues approximately 20 mm medial to the glenoid rim to enter the spinoglenoid notch. After exiting the spinoglenoid notch, it gives branches to innervate the infraspinatus (94,95).

Etiology

The most common reasons for primary suprascapular nerve dysfunction include compression by a ganglion cyst from the glenohumeral joint in patients with a labral tear, and repetitive traction microinjuries in certain sports such as volleyball, baseball, tennis, and weight lifting. Other less common reasons include direct blunt trauma, scapular fractures, and acute brachial neuritis (Parsonage-Turner syndrome). Idiopathic thickening of the superior transverse scapular ligament and progressive nerve distortion secondary to cuff retraction are possible additional etiologies not accepted by everyone.

Patient Evaluation

The clinical presentation will depend on the location of the injury. When the nerve is compressed more distally at the spinoglenoid notch, patients will develop painless atrophy of the infraspinatus with weakness in external rotation (Figure 6.34). When the nerve is compressed proximally at the suprascapular notch, pain is common and associated with atrophy of both the supraspinatus and infraspinatus with weakness in abduction, elevation, and external rotation.

EMG and nerve conduction studies may confirm the diagnosis by demonstrating fibrillation potentials and a delayed conduction velocity. Plain radiographs of the shoulder are typically complemented with advanced imaging studies (MRI or ultrasonography) to identify

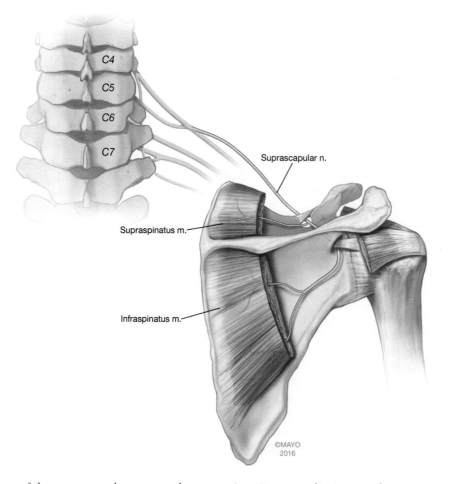

Figure 6.33 *Anatomy of the suprascapular nerve and compression sites. m. indicates muscle; n., nerve.*

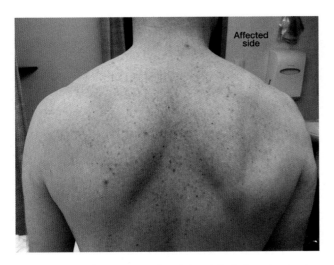

Figure 6.34 Selective atrophy of the right infraspinatus in a patient with distal suprascapular nerve compression.

associated pathology, especially labral tears and paralabral cysts (Figure 6.35). Selective atrophy of the infraspinatus or both the supra and infraspinatus is typically noted.

Treatment

A trial of nonoperative treatment including activity modifications, pain management modalities, and physical therapy can be tried for a few months in patients with neuropathy secondary to repetitive trauma, neuritis, or a recent injury. An injection of a local anesthetic with corticosteroids into the suprascapular notch under ultrasonography may be considered, especially in patients with severe pain. Patients with a ganglion cyst responsible for the compressive neuropathy are typically considered for a procedure

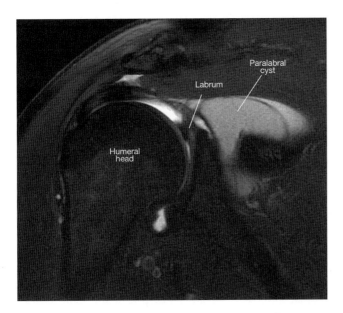

Figure 6.35 Paralabral cysts may compress the suprascapular nerve and are best seen on magnetic resonance imaging.

to decompress or eliminate the cyst. Patients with refractory symptoms after a trial of nonoperative treatment may be considered for suprascapular nerve decompression by dividing the superior transverse scapular ligament.

Compressive Neuropathy Secondary to Ganglion Cysts

There is some controversy regarding the ideal management of these patients. Since most cysts are secondary to a labral tear, some surgeons recommend labral repair (see chapter 7, Shoulder Instability and the Labrum); an attempt is made to decompress the cyst from the glenohumeral joint prior to fixing the labrum, but even if fluid is not seen to come out, if the labrum heals, most of the time the cyst disappears and the neuropathy resolves. Alternatively, aspiration of the cyst in the office setting under ultrasonography can be considered. The added value of formally decompressing the suprascapular nerve at the notch in patients with a decompressed cyst is unclear.

Suprascapular Nerve Decompression

Division of the superior transverse scapular ligament used to be performed through an open exposure. Currently, it is performed arthroscopically (⬤ Video 6.7) (96). There are several techniques described. My preference is to use 2 anterolateral subacromial portals, one for visualization and a second more anterior to dissect the subacromial bursa and adjacent tissue until the ligament, nerve, and vessels are visualized.

Identifying these structures can be a challenge. The key is to understand that the superior transverse scapular ligament is just medial to the base of the coracoid. The anterior aspect of the supraspinatus tendon and muscle can be followed medially until the coracoclavicular ligaments are visualized. The superior transverse scapular ligament will be located posterior and medial to the conoid and trapezoid ligaments. The artery and veins course superficial to the ligament, whereas the nerve courses underneath. An accessory superior portal 2 centimeters medial to the Neviaser portal (see chapter 2, Arthroscopic Shoulder Surgery) may be used to bluntly dissect the vessels and safely expose and divide the ligament (Figure 6.36).

Axillary Nerve and Its Branches

Traumatic injury to the axillary nerve can occur with severe fractures or anterior shoulder dislocation. Rarely, compressive neuropathy of the axillary nerve or its branches may affect the teres minor.

Quadrilateral Space Syndrome

Quadrilateral space syndrome arises from compression or mechanical injury to the axillary nerve and/or the posterior circumflex humeral artery (97). This space is defined by the long head of the triceps medially, the humerus laterally, the combined tendon of the teres major and

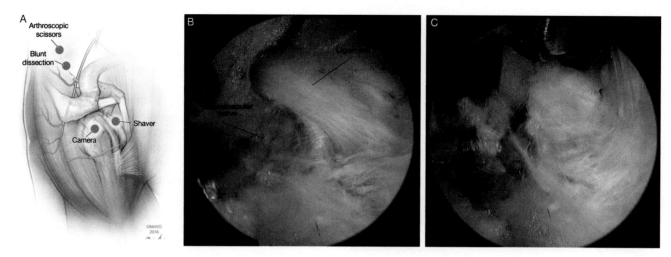

Figure 6.36 A, *Portals used for suprascapular nerve decompression.* **B,** *Arthroscopic view of the ligament, vessels, and nerve.* **C,** *Ligament being divided.*

latissimus dorsi inferiorly, and the teres minor or inferior glenohumeral joint capsule superiorly (Figure 6.37). It is most commonly reported in overhead athletes practicing volleyball, baseball, and swimming; it has occasionally been associated to yoga or window cleaning.

Neurogenic symptoms include pain and decreased sensation in the distribution of the axillary nerve, and weakness of the deltoid and teres minor. Vascular symptoms may include limb ischemia secondary to thromboembolism. When there is occlusion of the posterior circumflex humeral artery, the diagnosis may be established with digital substraction angiography, CT angiography, or magnetic resonance angiography. Otherwise, dynamic vascular studies in external rotation or teres minor EMG may help. Isolated atrophy of the teres minor with various degrees of deltoid atrophy may be observed.

Treatment should include activity modifications (avoid combined abduction and external rotation) and antiplatelet therapy for a few weeks to months. Patients with prominent vascular symptoms may require surgical ligation with thrombectomy if needed. Patients with prominent neurologic symptoms may require surgical decompression.

Isolated Teres Minor Atrophy

This entity is characterized by posterior shoulder pain, weakness of external rotation in abduction (occasionally Hornsblower sign), isolated atrophy of the teres minor, and isolated electromyographic changes in the teres minor. It is secondary to compression of the primary motor branch to the teres minor by a fascial sling. Surgical decompression of this motor branch can lead to complete resolution of the symptoms (98).

Biceps Tendon Pathology

Over time, the attributed importance of the biceps tendon in the field of shoulder surgery has ranged tremendously (5–8,99). To date, some surgeons believe the long head of the biceps is a pain generator in many patients, whereas others ignore this structure completely in the evaluation and management of the painful shoulder. Similarly, some surgeons have a very low threshold to perform a biceps tenotomy and believe that tenodesis is completely unnecessary, whereas others try to preserve, reconstruct, or tenodese the biceps at all cost.

Tenosynovitis and Partial Thickness Tendon Rupture

In theory, a formal diagnosis of tenosynovitis can be confirmed only with visual inspection of the long head of the biceps, typically at the time of arthroscopy (6–8). The biceps tendon can be pulled into the joint with a probe,

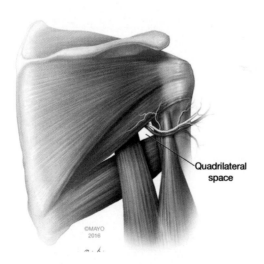

Figure 6.37 *The quadrilateral space of the shoulder.*

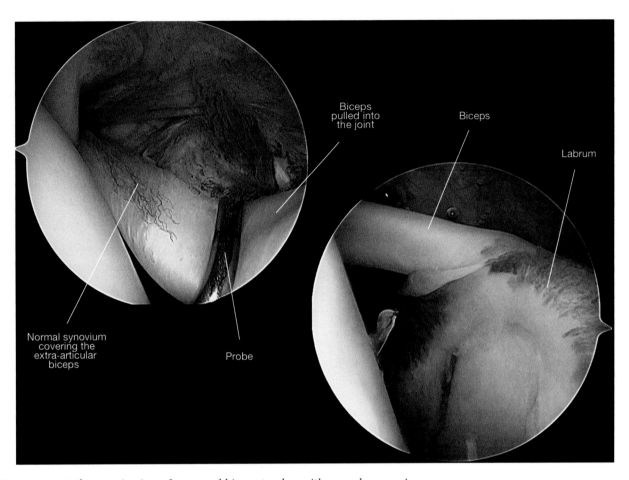

Figure 6.38 Arthroscopic view of a normal biceps tendon with some hyperemia.

although the lowest portion of the tendon cannot be visualized. Some vascularity in the portion of the biceps just distal to the joint is normal (Figure 6.38). Most individuals with excessive hyperemia and synovitis around the tendon also have rotator cuff pathology or glenohumeral joint degeneration. In some patients, inspection of the tendon demonstrates partial rupture (Figure 6.39). Alternatively, the tendon may hypertrophy and become incarcerated in the joint, developing an hourglass deformity that leads to a painful block in terminal elevation.

Establishing the diagnosis of tenosynovitis and partial rupture clinically can be difficult. The biceps tendon is suspected to contribute to patient symptoms when there is pain on direct palpation over the bicipital groove combined with positive Speed, Yergason, and upper cut tests (chapter 1, Evaluation of the Shoulder). However, the predictive value of these tests is questionable. Ultrasonography and magnetic resonance may show a thickened synovium, excessive peritendinous synovial fluid, or areas of partial thickness tears. Not uncommonly, patients feel that their pain radiates down to the muscle belly. Ultrasonography-guided injections in the bicipital tendon sheath are probably the best way to establish unequivocally that the biceps tendon contributes to the patient's symptoms.

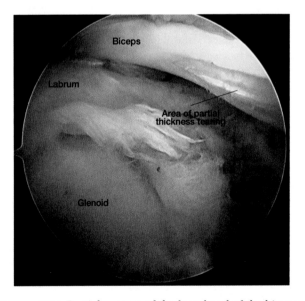

Figure 6.39 Partial rupture of the long head of the biceps.

Instability and Dislocation

As mentioned in the section on anatomy, the bicipital pulley stabilizes the biceps tendon in the groove. Fibers of the subscapularis tendon are the most important contributors to the bicipital pulley. The biceps tendon can subluxate, or completely dislocate, off the groove (6–8). Most commonly, the subluxation or dislocation is medial. In complete ruptures of the subscapularis, the tendon can dislocate into the glenohumeral joint. In partial ruptures, the tendon may sublux or dislocate deep to the subscapularis, in its substance (intratendinous), or rarely completely anterior. Lateral subluxation or dislocation is seen less commonly in some cuff tears involving the supraspinatus or after a proximal humerus fracture or dislocation.

Rarely, the tendon can demonstrate subluxation in and out of the groove with shoulder rotation. Most of the time, the subluxation or dislocation is permanent. Anterior shoulder pain is slightly more medial than in tenosynovitis, and biceps maneuvers may all be positive. The abnormal position of the biceps is confirmed with ultrasonography or MRI (Figure 6.11).

Rupture of the Long Head of the Biceps

Spontaneous rupture of the long head of the biceps is relatively common, especially in patients with rotator cuff disease (6–8). Some patients recall the rupture happening in the setting of an injury or heavy use of the shoulder, but it can also happen with a somewhat minor event. Most likely, all these patients have had a partial rupture for some time that all of a sudden gets completed.

Tendon rupture is typically felt as a pop followed by deformity and sometimes ecchymosis. Some patients experience pain for a few days, but interestingly many patients state that they were having moderate pain in the shoulder during the days or weeks preceding the rupture, and their pain has actually improved or it is completely gone after the rupture. The typical deformity involves dropping of the long head of the biceps, which looks lower and bulged (Popeye deformity, Figure 6.40). The deformity can be minimal in patients with an enlarged tendon that becomes trapped as it tries to exit the joint and becomes "autotenodesed" with scar tissue. An average loss of strength of 20% in elbow flexion and 20% in forearm supination has been reported. Imaging studies are seldom necessary to diagnose a rupture of the long head of the biceps, but should be considered to understand the status of the rotator cuff.

Without treatment, ruptures of the long head of the biceps seem to be well tolerated in most patients. The cosmetic aspect of the arm does not improve, but only a few individuals will complain of cramping in the biceps muscle belly area with repetitive use of the arm. Occasionally, some patients will complain of catching or pain if a large portion of retained biceps tendon is still in continuity with the labrum. Most patients are recommended to consider nonoperative treatment, but if they desire surgery for better cosmesis or to avoid any possibility of cramping, surgery should be done soon; otherwise retraction can make restoration of adequate length difficult.

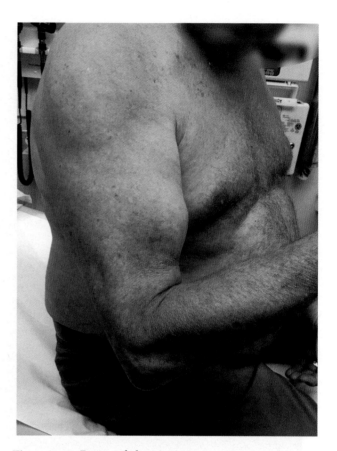

Figure 6.40 *Popeye deformity.*

Biceps Tenotomy and Tenodesis

Debate continues over the relative indications of the 2 main procedures used to deal with a symptomatic tendon of the long head of the biceps: tenotomy and tenodesis. Other procedures (synovectomy or tendon relocation with reconstruction of the pulley) have been tried without much success.

Tenotomy of the Long Head of the Biceps

Patients with tenosynovitis, a partial thickness tear, subluxation, or dislocation may be considered for biceps tenotomy, most commonly performed arthroscopically unless done in conjunction with an open cuff repair or an arthroplasty (Figure 6.41) (99). Tenotomy is very appealing because it is simple, quick, and requires no protection; it has been widely accepted partly due to the observation that most patients with a spontaneous rupture of the long head of the biceps experience improvement in pain and little dysfunction. The patient must be advised of the future cosmetic deformity and the possibility of cramping. Tenotomy has been used widely in the setting of arthroscopic cuff repair since the cuff repair portion of the procedure per se can be lengthy, and adding a tenodesis would increase surgical time even further.

Arthroscopic tenotomy is typically performed with the arthroscopic camera in the posterior portal. Instruments are

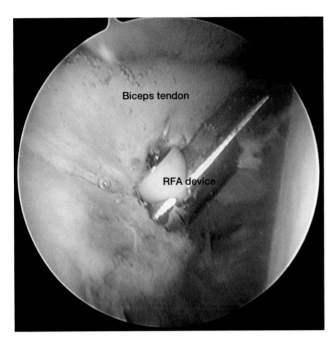

Figure 6.41 *Biceps tenotomy. RFA indicates radiofrequency ablation.*

introduced through an anterior portal. The biceps tendon is divided at its origin off the labrum. Tenotomy may be performed with arthroscopic scissors, an arthroscopic biter, or a radiofrequency ablation device. Some believe that use of an electrothermal device may slightly enlarge the biceps tendon and facilitate autotenodesis in the groove. The tenotomy also may be performed by dividing the labrum 5 to 10 mm (anteriorly and posteriorly) to the biceps anchor. The portions of the labrum still connected with the biceps tendon can then be trapped at the exit of the joint, facilitating autotenodesis. After surgery, patients use their shoulder as tolerated for comfort and may advance their activities as tolerated with no restrictions, provided no additional surgery was performed.

Tenodesis of the Long Head of the Biceps
Tenotomy of the long head of the biceps is estimated to be associated with cosmetic deformity in approximately 50% of the patients and an average decrease in elbow flexion strength and/or forearm supination strength of about 20%. The cosmetic deformity is much less noticeable in overweight patients. Surgeons commonly consider biceps tenodesis instead of tenotomy for younger patients as well as thin individuals who would be unsatisfied with the deformity, but the relative indications of one procedure over the other are not clearly established (5–8,99). As metioned earlier, when tenodesis is considered for a patient presenting after a spontaneous tendon rupture, surgery should be performed soon (first few weeks, ⊙ Video 6.8); otherwise the tendon may retract.

The benefits of tenodesis over tenotomy include restoration of the biceps contour and preservation of strength.

Possible disadvantages include longer surgical time, need for postoperative protection, as well as the fact that in some patients the tenodesis fails to heal. In addition, a number of individuals complain of pain at the tenodesis site for reasons that are not completely clear: some attribute the pain to sensitivity in the area of the bicipital groove; others believe it is secondary to intraosseous micromotion of the various devices used for tendon fixation.

Mutiple tenodesis sites and fixation techniques have been considered for the long head of the biceps (coracoid, transverse humeral ligament, pectoralis major tendon, greater tuberosity, bicipital groove). Currently, the most accepted location is the bicipital groove. Arthroscopic tenodesis is easier to perform at the proximal end of the bicipital groove, but some argue that performing a tenodesis in that location leaves some pathologic tendon in the groove below the tenodesis site. My preference is to perform a tenodesis in the lower end of the bicipital groove.

Tendon to bone fixation may be accomplished by creating a hole in the shape of a keyhole that will trap the tendon, using transosseous fixation, suture anchors, an interference screw, or a combination. Adequate fixation may be obtained with any of these techniques. Suture anchors and interference screws are easier to use in arthroscopic tenodesis. However, they increase the cost of the procedure substantially, and as mentioned before they have been blamed by some for persistent pain in the groove possibly related to micromotion. Care must be taken not to create a major cortical defect in the humerus, which is especially likely to happen with interference screws (enough space is required for both the screw and the tendon): postoperative fractures of the humeral shaft have been reported after biceps tenodesis when a very large stress riser was created at the tenodesis site.

Currently, my preference is to perform a biceps tenodesis in the lower portion of the bicipital groove using transosseous fixation (Figure 6.42). For an isolated biceps tenodesis or a tenodesis in the setting of an arthroscopic cuff repair, a tenotomy is first performed arthroscopically. Then, a 3-cm skin incision is placed over the location of the groove. The deltopectoral interval is developed bluntly and the biceps tendon sheath is divided. The biceps tendon is retrieved and approximately 4 centimeters of proximal tendon is resected. A heavy nonabsorbable suture is placed in the remaining biceps stump using a locking stitch configuration. A 4.0-mm bur is used to create a perforation in the anterior cortex just large enough to accommodate the biceps. Two 2.0-mm holes are created in the lateral cortex of the humerus communicating with the canal. The tendon and sutures are then introduced in the larger perforation and the sutures retrieved though the smaller lateral holes and tied over a bone bridge. Alternatively, when tenodesis is performed in the setting of arthroscopic cuff repair, the biceps tendon may be secured with sutures in the lateral row

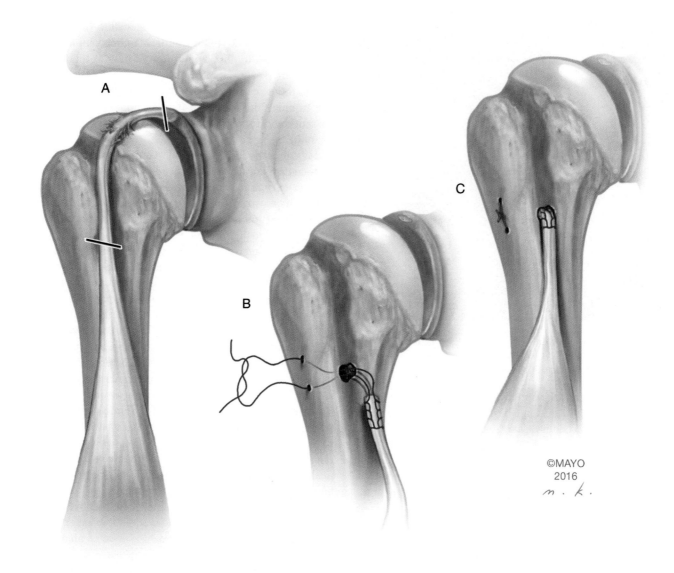

Figure 6.42 *Biceps tenodesis.* **A,** *Schematic.* **B,** *Tendon preparation.* **C,** *Biceps tenodesed.*

anchors. After surgery, patients are recommended use of a sling for 2 weeks and advised to avoid active elbow flexion against resistance for the first 6 postoperative weeks.

KEY POINTS

✓ Aging is the factor most commonly implicated in chronic rotator cuff disease; the correlation between the presence of a cuff tear and symptoms is not perfect, and many individuals have an asymptomatic cuff tear. Smoking, hypercholesterolemia, inflammatory joint disease, and a positive family history seem to predispose to cuff disease.

✓ Approximately 50% of individuals with asymptomatic cuff tears develop symptoms over 2 to

3 years. Approximately 50% of tendon tears increase in size over time. Increase in size correlates with muscle degeneration and symptoms.

✓ Major goals of the evaluation of patients with cuff disease are to identify risk factors correlated with poor healing potential and to distinguish acute traumatic tears from chronic tears with or without acute extension. True acute tears should be considered for surgery right away.

✓ Cuff tears present with pain and various degrees of weakness: active motion is typically worse than passive motion. Plain radiographs should always be obtained. Advanced imaging (MRI or ultrasonography) is extremely helpful, but may overdiagnose partial tears. Muscle atrophy and fatty infiltration on CT or MRI correlate with outcome after surgery.

✓ Nonoperative treatment can be successful in a large number of patients with a cuff tear. Strengthening of the inferior cuff seems to be most helpful. Corticosteroid injections may be used selectively.

✓ Open or arthroscopic cuff repair seems to provide improvements in pain and function for over 85% of patients; however, tendon healing does not occur in approximately 1 of every 4 patients.

✓ Tendon transfers may be considered for the salvage of an irreparable cuff tear. Anterosuperior tears have been classically salvaged with a pectoralis major transfer, but the latissimus dorsi may end up becoming a better option. Posterosuperior tears have been classically salvaged with a latissimus dorsi/teres major transfer, but transfer of the lower trapezius may end up being a better option.

✓ Reverse shoulder arthroplasty has become the standard of care for patients with cuff tear arthropathy, and it is commonly considered for the massive, irreparable cuff tear in elderly patients with pseudoparalysis.

✓ Acute episodes of pain in patients with calcifying tendinitis can be excruciating and respond to a corticosteroid injection with possible removal of part of the calcific deposit. Chronic cases may be helped with arthroscopic removal of the calcification.

✓ Suprascapular nerve decompression is considered by some as an adjunct to repair of large cuff tears and for primary neuropathy nonresponsive to conservative management. Compression secondary to a paralabral cyst seems to respond well to labral repair with or without cyst decompression.

✓ The biceps tendon may be responsible for symptoms secondary to tenosynovitis, rupture, subluxation, or dislocation. Biceps subluxation or dislocation is almost always associated to partial or complete disruption of the subscapularis.

✓ The relative indications of tenotomy versus tenodesis for management of the long head of the biceps are unclear. Tenotomy requires no protection and seems to provide consistent pain relief. Patients interested in avoiding cosmetic deformity or mild decrease in elbow and forearm strength may be considered for tenodesis.

REFERENCES

1. White JJ, Titchener AG, Fakis A, Tambe AA, Hubbard RB, Clark DI. An epidemiological study of rotator cuff pathology using The Health Improvement Network database. Bone Joint J. 2014 Mar;96-B(3):350–3.
2. Tashjian RZ. Epidemiology, natural history, and indications for treatment of rotator cuff tears. Clin Sports Med. 2012 Oct;31(4):589–604. Epub 2012 Aug 30.
3. Millett PJ, Warth RJ. Posterosuperior rotator cuff tears: classification, pattern recognition, and treatment. J Am Acad Orthop Surg. 2014 Aug;22(8):521–34.
4. Curtis AS, Burbank KM, Tierney JJ, Scheller AD, Curran AR. The insertional footprint of the rotator cuff: an anatomic study. Arthroscopy. 2006 Jun;22(6):609.e1.
5. Morag Y, Bedi A, Jamadar DA. The rotator interval and long head biceps tendon: anatomy, function, pathology, and magnetic resonance imaging. Magn Reson Imaging Clin N Am. 2012 May;20(2):229–59. Epub 2012 Feb 21.
6. Ahrens PM, Boileau P. The long head of biceps and associated tendinopathy. J Bone Joint Surg Br. 2007 Aug;89(8):1001–9.
7. McDonald LS, Dewing CB, Shupe PG, Provencher MT. Disorders of the proximal and distal aspects of the biceps muscle. J Bone Joint Surg Am. 2013 Jul 3;95(13):1235–45.
8. Elser F, Braun S, Dewing CB, Giphart JE, Millett PJ. Anatomy, function, injuries, and treatment of the long head of the biceps brachii tendon. Arthroscopy. 2011 Apr;27(4):581–92.
9. Lunn JV, Castellanos-Rosas J, Tavernier T, Barthelemy R, Walch G. A novel lesion of the infraspinatus characterized by musculotendinous disruption, edema, and late fatty infiltration. J Shoulder Elbow Surg. 2008 Jul-Aug;17(4):546–53. Epub 2008 Apr 18.
10. Benjamin M, Evans EJ, Copp L. The histology of tendon attachments to bone in man. J Anat. 1986 Dec;149:89–100.
11. Mannava S, Plate JF, Tuohy CJ, Seyler TM, Whitlock PW, Curl WW, et al. The science of rotator cuff tears: translating animal models to clinical recommendations using simulation analysis. Knee Surg Sports Traumatol Arthrosc. 2013 Jul;21(7):1610–9. Epub 2012 Jul 29.
12. Weeks KD 3rd, Dines JS, Rodeo SA, Bedi A. The basic science behind biologic augmentation of tendon-bone healing: a scientific review. Instr Course Lect. 2014;63:443–50.
13. Lorbach O, Baums MH, Kostuj T, Pauly S, Scheibel M, Carr A, et al. Advances in biology and mechanics of rotator cuff repair. Knee Surg Sports Traumatol Arthrosc. 2015 Feb;23(2):530–41. Epub 2015 Jan 9.
14. Moosmayer S, Tariq R, Stiris M, Smith HJ. The natural history of asymptomatic rotator cuff tears: a three-year follow-up of fifty cases. J Bone Joint Surg Am. 2013 Jul 17;95(14):1249–55.
15. Keener JD, Galatz LM, Teefey SA, Middleton WD, Steger-May K, Stobbs-Cucchi G, et al. A prospective evaluation of survivorship of asymptomatic degenerative rotator cuff tears. J Bone Joint Surg Am. 2015 Jan 21;97(2):89–98.
16. Familiari F, Gonzalez-Zapata A, Ianno B, Galasso O, Gasparini G, McFarland EG. Is acromioplasty necessary in the setting of full-thickness rotator cuff tears? A systematic review. J Orthop Traumatol. 2015 Sep;16(3):167–74. Epub 2015 May 24.
17. Unruh KP, Kuhn JE, Sanders R, An Q, Baumgarten KM, Bishop JY, et al; MOON Shoulder Group. The duration of symptoms does not correlate with rotator cuff tear severity or other patient-related features: a cross-sectional study of patients with atraumatic, full-thickness rotator cuff tears. J Shoulder Elbow Surg. 2014 Jul;23(7):1052–8. Epub 2014 Jan 8.
18. Dunn WR, Kuhn JE, Sanders R, An Q, Baumgarten KM, Bishop JY, et al. Symptoms of pain do not correlate with rotator cuff tear severity: a cross-sectional

study of 393 patients with a symptomatic atraumatic full-thickness rotator cuff tear. J Bone Joint Surg Am. 2014 May 21;96(10):793–800.

19. Sher JS, Uribe JW, Posada A, Murphy BJ, Zlatkin MB. Abnormal findings on magnetic resonance images of asymptomatic shoulders. J Bone Joint Surg Am. 1995 Jan;77(1):10–5.

20. Reuther KE, Thomas SJ, Tucker JJ, Sarver JJ, Gray CF, Rooney SI, et al. Disruption of the anterior-posterior rotator cuff force balance alters joint function and leads to joint damage in a rat model. J Orthop Res. 2014 May;32(5):638–44. Epub 2014 Jan 25.

21. Mesiha MM, Derwin KA, Sibole SC, Erdemir A, McCarron JA. The biomechanical relevance of anterior rotator cuff cable tears in a cadaveric shoulder model. J Bone Joint Surg Am. 2013 Oct 16;95(20):1817–24.

22. Thomopoulos S, Williams GR, Soslowsky LJ. Tendon to bone healing: differences in biomechanical, structural, and compositional properties due to a range of activity levels. J Biomech Eng. 2003 Feb;125(1):106–13.

23. Fuchs B, Weishaupt D, Zanetti M, Hodler J, Gerber C. Fatty degeneration of the muscles of the rotator cuff: assessment by computed tomography versus magnetic resonance imaging. J Shoulder Elbow Surg. 1999 Nov-Dec;8(6):599–605.

24. Goutallier D, Postel JM, Bernageau J, Lavau L, Voisin MC. Fatty muscle degeneration in cuff ruptures: pre- and postoperative evaluation by CT scan. Clin Orthop Relat Res. 1994 Jul;(304):78–83.

25. Collin P, Treseder T, Ladermann A, Benkalfate T, Mourtada R, Courage O, et al. Neuropathy of the suprascapular nerve and massive rotator cuff tears: a prospective electromyographic study. J Shoulder Elbow Surg. 2014 Jan;23(1):28–34. Epub 2013 Sep 30.

26. Shi LL, Boykin RE, Lin A, Warner JJ. Association of suprascapular neuropathy with rotator cuff tendon tears and fatty degeneration. J Shoulder Elbow Surg. 2014 Mar;23(3):339–46. Epub 2013 Sep 20.

27. Colvin AC, Egorova N, Harrison AK, Moskowitz A, Flatow EL. National trends in rotator cuff repair. J Bone Joint Surg Am. 2012 Feb 1;94(3):227–33.

28. Paloneva J, Lepola V, Aarimaa V, Joukainen A, Ylinen J, Mattila VM. Increasing incidence of rotator cuff repairs: a nationwide registry study in Finland. BMC Musculoskelet Disord. 2015 Aug 12;16:189.

29. Moor BK, Wieser K, Slankamenac K, Gerber C, Bouaicha S. Relationship of individual scapular anatomy and degenerative rotator cuff tears. J Shoulder Elbow Surg. 2014 Apr;23(4):536–41. Epub 2014 Jan 28.

30. Feeley BT, Gallo RA, Craig EV. Cuff tear arthropathy: current trends in diagnosis and surgical management. J Shoulder Elbow Surg. 2009 May-Jun;18(3):484–94. Epub 2009 Feb 8.

31. Roy JS, Braen C, Leblond J, Desmeules F, Dionne CE, MacDermid JC, et al. Diagnostic accuracy of ultrasonography, MRI and MR arthrography in the characterisation of rotator cuff disorders: a systematic review and meta-analysis. Br J Sports Med. 2015 Oct;49(20):1316–28. Epub 2015 Feb 11.

32. Sato EJ, Killian ML, Choi AJ, Lin E, Choo AD, Rodriguez-Soto AE, et al. Architectural and biochemical adaptations in skeletal muscle and bone following rotator cuff injury in a rat model. J Bone Joint Surg Am. 2015 Apr 1;97(7):565–73.

33. Chang EY, Chung CB. Current concepts on imaging diagnosis of rotator cuff disease. Semin Musculoskelet Radiol. 2014 Sep;18(4):412–24. Epub 2014 Sep 3.

34. Kissenberth MJ, Rulewicz GJ, Hamilton SC, Bruch HE, Hawkins RJ. A positive tangent sign predicts the repairability of rotator cuff tears. J Shoulder Elbow Surg. 2014 Jul;23(7):1023–7.

35. Lafosse L, Van Isacker T, Wilson JB, Shi LL. A concise and comprehensive description of shoulder pathology and procedures: the 4D code system. Adv Orthop. 2012;2012:930543. Epub 2012 Dec 4.

36. Matthewson G, Beach CJ, Nelson AA, Woodmass JM, Ono Y, Boorman RS, et al. Partial thickness rotator cuff tears: current concepts. Adv Orthop. 2015;2015:458786. Epub 2015 Jun 11.

37. Duncan NS, Booker SJ, Gooding BW, Geoghegan J, Wallace WA, Manning PA. Surgery within 6 months of an acute rotator cuff tear significantly improves outcome. J Shoulder Elbow Surg. 2015 Dec;24(12):1876–80. Epub 2015 Jul 7.

38. Loew M, Magosch P, Lichtenberg S, Habermeyer P, Porschke F. How to discriminate between acute traumatic and chronic degenerative rotator cuff lesions: an analysis of specific criteria on radiography and magnetic resonance imaging. J Shoulder Elbow Surg. 2015 Nov;24(11):1685–93. Epub 2015 Jul 31.

39. Pappou IP, Schmidt CC, Jarrett CD, Steen BM, Frankle MA. AAOS appropriate use criteria: optimizing the management of full-thickness rotator cuff tears. J Am Acad Orthop Surg. 2013 Dec;21(12):772–5.

40. Lambers Heerspink FO, van Raay JJ, Koorevaar RC, van Eerden PJ, Westerbeek RE, van 't Riet E, et al. Comparing surgical repair with conservative treatment for degenerative rotator cuff tears: a randomized controlled trial. J Shoulder Elbow Surg. 2015 Aug;24(8):1274–81.

41. Kukkonen J, Joukainen A, Lehtinen J, Mattila KT, Tuominen EK, Kauko T, et al. Treatment of non-traumatic rotator cuff tears: a randomised controlled trial with one-year clinical results. Bone Joint J. 2014 Jan;96-B(1):75–81.

42. Kuhn JE. How much benefit do we get from rotator cuff repair? J Bone Joint Surg Am. 2014 Sep 17;96(18):e162.

43. Frank JM, Chahal J, Frank RM, Cole BJ, Verma NN, Romeo AA. The role of acromioplasty for rotator cuff problems. Orthop Clin North Am. 2014 Apr;45(2):219–24. Epub 2014 Jan 16.

44. Lee BG, Cho NS, Rhee YG. Results of arthroscopic decompression and tuberoplasty for irreparable massive rotator cuff tears. Arthroscopy. 2011 Oct;27(10):1341–50. Epub 2011 Aug 27.

45. Cho CH, Jang HK, Bae KC, Lee SW, Lee YK, Shin HK, et al. Clinical outcomes of rotator cuff repair with arthroscopic capsular release and manipulation for rotator cuff tear with stiffness: a matched-pair comparative study between patients with and without stiffness. Arthroscopy. 2015 Mar;31(3):482–7. Epub 2014 Nov 1.

46. Cofield RH, Parvizi J, Hoffmeyer PJ, Lanzer WL, Ilstrup DM, Rowland CM. Surgical repair of chronic rotator cuff tears: a prospective long-term study. J Bone Joint Surg Am. 2001 Jan;83–A(1):71–7.

47. McElvany MD, McGoldrick E, Gee AO, Neradilek MB, Matsen FA 3rd. Rotator cuff repair: published evidence on factors associated with repair integrity and clinical

outcome. Am J Sports Med. 2015 Feb;43(2):491–500. Epub 2014 Apr 21.

48. Millett PJ, Warth RJ, Dornan GJ, Lee JT, Spiegl UJ. Clinical and structural outcomes after arthroscopic single-row versus double-row rotator cuff repair: a systematic review and meta-analysis of level I randomized clinical trials. J Shoulder Elbow Surg. 2014 Apr;23(4):586–97. Epub 2014 Jan 8.

49. Mascarenhas R, Chalmers PN, Sayegh ET, Bhandari M, Verma NN, Cole BJ, et al. Is double-row rotator cuff repair clinically superior to single-row rotator cuff repair: a systematic review of overlapping meta-analyses. Arthroscopy. 2014 Sep;30(9):1156–65. Epub 2014 May 10.

50. Lembach M, Mair S, Johnson DL. Surgical pearls and pitfalls for effective and reproducible arthroscopic rotator cuff repair. Orthopedics. 2014 Jul;37(7):472–6.

51. Kuntz AF, Raphael I, Dougherty MP, Abboud JA. Arthroscopic subscapularis repair. J Am Acad Orthop Surg. 2014 Feb;22(2):80–9.

52. Iyengar JJ, Samagh SP, Schairer W, Singh G, Valone FH 3rd, Feeley BT. Current trends in rotator cuff repair: surgical technique, setting, and cost. Arthroscopy. 2014 Mar;30(3):284–8. Epub 2014 Jan 24.

53. Fermont AJ, Wolterbeek N, Wessel RN, Baeyens JP, de Bie RA. Prognostic factors for successful recovery after arthroscopic rotator cuff repair: a systematic literature review. J Orthop Sports Phys Ther. 2014 Mar;44(3):153–63. Epub 2014 Jan 22.

54. Behrens SB, Bruce B, Zonno AJ, Paller D, Green A. Initial fixation strength of transosseous-equivalent suture bridge rotator cuff repair is comparable with transosseous repair. Am J Sports Med. 2012 Jan;40(1):133–40. Epub 2011 Nov 16.

55. Kim SJ, Jung M, Lee JH, Kim C, Chun YM. Arthroscopic repair of anterosuperior rotator cuff tears: in-continuity technique vs. disruption of subscapularis-supraspinatus tear margin: comparison of clinical outcomes and structural integrity between the two techniques. J Bone Joint Surg Am. 2014 Dec 17;96(24):2056–61.

56. Park YB, Koh KH, Shon MS, Park YE, Yoo JC. Arthroscopic distal clavicle resection in symptomatic acromioclavicular joint arthritis combined with rotator cuff tear: a prospective randomized trial. Am J Sports Med. 2015 Apr;43(4):985–90. Epub 2015 Jan 12.

57. Oh JH, Kim JY, Choi JH, Park SM. Is arthroscopic distal clavicle resection necessary for patients with radiological acromioclavicular joint arthritis and rotator cuff tears? A prospective randomized comparative study. Am J Sports Med. 2014 Nov;42(11):2567–73. Epub 2014 Sep 5.

58. Nho SJ, Delos D, Yadav H, Pensak M, Romeo AA, Warren RF, et al. Biomechanical and biologic augmentation for the treatment of massive rotator cuff tears. Am J Sports Med. 2010 Mar;38(3):619–29. Epub 2009 Sep 23.

59. Barbier O, Block D, Dezaly C, Sirveaux F, Mole D. Os acromiale, a cause of shoulder pain, not to be overlooked. Orthop Traumatol Surg Res. 2013 Jun;99(4):465–72. Epub 2013 May 2.

60. Spiegl UJ, Smith SD, Todd JN, Wijdicks CA, Millett PJ. Biomechanical evaluation of internal fixation techniques for unstable meso-type os acromiale. J Shoulder Elbow Surg. 2015 Apr;24(4):520–6. Epub 2014 Nov 28.

61. Johnston PS, Paxton ES, Gordon V, Kraeutler MJ, Abboud JA, Williams GR. Os acromiale: a review and an introduction of a new surgical technique for management. Orthop Clin North Am. 2013 Oct;44(4):635–44.

62. Harris JD, Griesser MJ, Jones GL. Systematic review of the surgical treatment for symptomatic os acromiale. Int J Shoulder Surg. 2011 Jan;5(1):9–16.

63. Ross D, Maerz T, Lynch J, Norris S, Baker K, Anderson K. Rehabilitation following arthroscopic rotator cuff repair: a review of current literature. J Am Acad Orthop Surg. 2014 Jan;22(1):1–9.

64. Keener JD, Galatz LM, Stobbs-Cucchi G, Patton R, Yamaguchi K. Rehabilitation following arthroscopic rotator cuff repair: a prospective randomized trial of immobilization compared with early motion. J Bone Joint Surg Am. 2014 Jan 1;96(1):11–9.

65. Henseler JF, Kolk A, van der Zwaal P, Nagels J, Vliet Vlieland TP, Nelissen RG. The minimal detectable change of the Constant score in impingement, full-thickness tears, and massive rotator cuff tears. J Shoulder Elbow Surg. 2015 Mar;24(3):376–81. Epub 2014 Sep 17.

66. Collin P, Abdullah A, Kherad O, Gain S, Denard PJ, Ladermann A. Prospective evaluation of clinical and radiologic factors predicting return to activity within 6 months after arthroscopic rotator cuff repair. J Shoulder Elbow Surg. 2015 Mar;24(3):439–45. Epub 2014 Oct 16.

67. Russell RD, Knight JR, Mulligan E, Khazzam MS. Structural integrity after rotator cuff repair does not correlate with patient function and pain: a meta-analysis. J Bone Joint Surg Am. 2014 Feb 19;96(4):265–71.

68. Namdari S, Donegan RP, Chamberlain AM, Galatz LM, Yamaguchi K, Keener JD. Factors affecting outcome after structural failure of repaired rotator cuff tears. J Bone Joint Surg Am. 2014 Jan 15;96(2):99–105.

69. Mall NA, Tanaka MJ, Choi LS, Paletta GA Jr. Factors affecting rotator cuff healing. J Bone Joint Surg Am. 2014 May 7;96(9):778–88.

70. Warth RJ, Dornan GJ, James EW, Horan MP, Millett PJ. Clinical and structural outcomes after arthroscopic repair of full-thickness rotator cuff tears with and without platelet-rich product supplementation: a meta-analysis and meta-regression. Arthroscopy. 2015 Feb;31(2):306–20. Epub 2014 Nov 14.

71. Valencia Mora M, Ruiz Iban MA, Diaz Heredia J, Barco Laakso R, Cuellar R, Garcia Arranz M. Stem cell therapy in the management of shoulder rotator cuff disorders. World J Stem Cells. 2015 May 26;7(4):691–9.

72. Nossov S, Dines JS, Murrell GA, Rodeo SA, Bedi A. Biologic augmentation of tendon-to-bone healing: scaffolds, mechanical load, vitamin D, and diabetes. Instr Course Lect. 2014;63:451–62.

73. Gerber C, Rahm SA, Catanzaro S, Farshad M, Moor BK. Latissimus dorsi tendon transfer for treatment of irreparable posterosuperior rotator cuff tears: long-term results at a minimum follow-up of ten years. J Bone Joint Surg Am. 2013 Nov 6;95(21):1920–6.

74. Elhassan BT. Feasibility of latissimus and teres major transfer to reconstruct irreparable subscapularis tendon tear: an anatomic study. J Shoulder Elbow Surg. 2015 Apr;24(4):e102–3. Epub 2015 Feb 18.

75. Boileau P, Chuinard C, Roussanne Y, Neyton L, Trojani C. Modified latissimus dorsi and teres major transfer through a single delto-pectoral approach for external

rotation deficit of the shoulder: as an isolated procedure or with a reverse arthroplasty. J Shoulder Elbow Surg. 2007 Nov-Dec;16(6):671–82.

76. Omid R, Heckmann N, Wang L, McGarry MH, Vangsness CT Jr, Lee TQ. Biomechanical comparison between the trapezius transfer and latissimus transfer for irreparable posterosuperior rotator cuff tears. J Shoulder Elbow Surg. 2015 Oct;24(10):1635–43. Epub 2015 Apr 3.

77. Elhassan B. Lower trapezius transfer for shoulder external rotation in patients with paralytic shoulder. J Hand Surg Am. 2014 Mar;39(3):556–62.

78. Hartzler RU, Barlow JD, An KN, Elhassan BT. Biomechanical effectiveness of different types of tendon transfers to the shoulder for external rotation. J Shoulder Elbow Surg. 2012 Oct;21(10):1370–6. Epub 2012 May 8.

79. Nelson GN, Namdari S, Galatz L, Keener JD. Pectoralis major tendon transfer for irreparable subscapularis tears. J Shoulder Elbow Surg. 2014 Jun;23(6):909–18. Epub 2014 Mar 20.

80. Ek ET, Neukom L, Catanzaro S, Gerber C. Reverse total shoulder arthroplasty for massive irreparable rotator cuff tears in patients younger than 65 years old: results after five to fifteen years. J Shoulder Elbow Surg. 2013 Sep;22(9):1199–208. Epub 2013 Feb 4.

81. Harreld KL, Puskas BL, Frankle MA. Massive rotator cuff tears without arthropathy: when to consider reverse shoulder arthroplasty. Instr Course Lect. 2012;61:143–56.

82. Mulieri P, Dunning P, Klein S, Pupello D, Frankle M. Reverse shoulder arthroplasty for the treatment of irreparable rotator cuff tear without glenohumeral arthritis. J Bone Joint Surg Am. 2010 Nov 3;92(15):2544–56.

83. Hirahara AM, Adams CR. Arthroscopic superior capsular reconstruction for treatment of massive irreparable rotator cuff tears. Arthrosc Tech. 2015 Nov 2;4(6):e637–41. Epub 2015 Dec.

84. Mihata T, Lee TQ, Watanabe C, Fukunishi K, Ohue M, Tsujimura T, Kinoshita M. Clinical results of arthroscopic superior capsule reconstruction for irreparable rotator cuff tears. Arthroscopy. 2013 Mar;29(3):459–70. Epub 2013 Jan 28.

85. Mihata T, McGarry MH, Kahn T, Goldberg I, Neo M, Lee TQ. Biomechanical effect of thickness and tension of fascia lata graft on glenohumeral stability for superior capsule reconstruction in irreparable supraspinatus tears. Arthroscopy. 2016 Mar;32(3):418–26. Epub 2015 Oct 30.

86. Mihata T, McGarry MH, Kahn T, Goldberg I, Neo M, Lee TQ. Biomechanical role of capsular continuity in superior capsule reconstruction for irreparable tears of the supraspinatus tendon. Am J Sports Med. 2016 Jun;44(6):1423–30. Epub 2016 Mar 4.

87. Parnes N, DeFranco M, Wells JH, Higgins LD, Warner JJ. Complications after arthroscopic revision rotator cuff repair. Arthroscopy. 2013 Sep;29(9):1479–86.

88. Hartzler RU, Sperling JW, Schleck CD, Cofield RH. Clinical and radiographic factors influencing the results of revision rotator cuff repair. Int J Shoulder Surg. 2013 Apr;7(2):41–5.

89. Shamsudin A, Lam PH, Peters K, Rubenis I, Hackett L, Murrell GA. Revision versus primary arthroscopic rotator cuff repair: a 2-year analysis of outcomes in 360 patients. Am J Sports Med. 2015 Mar;43(3):557–64. Epub 2014 Dec 19.

90. Kachewar SG, Kulkarni DS. Calcific tendinitis of the rotator cuff: a review. J Clin Diagn Res. 2013 Jul;7(7):1482–5. Epub 2013 Jul 1.

91. Louwerens JK, Sierevelt IN, van Hove RP, van den Bekerom MP, van Noort A. Prevalence of calcific deposits within the rotator cuff tendons in adults with and without subacromial pain syndrome: clinical and radiologic analysis of 1219 patients. J Shoulder Elbow Surg. 2015 Oct;24(10):1588–93. Epub 2015 Apr 11.

92. Balke M, Bielefeld R, Schmidt C, Dedy N, Liem D. Calcifying tendinitis of the shoulder: midterm results after arthroscopic treatment. Am J Sports Med. 2012 Mar;40(3):657–61. Epub 2011 Dec 8.

93. Seil R, Litzenburger H, Kohn D, Rupp S. Arthroscopic treatment of chronically painful calcifying tendinitis of the supraspinatus tendon. Arthroscopy. 2006 May;22(5):521–7.

94. Moen TC, Babatunde OM, Hsu SH, Ahmad CS, Levine WN. Suprascapular neuropathy: what does the literature show? J Shoulder Elbow Surg. 2012 Jun;21(6):835–46. Epub 2012 Mar 23. Erratum in: J Shoulder Elbow Surg. 2012 Oct;21(10):1442.

95. Boykin RE, Friedman DJ, Higgins LD, Warner JJ. Suprascapular neuropathy. J Bone Joint Surg Am. 2010 Oct 6;92(13):2348–64.

96. Shah AA, Butler RB, Sung SY, Wells JH, Higgins LD, Warner JJ. Clinical outcomes of suprascapular nerve decompression. J Shoulder Elbow Surg. 2011 Sep;20(6):975–82. Epub 2011 Feb 1.

97. Brown SA, Doolittle DA, Bohanon CJ, Jayaraj A, Naidu SG, Huettl EA, et al. Quadrilateral space syndrome: the Mayo Clinic experience with a new classification system and case series. Mayo Clin Proc. 2015 Mar;90(3):382–94. Epub 2015 Jan 31.

98. Kruse LM, Yamaguchi K, Keener JD, Chamberlain AM. Clinical outcomes after decompression of the nerve to the teres minor in patients with idiopathic isolated teres minor fatty atrophy. J Shoulder Elbow Surg. 2015 Apr;24(4):628–33. Epub 2014 Oct 29.

99. Ding DY, Garofolo G, Lowe D, Strauss EJ, Jazrawi LM. The biceps tendon: from proximal to distal: AAOS exhibit selection. J Bone Joint Surg Am. 2014 Oct 15;96(20):e176.

7 Shoulder Instability and the Labrum

The glenohumeral joint architecture allows for a very ample range of motion. This same architecture, so beneficial for shoulder mobility, also makes the glenohumeral joint particularly prone to instability. Damage to the glenoid labrum is present in many patients with shoulder instability, although the complexity of the pathology involved in shoulder instability goes beyond labral tears. The rotator cuff and the biceps tendon, discussed in chapter 6, The Rotator Cuff and Biceps Tendon, are intimately involved with instability and the labrum; some of the concepts described in chapter 6 will apply to the content of this chapter.

Basic Concepts

What Is Shoulder Instability?

In its simplest definition, joint *instability* is defined as excessive translation between 2 articulating ends leading to pain or other symptoms. By definition, instability interferes with function or generates pain; excessive *asymptomatic* translation of articulating ends is called *laxity*. The distinction between laxity and instability is not that important in highly constrained joints (like the hip), but is extremely relevant for the mobile shoulder joint. Some individuals will present with extremely loose shoulders, especially at a younger age, but they are completely pain free and can function normally, requiring no treatment. Occasionally, patients with laxity will eventually develop instability either secondary to an injury or progressively over time.

What Makes a Shoulder Stable or Unstable?

To understand the structural pathology of shoulder instability, picture the shoulder girdle as a vertical structure and add some elements to it (Figure 7.1). The scapula is the foundation of this structure, but it is a very

particular foundation, because it is suspended in space by the periscapular muscles and the clavicle-sternum complex. Lack of ability to maintain the suspended scapula in a proper position or to fine-tune its position to various activities may place the glenoid at an angle that facilitates shoulder instability: the ball will tend to fall off the socket. This has been compared to a trained seal constantly changing the position of its nose to keep a ball in equilibrium (Figure 7.1).

Additional structural elements involved in shoulder stability come into play in different circumstances. Some will resist instability in specific directions (anterior or posterior), whereas some will prevent instability in multiple directions. In the resting neutral position (arm by the side), the glenohumeral joint capsule and ligaments are lax (they need to be long enough to allow reaching terminal range of motion) and do not contribute much to stability; the balanced action of the cuff muscles is mostly responsible for stability in the mid range of motion through the so-called concavity-compression effect; negative intra-articular pressure also contributes to joint stability in the neutral position. On the contrary, at the terminal end of motion, the normal capsule and ligaments become progressively tight and thus responsible for stability (Figure 7.2). Obviously, bone loss over a certain threshold on the glenoid side, the humeral side, or both will also make it easier for subluxation or dislocation to occur.

Glenoid and Humeral Head

Bone abnormalities secondary to either developmental changes or trauma may contribute to shoulder instability.

Glenoid Dysplasia and Hypoplasia

Abnormal development of the glenoid can lead to a number of anomalies, including a shallow glenoid with a short glenoid neck, hypoplasia of the posterior glenoid rim, an enlarged posterior labrum, and excessive thickness of the

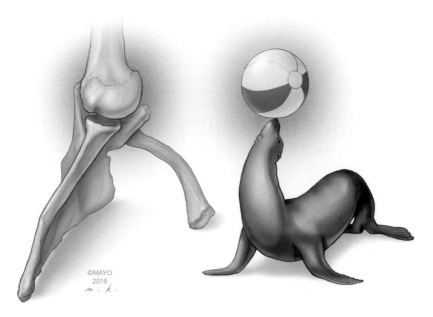

Figure 7.1 *The shoulder as a vertical structure with added layers. Fine-tuning of the scapula to maintain a stable joint has been compared to a seal maintaining a ball in equilibrium on its nose.*

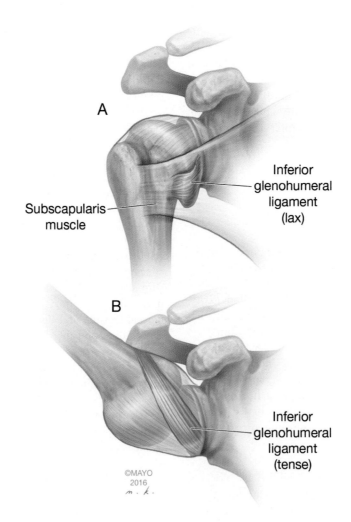

A

Subscapularis muscle

Inferior glenohumeral ligament (lax)

B

Inferior glenohumeral ligament (tense)

Figure 7.2 **A,** *In the resting position (mid-arc of motion) the capsule and ligaments are lax and the rotator cuff contraction maintains the humeral head in a stable position.* **B,** *The capsule and ligaments become tight and contribute to shoulder stability as terminal range of motion is approached.*

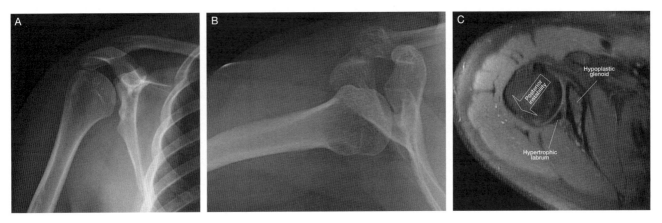

Figure 7.3 *Glenoid hypoplasia and dysplasia.* **A,** *Anteroposterior radiograph.* **B,** *Lateral radiograph.* **C,** *Magnetic resonance imaging.*

inferior articular cartilage (Figure 7.3) (1,2). These abnormalities predispose to shoulder instability, typically posterior or multidirectional. The role of glenoid hypoplasia and dysplasia in shoulder arthritis is discussed in chapter 9, Shoulder Arthritis and Arthroplasty.

Acquired Bone Loss (Trauma)

On the glenoid side, bone loss may occur as a consequence of fracture of part of the glenoid at the time of dislocation or progressive wear with recurrent instability episodes. In anterior shoulder dislocations, as the humeral head is

forced out of the joint at the time of trauma, it can shear off a portion of the anterior glenoid rim (Figure 7.4A–C). If the fractured glenoid rim develops a fibrous union or heals in a displaced position, the width of the articulating surface of the glenoid is decreased, facilitating recurrent instability. Also, once a fracture has happened, even if small, repeated subluxation or dislocation episodes will wear the anterior glenoid rim even further (Figure 7.4D–G). Posterior glenoid bone loss can also result from trauma, but is more commonly due to hypoplasia. The question is how much missing bone is enough to justify correcting instability by

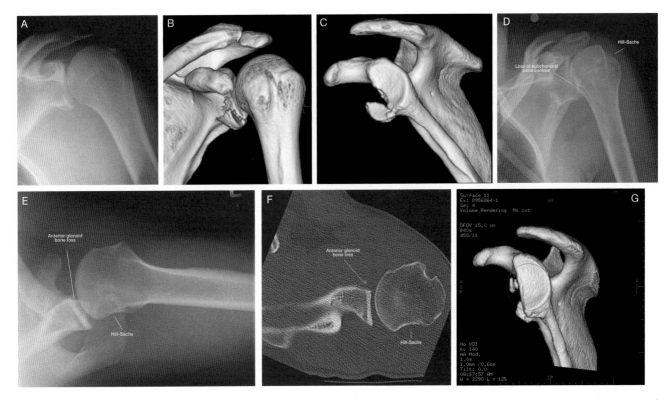

Figure 7.4 **A–C,** *Acute anterior glenoid rim fracture.* **D–G,** *Chronic anterior glenoid bone loss secondary to fracture and wear. The blue circle* **(G)** *helps understand the amount of bone missing.*

adding bone graft to the glenoid. Cadaver studies suggest that loss of approximately 20% of the glenoid width anteriorly increases instability substantially (3).

On the humeral side, bone loss in the setting of instability results from impaction fracture as the humeral head is forcefully driven into the glenoid rim. This injury creates an indentation similar to a dent created on a ping-pong ball by pushing with the thumb. In anterior dislocations, the humeral head defect is posterosuperior and known as a Hill-Sachs lesion (Figure 7.4D–F) (4). In posterior dislocations, the humeral head defect is anterior (reverse Hill-Sachs lesion, see Figure 7.11). The size of the defect is proportional to the magnitude of the injury and bone quality, but it will also tend to increase with repeated dislocation episodes. Reverse Hill-Sachs lesions are sometimes so large that they do not allow closed reduction of the posterior dislocation (locked posterior dislocation). This can also occur anteriorly (locked anterior dislocation). The management of locked dislocations is discussed in chapters 4, Proximal Humerus Fractures, and 9, Shoulder Arthritis and Arthroplasty.

Obviously, glenoid and humeral head bone loss interact, and the consequences of bone loss on both sides of the joint will potentially increase in stability even further. This interrelationship is best understood along the lines of the *glenoid track concept* (Figure 7.5) (5). This concept was developed trying to further understand when a Hill-Sachs lesion is large enough to engage in the anterior glenoid rim

and lead to recurrent anterior instability (engaging Hill-Sachs lesion).

Since the glenoid area is smaller than the humeral head area, in each shoulder position only a portion of the humeral head is in contact with the glenoid. The glenoid track was defined as the area of the humeral head that contacts the glenoid in maximal external rotation and horizontal abduction as the shoulder is elevated from neutral to full elevation (anterior shoulder instability typically recurs in this position of maximal combined abduction-external rotation). In cadaver studies, the glenoid track measures 84% of the width of the glenoid, measured from lateral to medial (from the cuff insertion into the articular cartilage) (5).

In patients with isolated humeral head bone loss (normal glenoid bone stock), the Hill-Sachs lesion will require surgical management (bone graft or remplissage, see later) if the area of the humeral head defect is beyond the glenoid track (i.e., larger than 84% of the glenoid width), since it will then engage in maximum abduction and external rotation and lead to recurrent instability. In patients with combined bone loss, since the glenoid is narrower, a smaller Hill-Sachs lesion will engage (Figure 7.5) (84% of a smaller width requires a smaller area of bone loss to engage). If the glenoid width can be built up to the point that the humeral head defect is smaller than the glenoid track, addressing glenoid bone loss will be enough to restore stability, and the humeral head defect can be

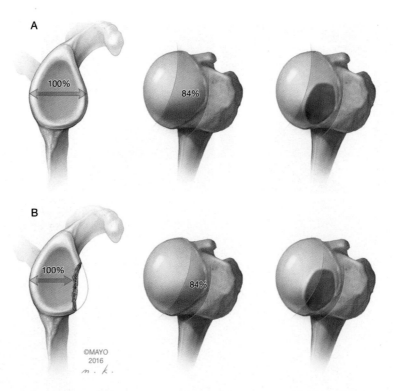

©MAYO
2016
m. k.

Figure 7.5 *The glenoid track concept.* **A,** *In the absence of glenoid bone loss, this Hill-Sachs lesion will not engage.* **B,** *In the presence of glenoid bone loss, the same Hill-Sachs lesion will engage.*

ignored. Alternatively, addressing the humeral head defect will be necessary if anterior glenoid bone loss is not reconstructed or if reconstructing the glenoid will still leave a Hill-Sachs lesion that engages (5–7).

Labrum, Biceps Tendon, Capsule, and Glenohumeral Ligaments

Damage to the labrum and glenohumeral ligaments contributes to shoulder instability in many individuals. The labrum is a fibrocartilaginous structure attached circumferentially to the glenoid rim (Figure 7.6). Inferiorly the labrum is round, elevated, and firmly attached to bone, whereas superiorly it is meniscal and more loosely attached. Table 7.1 summarizes the stabilizing functions of the labrum and some normal variants that may be confused with traumatic injuries (Figure 7.7).

Table 7.1 • **The Labrum: Mechanisms of Stability and Normal Variants**

Labrum stabilizing mechanisms

Bumper effect: the labrum doubles the anteroposterior depth of the glenoid from 2.5 to 5 mm and deepens the concavity to 9 mm

Increased contact area for the humeral head (glenoid + labrum)

Attachment site for the glenohumeral ligaments and capsule

Normal anatomical variants (see Figure 7.7)

Sublabral foramen: the labrum is completely separated from the anterosuperior glenoid margin (10%–20% of the population)

Buford complex: absence of the anterosuperior labrum and continuity of the labrum at this level with a cordlike middle glenohumeral ligament

---

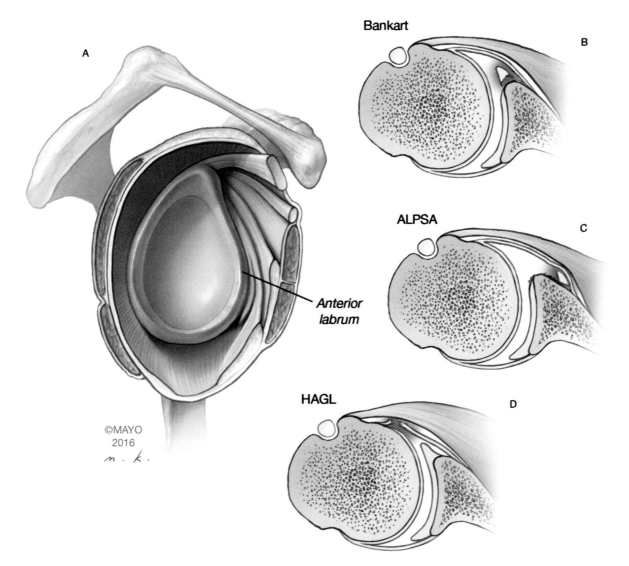

©MAYO
2016
m. k.

Figure 7.6 **A,** *Glenoid labrum, biceps, capsule, and glenohumeral ligaments.* **B,** *Bankart lesion.* **C,** *Anterior labrum and periosteal sleeve avulsion (ALPSA) lesion.* **D,** *Humeral avulsion of the inferior glenohumeral ligament (HAGL) lesion.*

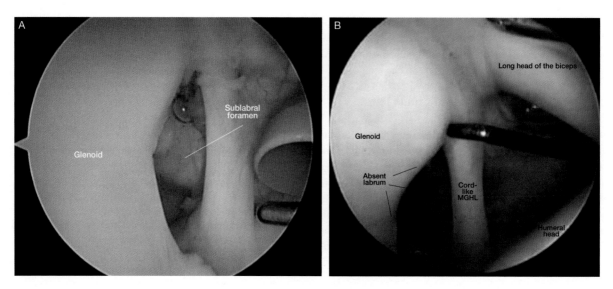

Figure 7.7 **A,** *Sublabral foramen.* **B,** *Buford complex. MGHL indicates middle glenohumeral ligament.*

The glenohumeral ligaments are specific portions of the capsule. Instead of acting as traditional ligaments carrying a pure tensile force, they become taut in various glenohumeral positions (Figure 7.6, Table 7.2). Anterior shoulder dislocations oftentimes result in disruption of the antero-inferior labrum and the anterior band of the inferior glenohumeral ligament. Several terms have been coined to define various patterns of injury (Table 7.3) (8,9). Normal variants described in Table 7.1 should not be confused with traumatic injuries.

In addition to all these traumatic discrete lesions described in Table 7.3, multiple episodes of subluxation or dislocation may lead to plastic deformation of the glenohumeral capsule and ligaments (10). The resultant elongated capsule has been shown to have poor tensile properties. The severity of this phenomenon is different from patient to patient based on the number of instability episodes, as well as individual factors. Surgical capsular plication is aimed to correct these abnormalities. Poor capsular properties may also be the consequence of some

Table 7.2 • Capsule and Glenohumeral Ligaments

	Anatomy	Tight In	Pathology
Superior glenohumeral ligament (SGHL)	Origin: Supraglenoid tubercle and labrum Insertion: Upper lesser tuberosity and bicipital groove	Adduction (prevents anterior and inferior instability)	Biceps tendon instability
Middle glenohumeral ligament (MGHL)	Origin: labrum Insertion: lesser tuberosity blended with subscapularis	Mid abduction and external rotation	Anterior instability
Inferior glenohumeral ligament (IGHL)			
Anterior band	Origin: labrum (type 1) or glenoid neck (type 2) Insertion: inferior humeral neck, 4–8 o'clock, V-shaped	Maximal abduction and external rotation	Anterior instability
Posterior band	Origin: glenoid neck and labrum 7–9 o'clock Insertion: humeral neck 4 o'clock	Flexion and internal rotation	Posterior instability
Rotator interval (RI)	Coracohumeral ligament + SGHL	External rotation in adduction	Anterior, posterior, and multidirectional instability

Table 7.3 • Various Patterns of Traumatic Disruption of the Labrum and Capsule

	Definition	Relevance
Bankart-Perthes lesion	Detachment of the anteroinferior glenoid labrum	Classic "essential lesion" in recurrent anterior shoulder instability. Leads to functional insufficiency of the IGHL. Poor healing potential
Bony Bankart lesion	Detachment of the anteroinferior glenoid labrum with a small fractured fragment of the glenoid rim	Leads to loss of labrum bumper effect, functional insufficiency of the IGHL and additional glenoid bone loss
Anterior labroligamentous periosteal sleeve avulsion (ALPSA)	Detachment of the labrum and periosteum off the glenoid neck in continuity	Tends to heal, but medially displaced. Associated with a higher failure rate after arthroscopic surgery, probably due to difficulty mobilizing tissue to the anatomical position
Humeral avulsion of the inferior glenohumeral ligament (HAGL)	Detachment of the anterior band of the IGHL on the humeral side (neck)	Easy to miss arthroscopically. Will lead to unexpected persistent anterior instability after surgery
Reverse humeral avulsion of the inferior glenohumeral ligament (reverse HAGL)	Detachment of the posterior band of the IGHL on the humeral side (neck)	Easy to miss arthroscopically. Will lead to unexpected persistent posterior instability after surgery
Glenolabral articular disruption (GLAD)	Anterior labral tear with adjacent cartilage disruption	Typically, it is not the result of a dislocation and tends not to facilitate recurrent instability, just pain and mechanical symptoms
Kim lesion	Posterior labral tear with intact superficial fibers	May be missed arthroscopically. When not addressed, it leads to recurrent posterior instability or persistent pain

Abbreviation: IGHL, inferior glenohumeral ligament.

connective tissue disorders, particularly Ehlers-Danlos syndrome.

Interestingly, individuals involved in throwing sports may be noted to have a deficit in glenohumeral internal rotation; although this has been attributed to changes in humeral torsion or a stiff posterior rotator cuff, some argue that glenohumeral internal rotation is the result of thickening and loss of elasticity of the posteroinferior capsule secondary to overload in patients with multiple posterior subluxation episodes (11).

Rotator Cuff

As mentioned in chapter 6, The Rotator Cuff and Biceps Tendon, contraction of the rotator cuff muscles contributes to keeping the humeral head centered on the glenoid during motion. The behavior of the glenohumeral joint with poor control of the rotator cuff can be compared with trying to run using loose shoes with the laces untied: the foot would move all over the place in the shoe, making it difficult to run. With poor control of the rotator cuff, the humeral head glides excessively all over the glenoid and makes it difficult for the prime movers (deltoid, pectoralis) to provide effective function secondary to this dynamic instability.

Poor coordination of the rotator cuff can contribute to instability. Full thickness cuff tears can also contribute to recurrent dislocation, especially in the elderly patient.

Older patients with a stiff and weakened rotator cuff may sustained a very large avulsion of the posterosuperior cuff and the posterior capsule that may facilitate recurrent dislocations due to lack of a posterior checkrein. The term *posterior mechanism of anterior instability* was coined to define this situation. Less commonly, a traumatic disruption of the subscapularis and anterior capsule facilitates anterior instability.

Scapula

As mentioned before, the scapula positions the glenoid in space. As discussed in detail in chapter 10, The Scapula, poor positioning of the scapula can be secondary to numerous reasons (e.g., bony injuries to the clavicle or scapula, disorders of the periscapular musculature, nerve injuries). In addition, patients with shoulder instability may have functional scapular dyskinesis, where there is poor control of the periscapular musculature without a specific structural pathology. Scapular dyskinesis may be the only abnormality responsible for shoulder instability (multidirectional) or it may be associated with other pathologic abnormalities described before.

Instability Classifications

Direction of Instability

As introduced in chapter 1, Evaluation of the Shoulder, glenohumeral instability may be classified based on the direction of excessive translation of the humeral head, respective to the glenoid, as anterior instability, posterior instability, or multidirectional instability. In general, these patterns of instability have a number of consistent features.

Anterior shoulder instability is almost always the result of substantial trauma leading to various degrees of soft-tissue disruption (anterior labrum and capsule) and/or bone injuries (bony Bankart, glenoid rim fracture, Hill-Sachs lesion). Patients may develop recurrent instability in the presence of substantial bone loss and/or persistent soft-tissue deficiency. Instability is most noticeable when the shoulder is placed in abduction and external rotation. Acute shoulder dislocations can also be associated with a subscapularis tear or a posterosuperior cuff tear.

Posterior shoulder instability can be secondary to 1 (or several) of the following factors: a substantial traumatic event leading to an acute posterior dislocation (oftentimes with a reverse Hill-Sachs lesion), traumatic disruption of the posterior labrum and capsule secondary to repetitive trauma (e.g., posteriorly directed force with the shoulder in flexion, adduction, and internal rotation, commonly seen in defensive linemen in American football), or glenoid dysplasia or hypoplasia.

The term *multidirectional instability* (MDI) is applied when there is instability in several directions (anterior, posterior, inferior). Typically, MDI affects younger patients with generalized hyperlaxity. This pattern of global instability is associated with a very large capsule with relatively poor tensile properties, a widened rotator interval, and poor coordination of the rotator cuff and the periscapular musculature. Sometimes, patients with MDI will state that they always knew they had a lax shoulder, but symptoms start later in life. Occasionally there is laxity in all directions but symptoms (instability) in only 1 direction. There are lax individuals who are able to translate the humeral head to a subluxed or dislocated position at will (voluntary shoulder instability). The labrum is oftentimes intact, but it may be found to be hypoplastic and after multiple subluxation episodes it may develop tearing. These 2 conditions are described in detail in the Multidirectional Instability section.

Severity of Translation and Chronology of Instability

Glenohumeral instability may lead to a complete anterior or posterior dislocation, subluxation, or a combination of both. As mentioned in chapter 1, Evaluation of the Shoulder, translation of the humeral head in the resting position is assessed in grades (Figure 7.8). For anterior instability, the first episode is oftentimes a complete dislocation; after reduction, some patients will never experience instability again, whereas others develop recurrent instability with multiple subsequent episodes of subluxation or dislocation. For posterior and MDI, subluxation episodes are more common than complete dislocation episodes, except for acute traumatic posterior dislocations.

End of Range of Motion versus Mid Range of Motion Instability

This concept has already been introduced to some extent. It summarizes the fact that any shoulder joint has some degree of translation in the resting position, but as the glenohumeral joint is positioned close to terminal range of motion, the static stabilizers (labrum, capsule, ligaments, interval region) tighten up, limiting additional translation and thus preventing instability.

In *end of range of motion instability*, the subluxation or dislocation episodes occur mostly secondary to insufficiency of the static stabilizers, anteriorly when the shoulder is placed in abduction and external rotation, or posteriorly when the shoulder is placed in adduction, flexion and internal rotation (Figure 7.9). This indicates structural damage that can reliably be repaired with surgery, and is oftentimes secondary to trauma. The acronym *TUBS* was coined to summarize the features of anterior end of range of motion instability: *T*raumatic in origin, *U*nilateral, associated with *B*ankart lesion, responds to *S*urgery.

In the *mid range of motion instability*, symptoms occur in the neutral position mostly due to lack of muscular control or a very loose joint with a large capsule. The term *AMBRI* was coined to summarize the features of mid range of motion instability: *A*traumatic in origin,

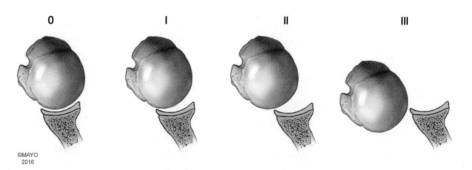

Figure 7.8 *Instability grading, where 0 indicates stable, I = <50%, II = 50%-99%, and III = 100%.*

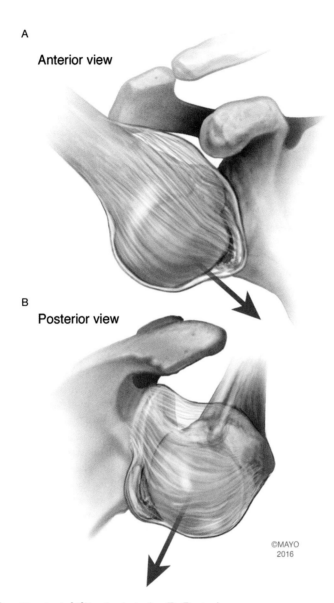

A

Anterior view

B

Posterior view

©MAYO
2016

Figure 7.9 *End of range of motion instability:* **A,** *Anterior.* **B,** *Posterior.*

*M*ultidirectional, *B*ilateral, requires *R*ehabilitation as a first line of treatment, and when treated surgically requires shift of the *I*nferior capsule.

Management of the Acute Glenohumeral Joint Dislocation

Every health care provider who participates in primary care, emergency medicine, or orthopedic surgery wants and needs to know how to help the patient with an acute glenohumeral joint dislocation. Patients oftentimes present with a somewhat dramatic clinical picture: sudden onset of severe pain after an injury, deformity, and inability to move the shoulder. Most of the time, care of these patients takes place in an emergency department setting;

occasionally, sports-related dislocations are managed in the field.

Anterior Dislocation

Shoulder dislocations account for approximately 45% of all dislocations seen in an emergency department, and more than 95% are anterior (12). The incidence of a first episode of anterior dislocation is approximately 8 per 100,000 population per year. Men are affected 3 times more often than women, and 90% of the patients are in their second decade of life, with a second incidence peak in the sixth decade.

Most of the time, anterior dislocations are the result of a substantial injury that forces the shoulder into combined abduction and external rotation; however, in patients with recurrent instability, anterior dislocations may occur with somewhat minor movements (turning to the back seat of the car, moving while sleeping). The dislocated shoulder is quite painful, held with the opposite hand in some abduction, and can barely be moved. The shoulder will appear squared off. The exception is the anterior dislocation where the humeral head rests under the glenoid with the arm in hyperabduction (*luxation erecta*). In every patient with a shoulder dislocation, the examination should include assessment of the axillary nerve and other terminal branches of the brachial plexus, as well as distal pulses and temperature and color of the fingers, to detect possible associated vascular injuries.

Whenever possible, radiographs should be obtained prior to attempted reduction in order to understand the magnitude of the injury and more importantly detect associated fractures of the tuberosities, shaft, or glenoid (Figure 7.10). Closed reduction without radiographs may be considered in the sports field if there are experienced personnel (13). The details of radiographic projections commonly used in trauma and the management of fracture-dislocations are summarized in chapter 4, Proximal Humerus Fractures. The management of the acute episode of anterior dislocation is discussed next.

Closed Reduction

Reduction is considered once the patient has received reassurance, information, and adequate pain relief. Intra-articular injection of a local anesthetic is a great way to provide pain relief and facilitate reduction (14). Oral or parenteral analgesia, sedation, or even general anesthesia may be considered as well. There are multiple maneuvers described for reduction of an anterior dislocation (Table 7.4). My preference is to use a traction-counter traction technique. The reduction is oftentimes felt by the patient as a clunk followed by improvement in comfort. Care must be taken to avoid forceful rotation of the arm, as it can lead to iatrogenic fracture.

Aftercare

Radiographs are obtained to confirm the adequacy of the reduction and assess for associated fractures. Computed tomography may be considered for certain fracture-dislocations (see chapter 4, Proximal Humerus Fractures). Patients who sustain a dislocation after the age of 40 have a relatively high risk of tearing their rotator cuff with their dislocation; if strength testing suggests the possibility of a cuff tear, advanced imaging studies (magnetic resonance imaging [MRI] or ultrasonography) should be considered. The neurovascular examination should be repeated after the adequacy of the reduction is confirmed. Injuries to the axillary or suprascapular nerve or the brachial plexus should be assessed using electromyography with nerve conduction studies 3 to 6 weeks after the dislocation. Most of these injuries are neurapraxias that will recover completely, but if no hint of recovery is noted by 6 months after the injury, consideration should be given to surgical treatment.

After successful closed reduction of an isolated anterior dislocation, the shoulder is immobilized for a period of time and physical therapy is then initiated to regain motion and strength. The position and length of immobilization are both controversial.

Traditionally, the shoulder has always been immobilized in adduction and internal rotation for comfort. However, some studies demonstrated that immobilization of the shoulder in approximately 30° to 45° of external

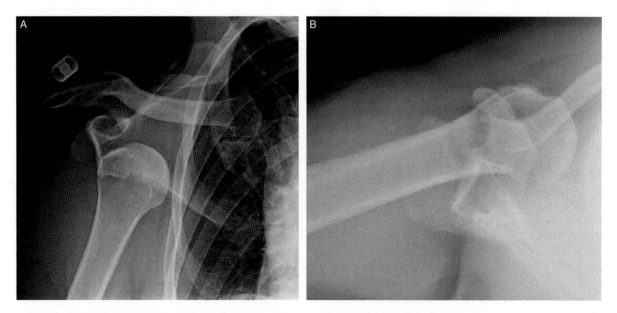

Figure 7.10 *Anterior shoulder dislocation.* **A,** *Anteroposterior view.* **B,** *Axillary view.*

Table 7.4 • Common Reduction Maneuvers for Anterior Shoulder Dislocation

	Description
Without axillary counter support	
Hippocratic maneuver	Simple traction in line with the arm
Kocher maneuver	Gradual external rotation and abduction followed by internal rotation and adduction
Stimson maneuver	Patient prone with the arm hanging down and a weight attached to the wrist
Milch maneuver	Gradual placement of the affected extremity in abduction with some external rotation
With axillary counter support	
Matsen maneuver	Traction in line with the arm with a folded sheet under the axilla
Chair maneuver	Traction in line with the arm by resting the weight of the provider on the forearm while the arm is hanging over the back of a chair

rotation led to less residual displacement of the capsulolabral injury secondary to tension on the subscapularis (15,16). In theory, this would facilitate healing in a more anatomic position and lead to lower persistent instability rates. However, immobilization in external rotation is less comfortable, and patients are less compliant. Various studies have failed to prove that immobilization in external rotation leads to a substantial reduction in recurrence rate (17).

Regarding length of immobilization, most surgeons base it on age. As detailed later, younger age is directly correlated with recurrence, and older age is correlated with residual stiffness. Younger patients are immobilized between 3 and 6 weeks, whereas older patients are immobilized 1 to 2 weeks (12).

Risk Assessment and Counseling for Persistent Instability

Most studies on the natural history of patients treated nonoperatively after a first anterior dislocation episode indicate that recurrence is more likely to happen in younger patients, those with substantial traumatic bone loss, and with longer follow-up.

In a prospective study of 229 anterior dislocations followed 25 years after nonoperative treatment, 43% had not redislocated. Of the 57% of shoulders that redislocated, 27% had undergone surgery for treatment of instability, 7% redislocated once, and 22% redislocated more than once. The rate of nonrecurrent instability was 28% in patients under 22 years, 44% in patients between 23 and 29 years, and 73% in patients between 30 and 40 years (18). In this study, associated fracture of the greater tuberosity was protective against instability, and use of immobilization after closed reduction did not change the outcome.

In a similar study of 252 anterior dislocations in patients between 15 and 35 years of age, recurrent instability developed in almost 60% at 2 years and 67% at 5 years. Significant factors for recurrence were younger age (>50% in patients younger than 20 versus 20% in patients over 30), male sex, hyperlaxity, and participation

in contact sports. Fracture of the greater tuberosity was again protective (19).

Based on available data, patients should be informed that the risk of an additional episode of dislocation for all age groups is probably around 40%. The risk is multiplied by 3 in men, by 3 in patients with hyperlaxity, and by 13 in patients under the age of 40. Patients under the age of 20 have a 50% to 70% chance of sustaining at least 1 additional dislocation episode. Participation in contact sports increases the risk even further (20).

Even in the absence of recurrent instability, some studies seem to indicate that a number of patients will not feel that their shoulder is ever normal again. In addition, radiographic evidence of arthritis develops in a number of patients. In the same cohort of 229 shoulders mentioned before (18), 223 were radiographically analyzed after 25 years. Radiographs were normal in 44%; arthritis was mild in 29%, moderate in 9%, and severe in 17%. Moderate or severe arthritis was 18% for shoulders with no recurrence, 26% for shoulders stabilized surgically, and 39% for shoulders with persistent instability. Other risk factors for arthritis included age over 25 at the time of the index dislocation, participation in contact sports, and alcohol abuse (21).

When to Consider Surgery Acutely

Surgical management immediately after an acute anterior shoulder dislocation can be considered in 3 circumstances.

Irreducible Dislocation

Closed reduction is successful in most patients with an anterior dislocation. However, in some patients a closed reduction may be impossible due to severe humeral head impaction or interposition of soft tissues. Open reduction then becomes necessary.

Management of Associated Injuries

Dislocations associated with a substantial fracture of the glenoid rim and persistent subluxation should be considered for internal fixation of the glenoid rim fracture.

As discussed in chapter 4, Proximal Humerus Fractures, surgery may also be necessary for patients with proximal humerus fracture-dislocations.

Prevention of Recurrence

Since the reported recurrence rate after nonoperative treatment is so high after a first episode of anterior dislocation, some surgeons argue that surgical stabilization of the shoulder joint should be considered at least for patients at high risk. In addition, recurrence also seems to increase the rate of late moderate or severe arthritis. Surgical stabilization after a first-time anterior dislocation is particularly appealing, since most of these surgeries can be performed arthroscopically with relatively little difficulty.

On one hand, several studies have demonstrated that surgery after a first anterior dislocation episode does reduce the rate of recurrent dislocation compared with nonoperative treatment, although not to zero: the rate of recurrent instability seems to be under 5% at 2 years and can escalate to about 15% after 10 years. On the other hand, some argue that if every patient with a first dislocation episode is operated on, many patients would undergo unnecessary surgery, since the risk of recurrence after nonoperative treatment is not 100%. It is important to note that successful restoration of stability does not seem to decrease the rate of late arthritis (22,23).

As in other aspects of orthopedic surgery, recommending and offering surgery is not the same. In my practice, I offer surgery after a first dislocation episode to ultrayoung patients (under 20 or 25) involved in contact sports, especially males or patients with hyperlaxity.

Posterior Dislocation

As noted before, acute posterior glenohumeral dislocations represent less than 5% of all shoulder dislocations. The reported prevalence rate is 1.1 per 100,000 population per year. Unfortunately, posterior dislocations are commonly missed when patients are first seen: the position of the arm is not particularly abnormal, and anteroposterior radiographs not obtained in the scapular plane may not look that abnormal either. Table 7.5 summarizes a number of features that should prompt you to think "this patient could have a posterior shoulder dislocation."

When evaluated, patients who have sustained a posterior dislocation as a consequence of a seizure or electrocution may not remember any details. After a posterior dislocation, patients tend to rest the arm on their lap in adduction and internal rotation. Lack of passive external rotation is the most obvious physical examination finding. Plain radiographs may not look that abnormal on the anteroposterior view (Figure 7.11); the axillary view or

---

Table 7.5 • Posterior Shoulder Dislocation

History
Traumatic injury with the shoulder in flexion and adduction
Shoulder pain after seizure
Shoulder pain after electrocution

Physical examination
Lack of passive external rotation
Difficulty performing supination
Fullness of the posterior shoulder with prominence of the coracoid in the front

Plain radiographs
Overlap of the contours of the humeral head and the glenoid on the anteroposterior view
Isolated fracture of the lesser tuberosity
Humeral head depression fracture anteromedially
The humeral head is posterior to the glenoid in axillary radiographs (and computed tomography)

---

computed tomography is extremely useful to confirm the diagnosis and important to identify associated fractures of the humeral neck and evaluate humeral head bone loss. Most posterior dislocations (>85%) have some degree of impaction fracture (reverse Hill-Sachs lesion) (24). Cuff tears are less common (15%), but 5 times more likely in those patients with a posterior dislocation and no fractures. Nerve injuries are also less common than in anterior dislocations.

Management

The management of acute posterior dislocations depends on the ease of reduction, presence of associated injuries, and magnitude of the reverse Hill-Sachs lesion. The management of fracture-dislocations is reviewed in chapter 4, Proximal Humerus Fractures. For the acute posterior dislocation with or without a reverse Hill-Sachs lesion but not other fractures, Figure 7.12 reviews my management algorithm.

Closed Reduction

Closed reduction of a posterior dislocation does require complete sedation or general anesthesia to minimize humeral head damage. As mentioned before, it is important to look for possible associated fractures, especially fractures of the surgical neck that could be further displaced with the reduction maneuver. Several maneuvers can be attempted. Simple traction in line with the upper extremity has been reported to be successful in one-third of patients (24,25). If traction is unsuccessful, the dislocation can be disimpacted by placing the shoulder in adduction, flexion, and internal rotation; under traction, the shoulder is then gently externally rotated as the humeral head is pushed anteriorly. Alternatively, the Stimson method, mentioned in Table 7.4, can be considered.

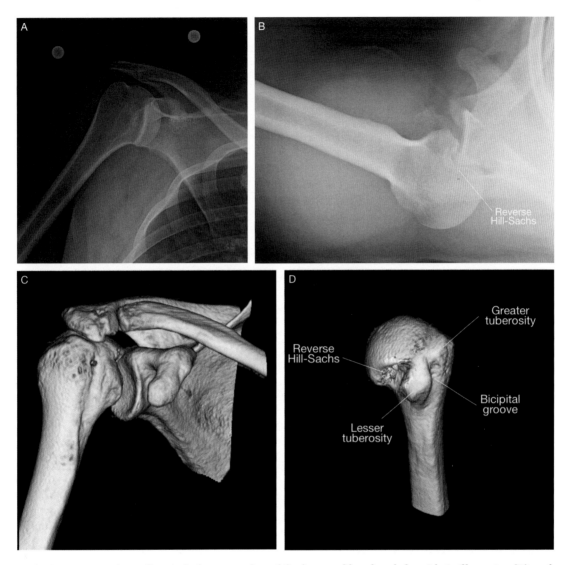

Figure 7.11 **A,** *Anteroposterior radiograph shows overlap of the humeral head and glenoid. Axillary view* **(B)** *and computed tomogram demonstrate the posterior dislocation* **(C)** *with a reverse Hill-Sachs lesion* **(D)**.

When closed reduction is successful, and gross instability with redislocation is not detected, patients are treated conservatively. The shoulder should be immobilized in external rotation for 4 to 6 weeks, followed by a program of physical therapy for range of motion and strengthening. On the other hand, if closed reduction is impossible or the joint redislocates, surgical management becomes necessary.

Labral Repair With or Without Capsular Shift
Repair of the posterior labrum with or without capsular shift is indicated for patients with recurrent posterior instability and minimal bone loss. Although this procedure was initially described using a posterior open approach to the shoulder joint, most surgeons currently perform this procedure arthroscopically (26–28). The details of this procedure are described later.

Disimpaction, Grafting, and Lesser Tuberosity Transfer
When the size of the humeral defect is greater than 20% of the humeral head diameter, the risk of recurrent instability is substantial if the defect is not corrected. Sometimes it is possible to elevate the area of impaction and fill the subchondral defect with bone graft or a substitute (24). Alternatively, the defect may be reconstructed with allograft or by transferring the lesser tuberosity to the area of deficiency.

Allograft reconstruction has been shown to restore stability and function with minimal pain (29,30). In a long-term study of 19 shoulders followed a minimum of 5 years, 2 patients eventually required a shoulder arthroplasty, and 4 had well-tolerated severe arthritis, with no to moderate radiographic changes in the remaining shoulders (29). All

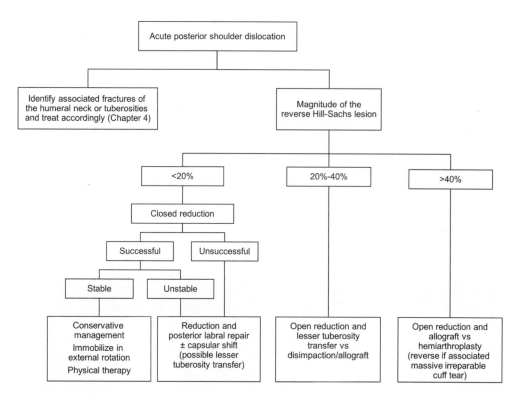

Figure 7.12 *Algorithm for management of acute posterior dislocations.*

patients had a defect involving at least 30% of the humeral head (mean involvement, 43%).

For relatively smaller defects, or when allograft is not available, transfer of the lesser tuberosity has also been reported to provide good results (Figure 7.13). McLaughlin first described transferring the subscapularis to the humeral head defect. Neer modified the procedure by transferring the subscapularis along with the lesser tuberosity. Alternatively, some authors anchor down the subscapularis to the defect without detaching it (reverse remplissage procedure). Transfer of the lesser tuberosity was reported to provide good or excellent results in a series of 7 patients with a humeral head defect measuring between 25% and 45%.

Arthroplasty

Humeral head replacement (anatomical hemiarthroplasty) is recommended in patients with substantial bone loss not deemed reconstructible with an allograft. Arthroplasty is particularly useful in patients treated late for a chronic posterior fracture-dislocation, since the size of the bone defect tends to enlarge over time and the remaining cartilage and bone are osteopenic and fragile. Shoulder arthroplasty is associated with improvements in pain and external rotation, but some shoulders may develop recurrent instability, and the clinical outcome has not been satisfactory in a number of individuals (31). As mentioned in chapter 9, Shoulder Arthritis and Arthroplasty, reverse

arthroplasty has emerged as an attractive alternative in patients with locked posterior dislocations.

Risk Assessment for Recurrent Instability

The risk of recurrent posterior instability after a documented posterior dislocation episode has not been investigated as much as for anterior dislocations. In 1 study including 120 posterior dislocations, close to 20% of the shoulders developed recurrent instability within 1 year (25). Risk factors for recurrent instability included age under 40, history of seizures, and a large (>1.5 cm³) reverse Hill-Sachs lesion.

Recurrent Anterior Instability

Evaluation

As mentioned before, recurrent instability develops in a substantial number of patients who sustain a first episode of anterior instability (typically a traumatic anterior dislocation). Their clinical presentation is quite characteristic (9): recurrent dislocation or subluxation episodes occur when the shoulder is placed in combined abduction and external rotation. Table 7.6 summarizes the key points of the evaluation for these patients. The hyperextension internal rotation test may be particularly useful, since it demonstrates insufficiency of the inferior glenohumeral ligament but does not create apprehension (32).

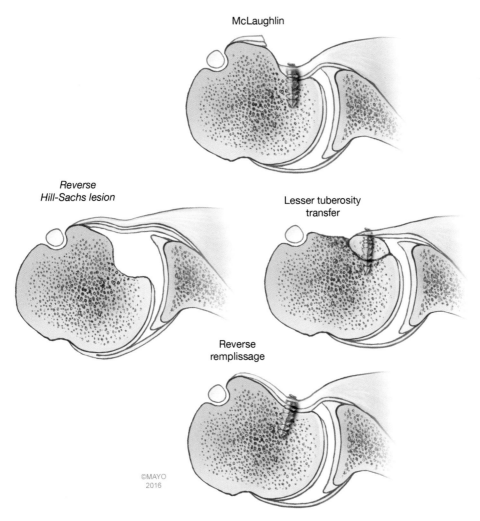

McLaughlin

Reverse Hill-Sachs lesion

Lesser tuberosity transfer

Reverse remplissage

©MAYO 2016

Figure 7.13 *Management options for reverse Hill-Sachs lesion: McLaughlin procedure, reverse remplissage, and lesser tuberosity transfer.*

Plain radiographs should be obtained in all patients. They can be normal, or demonstrate associated bone injuries on the glenoid or humeral head. Anteroinferior glenoid bone loss may be difficult to identify on radiographs; a subtle finding commonly seen in this situation is loss of the thicker subchondral bone as the glenoid contour is followed from superior to inferior (Figure 7.4D and E). Smaller Hill-Sachs lesions are seen only in internal rotation, whereas larger ones are seen in both internal and external rotation. Axillary views provide a better projection of Hill-Sachs lesions.

Some surgeons recommend use of a specific radiographic projection, the Bernageau view, to assess for glenoid bone loss (33). The radiograph is obtained with the patient standing, the axilla resting on the cassette, and the arm in hyperabduction (Figure 7.14). The radiographic beam is angled 15° caudal. This can be a useful screening radiograph for both anterior and posterior instability.

Computed tomography with 3-dimensional reconstruction is the best imaging study to analyze bone loss in recurrent instability (9). Most surgeons assess glenoid bone loss on the 3-dimensional view of the face of the glenoid by digitally tracing a circle that will best fit the dimensions of the glenoid (Figure 7.15). Bone loss can be estimated in millimeters (distance between the edge of the circle anteriorly and the rim of the glenoid defect) or as percentage area. Humeral head defects are measured on the 2-dimensional axial, sagittal, and coronal cuts that capture the largest portion of the defect (Figure 7.16). The magnitude of the defect can then be compared with the width of the glenoid track (84% of the glenoid width, see Figure 7.5) (5).

MRI is best for evaluation of soft tissue injuries and cartilage damage. Intra-articular gadolinium is commonly considered, although not necessary if the person reading the images has some experience. MRI will identify the presence and extent of labral tears. It is particularly

Table 7.6 • **Evaluation of Patients With Recurrent Anterior Shoulder Instability**

History

What was the nature of the initial injury leading to the first instability episode?

Have any of the dislocation episodes been documented on radiographs?

Does instability occur in abduction and external rotation?

Previous treatment attempts?

Pain at rest, at night, or when the joint is not unstable?

History of hyperlaxity

Occupation/sports planned to be performed

Physical examination

Increased passive external rotation (in some)—Decreased external rotation less common (ALPSA; see Table 7.3)

Apprehension/relocation/surprise (see chapter 1)

Hyperextension internal rotation (HERI) test

Examine for posterior/multidirectional instability

Examine for painful superior labrum (dynamic labral shear test, O'Brien test, see chapter 1)

Examine for hyperlaxity

Examine the scapula

Examine the rotator cuff (especially in patients over 40)

Axillary nerve and brachial plexus

Additional investigations

Plain radiographs (joint position, glenoid rim, Hill-Sachs lesion, arthritis)

MRI (with or without intra-articular gadolinium) to assess labrum and capsule (and cuff in older patients)

CT with 3D reconstruction to assess bone loss

Genetic testing if Ehlers-Danlos syndrome suspected

EMG if neurologic abnormalities suspected

Abbreviations: ALPSA, anterior labroligamentous periosteal sleeve avulsion; CT, computed tomography; EMG, electromyography; MRI, magnetic resonance imaging; 3D, 3-dimensional.

important to detect humeral avulsions of the inferior glenohumeral ligament (HAGL lesions) (9,34). It is also very useful to detect associated tears of the rotator cuff in older patients.

Treatment Options

Since most patients with anterior recurrent instability present with substantial structural pathology, conservative treatment has a low chance of success, although a small

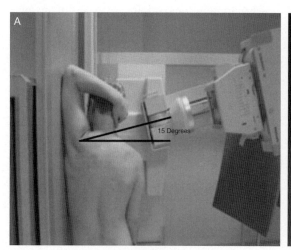
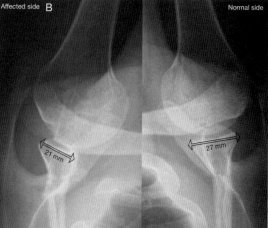

Figure 7.14 *Bernageau position* **(A)** *and view* **(B)**.

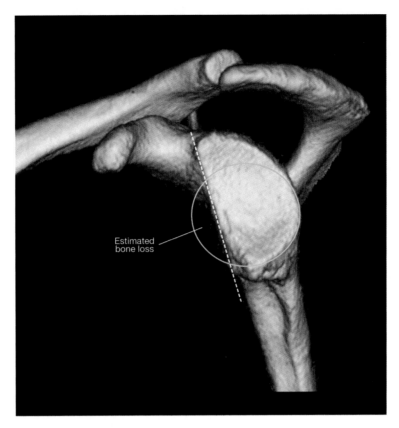

Figure 7.15 *Bone loss can be estimated using 3-dimensional reconstructions of the glenoid face.*

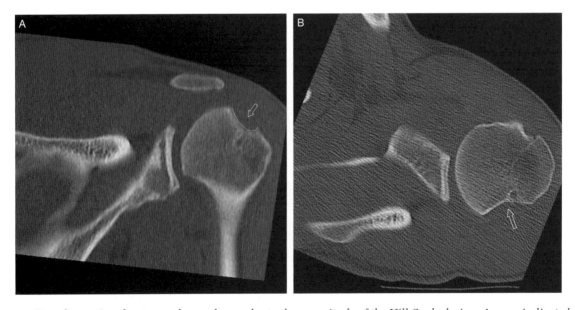

Figure 7.16 *Two-dimensional cuts may be used to evaluate the magnitude of the Hill-Sachs lesion. Arrows indicate location and size of Hill-Sachs lesion.* **A,** *Coronal,* **B,** *Axial.*

Table 7.7 • Surgical Procedures for Recurrent Anterior Shoulder Instability

Procedure	Description	Advantages	Disadvantages
Repair of labrum and capsule			
Open Bankart repair and capsular shift	Open exposure for anchoring the labrum to the glenoid rim and capsuloplasty	Allows substantial capsuloplasty Can be easily converted to bone block procedure	Violates the subscapularis Difficult management of the superior labrum
Arthroscopic Bankart repair and capsular shift	Arthroscopic reattachment of the labrum to the glenoid rim with capsular plication	Less invasive Preserves subscapularis Allows repair of the superior and posterior structures if needed	Does not allow as much capsuloplasty
HAGL repair	Open or arthroscopic reattachment of the capsule to the humeral neck	Avoids bone block procedures in patients with an isolated soft-tissue injury	Difficult to perform, especially arthroscopically
Glenoid bone block procedures			
Latarjet	Sideways transfer of the coracoid process and conjoined tendon to the glenoid rim	Widens the glenoid Bony bumper effect Hammock effect conjoined tendon Autograft (healing)	Difficult Higher complication rate If poorly performed, can lead to arthritis
Bristow	Standing transfer of the coracoid process and conjoined tendon to the glenoid rim	Widens the glenoid Bony bumper effect Hammock effect conjoined tendon Autograft (healing)	Difficult Higher complication rate If poorly performed, can lead to arthritis
Structural graft	Iliac crest autograft or allograft from glenoid, distal tibia, or other location	Widens the glenoid Bony bumper effect Allows management of osteoarticular defects	Allograft may not heal reliably Difficult Does not provide conjoined tendon effect
Hill-Sachs management			
Remplissage	Medialization of the insertion of the infraspinatus on the bed of a Hill-Sachs lesion	Minimally invasive management of humeral bone loss	Can limit external rotation
Bone grafting	Reconstruction of the defect with humeral or femoral head allograft	Restores anatomical bone stock	More invasive Potential for nonunion or collapse

Abbreviation: HAGL, humeral avulsion of the inferior glenohumeral ligament.

number of patients will not suffer additional dislocation episodes after a while (18). Physical therapy can be helpful prior to surgery for patients with stiffness or scapular dyskinesia.

Table 7.7 summarizes the main procedures commonly considered in the surgical management of recurrent anterior shoulder instability. Many shoulders with anterior instability can be rendered stable with surgical repair of the labrum, with or without capsular shift. However, the success rate of this procedure is not universal, and some patients will have a relatively high recurrence rate after surgery. The practice of contact sports, hyperlaxity, and bone loss are the main risk factors for failure of repair of the labrum and capsule. In patients with a high risk of failure after a soft-tissue procedure, many surgeons currently consider so-called bone block procedures a better alternative. The Instability

Severity Index Score (ISIS) was developed in order to determine which patients would have a high risk of recurrence after repair of the labrum and capsule, and should thus be considered for alternative interventions (Table 7.8) (35). In the first report describing the ISIS, a score of 6 or more points was correlated with poor outcome after arthroscopic stabilization (35). Other studies have suggested a high failure rate with an ISIS greater than 3 to 4 (36,37).

Comparing the outcomes of the various procedures that will be described next is extremely difficult for several reasons (Table 7.9). Bearing in mind these limitations, some studies seem to show the same recurrent instability rates with open and arthroscopic Bankart repair (38,39), whereas others show higher recurrence rate with arthroscopic techniques (40,41). The Latarjet procedure seems to be associated with lower recurrent instability rates and better

Table 7.8 • Instability Severity Index Score (ISIS)

Prognostic Factors	Points
Age at surgery (yrs)	
≤20	2
>20	0
Degree of sport participation (preoperative)	
Competitive	2
Recreational or none	0
Type of sport (preoperative)	
Contact or forced overhead	1
Other	0
Shoulder hyperlaxity	
Shoulder hyperlaxity (anterior or inferior)	1
Normal laxity	0
Hill-Sachs lesion on anteroposterior radiograph	
Visible in external rotation	2
Not visible in external rotation	0
Glenoid loss of contour on anteroposterior radiograph	
Loss of contour	2
No lesion	0
Total (points)	10

Adapted from Balg and Boileau (35). Used with permission.

function than arthroscopic Bankart repairs (37). The rate of recurrent instability in patients undergoing arthroscopic Bankart repair in the presence of an engaging Hill-Sachs lesion seems to improve by adding an arthroscopic advancement of the infraspinatus (remplissage) (42). Based on this data, my current treatment algorithm for patients with recurrent anterior instability is summarized in Figure 7.17. The management of patients with instability and a rotator cuff tear is discussed later.

Table 7.9 • Challenges When Comparing the Outcome of Various Surgical Techniques for Recurrent Anterior Instability

How is failure defined?
Recurrent dislocation
Recurrent dislocation or subluxation
Functional scores
Return to sports and other activities

Various lengths of follow-up
The rate of recurrent instability increases with follow-up

Mixed underlying pathology
Presence and magnitude of bone loss
Severity of soft-tissue injuries (i.e., Bankart vs ALPSA)
No. of patients with hyperlaxity

Abbreviation: ALPSA, anterior labroligamentous periosteal sleeve avulsion.

Repair of the Labrum and Capsule

Repair of the labrum with various degrees of capsular shift is the procedure of choice for patients with no or minimal glenoid bone loss (<20%) and an ISIS of 4 points or less. The procedure can be performed open or arthroscopically. In patients with a HAGL lesion, reattachment of the capsule to the humeral neck can also be performed either open or arthroscopically.

Open Bankart Repair and Capsular Shift

Exposure is obtained through a low deltopectoral approach (chapter 3, Surgical Exposures). The 2 most difficult steps of the operation are to dissect the subscapularis from the capsule and to anchor the labrum to the glenoid rim. The joint is exposed through a subscapularis tenotomy. The plane between the subscapularis and capsule is best identified in the lower third, where the subscapularis is more muscular; finding the right plane is more difficult proximally since the tendon fibers of the subscapularis and capsule merge, and the capsule in patients with recurrent anterior instability can be extremely stretched and thinned out (⬤ Video 7.1).

My preference is to detach the capsule laterally along the margin of the anatomic humeral neck (Figure 7.18). The capsule is then divided horizontally in preparation for later shift. The glenoid neck is exposed and prepared to bleeding bone with a bur, and the labrum is anchored using drill holes or suture anchors. The capsule is then shifted so that the inferior capsular flap is repaired as proximal as possible and the superior capsular flap covers the inferior flap anteriorly. This shift reduces the capsular volume and doubles the thickness of the anterior capsule. The position of the capsular flaps is determined with the arm in 45° of abduction and 20° of external rotation. The subscapularis tenotomy is then repaired anatomically. After surgery, the shoulder is immobilized in internal rotation for 3 to 4 weeks. Physical therapy starts then, with active assisted motion exercises followed by strengthening and scapular stabilizing exercises.

The long-term outcome of open Bankart repair and capsular shift has been documented in a number of studies. The recurrence instability rate at 2 years seems to be around 10% (41). A recent study reported the 20-year outcome of this procedure in 47 patients with minimal or no glenoid bone loss. The recurrence rate was approximately 17%, and a number of recurrences occurred 8 years after the index procedure (43).

Arthroscopic Bankart Repair and Capsular Shift

This procedure can be performed in the lateral or beach chair position (⬤ Video 7.2) (chapter 2, Arthroscopic Shoulder Surgery). I typically use a posterior glenohumeral portal and 2 or 3 anterior portals. Anteriorly, cannulas are placed in a lower medial portal just proximal to

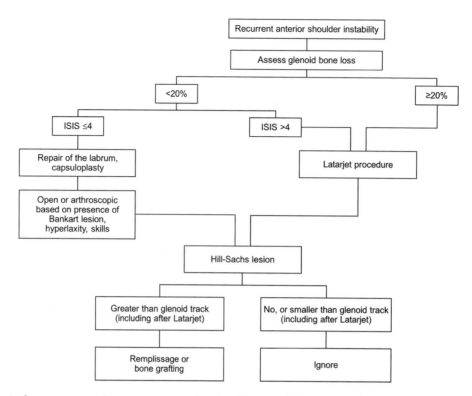

Figure 7.17 *Surgical management for recurrent anterior shoulder instability. ISIS indicates Instability Severity Index Score.*

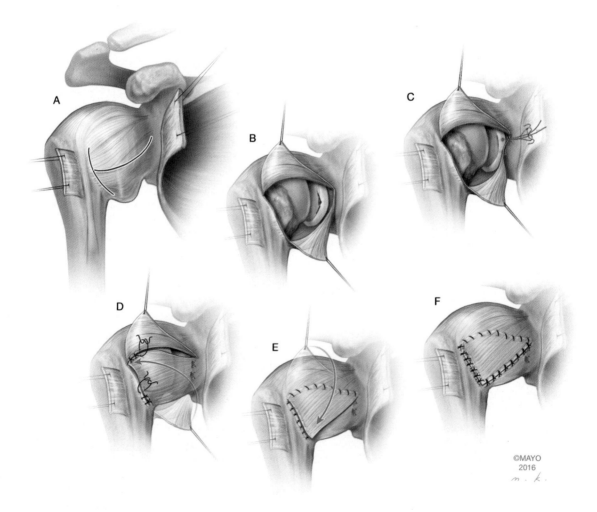

Figure 7.18 *Open Bankart repair and capsular shift.* **A,** *Capsulotomy.* **B,** *Glenoid exposure.* **C,** *Labrum repair.* **D,** *Inferior to superior shift.* **E,** *Superior to inferior shift.* **F,** *Final reconstruction.*

Table 7.10 • Strategies for Successful Arthroscopic Bankart Repair and Capsular Shift

---

Visualization and working space
Arm holder or distraction
Placement of a bump under the axilla

Anterior cannula placement
Avoid crowding

Mobilization of capsule and labrum anteriorly
Visualize from anterosuperior portal
Mobilize tissue until subscapularis muscle fibers are
    visualized
Prepare the anterior glenoid rim to bleeding bone

Anchor placement
Place inferior anchors low enough
Anchors should be at the very rim
    Anchors on the medial glenoid neck will not help restore
        bumper effect
    Anchors on the glenoid face can lead to cartilage damage
Use enough anchors: 3 are commonly required, 4 if superior
    labrum is repaired
Consider double-loaded anchors

Labrum repair and capsular shift
Consider placement of traction sutures
Shift the capsule from distal to proximal
Consider plication (commensurate with abnormal laxity as
    determined in examination under anesthesia)

---

the subscapularis tendon, and a higher more lateral portal over the biceps tendon. A third anterior portal with no cannula is used for placement of the lowest 1 or 2 anchors. A number of elements are key for the successful performance of an arthroscopic Bankart repair and capsular shift (Table 7.10, Figure 7.19). The postoperative management is similar to the program used after open Bankart repair.

The outcome of arthroscopic repair has continued to improve over time. When arthoscopic techniques were first introduced, the recurrence rate was higher than with open Bankart repair. Currently, some studies suggest than open repair is associated with a lower recurrence rate (41), whereas others indicate that with proper patient selection and surgical technique, the outcome is equivalent (38,39). Unfortunately, recent studies continue to report recurrence instability rates as high as 25% to 30% with arthroscopic Bankart repair and capsular shift (39,41). Hopefully, these rates will continue to go down as patient selection and surgical techniques are both improved.

Repair of a HAGL Lesion
A HAGL lesion is uncommon and can be easily missed. It can be associated with an injury to the glenoid labrum, and if not carefully looked for at the time of soft-tissue stabilization, it can be missed and not repaired, leading

to failed surgery. This diagnosis can be made on preoperative MRI (Figure 7.20), or at the time of surgery (9,34). Repair can be performed through an open exposure, gaining access to the capsule and the humeral neck through a subscapularis tenotomy or by elevating the subscapularis muscle fibers off the capsule from inferior to superior. It can also be performed arthroscopically using dedicated inferior portals.

Bone Block Procedures
Bone block procedures are considered when the magnitude of bone loss (either an isolated glenoid defect or a combined glenoid-humeral head defect) is severe enough to generate instability on its own, and in patients with a substantial risk of failure with soft-tissue repair techniques (i.e., ISIS >4–6 points).

The common underlying feature of bone block procedures for recurrent anterior shoulder instability is placement of a bone graft on the anteroinferior glenoid rim. Options include use of a free autograft (typically from the iliac crest), use of allograft (either bone without cartilage or a segmental osteoarticular allograft), or transferring a segment of the coracoid process with the origin of the conjoined tendon attached. The transferred coracoid can be secured to the glenoid rim "standing," so that the base of the osteotomized coracoid rests on the glenoid neck (Bristow procedure). Alternatively, it can be placed "lying" so that the inferior cortex of the coracoid rests on the glenoid rim (Latarjet procedure).

Currently, the Latarjet procedure is the most commonly used bone block procedure, and my preferred surgical technique as well (44). In contrast to the Bristow procedure, the Latarjet procedure provides more contact area for healing by placing the graft on the side, and 2 screws may be used for stable fixation. As mentioned in Table 7.7, the Latarjet procedure stabilizes the shoulder though several mechanisms: it widens the glenoid on the anteroposterior dimension, it provides a bumper effect, and the transferred conjoined tendon supports the humeral head when it tries to escape anteroinferiorly in abduction and external rotation (Figure 7.21). In addition, some surgeons repair the coracoacromial ligament to the capsule, which may add stability at the end of range of motion. In the mid arc of motion, the transferred bone and the conjoined tendon seem to each contribute approximately 50% to shoulder stability. At the end of range of motion (abduction and external rotation), the conjoined tendon seems responsible for at least 75% of the benefit of the procedure (45).

Reconstruction of the anteroinferior glenoid rim with allograft is mostly considered instead of a Latarjet procedure in patients with previous failed coracoid transfer procedures or extensive bone loss with need to provide articular cartilage as well. Ideally, a matched glenoid allograft is used

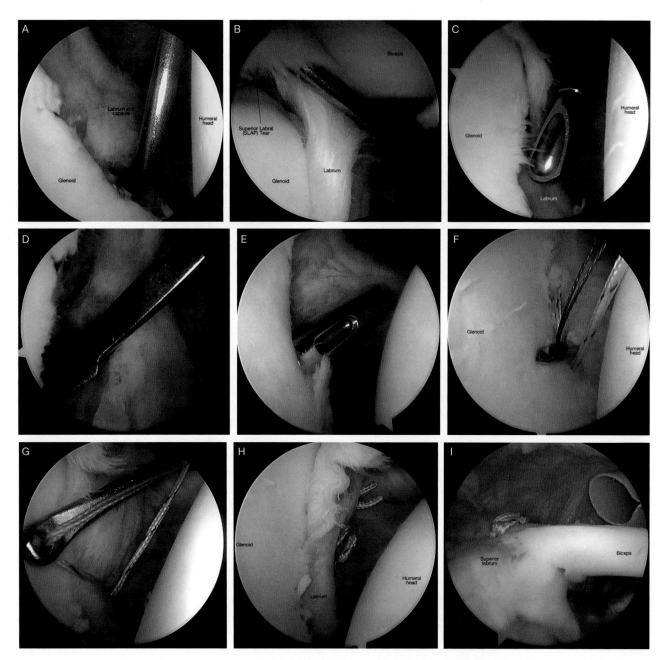

Figure 7.19 *Arthroscopic Bankart repair.* **A,** *Detachment of the anterior labrum and capsule.* **B,** *Associated superior labral tear.* **C,** *Preparation of the bone surface.* **D,** *Mobilization of the labrum and capsule.* **E,** *Anchor placement.* **F,** *Suture passing.* **G,** *Suture tying.* **H,** *Finalized repair with horizontal mattress sutures and restoration of the so-called bumper effect of the labrum.* **I,** *Repair of the superior labrum as well (when needed).*

in these circumstances. However, glenoid allografts can be difficult to obtain; alternatively, the distal tibial plafond geometry seems to fit well with the glenoid overall morphology (46,47).

Open Latarjet Procedure
Exposure is obtained through a low deltopectoral approach (chapter 3, Surgical Exposures) (⬤ Video 7.3). Osteotomy of the base of the coracoid, performed as a first step,

provides great exposure to the anterior aspect of the glenohumeral joint (Figure 7.22). Once the coracoid is identified and delineated, the coracoacromial ligament is detached from the lateral side, the pectoralis tendon is detached from the medial side, and a 90° angle blade is used to perform the osteotomy at the coracoid base. Care must be taken to obtain as much graft as possible without violating the glenoid cavity or fracturing the glenoid or the graft. The conjoined tendon is mobilized distally, taking care not to

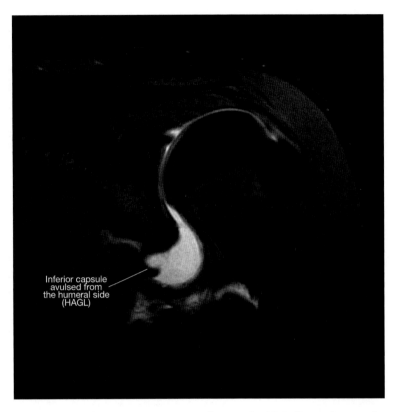

Figure 7.20 *Magnetic resonance image demonstrates a HAGL lesion. HAGL indicates humeral avulsion of the inferior glenohumeral ligament.*

damage the musculocutaneous nerve. The inferior cortex of the coracoid is then lightly freshened to remove fibrous tissue and expose bleeding bone.

Deep exposure may be performed through a subscapularis tenotomy, but my preference is to expose the glenoid splitting the subscapularis muscle horizontally in its midportion or at the junction of the superior two-thirds and the inferior third. The capsule is then divided vertically close to the glenoid rim and a posterior humeral head retractor inserted in the joint. The anteroinferior aspect of the glenoid neck is prepared by removing fibrous tissue and exposing bleeding bone, and the coracoid is fixed to the glenoid with 2 compression bicortical screws. Care must be taken to place the graft so that it is flush with

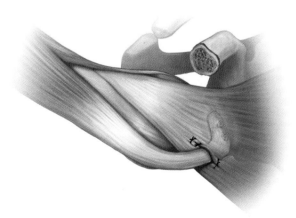

Figure 7.21 *Latarjet procedure: hammock effect of the conjoined tendon in abduction and external rotation.*

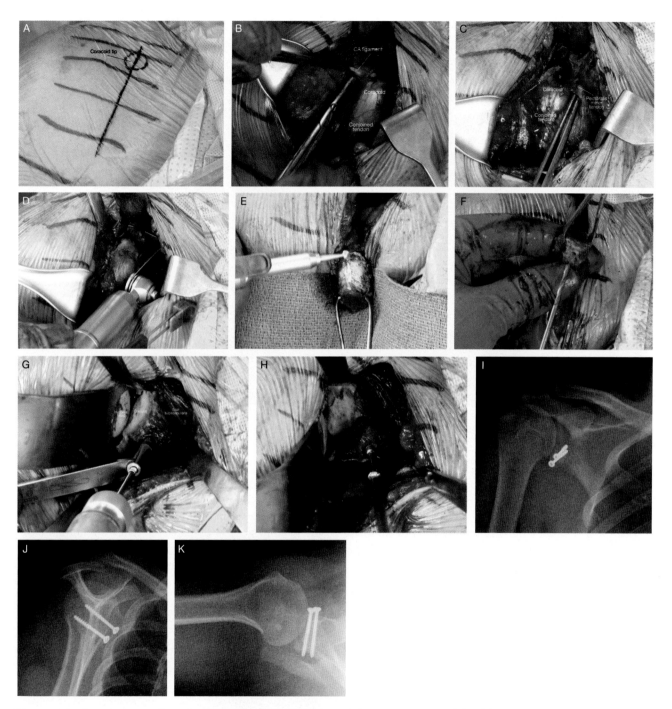

Figure 7.22 *Latarjet procedure.* **A,** *Skin incision.* **B,** *Division of the coracoacromial (CA) ligament.* **C,** *Detachment of the pectoralis minor.* **D,** *Coracoid osteotomy,* **E,** *Coracoid preparation.* **F,** *Drilling of the coracoid.* **G,** *Drilling of the glenoid.* **H,** *Screw fixation.* **I,** *Anteroposterior radiograph.* **J,** *Lateral radiograph.* **K,** *Axillary radiograph.*

the glenoid concavity: a graft placed too medial may not restore stability, whereas a graft placed too lateral may impinge with the humeral head and lead to early osteoarthritis. It is also important to achieve stable fixation of the coracoid while avoiding screw damage to the glenoid or the suprascapular nerve branches, which might be injured posteriorly if the screw tips are too prominent. The lateral

aspect of the capsule can be repaired to the coracoacromial ligament stump.

The reported outcome of the Latarjet procedure is quite good. In a study of 68 shoulders followed for a minimum of 20 years, the recurrence instability rate was 6%, and the average subjective shoulder value was 90% (44). Some studies seem to indicate that the rate of recurrent instability overall is more favorable for the Latarjet procedure when compared with repair of the labrum and capsule (37,48), with similar long-term osteoarthritis rates (48). The long-term rate of osteoarthritis has been reported to be 30% at 20 years: Twenty percent of the patients with no arthritis at the time of the Latarjet procedure developed arthritis, and 50% of the patients with arthritis experienced worsening of arthritis. The grade of osteoarthritis was moderate in only approximately 10% (44). However, the reported complication rate of the Latarjet procedure has varied between 15% and 30% (49–51).

Arthroscopic Latarjet Procedure

The Latarjet procedure can also be performed arthroscopically, although the degree of difficulty is substantial and the learning curve steep (52). Visualization may be performed through a standard posterior portal for some parts of the procedure, and through an anterosuperior portal for other parts of the procedure. The steps include preparation and osteotomy of the coracoid, transfer of the coracoid, and fixation. Guides have been developed to facilitate the procedure (53,54). Most reported complications of the Latarjet procedure performed arthroscopically are related to poor positioning of the graft, problems with screw fixation, and neurovascular complications. Use of cortical buttons instead of screws may help address some of these concerns (53). In experienced hands, the Latarjet procedure performed arthroscopically has been reported to provide low (1%–2%) recurrence rates (53,55).

Management of the Hill-Sachs Lesion

As mentioned previously, posterosuperior humeral head bone loss (Hill-Sachs lesion) may need to be addressed in order to prevent recurrent instability. The decision to address an associated Hill-Sachs lesion at the time of surgery may be made preoperatively (based on the glenoid track concept) or intraoperatively (based on engagement of the humeral head defect on the anterior glenoid rim during dynamic evaluation under arthroscopic visualization). Two techniques are commonly considered for surgical management of an engaging Hill-Sachs lesion: remplissage and grafting.

Remplissage

This procedure involves advancement of the infraspinatus and posterior capsule to the osseous surface of the Hill-Sachs lesion (in French, *remplissage* means "to fill in") (42). Some advocate advancement of the capsule only in selected patients (56). If the soft tissues heal in the new transferred position, stability improves through 2 mechanisms: the bone defect is no longer intra-articular (capsule and cuff will prevent the defect from contacting the glenoid rim), and the infraspinatus tenodesis serves as a checkrein against anterior translation of the humeral head (Figure 7.23). This technique is attractive because

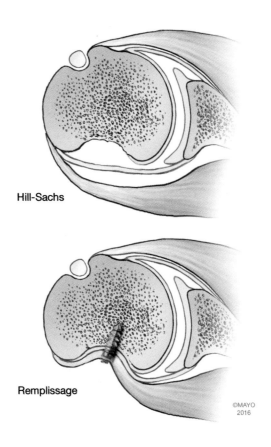

Figure 7.23 *Management of Hill-Sachs lesion: Remplissage.*

it can be added to an arthroscopic repair of the capsule and labrum relatively easily. Its main disadvantage is the potential for limited external rotation. The magnitude of a Hill-Sachs lesion that can be managed with remplissage remains unclear. Most studies on the outcome of this technique have included patients with no or minimal glenoid bone loss and defects involving up to 25% of the humeral head.

The remplissage portion of the procedure is performed prior to repair of the anterior labrum and capsule in order to allow anterior humeral head subluxation while working on the posterosuperior humeral head. With the arthroscope in the anterosuperior portal, an accessory posterolateral portal is created. Once the bone surface of the defect is prepared, 1 or 2 anchors loaded with multiple sutures are inserted in the defect (Figure 7.24), the capsule and infraspinatus are pierced to retrieve the sutures, and as sutures are tied, the bone defect is filled with the transferred soft tissues. Repair of the anterior labrum and capsule is then performed. When remplissage is added to a Bankart procedure, patients are immobilized in slight external rotation.

A number of authors have reported on the outcome of arthroscopic repair of the labrum and capsule combined with remplissage (42). The reported recurrence rate at

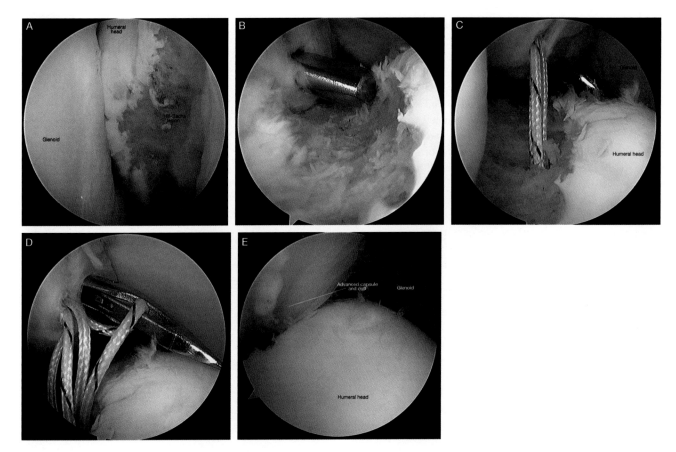

Figure 7.24 *Arthroscopic pictures of remplissage.* **A,** *Engaging Hill-Sachs.* **B,** *Preparation of the defect.* **C,** *Anchor placement.* **D,** *Suture passing.* **E,** *Final remplissage.*

2 years is approximately 5%. Some studies have reported isolated cases of substantial loss of external rotation, but the average loss of external rotation has been only approximately 10°. Most patients included in these studies achieved satisfactory outcome scores, with a high rate of return to sports (42).

Bone Grafting

Extremely large Hill-Sachs lesions may not be amenable to remplissage. Structural osteoarticular allografts are considered in these circumstances. The average size of the Hill-Sachs lesion in studies on allograft reconstruction has been approximately 40% (57). Most surgeons use femoral head or humeral head osteoarticular allografts fixed with screws. Interestingly, whereas reported outcomes after allograft reconstruction of humeral head defects in locked posterior dislocations have been very good (29,30), the outcome in recurrent anterior dislocation has been less predictable. A meta-analysis of published studies found that allograft reconstruction does restore stability and function, but the reoperation rate is approximately 25%, with arthroplasty being required in 50% of the patients followed over 5 years (57).

Recurrent Posterior Instability and Posterior Labral Tears

Recurrent unidirectional posterior instability is less common and more difficult to diagnose than anterior instability. However, the rate of posterior instability is relatively high in younger active patients involved in sports (58). Excluding patients with locked posterior dislocations, most patients with posterior instability present with somewhat vague symptoms related to multiple subluxation episodes; dysplasia and hypermobility syndrome (e.g., Ehlers-Danlos syndrome) are also more common than in anterior instability.

Evaluation

Although some patients with posterior instability do complain of repeated episodes of subjective subluxation or dislocation, many will complain of vague posterior shoulder pain and inability to participate in sports. Occasionally, patients will be able to identify a specific high-energy traumatic event sustained with the shoulder in flexion, adduction, and internal rotation that initiated the onset of symptoms. More commonly, patients are involved in

Table 7.11 • **Activities Commonly Practiced by Patients With Recurrent Posterior Instability**

American football (defensive linemen constantly stopping offensive players with the hands forward and their shoulders in flexion and internal rotation)

Baseball (repetitive overhead in pitchers, repetitive follow-through in batters)

Racket sports (backhand stroke)

Golf (follow-through)

Swimming (pull-through)

activities that result in microtraumatic injuries to the posterior labrum and elongation of the posterior capsule (Table 7.11).

At the time of evaluation, most patients state that their shoulder bothers them only when placed in flexion with varying degrees of adduction and internal rotation, or more indistinctly during sports. Special attention should be paid to examination of the scapula to detect associated scapular dyskinesia. Patients should also be assessed for poor rotator cuff function and generalized hypermobility.

Physical examination maneuvers specifically aimed to identify posterior instability include excessive translation of the humeral head to or over the posterior glenoid rim with forced flexion, adduction, and internal rotation, as well as the posterior apprehension test and the jerk test (see chapter 1, Evaluation of the Shoulder). The Whipple test was described to assess supraspinatus strength (59). However, it has been noted to be very useful in patients with posterior instability: The patient is standing or sitting, with the shoulder in 90° of flexion, the palm facing the floor and at the level of the opposite acromioclavicular joint, and the elbow in full extension or in 90° of flexion; as the examiner applies downward pressure, the humeral head subluxes or dislocates posteriorly (Figure 7.25).

Plain radiographs may be normal, or may show posterior subluxation, blunting of the posterior glenoid rim, or glenoid dysplasia. The Bernageau view may be helpful in screening for glenoid bone loss. MRI may show static subluxation, a torn or attenuated posterior labrum, elongation of the posterior capsule, glenoid dysplasia, and/or a reverse Hill-Sachs lesion. Computed tomography is typically obtained in patients with unidirectional posterior instability when bone procedures are being considered for the glenoid, the humeral side, or both.

Nonoperative Treatment

A trial of nonoperative treatment is warranted in many patients with posterior shoulder subluxation, minimal dysplasia, and a relatively preserved posterior labrum, especially if hypermobility, cuff dysfunction, or scapular dyskinesia are detected during evaluation. Patients are

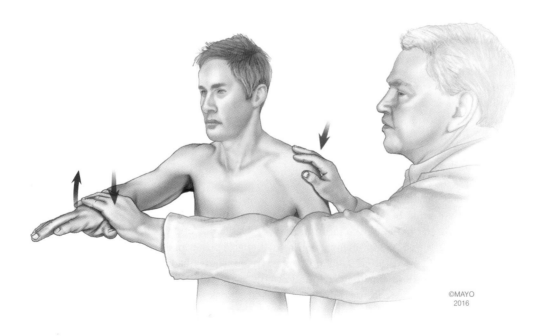

©MAYO 2016

Figure 7.25 Whipple test.

educated about avoidance of combined flexion, adduction, and internal rotation of the shoulder during the practice of sports. They may be counseled to discontinue the practice of activities responsible for posterior instability (Table 7.11). Physical therapy is focused on strengthening the cuff and scapular stabilizers, and patients may be re-evaluated in 3 to 6 months.

Surgical Treatment

Surgical treatment is considered for patients with substantial pathology (large traumatic labral tears, marked dysplasia), as well as those who fail a good program of nonoperative treatment. Repair of the posterior labrum with various degrees of posterior capsular plication is considered for patients with minor bony abnormalities. Posterior bone block procedures and glenoid osteotomy are considered for patients with marked bony pathology and those who fail a posterior soft-tissue procedure.

Repair of the Posterior Labrum and Capsule

Although the posterior labrum and capsule may be addressed through an open posterior approach (chapter 3, Surgical Exposures), currently this procedure is most commonly performed arthroscopically. The procedure mirrors repair of the anterior labrum and capsular shift for recurrent anterior instability.

Examination under anesthesia is important in order to confirm the diagnosis and understand the magnitude of capsular plication required to render the shoulder stable. Many surgeons prefer the lateral decubitus position for arthroscopic management of posterior shoulder instability, even if their preferred position for most other procedures is beach chair (chapter 2, Arthroscopic Shoulder Surgery).

After standard evaluation of the glenohumeral joint with the camera in a posterior portal, portals are switched and the shoulder is visualized from an anterior portal. Posterior portals used for repair of the posterior labrum and capsule need to be placed relatively lateral, so at the beginning of the procedure it is not a bad idea to place the standard posterior portal more lateral than usual.

The posterior labrum may be found to be detached or attenuated (Figure 7.26). Care must be taken not to miss a Kim lesion (Table 7.3). In some patients, the labrum is completely intact and the only pathologic element contributing to instability is an enlarged, attenuated posterior capsule. Suture anchor repair and capsular plication are performed as needed in order to address soft-tissue pathology (Figure 7.27). Some surgeons favor suture closure of the posterior portals. The rotator interval may also be plicated with sutures in some patients. After surgery, the shoulder is immobilized in external rotation for 4 to 6 weeks.

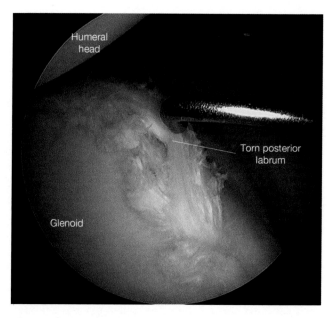

Figure 7.26 *Arthroscopic view of a posterior labral tear.*

Several recent publications have reported good outcomes when arthroscopic repair of the posterior labrum and capsule are performed in patients with unidirectional posterior instability (26–28,60). Outcomes seem to be best in contact athletes as compared with overhead athletes (27,28,60). Use of suture anchors also seems to provide better outcomes when compared with isolated suture plication of the capsule (27,28). However, long-term outcomes have not been universally good.

Bone Block Procedures

Placement of a bone graft attached to the posterior glenoid rim has been described for selected patients with posterior instability (Figure 7.28). There is no consensus in the literature regarding the indications for this procedure. Most surgeons consider it as a salvage procedure only after failed soft-tissue repair. Others will recommend a posterior bone block procedure as a first line of surgical treatment for patients with symptomatic posterior instability in the setting of traumatic bone loss, glenoid hypoplasia, hyperlaxity, or voluntary instability.

Open posterior bone block procedures are performed though a posterior approach (chapter 3, Surgical Exposures). The graft may be obtained from the posterior iliac crest or the scapular spine or acromion; use of a pedicle acromial bone block with rotation of a portion of the deltoid muscle has also been described in an attempt to provide not only the bone block effect but also a sling effect by the deltoid fibers similar to the conjoined tendon sling effect in the Latarjet procedure. Some recommend use of allograft (61). The procedure can also be performed arthroscopically (62).

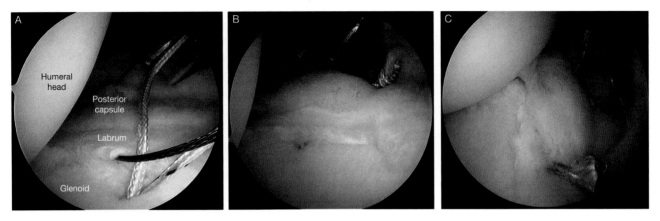

Figure 7.27 *Repair of the posterior labrum and posterior capsular plication.* **A,** *Suture management.* **B and C,** *Final repair.*

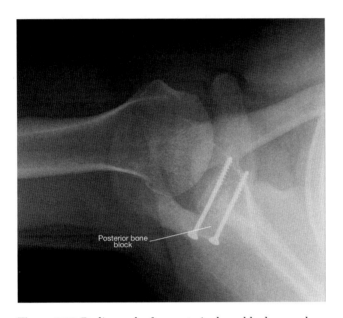

Figure 7.28 *Radiograph after posterior bone block procedure.*

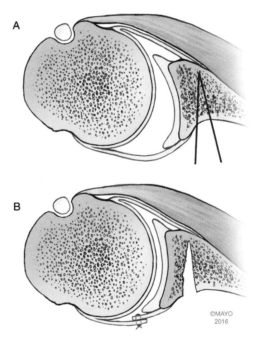

Figure 7.29 *Glenoid osteotomy.* **A,** *Planned wedge.* **B,** *Correction and capsular plication.*

As with anterior bone block procedures, care must be taken to place the bone graft in continuity with the glenoid articular arch, and to avoid inadvertent intra-articular screw penetration (◉ Video 7.4).

Since this is an uncommon procedure, most reports include just a few shoulders. Servien et al (63) reported on 21 patients with traumatic posterior instability, with restoration of stability and function in most cases at 6 years of follow-up. However, results may deteriorate at longer follow-up: Meuffels et al (64) reported on 11 patients followed for an average of 18 years; 4 (36%) experienced recurrent posterior dislocation, and all had moderate shoulder scores and radiographic evidence of osteoarthritis. Arthroscopic posterior bone block procedures have been reported to provide good stability rates but a very high complication and reoperation rate related to graft prominence and hardware problems (62).

Glenoid Osteotomy

Glenoid osteotomy has been considered as an alternative to a posterior bone block procedure for patients with marked posterior glenoid version and posterior instability, either as a primary procedure or as salvage after failed soft-tissue stabilization. The posterior aspect of the glenoid is exposed through a posterior approach, and an opening wedge osteotomy is performed to antevert the glenoid (Figure 7.29). Although some have reported relatively good results with this procedure (65), severe complications (intra-articular fracture, graft extrusion, avascular necrosis, and progressive osteoarthritis) have also been reported (65,66).

Improvement in imaging studies and 3-dimensional computer-assisted planning may translate in the future to reproducible results, but at the present time I favor posterior bone block procedures over glenoid osteotomy when correction of abnormal glenoid retroversion is considered necessary to render the shoulder stable.

Multidirectional Instability

The concepts of MDI and voluntary instability were introduced at the beginning of this chapter. MDI was coined to describe those patients with anterior and posterior instability associated with involuntary inferior subluxation or dislocation (67). Most surgeons use this term for patients with symptoms of instability in at least 2 directions, but diagnostic criteria for MDI do not exist, which explains discrepancies in reported rates and probably in reported outcomes as well (68). When the term *MDI* is mentioned, most of us automatically think that 1 or both of the following elements are involved: generalized soft-tissue hyperlaxity (with or without a formal diagnosis of Ehlers-Danlos syndrome) and poor coordination of the rotator cuff and/or periscapular muscles, both contributing to instability in the mid range. Bone dysplasia or hypoplasia may be seen as well in patients with MDI (69).

The term *voluntary instability* refers to those individuals who are able to subluxate or dislocate their glenohumeral joint at will by either muscle contraction or by placing the shoulder girdle in specific positions. Some individuals will demonstrate voluntary instability in only 1 direction, whereas others can excessively translate the humeral head at will in several directions. In some circumstances, these excessive translations are painful in 1 direction or more, but sometimes there is no pain or functional limitations. Commonly, patients with voluntary instability report that they have been able to dislocate their shoulders at will since they were little, but only later in life their shoulder became painful and interferes with activity. Traditionally, many patients with voluntary instability have been considered to have psychologic abnormalities or to be looking for secondary gains (mostly attention), but that is not always the case.

Evaluation

Most patients with MDI present with insidious onset of activity-related symptoms in the second to third decade of life. Symptoms include subjective sense of instability, pain, a perception of decreased strength, worsening athletic performance, and occasionally paresthesias. The prevalence of MDI is higher in individuals involved in certain sports (e.g., swimming, gymnastics, volleyball). Patients should be asked regarding which positions facilitate instability episodes. A distinction needs to be made between those patients who can demonstrate instability in specific positions (*positional* instability) but attempt to avoid these positions, versus those patients who constantly seek placing the shoulder girdle in positions that

Table 7.12 • Beighton Criteria: A Score of ≥4 Points on a 9-Point Scale Is Considered Highly Suggestive of Generalized Ligamentous Laxity

Passive dorsiflexion of the little finger beyond 90°	1 point for each hand
Passive apposition of the thumb to the ipsilateral forearm	1 point for each hand
Active hyperextension of the elbow beyond 10°	1 point for each elbow
Active hyperextension of the knee beyond 10°	1 point for each knee
Forward flexion of the trunk with the knees fully extended so that the palms of the hands rest flat on the floor	1 point

Adapted from Beighton P, Solomon L, Soskolne CL. Articular mobility in an African population. Ann Rheum Dis. 1973 Sep;32(5):413–8. Used with permission.

favor dislocation (*voluntary* instability). Marked shoulder laxity is present in both shoulders for most patients with MDI, but commonly symptoms are present on only 1 side.

On physical examination, most patients with MDI will demonstrate normal or even excessive range of motion. It is useful to ask the patient to demonstrate the position of the arm that generates symptoms and instability. Physical examination maneuvers helpful in the evaluation of MDI are described in chapter 1, Evaluation of the Shoulder, and include the load and shift test, anterior and posterior drawer tests in various degrees of rotation, and the inferior sulcus sign. These tests are useful to confirm and grade the presence of instability in more than 1 direction (anterior, posterior, inferior). Laxity of the inferior capsule can also be assessed with the hyperabduction test: Passive abduction greater than 105° is considered indicative of excessive inferior capsular laxity (70). The condition of the rotator cuff and scapula should also be examined. Finally, patients should be assessed for generalized ligamentous laxity (see chapter 1, Evaluation of the Shoulder), and consideration should be given to genetic testing for patients who could have Ehlers-Danlos syndrome, Marfan syndrome, or other collagenopathies (Table 7.12) (71).

Plain radiographs in patients with MDI may be completely normal or may show dysplastic changes or blunting of the glenoid rim. The dominant pathologic feature is enlargement of the shoulder capsule. This is best appreciated in MRI with intra-articular contrast, which typically demonstrates a very large inferior capsular recess, an enlarged interval region, and large anterior and posterior capsular spaces as well. The labrum is oftentimes completely normal, but occasionally patients will have developed tearing of the anterior or posterior labrum secondary to microtrauma. Some patients may have a concealed lesion of the labrum that can be difficult to appreciate at the time of arthroscopy (Kim lesion) (8).

Table 7.13 • Management of Patients With Multidirectional Instability

Rule out pathologic generalized ligamentous laxity (i.e., Ehlers-Danlos syndrome)

Patient counseling and education

Physical therapy
Scapular stabilizing exercises
Rotator cuff strengthening
Core strengthening

External bracing (proprioception)

Management

Conservative management represents the first line of treatment for most patients with MDI (Table 7.13) (69,72). Interestingly, the effectiveness of exercises for patients with MDI has been difficult to prove (73,74). When conservative management fails, consideration can be given to surgical procedures directed to decrease the capsular volume.

Nonoperative Management

Patient education and counseling are major elements of nonoperative management for patients with MDI. Patients with voluntary instability should be counseled to make a real effort to stop their dislocations at will, since eventually they can create secondary damage to the labrum and articular cartilage. Patients with positional instability should be counseled to learn to avoid the provoking positions. If psychologic abnormalities or seeking for a secondary gain are detected, they should be addressed accordingly.

Physical therapy is the mainstay of nonoperative management. The goal is to provide the patient with such coordinated muscular control of scapular position and humeral head position that the humeral head remains centered at all times despite an ample capsular space. Scapular stabilizing and rotator cuff strengthening exercises are useful for most patients (see chapter 12, Rehabilitation and Injections); more emphasis may be placed on some exercises compared with others based on the outcome of the physical examination.

Surgical Management

Surgery may be considered selectively in patients with MDI that have clearly failed a good program of nonoperative management. Surgery is perceived to have a higher failure rate in patients with voluntary instability or pathologic generalized ligamentous hyperlaxity, and some surgeons consider these 2 conditions a contraindication for surgery (69,72). Very few studies have reported on the outcome of surgery for Ehlers-Danlos syndrome, but some seem to suggest that patients feel they benefit

from surgery, even though up to 50% may continue to experience instability to some extent (75). Better results could theoretically be obtained in these patients with abnormal collagen by augmenting their capsule with allograft from a healthy donor (76).

Some patients with MDI are found to have a primary scapular disorder that requires a specific surgical procedure (see chapter 10, The Scapula). However, in most patients, surgery is directed to decrease the volume of the shoulder capsule. This can be accomplished by shifting or plicating the capsule in various directions using either an open procedure or arthroscopic techniques. Some surgeons add closure or plication or the interval region, but the added value of interval closure is controversial (72).

Thermal capsulorrhaphy was used a fair amount for patients with MDI a few years ago. In this procedure, thermal energy was applied arthroscopically to the capsule using either laser or radiofrequency in order to disrupt the molecular bonds that stabilize collagen, decreasing the molecule length with resultant capsular shrinkage (77). Unfortunately, this technique was associated with a high complication and failure rate (78,79). In addition, changes in the material properties of the capsule made revision surgery extremely challenging (80). This procedure has been largely abandoned.

Open Capsular Shift

This procedure is typically performed through an anterior inferior approach as described in Chapter 3, Surgical Exposures, and discussed and demonstrated in the section Open Bankart Repair and Capsular Shift (⬤ Video 7.1) (67,69). In patients with extreme posterior capsular redundancy, it may be best to perform the procedure through a posterior approach, and very rarely the shoulder needs to be approached from both sides.

The dissecting plane between the subscapularis and capsule can be extremely difficult to develop due to capsular thinning, especially in patients with generalized ligamentous hyperlaxity. Once the anterior capsule is fully exposed, it is divided in a T fashion, detaching it circumferentially from the humeral neck first, and then dividing the capsule horizontally to the glenoid rim (Figure 7.30). The inferior capsular flap is then advanced superiorly and the superior flap advanced inferiorly. The interval region can also be plicated if needed. Shift of the capsule and interval closure are performed with the arm in approximately 30° of abduction and external rotation to avoid postoperative stiffness. After surgery, patients are immobilized for 6 weeks and active assisted and motion exercises are then started. Slow progress with therapy is emphasized, especially in patients with poor collagen. Several studies have documented a high rate of satisfactory results, ranging from 80% to 95% (67,69,72,81).

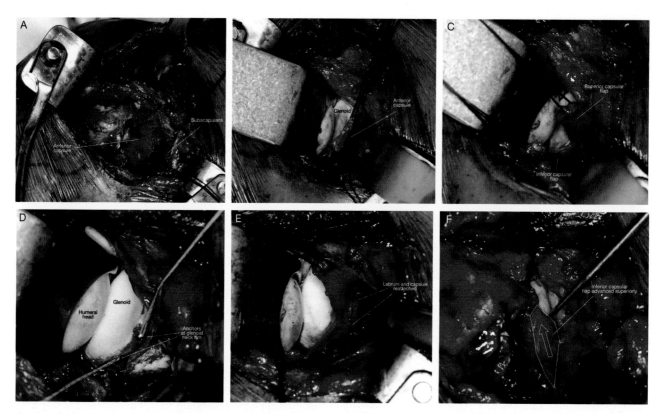

Figure 7.30 *Open capsular shift.* **A,** *Finding the plane between subscapularis and capsule.* **B,** *Arthrotomy.* **C,** *Capsular split.* **D,** *Anchor placement.* **E,** *Glenoid reattachment of the capsule.* **F,** *Capsular shift.*

Arthroscopic Capsular Shift and Plication

The excessive capsular volume of the glenohumeral joint can also be addressed arthroscopically. Although the capsule can also be physically divided and shifted arthroscopically, most surgeons prefer to plicate the capsule. Sutures are passed through the capsule and reattached in a plicated fashion to either the labrum or suture anchors placed on the glenoid (Figure 7.31). The number of horizontal mattress plicating stitches placed anteriorly and posteriorly is proportional to the severity of capsular laxity in each individual.

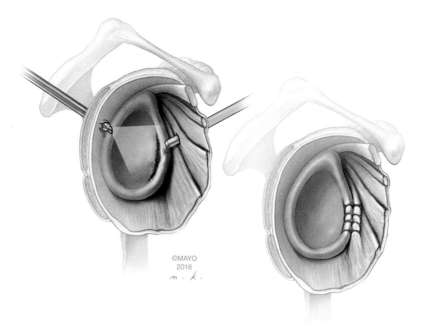

Figure 7.31 *Arthroscopic capsular plication.*

Table 7.14 • Clinical Scenarios Associated With Superior Labral Tears

	Etiology	Clinical Features	Surgical Management
Isolated superior labral tear	Acute traumatic event Repetitive microtrauma	Pain Mechanical symptoms	Repair of the labrum **vs** biceps tenotomy and tenodesis
Labral tear with associated paralabral cyst		Pain Mechanical symptoms Suprascapular neuropathy	Repair of the labrum with or without biceps tenotomy or tenodesis
Labral tear in the setting of shoulder instability	Acute traumatic event	Instability (recurrent subluxation or dislocation)	Repair of the labrum
Degenerative labral tear	Aging, generalized joint degeneration	Pain Commonly associated with biceps symptoms	Ignore **vs** biceps tenotomy or tenodesis

The interval region may be plicated as well. Postoperative management is similar to what I just described for open capsular shift. The recurrence rates seem to be similar for both open and arthroscopic techniques (78,79).

Superior Labral Tears

The superior portion of the labrum can contribute to patients' symptoms in a number of ways. The first reports on symptomatic tears of the superior labrum were published in the mid 1980s and early 1990s (82,83). Superior labral injuries were initially described in baseball pitchers and other throwing athletes (82). We now know that superior labral tears can contribute to symptoms in various clinical scenarios (Table 7.14). We also know that MRI will be interpreted as consistent with the presence of a labral tear in individuals with no symptoms or other reasons for shoulder pain, especially in middle-aged individuals (84). Labral repairs performed on the basis of only imaging studies carry the risk of a poor outcome, not only because the primary reason for symptoms would not be addressed but also because repair of a nonpathologic labrum can lead to pain and stiffness. Every effort should be made to base treatment decisions on the patient's history and physical examination, using imaging studies and surgical findings to confirm.

The Superior Labrum: What Is Normal and Abnormal?

As mentioned at the beginning of this chapter, the superior aspect of the labrum is triangular or meniscoid, and not as closely attached to the articular margin of the glenoid cartilage as on the lower portions of the joint. The biceps tendon typically originates partly from the supraglenoid tubercle and partly from the superior labrum. Since the superior labrum is somewhat mobile, determining the presence of a detached superior labrum can be somewhat subjective. In addition, normal variants can be confused with a labral tear (Table 7.1).

Overall Management Strategy

When superior labral tears were first described, the term *SLAP* (superior labrum from anterior to posterior) tear was coined and these tears were classified in 4 categories (Figure 7.32): degenerative labral fraying (I), labral detachment (II), bucket-handle tear with a stable biceps (III), and bucket-handle tear with extension into the biceps (IV). A damaged labrum can create symptoms through 4 different mechanisms: instability, poor joint seal, mechanical symptoms, and degenerative symptoms.

In patients with anterior or posterior instability secondary to an anterior or posterior Bankart lesion, extension of the anterior or posterior labral tear superiorly can contribute to instability. When the superior labral tear allows escape of intra-articular fluid in-between the labrum and the glenoid rim, ganglion cysts may form. Depending on the location and size of these cysts, they can contribute to entrapment of the suprascapular nerve, which may present as pain with or without weakness and neurogenic muscle atrophy. An unstable labrum may be responsible for episodes of mechanical pain, typically felt posterosuperiorly and reproduced with specific tests (see dynamic labral shear test and active compression test in chapter 1, Evaluation of the Shoulder). A frayed or torn labrum can also contribute to symptoms in patients with early degenerative joint disease or cuff tears. In arthritis and cuff tears, it is challenging to understand how much of the patient's pain can be attributed to the labral tear.

It is interesting to review how the management of the superior labrum has evolved over time. When superior labral tears were first recognized, it made sense to apply the same repair techniques to the superior labrum that were already developed for the anterior and posterior labrum. Arthroscopic labral repair quickly became the treatment of choice (except for areas of fraying or detached fragments of labrum, which were treated with arthroscopic débridement) (83,85,86).

Although the outcome of repair of the superior labrum was satisfactory in well-selected patients (87–90), a number of individuals did not do well, with pain, stiffness, and difficulty returning to the practice of sports (85). Poor

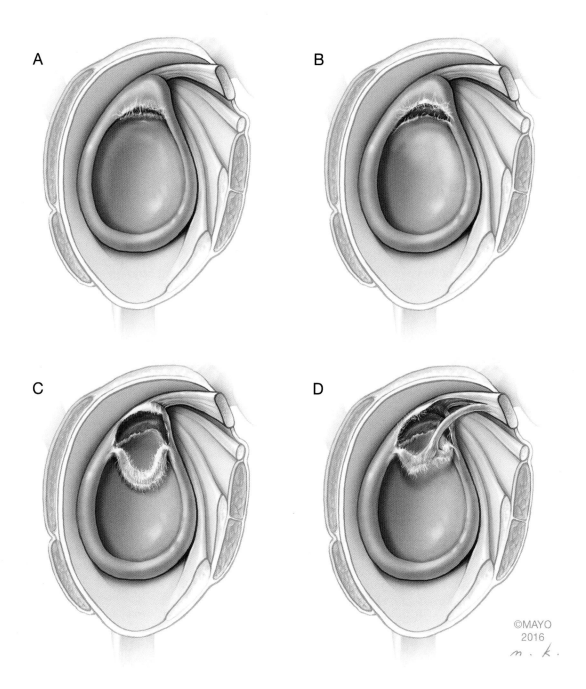

Figure 7.32 *Types of superior labral tears.* **A,** *Degenerative labral fraying.* **B,** *Labral detachment.* **C,** *Bucket-handle tear with stable biceps.* **D,** *Bucket-handle tear with extension into biceps.*

outcomes after repair of the superior labrum can be due to a number of reasons (Table 7.15). Since the long head of the biceps is in continuity with the labrum, and biceps pathology is commonly observed at the time of arthroscopy in many patients, biceps tenotomy or tenodesis was recommended for the management of failed repairs of the superior labrum (91), or as a primary treatment modality for patients with a superior labral tear (85,92,93).

Currently, the controversy continues regarding the relative indications of labral repair versus biceps tenotomy or tenodesis for the management of symptomatic labral tears. In my practice, the management of tears of the superior labrum depends on the clinical presentation, age, and activities performed by the patient, and associated pathology (Figure 7.33). Considerations regarding biceps tenodesis techniques as well as the surgical management of suprascapular nerve

Table 7.15 • **Reasons That Can Contribute to a Poor Outcome After Repair of the Superior Labrum Anterior to Posterior (SLAP)**

Wrong diagnosis
Repair performed on the basis of MRI findings without clinical correlation
Subjective assessment of the superior labrum at the time of arthroscopy

Ignoring associated biceps pathology in a patient with a superior labral tear

Repair of the labrum in patients with "aging" conditions (cuff tears, osteoarthritis)

Residual stiffness severe enough to interfere with throwing

Intra-articular prominence of sutures (especially knots)

Abbreviation: MRI, magnetic resonance imaging.

entrapment in the setting of a labral tear with a paralabral cyst are discussed in chapter 6, The Rotator Cuff and Biceps Tendon. The technique for arthroscopic repair of the superior labrum, when indicated, is discussed below.

Superior Labral Tears in the Setting of Recurrent Instability

Most of the time superior labral tears are fully identified at the time of arthroscopic shoulder surgery for the management of recurrent anterior (less commonly, posterior)

instability. Some studies have reported a rate of superior labral tears close to 20% to 25% in patients undergoing arthroscopic labral repair for recurrent anterior instability (94). The consensus in this situation is to extend the repair of the anterior or posterior labrum to the superior labrum using additional suture anchors. When the superior extension of the labrum is properly repaired, the outcome of the instability surgery is equivalent to those patients without superior extension of the anterior labral tear (94).

Labral Tears Associated With Paralabral Cysts

Pain in patients with a superior labral tear and an associated paralabral cyst can be related to the presence of the tear, the mass effect of the cyst, compression on the suprascapular nerve, or a combination. As mentioned before, the labral tear is thought to behave as a valve, allowing articular fluid to collect in the adjacent paralabral space. In some individuals, compression of the suprascapular nerve will lead to atrophy and weakness of the infraspinatus or both the supraspinatus and infraspinatus.

Repair of the superior labrum has been proved to lead to spontaneous resolution of the cyst and recovery of muscle strength (95). Many surgeons opt to also decompress the cyst by using a blunt instrument or a shaver terminal intra-articularly to evacuate or aspirate the content of the cyst. The added benefit of cyst decompression is controversial, with some studies showing no difference (95), and others showing better recovery of strength when cyst decompression is

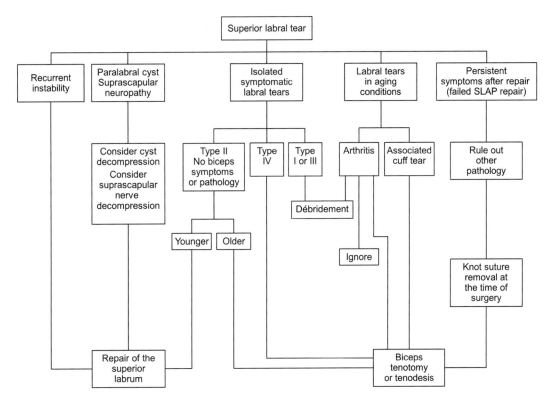

Figure 7.33 *Algorithm for management of superior labral tears. SLAP, superior labrum from anterior to posterior.*

added (96). The additional benefit of releasing the suprascapular or spinoglenoid ligaments to fully decompress the suprascapular nerve is largely unknown, since most of the reports on arthroscopic suprascapular nerve decompression do not report on patients with cysts (97).

In my practice, I repair the labrum and attempt to decompress the cyst in all patients with a SLAP tear and an associated cyst; if the biceps tendon itself has separate pathology, both a labral repair and a biceps tenotomy or tenodesis may be considered. I add arthroscopic decompression of the suprascapular nerve for patients with clear atrophy and weakness. Even though I realize that the added value of these 2 additional gestures (cyst decompression, nerve decompression) has not been proven, they add very little to no morbidity and I prefer to add them in case they do end up leading to better outcomes in some patients.

Symptomatic Isolated Labral Tears

This is probably the most challenging category of patient with a SLAP tear. Part of the challenge resides in confirming that a superior labral tear is the main or only reason for shoulder pain. The fact that MRI studies tend to overdiagnose superior labral tears makes the whole situation more complicated.

In my practice, the history and physical examination are critical to consider surgical management. Symptomatic isolated labral tears are commonly secondary to either a substantial injury or repetitive overhead activity; if a patient is sent for treatment based on the MRI finding of a SLAP tear, and there is no history of trauma or overuse, I am extremely cautious. On the other hand, patients who clearly demonstrate posterosuperior shoulder pain after an injury or overuse, and whose symptoms are clearly reproduced by the dynamic labral shear test or the active compression test, can be helped by addressing the labral tear.

Once it is decided that the patient will benefit from treatment of a superior labral tear, conservative management may be occasionally successful, including 1 intraarticular glenohumeral injection and physical therapy (98). When conservative treatment fails, the question is when to perform a labral repair and when to consider a biceps tenotomy or tenodesis. The pluses and minuses of these 2 options need to be carefully discussed with the patient. Repair of the superior labrum is a more anatomic solution with good reported outcomes; however, persistent pain and lingering stiffness can happen. Biceps tenotomy or tenodesis will typically resolve shoulder pain without risk of stiffness, but cramping pain and abnormal cosmetics can occur after either a tenotomy or even tenodesis, and some patients develop discomfort at the tenodesis site. In general, repair of the labrum is considered for younger patients with a true type II labral tear, no biceps symptoms, and a pristine biceps at the time of surgery. Biceps tenotomy or tenodesis is favored in the remaining patients (Figure 7.33).

Labral Tears in the Setting of Rotator Cuff Disease

The presence of labral tears in patients with rotator cuff disease is not uncommon. Partial thickness tears of the articular side of the supraspinatus tendon are commonly seen in overhead athletes with a superior labral tear. Similarly, labral tears may be seen in patients undergoing surgery for a full-thickness rotator cuff tear.

Some surgeons have argued that repair of the labrum in the setting of a rotator cuff repair may increase the risk of stiffness. Some studies have reported good outcomes in patients undergoing combined repair of the rotator cuff and superior labrum (99). Others have reported better outcomes combining a biceps tenotomy or tenodesis with cuff repair as compared with repairing the superior labrum (100). Part of the problem resides with the fact that many patients with rotator cuff tears are older, their labrum does show degenerative changes, and the diagnosis of a superior labral tear is very subjective. In addition, the biceps tendon shows degenerative changes too.

In general, except in the younger patient with a small cuff tear and a clearly symptomatic labral tear, if I feel that the labrum needs to be addressed at the time of cuff repair, I favor a biceps tenotomy or tenodesis. Many surgeons argue in favor of addressing the biceps with tenotomy or tenodesis at the time of cuff repair in every single shoulder since it facilitates visualization and eliminates 1 more potential pain generator (see chapter 6, The Rotator Cuff and Biceps Tendon).

Labral Tears in Degenerative Joint Disease

Another challenging category of patients are those with mild to moderate glenohumeral osteoarthritis, minimal radiographic changes, and evidence on MRI of cartilage loss and a degenerative labral tear. As patients and nonorthopedic health care providers realize that the MRI shows a superior labral tear, their thought process leads them to assume that all symptoms are related to the labral tear, which needs to be fixed. These patients benefit the most from reassurance and conservative treatment. Repair of a degenerative labrum carries the risk of tightening the joint, which will aggravate symptoms of osteoarthritis. Only if a patient with moderate osteoarthritis is considered for an arthroscopic débridement (chapter 9, Shoulder Arthritis and Arthroplasty) should a biceps tenotomy or tenodesis be considered, depending on intraoperative assessment of the labrum and the biceps.

Arthroscopic Repair of a Superior Labral Tear

Arthroscopic repair of a superior labral tear is performed in my practice in the beach chair position (◉ Video 7.5). The arthroscopic camera is placed in the standard posterior glenohumeral portal. An anterosuperior portal is established and the presence of a superior labral tear is confirmed using a probe. As mentioned several times, the normal labrum does have some mobility superiorly, and normal anatomic variants need to be identified in order to avoid fixing a normal labrum, which will tighten the joint excessively and

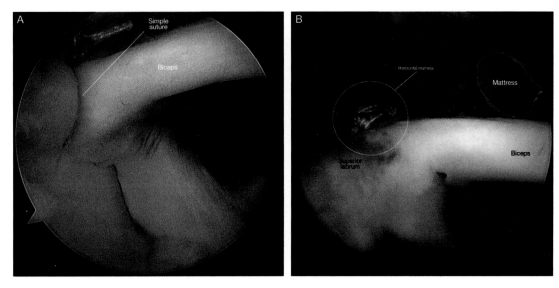

Figure 7.34 *Arthroscopic view of repair of the superior labrum.* **A,** *Simple suture.* **B,** *Horizontal mattress.*

lead to stiffness and pain. The biceps tendon should also be pulled into the joint with a probe and carefully evaluated. If a paralabral cyst was identified preoperatively, the cyst can be accessed from the joint and decompressed with a blunt instrument or a shaver terminal.

Provided the need to fix the labrum to the superior glenoid rim is confirmed, a cannula is placed in the anterior portal. Multiple suture and suture anchor configurations have been described. The number of anchors used depends on the extent of the tear. Most of the time, I end up placing the first anchor in the superior glenoid neck just posterior to the biceps take-off point. This anchor is best introduced percutaneously through the rotator cuff (Willmington portal, see chapter 2, Arthroscopic Shoulder Surgery). A second anchor may need to be placed in the anterosuperior glenoid for larger tears. It is essential not to leave prominent suture knots close to the humeral head, so either the knots are tied on the nonarticular side of the labrum for simple sutures or a horizontal mattress configuration is used (Figure 7.34). If deemed necessary, decompression of the suprascapular nerve can be performed arthroscopically as well (see chapter 6, The Rotator Cuff and Biceps Tendon). After surgery, patients are immobilized for 3 to 4 weeks and then rehabilitation starts.

Rotator Cuff Tears and Shoulder Instability

Rotator cuff pathology is fully addressed in chapter 6, The Rotator Cuff and Biceps Tendon. The presence of a full-thickness rotator cuff tear in patients with recurrent instability should prompt 2 questions to the treating orthopedic surgeon: Is the size and location of the cuff tear such that if the cuff is not fixed, recurrent instability will not be corrected with a capsulolabral or bone procedure? and, For smaller tears, should surgical management combine

addressing instability and repairing the cuff, or should these procedures be staged?

Cuff Insufficiency as a Contributor to Instability

The fibers of the rotator cuff can become disrupted as a consequence of an anterior dislocation episode. This is more likely to happen in patients over the age of 40, who may have a stiffer cuff or areas of asymptomatic tendinopathy at the time of the dislocation. The location and extent of the tear vary. In some patients the tear is anterosuperior (subscapularis with various degrees of extension into the interval and supraspinatus), in others it is posterosuperior (avulsion of the supraspinatus and infraspinatus, rarely the teres minor, as the head is forcefully displaced forward and the cuff is left behind), and occasionally the whole cuff is torn.

Large subscapularis tears facilitate recurrent anterior instability since they do not contain the humeral head in place; they may or may not be associated with a capsulolabral injury or bone loss. This is more common in middle-aged patients. Large posterosuperior tears facilitate recurrent anterior instability since they do not function as a checkrein against anterior translation, and this is more common in older (elderly) patients; as mentioned previously, the term *posterior mechanism of anterior dislocation* was coined to refer to this second situation.

The key for management of these situations is to diagnose the rotator cuff tear (see chapter 6, The Rotator Cuff and Biceps Tendon). It is wise to perform manual strength testing gently in all patients with a single episode of dislocation or recurrent instability, especially if they are older than 35 or 40. Weakness of physical examination in the absence of an associated nerve injury should prompt obtaining advanced imaging studies. If a large traumatic cuff tear is confirmed, the cuff should be repaired to add stability and provide the best possible functional outcome (101).

Disruptions of the capsulolabral structure and areas of substantial bone loss should also be addressed. If the tear is so large that it is considered not repairable, tendon transfers or reverse arthroplasty may be necessary.

Management of Small Cuff Tears in Patients Requiring Instability Surgery

Occasionally, patients with recurrent anterior instability will also be found to have a small to medium-size supraspinatus tear that may not clearly contribute to instability but may be symptomatic. Management of this combination of abnormalities was controversial in the past for 2 reasons. First, before the widespread application of arthroscopic cuff repair, many surgeons did not like the idea of being able to repair the labrum and capsule arthroscopically and then require an open exposure to fix the cuff. Second, the physical therapy programs used to be very different (no motion after Bankart repair for a few weeks vs passive motion right away for an open rotator cuff tear), and it was felt that adding a cuff repair could lead to a higher rate of postoperative stiffness. Some surgeons chose to stage these 2 procedures.

Currently, there is evidence to suggest that the outcome of concomitant repair of the capsulolabral injury and an associated supraspinatus tear arthroscopically provides good outcomes and does not increase the risk of stiffness substantially. As mentioned in chapter 6, The Rotator Cuff and Biceps Tendon, not all cuff repairs can be proven to have healed with imaging studies, but the outcome of the combined procedure does not seem to be affected by incomplete tendon healing (102,103).

Failed Instability Surgery and Salvage Procedures

The management of patients with continued instability after surgery, as well as those deemed to be unreconstructable, may be a challenge. Salvage procedures are considered for those patients with such compromise of their capsule and labrum, rotator cuff, deltoid, bone structure, and/or joint surface that all procedures described throughout this chapter would not be successful. Salvage procedures include soft-tissue augmentation, arthrodesis, and reverse arthroplasty.

Special care should be taken to carefully evaluate patients with failed instability surgery before resorting to salvage procedures. Common reasons for failure include poor surgical technique for arthroscopic soft-tissue procedures, substantial bone loss not addressed at the time of primary surgery, lack of compliance, undetected hyperlaxity, or the practice of contact sports or risky activities. Physical examination, advanced imaging studies, and review of operative records can be used to understand which elements are contributing to persistent instability after surgery. The Latarjet procedure is now commonly considered the revision procedure of choice after a failed soft-tissue procedure, even in patients without bone loss (104). However, revision arthroscopic or open soft-tissue repairs may be considered for a few patients.

Soft-tissue Augmentation Procedures

This salvage procedure is mostly considered for patients with abnormal collagen, most commonly Elhers-Danlos syndrome (75). When these individuals are considered for surgery, especially if a previous conventional soft-tissue procedure has failed, allograft tissue may be used to reconstruct the capsule anteriorly, posteriorly, or both (Figure 7.35). Most commonly, Achilles tendon allograft is used, since it is long and wide enough to provide plenty of healthy collagen. Soft-tissue augmentation can also be considered for patients with very poor soft-tissue quality after thermal capsulorraphy, which as mentioned before is no longer used for the most part (79).

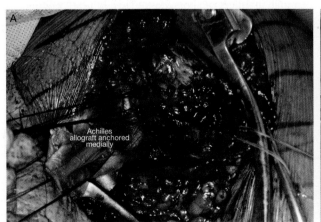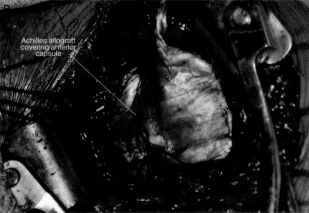

Figure 7.35 *Achilles allograft augmentation used in a patient with Ehlers-Danlos syndrome.* **A,** *Achilles allograft fixed to glenoid rim.* **B,** *Lateral allograft fixation to reconstruct or augment the anterior capsule.*

Arthrodesis

As mentioned in chapter 11, Salvage Procedures, failed instability surgery has become the most common indication for shoulder arthrodesis. Fusion of the glenohumeral joint is uncommonly performed currently. It can be considered for the ultrayoung patient with a hyperlaxity syndrome and multiple failed attempts to stabilize the joint, as well as patients with iatrogenic damage to the articular surface in the presence of an irreparable subscapularis, irreconstructible glenoid bone loss, absent deltoid function, or uncontrolled epilepsy (105,106). Care must be taken when arthrodesis is considered for patients with Ehlers-Danlos syndrome, since once their glenohumeral joint is fused, their scapulothoracic joint may become very symptomatic.

Reverse Shoulder Arthroplasty

Reverse shoulder arthroplasty is most commonly considered for elderly patients with recurrent anterior instability secondary to massive, irreparable cuff tearing, especially if the articular surface is damaged or there is marked bone loss. It can also be considered for patients with a well-functioning deltoid when arthrodesis is the only other alternative. Reverse arthroplasty is discussed fully in chapter 9, Shoulder Arthritis and Arthroplasty.

KEY POINTS

✓ Instability and laxity must be distinguished: Laxity is defined as excessive *asymptomatic* glenohumeral joint translation, whereas instability requires the presence of pain or other symptoms.

✓ The glenohumeral joint may become unstable secondary to one or more factors, including poor scapular function, bone loss on the glenoid and/or humeral head, damage to the capsule and labrum, and rotator cuff tearing or poor cuff coordination.

✓ Closed reduction is the treatment of choice for most patients presenting with an acute anterior shoulder dislocation; however, recurrence is common, especially in younger patients, males, those with hyperlaxity, and those involved in the practice of contact sports.

✓ Posterior dislocations can easily be missed and are commonly associated with impaction fractures of the anterior humeral head; management is largely based on the magnitude of the associated area of bone impaction, and may range from closed reduction to arthroplasty.

✓ Recurrent anterior instability oftentimes requires surgery. The key for success is to individualize treatment strategies to each patient. Arthroscopic repair of the capsule and labrum is the most common procedure performed for this condition in North America, but glenoid bone block procedures (Latarjet) and management of a Hill-Sachs lesion with remplissage have increased in popularity, especially for high-risk patients and, of course, those with substantial bone loss.

✓ Isolated posterior labral tears oftentimes manifest as pain more than subjective instability and respond well to arthroscopic repair.

✓ True recurrent posterior dislocation should prompt assessment for multidirectional instability, hyperlaxity, or dysplasia.

✓ Conservative management represents the first line of treatment for patients with multidirectional instability. However, those who fail can be helped by an arthroscopic or open capsular shift or plication.

✓ MRI overdiagnoses SLAP tears and has led to unnecessary surgery in the past, which leads to pain, stiffness, and poor outcomes.

✓ Superior labral tears may present in very different situations, from the isolated SLAP tear with mechanical symptoms to those associated with paralabral cyst with or without suprascapular neuropathy, or those that contribute to instability.

✓ Controversy remains regarding the relative indications of arthroscopic SLAP repair versus biceps tenotomy or tenodesis in patients with a superior labral tear.

✓ Cuff tears are not uncommonly seen in patients requiring surgery for instability; cuff repair in these circumstances is added to other procedures as needed to render the joint stable and provide the best possible function.

✓ Patients with failed instability surgery should be carefully evaluated and can oftentimes be managed with standard revision instability procedures; occasionally salvage may be necessary with allograft augmentation, arthrodesis, or reverse arthroplasty.

REFERENCES

1. Theodorou SJ, Theodorou DJ, Resnick D. Hypoplasia of the glenoid neck of the scapula: imaging findings and report of 16 patients. J Comput Assist Tomogr. 2006 May-Jun;30(3):535–42.
2. Wirth MA, Lyons FR, Rockwood CA Jr. Hypoplasia of the glenoid: a review of sixteen patients. J Bone Joint Surg Am. 1993 Aug;75(8):1175–84.
3. Itoi E, Lee SB, Berglund LJ, Berge LL, An KN. The effect of a glenoid defect on anteroinferior stability of the shoulder after Bankart repair: a cadaveric study. J Bone Joint Surg Am. 2000 Jan;82(1):35–46.
4. Provencher MT, Frank RM, Leclere LE, Metzger PD, Ryu JJ, Bernhardson A, et al. The Hill-Sachs lesion: diagnosis, classification, and management. J Am Acad Orthop Surg. 2012 Apr;20(4):242–52.
5. Yamamoto N, Itoi E, Abe H, Minagawa H, Seki N, Shimada Y, et al. Contact between the glenoid and the humeral head in abduction, external rotation, and horizontal extension: a new concept of glenoid track. J Shoulder Elbow Surg. 2007 Sep-Oct;16(5):649–56. Epub 2007 Jul 23.

6. Trivedi S, Pomerantz ML, Gross D, Golijanan P, Provencher MT. Shoulder instability in the setting of bipolar (glenoid and humeral head) bone loss: the glenoid track concept. Clin Orthop Relat Res. 2014 Aug;472(8):2352–62.

7. Omori Y, Yamamoto N, Koishi H, Futai K, Goto A, Sugamoto K, et al. Measurement of the glenoid track in vivo as investigated by 3-dimensional motion analysis using open MRI. Am J Sports Med. 2014 Jun;42(6):1290–5. Epub 2014 Mar 28.

8. Kim SH, Ha KI, Yoo JC, Noh KC. Kim's lesion: an incomplete and concealed avulsion of the posteroinferior labrum in posterior or multidirectional posteroinferior instability of the shoulder. Arthroscopy. 2004 Sep;20(7):712–20.

9. Streubel PN, Krych AJ, Simone JP, Dahm DL, Sperling JW, Steinmann SP, et al. Anterior glenohumeral instability: a pathology-based surgical treatment strategy. J Am Acad Orthop Surg. 2014 May;22(5):283–94.

10. Browe DP, Voycheck CA, McMahon PJ, Debski RE. Changes to the mechanical properties of the glenohumeral capsule during anterior dislocation. J Biomech. 2014 Jan 22;47(2):464–9. Epub 2013 Nov 19.

11. Takenaga T, Sugimoto K, Goto H, Nozaki M, Fukuyoshi M, Tsuchiya A, et al. Posterior shoulder capsules are thicker and stiffer in the throwing shoulders of healthy college baseball players: a quantitative assessment using shear-wave ultrasound elastography. Am J Sports Med. 2015 Dec;43(12):2935–42. Epub 2015 Oct 15.

12. Khiami F, Gerometta A, Loriaut P. Management of recent first-time anterior shoulder dislocations. Orthop Traumatol Surg Res. 2015 Feb;101(1 Suppl):S51–7. Epub 2015 Jan 14.

13. Norte GE, West A, Gnacinski M, van der Meijden OA, Millett PJ. On-field management of the acute anterior glenohumeral dislocation. Phys Sportsmed. 2011 Sep;39(3):151–62.

14. Jiang N, Hu YJ, Zhang KR, Zhang S, Bin Y. Intra-articular lidocaine versus intravenous analgesia and sedation for manual closed reduction of acute anterior shoulder dislocation: an updated meta-analysis. J Clin Anesth. 2014 Aug;26(5):350–9. Epub 2014 Jul 25.

15. Itoi E, Sashi R, Minagawa H, Shimizu T, Wakabayashi I, Sato K. Position of immobilization after dislocation of the glenohumeral joint: a study with use of magnetic resonance imaging. J Bone Joint Surg Am. 2001 May;83-A(5):661–7.

16. Itoi E, Hatakeyama Y, Urayama M, Pradhan RL, Kido T, Sato K. Position of immobilization after dislocation of the shoulder. A cadaveric study. J Bone Joint Surg Am. 1999 Mar;81(3):385–90.

17. Whelan DB, Kletke SN, Schemitsch G, Chahal J. Immobilization in external rotation versus internal rotation after primary anterior shoulder dislocation: a meta-analysis of randomized controlled trials. Am J Sports Med. 2016 Feb;44(2):521–32. Epub 2015 Jun 26.

18. Hovelius L, Olofsson A, Sandstrom B, Augustini BG, Krantz L, Fredin H, et al. Nonoperative treatment of primary anterior shoulder dislocation in patients forty years of age and younger: a prospective twenty-five-year follow-up. J Bone Joint Surg Am. 2008 May;90(5):945–52.

19. Robinson CM, Howes J, Murdoch H, Will E, Graham C. Functional outcome and risk of recurrent instability after primary traumatic anterior shoulder dislocation in young patients. J Bone Joint Surg Am. 2006 Nov;88(11):2326–36.

20. Olds M, Ellis R, Donaldson K, Parmar P, Kersten P. Risk factors which predispose first-time traumatic anterior shoulder dislocations to recurrent instability in adults: a systematic review and meta-analysis. Br J Sports Med. 2015 Jul;49(14):913–22. Epub 2015 Apr 21.

21. Hovelius L, Saeboe M. Neer Award 2008: arthropathy after primary anterior shoulder dislocation: 223 shoulders prospectively followed up for twenty-five years. J Shoulder Elbow Surg. 2009 May-Jun;18(3):339–47. Epub 2009 Feb 28.

22. Plath JE, Aboalata M, Seppel G, Juretzko J, Waldt S, Vogt S, et al. Prevalence of and risk factors for dislocation arthropathy: radiological long-term outcome of arthroscopic bankart repair in 100 shoulders at an average 13-year follow-up. Am J Sports Med. 2015 May;43(5):1084–90. Epub 2015 Mar 2.

23. Gordins V, Hovelius L, Sandstrom B, Rahme H, Bergstrom U. Risk of arthropathy after the Bristow-Latarjet repair: a radiologic and clinical thirty-three to thirty-five years of follow-up of thirty-one shoulders. J Shoulder Elbow Surg. 2015 May;24(5):691–9. Epub 2014 Oct 30.

24. Rouleau DM, Hebert-Davies J, Robinson CM. Acute traumatic posterior shoulder dislocation. J Am Acad Orthop Surg. 2014 Mar;22(3):145–52. Erratum in: J Am Acad Orthop Surg. 2014 Jun;22(6):401.

25. Robinson CM, Seah M, Akhtar MA. The epidemiology, risk of recurrence, and functional outcome after an acute traumatic posterior dislocation of the shoulder. J Bone Joint Surg Am. 2011 Sep 7;93(17):1605–13.

26. Leivadiotou D, Ahrens P. Arthroscopic treatment of posterior shoulder instability: a systematic review. Arthroscopy. 2015 Mar;31(3):555–60. Epub 2014 Dec 25.

27. DeLong JM, Jiang K, Bradley JP. Posterior instability of the shoulder: a systematic review and meta-analysis of clinical outcomes. Am J Sports Med. 2015 Jul;43(7):1805–17. Epub 2015 Apr 10.

28. Bradley JP, McClincy MP, Arner JW, Tejwani SG. Arthroscopic capsulolabral reconstruction for posterior instability of the shoulder: a prospective study of 200 shoulders. Am J Sports Med. 2013 Sep;41(9):2005–14. Epub 2013 Jun 26.

29. Gerber C, Catanzaro S, Jundt-Ecker M, Farshad M. Long-term outcome of segmental reconstruction of the humeral head for the treatment of locked posterior dislocation of the shoulder. J Shoulder Elbow Surg. 2014 Nov;23(11):1682–90. Epub 2014 Jun 12.

30. Diklic ID, Ganic ZD, Blagojevic ZD, Nho SJ, Romeo AA. Treatment of locked chronic posterior dislocation of the shoulder by reconstruction of the defect in the humeral head with an allograft. J Bone Joint Surg Br. 2010 Jan;92(1):71–6.

31. Wooten C, Klika B, Schleck CD, Harmsen WS, Sperling JW, Cofield RH. Anatomic shoulder arthroplasty as treatment for locked posterior dislocation of the shoulder. J Bone Joint Surg Am. 2014 Feb 5;96(3):e19.

32. Lafosse T, Fogerty S, Idoine J, Gobezie R, Lafosse L. Hyper extension-internal rotation (HERI): a new test for anterior gleno-humeral instability. Orthop Traumatol Surg Res. 2016 Feb;102(1):3–12.

33. Pansard E, Klouche S, Billot N, Rousselin B, Kraus TM, Bauer T, et al. Reliability and validity assessment of a glenoid bone loss measurement using the Bernageau profile view in chronic anterior shoulder instability. J Shoulder Elbow Surg. 2013 Sep;22(9):1193–8. Epub 2013 Mar 6.

34. George MS, Khazzam M, Kuhn JE. Humeral avulsion of glenohumeral ligaments. J Am Acad Orthop Surg. 2011 Mar;19(3):127–33.

35. Balg F, Boileau P. The instability severity index score: a simple pre-operative score to select patients for arthroscopic or open shoulder stabilisation. J Bone Joint Surg Br. 2007 Nov;89(11):1470–7.

36. Phadnis J, Arnold C, Elmorsy A, Flannery M. Utility of the instability severity index score in predicting failure after arthroscopic anterior stabilization of the shoulder. Am J Sports Med. 2015 Aug;43(8):1983–8. Epub 2015 Jun 29.

37. Bessiere C, Trojani C, Carles M, Mehta SS, Boileau P. The open latarjet procedure is more reliable in terms of shoulder stability than arthroscopic bankart repair. Clin Orthop Relat Res. 2014 Aug;472(8):2345–51.

38. Chalmers PN, Mascarenhas R, Leroux T, Sayegh ET, Verma NN, Cole BJ, et al. Do arthroscopic and open stabilization techniques restore equivalent stability to the shoulder in the setting of anterior glenohumeral instability? A systematic review of overlapping meta-analyses. Arthroscopy. 2015 Feb;31(2):355–63. Epub 2014 Sep 10.

39. Owens BD, Cameron KL, Peck KY, DeBerardino TM, Nelson BJ, Taylor DC, et al. Arthroscopic versus open stabilization for anterior shoulder subluxations. Orthop J Sports Med. 2015 Jan 23;3(1):2325967115571084. Epub 2015 Jan.

40. Chen L, Xu Z, Peng J, Xing F, Wang H, Xiang Z. Effectiveness and safety of arthroscopic versus open Bankart repair for recurrent anterior shoulder dislocation: a meta-analysis of clinical trial data. Arch Orthop Trauma Surg. 2015 Apr;135(4):529–38. Epub 2015 Mar 6.

41. Mohtadi NG, Chan DS, Hollinshead RM, Boorman RS, Hiemstra LA, Lo IK, et al. A randomized clinical trial comparing open and arthroscopic stabilization for recurrent traumatic anterior shoulder instability: two-year follow-up with disease-specific quality-of-life outcomes. J Bone Joint Surg Am. 2014 Mar 5;96(5):353–60.

42. Buza JA 3rd, Iyengar JJ, Anakwenze OA, Ahmad CS, Levine WN. Arthroscopic Hill-Sachs remplissage: a systematic review. J Bone Joint Surg Am. 2014 Apr 2;96(7):549–55.

43. Moroder P, Odorizzi M, Pizzinini S, Demetz E, Resch H, Moroder P. Open Bankart repair for the treatment of anterior shoulder instability without substantial osseous glenoid defects: results after a minimum follow-up of twenty years. J Bone Joint Surg Am. 2015 Sep 2;97(17):1398–405.

44. Mizuno N, Denard PJ, Raiss P, Melis B, Walch G. Long-term results of the Latarjet procedure for anterior instability of the shoulder. J Shoulder Elbow Surg. 2014 Nov;23(11):1691–9. Epub 2014 May 14.

45. Yamamoto N, Muraki T, An KN, Sperling JW, Cofield RH, Itoi E, et al. The stabilizing mechanism of the Latarjet procedure: a cadaveric study. J Bone Joint Surg Am. 2013 Aug 7;95(15):1390–7.

46. Sayegh ET, Mascarenhas R, Chalmers PN, Cole BJ, Verma NN, Romeo AA. Allograft reconstruction for glenoid bone loss in glenohumeral instability: a systematic review. Arthroscopy. 2014 Dec;30(12):1642–9. Epub 2014 Jul 4.

47. Gupta AK, Forsythe B, Lee AS, Harris JD, McCormick F, Abrams GD, et al. Topographic analysis of the glenoid and proximal medial tibial articular surfaces: a search for the ideal match for glenoid resurfacing. Am J Sports Med. 2013 Aug;41(8):1893–9. Epub 2013 Jul 15.

48. Longo UG, Loppini M, Rizzello G, Ciuffreda M, Maffulli N, Denaro V. Latarjet, Bristow, and Eden-Hybinette procedures for anterior shoulder dislocation: systematic review and quantitative synthesis of the literature. Arthroscopy. 2014 Sep;30(9):1184–211. Epub 2014 Jun 4.

49. Gupta A, Delaney R, Petkin K, Lafosse L. Complications of the Latarjet procedure. Curr Rev Musculoskelet Med. 2015 Mar;8(1):59–66.

50. Griesser MJ, Harris JD, McCoy BW, Hussain WM, Jones MH, Bishop JY, et al. Complications and re-operations after Bristow-Latarjet shoulder stabilization: a systematic review. J Shoulder Elbow Surg. 2013 Feb;22(2):286–92.

51. Shah AA, Butler RB, Romanowski J, Goel D, Karadagli D, Warner JJ. Short-term complications of the Latarjet procedure. J Bone Joint Surg Am. 2012 Mar 21;94(6):495–501.

52. Cunningham G, Benchouk S, Kherad O, Ladermann A. Comparison of arthroscopic and open Latarjet with a learning curve analysis. Knee Surg Sports Traumatol Arthrosc. 2016 Feb;24(2):540–5. Epub 2015 Dec 12.

53. Boileau P, Gendre P, Baba M, Thelu CE, Baring T, Gonzalez JF, et al. A guided surgical approach and novel fixation method for arthroscopic Latarjet. J Shoulder Elbow Surg. 2016 Jan;25(1):78–89. Epub 2015 Aug 7.

54. Rosso C, Bongiorno V, Samitier G, Dumont GD, Szollosy G, Lafosse L. Technical guide and tips on the all-arthroscopic Latarjet procedure. Knee Surg Sports Traumatol Arthrosc. 2016 Feb;24(2):564–72. Epub 2014 May 10.

55. Dumont GD, Fogerty S, Rosso C, Lafosse L. The arthroscopic latarjet procedure for anterior shoulder instability: 5-year minimum follow-up. Am J Sports Med. 2014 Nov;42(11):2560–6. Epub 2014 Aug 12.

56. Camp CL, Dahm DL, Krych AJ. Arthroscopic remplissage for engaging hill-sachs lesions in patients with anterior shoulder instability. Arthrosc Tech. 2015 Sep 28;4(5):e499–502. Epub 2015 Oct.

57. Saltzman BM, Riboh JC, Cole BJ, Yanke AB. Humeral head reconstruction with osteochondral allograft transplantation. Arthroscopy. 2015 Sep;31(9):1827–34. Epub 2015 May 13.

58. Song DJ, Cook JB, Krul KP, Bottoni CR, Rowles DJ, Shaha SH, et al. High frequency of posterior and combined shoulder instability in young active patients. J Shoulder Elbow Surg. 2015 Feb;24(2):186–90. Epub 2014 Sep 11.

59. Savoie FH 3rd, Field LD, Atchinson S. Anterior superior instability with rotator cuff tearing: SLAC lesion. Orthop Clin North Am. 2001 Jul;32(3):457–61.

60. Arner JW, McClincy MP, Bradley JP. Arthroscopic stabilization of posterior shoulder instability is

successful in american football players. Arthroscopy. 2015 Aug;31(8):1466–71. Epub 2015 Apr 14.

61. Chalmers PN, Hammond J, Juhan T, Romeo AA. Revision posterior shoulder stabilization. J Shoulder Elbow Surg. 2013 Sep;22(9):1209–20. Epub 2013 Feb 15.

62. Schwartz DG, Goebel S, Piper K, Kordasiewicz B, Boyle S, Lafosse L. Arthroscopic posterior bone block augmentation in posterior shoulder instability. J Shoulder Elbow Surg. 2013 Aug;22(8):1092–101. Epub 2013 Jan 20.

63. Servien E, Walch G, Cortes ZE, Edwards TB, O'Connor DP. Posterior bone block procedure for posterior shoulder instability. Knee Surg Sports Traumatol Arthrosc. 2007 Sep;15(9):1130–6.

64. Meuffels DE, Schuit H, van Biezen FC, Reijman M, Verhaar JA. The posterior bone block procedure in posterior shoulder instability: a long-term follow-up study. J Bone Joint Surg Br. 2010 May;92(5):651–5.

65. Graichen H, Koydl P, Zichner L. Effectiveness of glenoid osteotomy in atraumatic posterior instability of the shoulder associated with excessive retroversion and flatness of the glenoid. Int Orthop. 1999;23(2):95–9.

66. Hawkins RH. Glenoid osteotomy for recurrent posterior subluxation of the shoulder: assessment by computed axial tomography. J Shoulder Elbow Surg. 1996 Sep-Oct;5(5):393–400.

67. Neer CS 2nd, Foster CR. Inferior capsular shift for involuntary inferior and multidirectional instability of the shoulder: a preliminary report. J Bone Joint Surg Am. 1980 Sep;62(6):897–908.

68. McFarland EG, Kim TK, Park HB, Neira CA, Gutierrez MI. The effect of variation in definition on the diagnosis of multidirectional instability of the shoulder. J Bone Joint Surg Am. 2003 Nov;85-A(11):2138–44.

69. Johnson SM, Robinson CM. Shoulder instability in patients with joint hyperlaxity. J Bone Joint Surg Am. 2010 Jun;92(6):1545–57.

70. Gagey OJ, Gagey N. The hyperabduction test. J Bone Joint Surg Br. 2001 Jan;83(1):69–74.

71. Beighton P, Horan F. Orthopaedic aspects of the Ehlers-Danlos syndrome. J Bone Joint Surg Br. 1969 Aug;51(3):444–53.

72. Gaskill TR, Taylor DC, Millett PJ. Management of multidirectional instability of the shoulder. J Am Acad Orthop Surg. 2011 Dec;19(12):758–67.

73. Warby SA, Pizzari T, Ford JJ, Hahne AJ, Watson L. Exercise-based management versus surgery for multidirectional instability of the glenohumeral joint: a systematic review. Br J Sports Med. 2016 Sep;50(18):1115–23. Epub 2015 Dec 23.

74. Warby SA, Pizzari T, Ford JJ, Hahne AJ, Watson L. The effect of exercise-based management for multidirectional instability of the glenohumeral joint: a systematic review. J Shoulder Elbow Surg. 2014 Jan;23(1):128–42.

75. Vavken P, Tepolt FA, Kocher MS. Open inferior capsular shift for multidirectional shoulder instability in adolescents with generalized ligamentous hyperlaxity or Ehlers-Danlos syndrome. J Shoulder Elbow Surg. 2016 Jun;25(6):907–12. Epub 2016 Jan 14.

76. Chaudhury S, Gasinu S, Rodeo SA. Bilateral anterior and posterior glenohumeral stabilization using Achilles tendon allograft augmentation in a patient with Ehlers-Danlos syndrome. J Shoulder Elbow Surg. 2012 Jun;21(6):e1–5. Epub 2012 Feb 10.

77. Wallace AL, Hollinshead RM, Frank CB. The scientific basis of thermal capsular shrinkage. J Shoulder Elbow Surg. 2000 Jul-Aug;9(4):354–60.

78. Longo UG, Rizzello G, Loppini M, Locher J, Buchmann S, Maffulli N, et al. Multidirectional instability of the shoulder: a systematic review. Arthroscopy. 2015 Dec;31(12):2431–43. Epub 2015 Jul 21.

79. Chen D, Goldberg J, Herald J, Critchley I, Barmare A. Effects of surgical management on multidirectional instability of the shoulder: a meta-analysis. Knee Surg Sports Traumatol Arthrosc. 2016 Feb;24(2):630–9. Epub 2015 Dec 12.

80. Park HB, Yokota A, Gill HS, El Rassi G, McFarland EG. Revision surgery for failed thermal capsulorrhaphy. Am J Sports Med. 2005 Sep;33(9):1321–6. Epub 2005 Jul 7.

81. Pollock RG, Owens JM, Flatow EL, Bigliani LU. Operative results of the inferior capsular shift procedure for multidirectional instability of the shoulder. J Bone Joint Surg Am. 2000 Jul;82-A(7):919–28.

82. Andrews JR, Carson WG Jr, McLeod WD. Glenoid labrum tears related to the long head of the biceps. Am J Sports Med. 1985 Sep-Oct;13(5):337–41.

83. Snyder SJ, Karzel RP, Del Pizzo W, Ferkel RD, Friedman MJ. SLAP lesions of the shoulder. Arthroscopy. 1990;6(4):274–9.

84. Schwartzberg R, Reuss BL, Burkhart BG, Butterfield M, Wu JY, McLean KW. High prevalence of superior labral tears diagnosed by MRI in middle-aged patients with asymptomatic shoulders. Orthop J Sports Med. 2016 Jan 5;4(1):2325967115623212. Epub 2016 Jan.

85. Burns JP, Bahk M, Snyder SJ. Superior labral tears: repair versus biceps tenodesis. J Shoulder Elbow Surg. 2011 Mar;20(2 Suppl):S2–8.

86. Keener JD, Brophy RH. Superior labral tears of the shoulder: pathogenesis, evaluation, and treatment. J Am Acad Orthop Surg. 2009 Oct;17(10):627–37.

87. McCormick F, Bhatia S, Chalmers P, Gupta A, Verma N, Romeo AA. The management of type II superior labral anterior to posterior injuries. Orthop Clin North Am. 2014 Jan;45(1):121–8. Epub 2013 Oct 1.

88. Fedoriw WW, Ramkumar P, McCulloch PC, Lintner DM. Return to play after treatment of superior labral tears in professional baseball players. Am J Sports Med. 2014 May;42(5):1155–60. Epub 2014 Mar 27. Erratum in: Am J Sports Med. 2015 Dec;43(12):NP46.

89. Sayde WM, Cohen SB, Ciccotti MG, Dodson CC. Return to play after Type II superior labral anterior-posterior lesion repairs in athletes: a systematic review. Clin Orthop Relat Res. 2012 Jun;470(6):1595–600.

90. Neuman BJ, Boisvert CB, Reiter B, Lawson K, Ciccotti MG, Cohen SB. Results of arthroscopic repair of type II superior labral anterior posterior lesions in overhead athletes: assessment of return to preinjury playing level and satisfaction. Am J Sports Med. 2011 Sep;39(9):1883–8. Epub 2011 Jul 7.

91. McCormick F, Nwachukwu BU, Solomon D, Dewing C, Golijanin P, Gross DJ, et al. The efficacy of biceps tenodesis in the treatment of failed superior labral anterior posterior repairs. Am J Sports Med. 2014 Apr;42(4):820–5. Epub 2014 Feb 11.

92. Werner BC, Brockmeier SF, Gwathmey FW. Trends in long head biceps tenodesis. Am J Sports Med. 2015 Mar;43(3):570–8. Epub 2014 Dec 12.

93. Creech MJ, Yeung M, Denkers M, Simunovic N, Athwal GS, Ayeni OR. Surgical indications for long head biceps tenodesis: a systematic review. Knee Surg Sports Traumatol Arthrosc. 2016 Jul;24(7):2156–66. Epub 2014 Nov 23.

94. Gaudelli C, Hebert-Davies J, Balg F, Pelet S, Djahangiri A, Godbout V, et al. The impact of superior labral anterior to posterior lesions on functional status in shoulder instability: a multicenter cohort study. Orthop J Sports Med. 2014 Oct 29;2(10):2325967114554195. Epub 2014 Oct.

95. Kim DS, Park HK, Park JH, Yoon WS. Ganglion cyst of the spinoglenoid notch: comparison between SLAP repair alone and SLAP repair with cyst decompression. J Shoulder Elbow Surg. 2012 Nov;21(11):1456–63. Epub 2012 Apr 26.

96. Pillai G, Baynes JR, Gladstone J, Flatow EL. Greater strength increase with cyst decompression and SLAP repair than SLAP repair alone. Clin Orthop Relat Res. 2011 Apr;469(4):1056–60.

97. Lafosse L, Tomasi A, Corbett S, Baier G, Willems K, Gobezie R. Arthroscopic release of suprascapular nerve entrapment at the suprascapular notch: technique and preliminary results. Arthroscopy. 2007 Jan;23(1):34–42.

98. Edwards SL, Lee JA, Bell JE, Packer JD, Ahmad CS, Levine WN, et al. Nonoperative treatment of superior labrum anterior posterior tears: improvements in pain, function, and quality of life. Am J Sports Med. 2010 Jul;38(7):1456–61. Epub 2010 Jun 3.

99. Forsythe B, Guss D, Anthony SG, Martin SD. Concomitant arthroscopic SLAP and rotator cuff repair. J Bone Joint Surg Am. 2010 Jun;92(6):1362–9.

100. Franceschi F, Longo UG, Ruzzini L, Rizzello G, Maffulli N, Denaro V. No advantages in repairing a type II superior labrum anterior and posterior (SLAP) lesion when associated with rotator cuff repair in patients over age 50: a randomized controlled trial. Am J Sports Med. 2008 Feb;36(2):247–53. Epub 2007 Oct 16.

101. Gombera MM, Sekiya JK. Rotator cuff tear and glenohumeral instability: a systematic review. Clin Orthop Relat Res. 2014 Aug;472(8):2448–56. Erratum in: Clin Orthop Relat Res. 2015 Feb;473(2):751. Gomberawalla, M Mustafa [corrected to Gombera, Mufaddal Mustafa].

102. Shields E, Mirabelli M, Amsdell S, Thorsness R, Goldblatt J, Maloney M, et al. Functional and imaging outcomes of arthroscopic simultaneous rotator cuff repair and bankart repair after shoulder dislocations. Am J Sports Med. 2014 Nov;42(11):2614–20. Epub 2014 Sep 26.

103. Voos JE, Pearle AD, Mattern CJ, Cordasco FA, Allen AA, Warren RF. Outcomes of combined arthroscopic rotator cuff and labral repair. Am J Sports Med. 2007 Jul;35(7):1174–9. Epub 2007 Mar 26.

104. Schmid SL, Farshad M, Catanzaro S, Gerber C. The Latarjet procedure for the treatment of recurrence of anterior instability of the shoulder after operative repair: a retrospective case series of forty-nine consecutive patients. J Bone Joint Surg Am. 2012 Jun 6;94(11):e75.

105. Thangarajah T, Alexander S, Bayley I, Lambert SM. Glenohumeral arthrodesis for the treatment of recurrent shoulder instability in epileptic patients. Bone Joint J. 2014 Nov;96-B(11):1525–9.

106. Diaz JA, Cohen SB, Warren RF, Craig EV, Allen AA. Arthrodesis as a salvage procedure for recurrent instability of the shoulder. J Shoulder Elbow Surg. 2003 May-Jun;12(3):237–41.

8 Adhesive Capsulitis

Some individuals experience a condition characterized by spontaneous shoulder pain and stiffness due to synovitis, fibrosis, and loss of capsule elasticity without a clear-cut inciting cause. Most commonly, this condition is named *adhesive capsulitis* or *frozen shoulder*, terms applied only when shoulder radiographs are essentially normal and other reasons for shoulder pain and stiffness (e.g., cuff disease, fractures, dislocations, and arthritis) can be excluded. Although this condition resolves spontaneously in many patients, its course is protracted and a number of individuals may experience permanent restrictions in motion and function.

Terminology

There is some confusion regarding the terminology used to describe this condition. The term *frozen shoulder* implies loss of shoulder motion in all planes (Table 8.1). The term *primary frozen shoulder* is used for those individuals for whom associated underlying pathology cannot be identified in the shoulder joint. The term *adhesive capsulitis* is somewhat misleading, since in this condition the capsule does not adhere to other structures; however, most accept the term *adhesive capsulitis* to be synonymous with *primary frozen shoulder*. A number of conditions have been associated with adhesive capsulitis, as detailed later (see Pathogenesis); when none of these conditions can be identified, patients are diagnosed with *idiopathic primary frozen shoulder* (*idiopathic adhesive capsulitis*). The term *secondary frozen shoulder* is applied when capsular fibrosis restricting motion in all planes develops after a fracture, surgery, or as a consequence of rotator cuff problems or neuromuscular dysfunction.

Epidemiology

The prevalence of frozen shoulder is difficult to determine accurately due to the various terms used to describe

Table 8.1 • Conditions Presenting with Shoulder Stiffness

Frozen shoulder (capsular fibrosis is the main reason for stiffness)
Primary frozen shoulder (adhesive capsulitis)
  Idiopathic (no predisposing condition can be identified)
  Associated with hormone disorders, drugs, and other causes (Table 8.2)
Secondary frozen shoulder: capsular fibrosis induced by 1 of the following:
  Cuff disease
  Calcifying tendinitis
  Fractures (despite union in good position)
  Surgical procedures
  Lack of use secondary to neuromuscular conditions
  Other

Stiffness as a symptom of other shoulder conditions
Osteoarthritis
Inflammatory arthritis
Fracture malunion or nonunion
Avascular necrosis
Malignancy
Other

subcategories of the condition and the absence of a strict definition. It is estimated that frozen shoulder affects 2% of the general population, with a cumulative incidence of 2.4 per 1,000 persons per year (1). Adhesive capsulitis typically affects patients between 40 and 60 years of age, and is slightly more common in women (2–4). Recurrence in the same shoulder is rare, but approximately 20% of patients with adhesive capsulitis develop the same condition on the opposite shoulder (2). Some patients present with simultaneous bilateral involvement.

Pathogenesis

Pain and stiffness in patients with adhesive capsulitis are secondary to a combination of synovitis and capsular

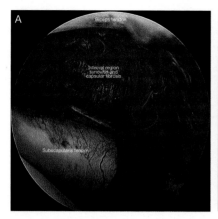
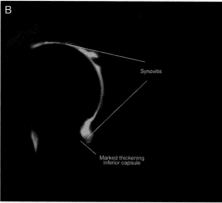
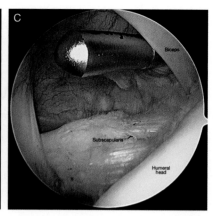

Figure 8.1 *Adhesive capsulitis is characterized by marked synovitis* **(A)** *and capsular thickening* **(B)**. *These features are in contrast with the mildly hyperemic, nonfibrotic shoulder, as in the example shown in* **C** *from a patient with a partial-thickness subscapularis tear.*

fibrosis (Figure 8.1). However, it is still unclear *why* this process starts and *what* drives the process at the cellular and molecular level.

Areas of the Joint Involved

The synovitis and fibrosis characteristic of adhesive capsulitis primarily involve the rotator interval region and the anterior and inferior capsule. Fibrosis of the interval region contributes substantially to limited external rotation in adduction, whereas fibrosis of the anteroinferior capsule limits elevation as well as external rotation in abduction. When the posterior capsule is affected as well, it limits internal rotation.

Conditions Associated With Adhesive Capsulitis

As mentioned before, primary frozen shoulder may be idiopathic, but it can also be associated with certain conditions with a higher likelihood of developing adhesive capsulitis compared to the general population (Table 8.2) (3). Diabetes mellitus is the condition most commonly associated with adhesive capsulitis: approximately 10% of patients with type I and 20% of patients with type II diabetes mellitus develop capsulitis, which translates into 2 to 4 times the risk of the general population (5,6).

Cells and Pathways Involved

The intimate mechanisms leading to spontaneous synovitis and fibrosis are not clearly understood. Histologically, samples obtained from patients with capsulitis are composed of a dense matrix of compact, mature type-III collagen containing fibroblasts, myofibroblasts, and chronic inflammatory cells (2).

The process that triggers the deposition of this tissue is likely different depending on the associated conditions.

Table 8.2 • Conditions Known to Carry a Higher Risk of Developing Adhesive Capsulitis Compared With General Population

Source of Condition	Condition
Hormonal/ homeostatic	Diabetes mellitus Thyroid (both hypothyroidism and hyperthyroidism) Adrenocorticotropic hormone (ACTH) deficiency Hyperlipidemia (triglycerides and/or cholesterol)
Cardiac	Cardiac surgery Ischemic heart disease
Neurologic	Stroke Parkinson disease Neurosurgery (especially acute aneurysm surgery)
Trauma	Not including shoulder fracture or dislocation or cuff tear
Drug-induced or drug-related	Matrix metalloproteinase inhibitor for gastric carcinoma Antiretrovirals Fluoroquinolones Pneumococcal vaccine
Fibrotic conditions	Dupuytren contracture La Peyronie disease
Other	Chronic obstructive pulmonary disease Radical neck dissection Malignancy

For example, in diabetic patients it has been proposed that adhesive capsulitis may be mediated by either microvascular disease or peripheral neuropathy. The fact that adhesive capsulitis results from the administration of a metalloproteinase inhibitor may indicate that in idiopathic capsulitis there is an imbalance between metalloproteinases (which degrade the connective tissue matrix) and their inhibitors. Capsular contracture in patients with a stroke or other neurologic abnormalities suggests a neuropathic pathway in these individuals. Some individuals may be genetically predetermined to fibrosis in multiple locations or after trauma. In summary, there is not a single convincing pathophysiologic pathway that explains adhesive capsulitis, idiopathic or otherwise.

Natural History

Phases of the Disease

In most patients with adhesive capsulitis, the disease courses in 3 sequential phases (Table 8.3). It begins with the *freezing* or *painful phase*, characterized by insidious progressive onset of pain and stiffness. Typically, patients note pain first with activities and at night, but eventually pain is constant. Most of the time, pain precedes stiffness, but in some patients stiffness is the first symptom. The next phase (*frozen* or *stiff*) is characterized by less severe pain and a plateau in the progression of motion loss. The last phase *(thawing* or *recovery)* is characterized by gradual spontaneous improvement in pain and motion. The mean duration of all 3 phases without treatment is 30 months.

Long-Term Outcome Without Intervention

For years, many surgeons believed that adhesive capsulitis was always a self-resolving condition and all patients recover satisfactory, pain-free shoulder motion and function. However, the information provided by studies on the natural history of capsulitis is contradictory, and may be biased by a number of factors, such as exclusion of the most severe cases (in which intervention is offered without providing an opportunity for spontaneous resolution), as well as various definitions of complete versus functional recovery of motion. A frequently quoted study that followed 62 patients over 7 years reported persistent pain in 50% and persistent stiffness in 60% of shoulders. It is now accepted that 7% to 15% of patients will

have some degree of permanent loss of motion without intervention, although few have persistent functional limitations (3,4).

Patient Evaluation

When a patient presents with the symptoms consistent with adhesive capsulitis, the evaluation should have 4 goals: exclude other conditions that may present with shoulder stiffness, identify possible associated predisposing factors, explain the natural history to the patient, and formulate a treatment plan. Table 8.4 summarizes the clinical features of adhesive capsulitis.

History

Pain and stiffness without a clearly identifiable explanation are the hallmarks of adhesive capsulitis. Most patients complain of severe, deep-seated, burning pain felt diffusely around the shoulder region. Oftentimes, pain at night interferes with sleep. Loss of external rotation is almost universally present, and loss of motion in elevation and internal rotation is very common as well. Most patients present in the freezing or frozen phase, and confirmation of the phasic nature of the symptoms reinforces the diagnosis. Patients should be questioned about prior injuries or surgery to the shoulder to identify instances of secondary frozen shoulder. In addition, patients should be questioned about conditions known to carry a higher risk of adhesive capsulitis (Table 8.2).

Physical Examination

The key finding on physical examination is loss of passive glenohumeral motion. In patients with frozen shoulder,

Table 8.3 • Clinical Phases of Adhesive Capsulitis

Phase	Characteristic Features	Average Duration
Freezing	Severe pain Progressive loss of motion	10–36 weeks
Frozen	Pain improves Motion plateaus or worsens	4–12 months
Thawing	Gradual recovery of motion	5–26 months

Table 8.4 • Clinical Features of Adhesive Capsulitis

History and physical examination
Generalized shoulder pain (deep, burning)
Progressive loss of motion in most or all planes
Secondary pain at
   Periscapular region
   Acromioclavicular joint
Normal cuff and deltoid strength
Inquire for possible reasons for:
   Nonidiopathic adhesive capsulitis
   Secondary frozen shoulder

Imaging studies
Plain radiographs appear normal
Magnetic resonance imaging shows:
   Reduced joint capacity
   Thickened capsule
   Interval region narrow and thick
   Occasional synovitis

motion may be somewhat limited by pain, but firm end points resisting motion are easily identified. Passive motion in elevation, external rotation, and internal rotation should be accurately measured and recorded to understand how severe the contracture is and to monitor motion gains or losses over time.

Other findings on physical examination may include pain at the acromioclavicular joint (attributed to forced compensatory acromioclavicular joint overload), periscapular and neck pain (attributed to compensatory scapulothoracic motion), and generalized muscle wasting in patients with longstanding symptoms. Strength should also be examined carefully, since rotator cuff tears may lead to secondary stiffness. The presence of swelling or erythema should prompt consideration of an alternative diagnosis, such as infection, malignancy, or neuropathic arthropathy. It is important to realize that in patients with adhesive capsulitis, examination maneuvers for impingement and labral tears cannot be performed reliably.

Imaging Studies and Other Tests

Plain radiographs are normal in patients with adhesive capsulitis (Figure 8.2). However, they should be obtained routinely to rule out other reasons for shoulder stiffness, mainly glenohumeral joint arthritis, calcifying tendinitis, a missed locked posterior dislocation, or malignancy.

Advanced imaging studies, such as magnetic resonance or ultrasonography, are not obtained routinely unless the physical examination suggests the possibility of an underlying rotator cuff tear. However, by the time patients are referred to the orthopedic surgeon, many have already undergone advanced imaging. The most typical findings in these studies include capsular thickening in the interval region, anterior capsule, and inferior axillary recess, as well as thickening of the coracohumeral ligament (Figures 8.1 and 8.3). Magnetic resonance should be obtained when the presentation is consistent with a rotator cuff tear or when there are concerns about the possibility of avascular necrosis, osteomyelitis, or malignancy.

Due to the high prevalence of diabetes mellitus, subclinical hyperglycemia, or intolerance to glucose in patients with adhesive capsulitis, some surgeons order fasting glucose testing in all patients presenting with idiopathic frozen shoulder. Further evaluation of underlying endocrinopathies is best completed with the help of the patient's primary care physician or through referral to the appropriate specialist.

Most Common Mistakes

Failure to Identify Underlying Pathology

Unfortunately, I have witnessed misdiagnosis of adhesive capsulitis in patients with both osteoarthritis and a locked posterior shoulder dislocation. In these circumstances, patients had been sent to therapy for shoulder stretching for weeks until lack of improvement prompted evaluation with plain radiographs. Radiographs are safe and relatively inexpensive, and as mentioned earlier, they should be considered routinely in patients suspected of having adhesive

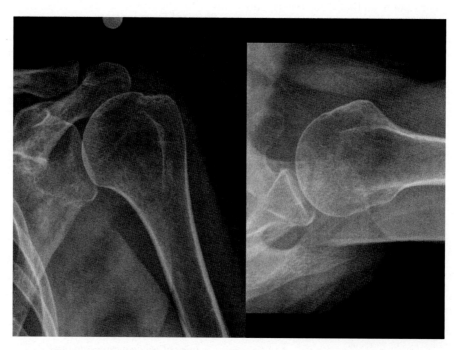

Figure 8.2 *Radiographs in patients with suspected adhesive capsulitis are almost always normal but always should be obtained to exclude other reasons for shoulder stiffness, most commonly primary osteoarthritis or undiagnosed inflammatory arthritis.*

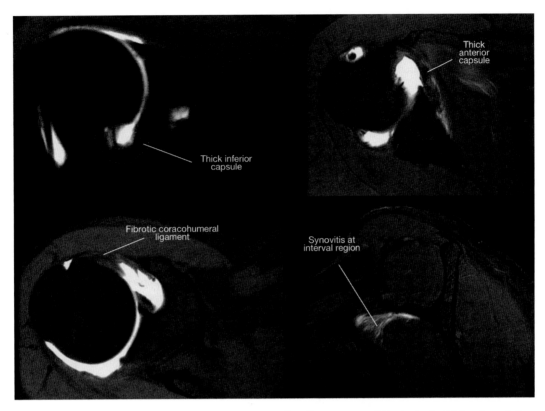

Figure 8.3 *Classic magnetic resonance findings in patients with adhesive capsulitis include thickening of the capsule and interval region as well as synovitis. Magnetic resonance may also be interpreted as consistent with labral tears or partial-thickness cuff tears, but those findings are seldom clinically significant in classic adhesive capsulitis.*

capsulitis. They will help identify several of the conditions summarized in Table 8.1.

Attribution of Symptoms to Labral or Cuff Pathology

Signal changes in the labrum and/or rotator cuff are very commonly visualized in magnetic resonance studies of patients with no shoulder symptoms (*see* chapter 6, Rotator Cuff and Labrum). When patients with adhesive capsulitis do undergo magnetic resonance evaluation, the report often contains the words "labral tear" and/or "partial-thickness rotator cuff tear." Current access to information by patients (both their reports and websites with medical information) can easily lead to the misunderstanding that the shoulder is painful and stiff because there is a tear that needs to be fixed surgically. Although some high-grade, partial-thickness supraspinatus tears may present with pain and stiffness, most patients with true adhesive capsulitis will improve without addressing these magnetic resonance changes surgically.

Correlation of the magnetic resonance findings with the history and physical examination is essential to really understand where the pain and stiffness are coming from. Avoidance of advanced imaging studies in patients with classic findings of adhesive capsulitis and negative

radiographs will save an unnecessary expense and decrease confusion in patients and providers. Having said that, some patients with pain and stiffness do need to be evaluated with magnetic resonance or other advanced imaging studies, as detailed before.

Overtreatment of the Acromioclavicular Joint

As mentioned before, a number of patients with adhesive capsulitis will have pain on deep palpation over the acromioclavicular joint. This seems to be secondary to overload and improves as the capsulitis resolves (7). Unnecessary resections of the distal end of the clavicle should be avoided in patients with adhesive capsulitis, although they may be beneficial in patients with truly symptomatic associated pathology at the acromioclavicular joint.

Treatment

Once the diagnosis of adhesive capsulitis is clearly established, treatment recommendations are oftentimes influenced by the surgeon's interpretation of the natural history of this condition; the phase, duration, and severity of symptoms; the presence of underlying predisposing conditions; access to health care; prior treatment attempts; and patient and surgeon preferences.

If the patient is averse to surgery, the surgeon has limited operating room availability, there are no predisposing conditions such as diabetes mellitus, and/or symptoms are mild to moderate, a trial of nonoperative treatment is oftentimes recommended, especially if the patient has never tried stretching exercises. On the other hand, our society is now used to finding a relatively quick solution to problems, and even when patients are told that they do have a high chance of getting better without surgery, they do opt for surgical treatment when they are informed that the average timeframe to recovery can be over 2 years.

What would you do if the patient were you? Would you rather wait for quite some time in an effort to avoid surgery, or would you prefer to get surgery in order to get better sooner? Clearly, this is 1 condition where the surgeon should explain to the patient what is known about the natural history of adhesive capsulitis, discuss treatment alternatives, and let the patient decide. Figure 8.4 summarizes my overall approach to the management of adhesive capsulitis.

Nonoperative Treatment

Most patients are treated at least initially with a combination of pain management modalities, physical therapy, and 1 or 2 intra-articular corticosteroid injections. Since the course of the disease seems to be self-resolving in many patients, and these treatment strategies are used in combination, it has been difficult to prove their benefit definitively. However, even if nonoperative treatment does not change the final outcome, it certainly helps during the symptomatic phases and may shorten the overall duration of the condition.

Pain Management and Physical Therapy

Since adhesive capsulitis is a painful condition, pain management is an important element of nonoperative treatment. My preference is to combine acetaminophen and a nonsteroidal anti-inflammatory drug; I avoid use of narcotic pain medications due to their adverse effects. Anecdotally, moist heat seems to help some patients. A short course of oral corticosteroids is recommended by some for patients with severe pain, especially during the freezing phase. When pain cannot be addressed properly with any of these modalities, consideration should be given to intra-articular injections, a suprascapular nerve block, or surgery (see later in this chapter).

Physical therapy is directed mostly to gentle, progressive stretching of the shoulder in all directions (see chapter 12, Rehabilitation and Injections). Physical therapy may really

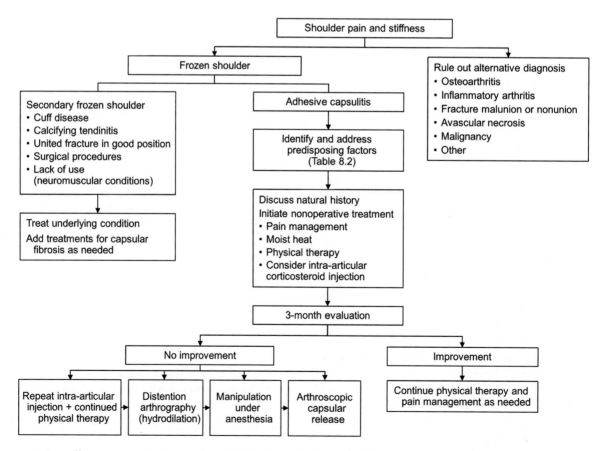

Figure 8.4 *Overall management strategy for patients with adhesive capsulitis.*

aggravate the condition when initiated in the freezing phase, but if possible it should be instituted as soon as the diagnosis is established. Patients may regain motion successfully stretching on their own, or they may need the help of a physical therapist. Most surgeons agree on trying therapy for at least 3 months before considering manipulation under anesthesia or surgery.

Intra-articular Corticosteroid Injections

The rationale for use of corticosteroid injections is the known presence of synovitis in adhesive capsulitis. Intra-articular injections have the added benefit of providing some pain relief, facilitating physical therapy by making it less painful. Since the injection needs to be placed intra-articularly, the capsule to be pierced with the needle is thickened, and the joint volume is decreased, it is probably best to administer these injections with image guidance, most commonly ultrasonography. Otherwise it may be difficult to ensure that the injection is truly intra-articular.

When to use injections and how many to use is based more on common sense than scientific data. Most surgeons recommend using 1 injection, and repeating the injection at the most 2 more times 3 months apart if the first injection was beneficial but the condition does not seem to be resolving. In my practice, I offer an injection in the first consultation for patients with severe pain who are thought to be unable to initiate physical therapy otherwise, as well as for those who have already tried physical therapy for weeks and do not seem to be making much progress.

Distention Arthrography (Hydrodilatation)

The goal of this procedure is to distend the glenohumeral joint with saline injected under pressure sufficient enough to cause capsular rupture. The joint is first injected with local anesthesia so that the procedure is less painful. Next, saline is injected until the pressure necessary to continue to inject suddenly decreases. Not uncommonly, the procedure is completed by also injecting corticosteroids at the end. Intensive physical therapy starts right after. Although some authors have reported good outcome with this treatment modality (8), I seldom use it in my practice. It is difficult to determine whether patients subjected to distention arthrography improve because of the capsular rupture, the corticosteroid injection, the program of physical therapy that follows, or a combination.

Manipulation Under Anesthesia

This procedure involves placing the patient under anesthesia, typically with muscle relaxation, and forcefully moving the shoulder in a controlled fashion in order to rupture the capsule until a full arc of motion is regained. The main risks of this procedure are shoulder dislocation or a fracture of the proximal humerus; other potential complications include tears of the rotator cuff or the labrum as well as glenoid rim fractures. Some studies have confirmed that most patients subjected to a manipulation under anesthesia maintain a good arc of motion at long-term follow-up (9). However, comparative studies have failed to demonstrate a superior outcome using manipulation under anesthesia versus conservative treatment modalities (10).

Most surgeons recommend working sequentially, starting with forward flexion, then external rotation in adduction, external rotation in abduction, and, last, internal rotation. After the manipulation is completed, the shoulder may be injected with corticosteroids. Postmanipulation radiographs should be obtained to confirm that complications have not occurred. As with other interventions, postmanipulation physical therapy is extremely important to maintain the range of motion obtained with the manipulation.

Arthroscopic Capsular Release

This procedure has become my treatment of choice for patients not responding to a course of nonoperative treatment (⬤ Video 8.1). Table 8.5 summarizes why arthroscopic capsular release is an attractive treatment option for adhesive capsulitis.

Indications

Surgery is considered for patients whose program of nonoperative treatment has clearly failed and who do not want to wait the time it may take for the condition to resolve spontaneously, if it does.

Technique

My preference is to perform this procedure in the beach chair position under general anesthesia. Brachial plexus blockade with a long-acting local anesthetic helps with postoperative pain control and allows the surgeon to

---

Table 8.5 • Advantages of Arthroscopic Capsular Release

Allows identification of associated or underlying conditions (e.g., early osteoarthritis)

Carries less risk of complications (such as fracture or dislocation) because procedure is performed in a controlled fashion

Allows not only division of tissue but also its removal (selective areas of capsulectomy such as interval region)

Minimizes residual intra-articular hematoma that could contribute to recurrence

Allows addressing biceps involvement if present

Allows release of the subdeltoid/subacromial space in cases of frozen shoulder secondary to fracture

Resolves pain and stiffness very quickly

Is minimally invasive

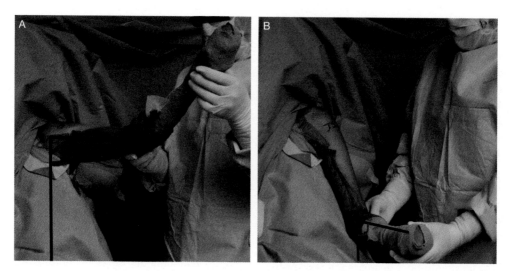

Figure 8.5 *Range of motion is documented with the patient under anesthesia.* **A,** *Limited abduction.* **B,** *Limited external rotation.*

show the patient that surgery has restored motion while the block is still effective. Prior to starting the procedure, shoulder motion under anesthesia is measured and documented (Figure 8.5).

Care should be taken when the posterior glenohumeral portal is established, since the contracted joint makes it more difficult to place the arthroscopic camera in the joint, with risk of cartilage damage or inadvertent interosseous placement of instrumentation. Joint distraction by an assistant or use of traction devices may help.

As soon as the camera is in the joint, it is easy to recognize the inflamed synovium (Figure 8.1). An anterior portal is established and a complete diagnostic arthroscopy is performed (chapter 2, Arthroscopic Shoulder Surgery). Special attention is paid to the biceps; rarely, I have operated on patients with long-standing contractures where the fibrosis did involve the biceps and motion could not be restored until the biceps was tenotomized. If a biceps tenotomy is necessary, my preference is to tenodese the biceps (chapter 6, The Rotator Cuff and Biceps Tendon).

The contracted interval region, anterior, posterior, and inferior capsule are then addressed systematically. I first use either a thermal (radiofrequency) ablation device or a mechanical tissue shaver to completely remove all tissue in the interval region, including not only the capsule and superior glenohumeral ligament but also the coracohumeral ligament (Figure 8.6A). I then continue dividing and removing a strip of anterior capsule just deep to the subscapularis, getting as low as possible (Figure 8.6B). As the surgeon tries to reach inferiorly, close to the axillary recess, it may be helpful to switch to an arthroscopic punch, since it may reach further and will decrease the risk of thermal injury to the axillary nerve.

Once the rotator cuff interval and anterior capsule have been addressed, portals are switched (Figures 8.6C and D). With the camera in the anterior portal and instruments introduced posteriorly, a strip of posterior capsule is divided and removed (Figures 8.6E and F). Identification of the transverse muscular fibers of the infraspinatus through the capsular division allows confirmation of complete division of the capsule. The release continues inferiorly until the inferior capsule can be divided and the posterior release fully connects with the anterior release. Again, care is taken to avoid iatrogenic injury to the axillary nerve by maintaining adequate visualization, paying close attention to unexpected contractions of the deltoid when using a thermal device, or using a punch inferiorly. A main obstacle to a successful complete release of the capsule may be access and visualization. Table 8.6 summarizes a few strategies that may improve proficiency when performing this procedure.

Arthroscopic evaluation of the subacromial space with possible bursectomy and acromioplasty is recommended in patients with frozen shoulder secondary to fracture or after a prior surgical procedure, since in these patients adhesions in the subacromial and subdeltoid space may contribute to stiffness. This is rarely required in adhesive capsulitis.

Once the procedure is finalized, I typically inject the glenohumeral joint with corticosteroids. Portals are closed, and range of motion after release is determined and documented; photographic documentation of the motion achieved may be considered (Figure 8.7). If full motion has not been achieved, gentle manipulation of the shoulder may be added. Some surgeons favor manipulating the shoulder prior to performing the capsular release. The benefits are restoration of motion when the shoulder tissues are not infiltrated by arthroscopic fluid and potentially an easier access to an already released joint; however, tissue ruptures in a more uncontrolled fashion and the hematoma

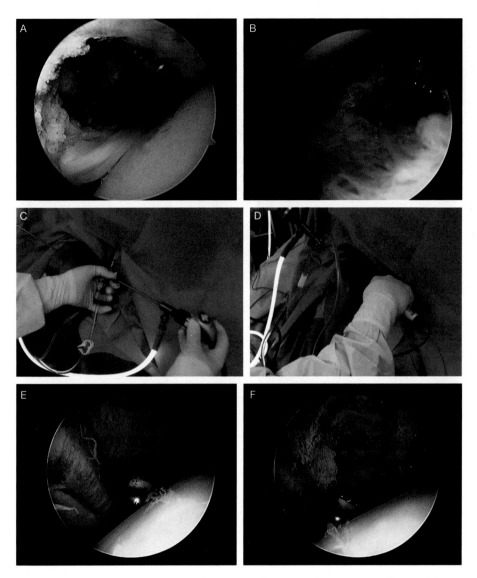

Figure 8.6 *Arthroscopic release.* **A,** *Wide release of all layers at the interval region.* **B,** *Release of the anterior-inferior capsule.* **C and D,** *Switching portals to release the posteroinferior capsule.* **E,** *Posterior capsule and synovium.* **F,** *Posterior capsule released.*

Table 8.6 • Strategies to Improve Access to the Capsule During Arthroscopic Release

Joint distraction by an assistant or mechanical traction

Using the scope as a joint distractor by keeping the camera in between the humeral head and the glenoid

Complete release of the interval region prior to dividing the rest of the capsule

Change in abduction and rotation of the shoulder for different portions of the procedure

Use of an axillary roll to distract the joint inferiorly

Use of an accessory posterior-inferior portal for division of the inferior capsule

---

that occurs with closed manipulation may obscure the arthroscopic view.

Postoperative Management

When patients are seen on rounds just after surgery, the pain relief provided by the interscalenic brachial plexus block offers an opportunity to show the patient the range of motion restored. I move the shoulder into full passive elevation and full passive external rotation to motivate the patient about the fact that all mechanical blocks to motion have been removed. A sling is used for a few days after surgery mainly for comfort. Postoperative pain management is important so that patients can start an intensive program of physical therapy right away. I recommend physical therapy for 2 to 3 months, and evaluate the patients at weeks 2, 6, and 12.

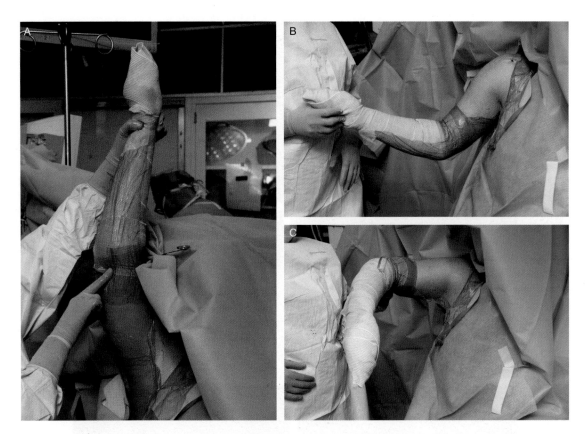

Figure 8.7 *Range of motion at the end of the procedure, with adequate restoration of elevation* **(A)**, *external rotation* **(B)**, *and internal rotation* **(C)**.

Outcome

Comparative studies and systematic reviews have failed to definitely prove that arthroscopic capsular release is superior to continued nonoperative treatment or waiting until the condition resolves; however, my analysis of the literature does show that arthroscopic contracture release leads to a very quick improvement in pain and recovery of motion, which seem to be maintained in a large proportion of patients at long-term follow-up (3,4,11–14). Most patients experience major improvement in pain and motion within 2 weeks of the procedure. Long-term follow-up seems to demonstrate restoration of motion to the same arc as the opposite noninvolved shoulder; however, some studies on the natural history have documented some degree of motion restriction in a number of patients (3,4,14).

Dealing With Failures

Unfortunately, a few patients are not able to maintain the motion regained with an arthroscopic capsular release. When that happens, a second attempt to release the joint arthroscopically may be warranted. In these circumstances, it is extremely important to identify factors that may explain why surgery did not work the first time around (Table 8.7). Obviously, any of these factors would need to be addressed properly for a second attempt to have higher

Table 8.7 • Questions to be Asked Before Revision Arthroscopic Capsular Release

Was the initial diagnosis wrong?

Are there predisposing conditions with suboptimal control? (e.g., uncontrolled diabetes mellitus)

Was the previous surgical release incomplete?

Were there issues with patient compliance regarding postoperative physical therapy?

Did the initial treatment succeed, and the patient presents with a true new recurrence?

chances of success. There are individuals clearly predisposed to recurrent fibrosis, and in those circumstances I have used empirically a single dose of radiation therapy in an attempt to mitigate the exuberant fibrotic response.

Open Release

Prior to the development of arthroscopy, open release of adhesions was the only surgical alternative to conservative treatment. Currently, open release is mostly abandoned. The only exception may be patients with heterotopic ossification limiting motion, as well as those with secondary frozen shoulder when hardware used for previous fracture fixation may be removed; and even in these circumstances, many surgeons would consider an arthroscopic capsular release followed by limited open exposure to remove hardware. When hardware is being removed, it is important to avoid any manipulation afterward, since empty screw holes can act as stress risers and facilitate fracture: first obtain a complete arc of motion with or without manipulation, and then remove the hardware.

KEY POINTS

✓ Adhesive capsulitis is characterized by painful stiffness in patients with normal radiographs and without a clear-cut inciting reason.

✓ Certain conditions carry a higher risk for the development of adhesive capsulitis; diabetes mellitus is the most common of these conditions.

✓ Adhesive capsulitis evolves in 3 phases: freezing, frozen, and thawing.

✓ Although this condition is self-resolving in many individuals, the average time to resolution without treatment is 30 months, and some patients will experience permanent reductions in motion of varying severity.

✓ Nonoperative treatment represents the first line of treatment and typically combines pain management modalities with physical therapy and the occasional use of intra-articular corticosteroid injections.

✓ Surgery is considered for patients not responding to conservative treatment and unwilling to wait several months to see if their condition will resolve spontaneously.

✓ Arthroscopic capsular release is the surgical procedure of choice for patients with adhesive capsulitis; it seems to provide very quick resolution of symptoms and the improvements in motion are maintained over time.

✓ Manipulation under anesthesia and distention arthrography are alternative procedures that may be considered prior to arthroscopic capsular release.

REFERENCES

1. van der Windt DA, Koes BW, de Jong BA, Bouter LM. Shoulder disorders in general practice: incidence, patient characteristics, and management. Ann Rheum Dis. 1995 Dec;54(12):959–64.
2. Hand GC, Athanasou NA, Matthews T, Carr AJ. The pathology of frozen shoulder. J Bone Joint Surg Br. 2007 Jul;89(7):928–32.
3. Hsu JE, Anakwenze OA, Warrender WJ, Abboud JA. Current review of adhesive capsulitis. J Shoulder Elbow Surg. 2011 Apr;20(3):502–14.
4. Robinson CM, Seah KT, Chee YH, Hindle P, Murray IR. Frozen shoulder. J Bone Joint Surg Br. 2012 Jan;94(1):1–9.
5. Arkkila PE, Kantola IM, Viikari JS, Ronnemaa T. Shoulder capsulitis in type I and II diabetic patients: association with diabetic complications and related diseases. Ann Rheum Dis. 1996 Dec;55(12):907–14.
6. Tighe CB, Oakley WS Jr. The prevalence of a diabetic condition and adhesive capsulitis of the shoulder. South Med J. 2008 Jun;101(6):591–5.
7. Anakwenze OA, Hsu JE, Kim JS, Abboud JA. Acromioclavicular joint pain in patients with adhesive capsulitis: a prospective outcome study. Orthopedics. 2011 Sep 9;34(9):e556–60.
8. Rizk TE, Gavant ML, Pinals RS. Treatment of adhesive capsulitis (frozen shoulder) with arthrographic capsular distension and rupture. Arch Phys Med Rehabil. 1994 Jul;75(7):803–7.
9. Farrell CM, Sperling JW, Cofield RH. Manipulation for frozen shoulder: long-term results. J Shoulder Elbow Surg. 2005 Sep-Oct;14(5):480–4.
10. Kivimaki J, Pohjolainen T, Malmivaara A, Kannisto M, Guillaume J, Seitsalo S, et al. Manipulation under anesthesia with home exercises versus home exercises alone in the treatment of frozen shoulder: a randomized, controlled trial with 125 patients. J Shoulder Elbow Surg. 2007 Nov-Dec;16(6):722–6.
11. Uppal HS, Evans JP, Smith C. Frozen shoulder: a systematic review of therapeutic options. World J Orthop. 2015 Mar 18;6(2):263–8. Epub 2015 Mar 18.
12. Smitherman JA, Struk AM, Cricchio M, McFadden G, Dell RB, Horodyski M, et al. Arthroscopy and manipulation versus home therapy program in treatment of adhesive capsulitis of the shoulder: a prospective randomized study. J Surg Orthop Adv. 2015 Spring;24(1):69–74.
13. Grant JA, Schroeder N, Miller BS, Carpenter JE. Comparison of manipulation and arthroscopic capsular release for adhesive capsulitis: a systematic review. J Shoulder Elbow Surg. 2013 Aug;22(8):1135–45.
14. Le Lievre HM, Murrell GA. Long-term outcomes after arthroscopic capsular release for idiopathic adhesive capsulitis. J Bone Joint Surg Am. 2012 Jul 3;94(13):1208–16.

9 Shoulder Arthritis and Arthroplasty

Progressive degeneration of the articular cartilage and other articular structures is the hallmark of glenohumeral arthritis. These structural changes may occur primarily or they may be a consequence of a number of conditions, including dysplasia, inflammatory conditions, trauma, avascular necrosis (AVN), instability, infection, and prior surgery. The pathology underlying various arthritic conditions is different, and these differences have direct practical implications on treatment. Shoulder arthroplasty is the surgical treatment of choice for most patients with advanced symptomatic arthritis (1).

Structural Pathology in Shoulder Arthritis

Primary Glenohumeral Osteoarthritis

Primary glenohumeral osteoarthritis, like osteoarthritis of other joints such as the hip and the knee, is probably due in most patients to a combination of genetic predisposition and heavy use of the joint. Cartilage degeneration is oftentimes associated with osteophytes, intraosseous cysts, loose bodies, degenerative changes of the labrum and biceps tendon, capsular fibrosis, and various degrees of bone loss (Figure 9.1). In some individuals, dysplastic changes may be appreciated, and it may be difficult to distinguish mild dysplasia leading to arthritis from primary osteoarthritis. All these changes result in shoulder pain and stiffness. Interestingly, *the rotator cuff is intact in most patients with primary osteoarthritis* (2), although some patients do develop progressive cuff tears either before or after arthroplasty (3).

Two major patterns of primary osteoarthritis are seen in practice. In some patients, the humeral head remains relatively centered on the glenoid and any bone loss occurs directly medially. In these circumstances, bone loss and soft tissue contractures are symmetric (Figure 9.2A). A second classic pattern of osteoarthritis combines various

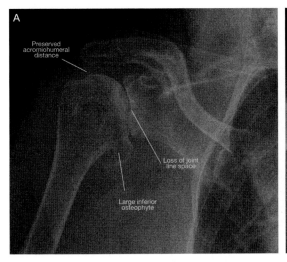
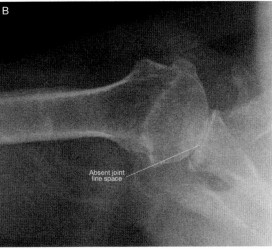

Figure 9.1 Anteroposterior (**A**) and axillary (**B**) radiographs of a patient with primary glenohumeral osteoarthritis.

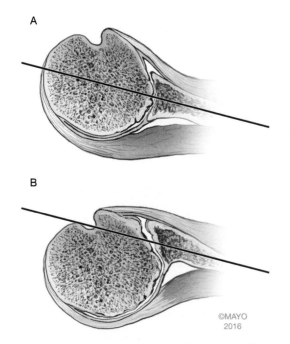

A

B

©MAYO
2016

*Figure 9.2 Two major patterns of glenohumeral osteoarthritis: concentric **(A)** and eccentric **(B)**.*

degrees of posterior subluxation and selective bone loss on the posterior aspect of the glenoid (Figure 9.2B). Some argue that posterior subluxation may be the first pathologic change in these patients, leading to cartilage edge loading and progressive osteoarthritis. Posterior subluxation is associated with progressive stretching of the posterior capsule and rotator cuff; this soft-tissue imbalance needs to be corrected at the time of anatomic arthroplasty. Various methods of rebalancing eccentric glenohumeral joints are discussed later.

In primary glenohumeral osteoarthritis, humeral bone loss is less pronounced than glenoid bone loss and, most of the time, less relevant at the time of surgery. Most commonly, the humeral head becomes flattened, which may complicate surgical dislocation and also needs to be considered at the time of humeral head sizing during arthroplasty.

Glenoid bone loss is of greater concern: the human glenoid is relatively small to begin with, and moderate bone loss can complicate shoulder arthroplasty to a great extent. Glenoid bone loss may be appreciated on radiographs. On the anteroposterior view, it translates into loss of offset (Figure 9.3A): the humerus is more medial compared with the rest of the scapula, such that the lateral humeral cortex may be at the level of, or medial to, the lateral aspect of the acromion. On the axillary radiograph, the glenoid vault is shortened, although the face of the glenoid may look wider in patients with extensive osteophytes (Figure 9.3B).

Glenoid bone loss patterns are best appreciated on axial computed tomography (CT) (Figure 9.3C). The Walch classification is used most commonly to categorize glenoid

morphology (Figure 9.4) (4). In this classification system, shoulders are categorized as A if there is no posterior subluxation, B if there is posterior subluxation, and C if there is primary glenoid dysplasia. Type C glenoids are characterized further in the section on shoulder dysplasia. The degree of subluxation is calculated on CT scans as described in Figure 9.5.

Shoulder types A and B are divided into 2 subtypes: subtype 1 if there is no bone loss, and subtype 2 if there is bone loss. Thus, A1 describes a concentric joint with no bone loss; A2, a concentric joint with medial bone loss; B1, an eccentric joint with no bone loss; and B2, an eccentric joint with posterior asymmetric bone loss (so-called biconcave glenoid). In a B2 glenoid pattern, the humeral head articulates with the area where bone loss has occurred (neoglenoid) and not with the healthier anterior glenoid (paleoglenoid). As asymmetric glenoid bone loss continues, the paleoglenoid becomes larger and the neoglenoid may completely disappear. The term *B3 glenoid* is used to define this situation, where most of the neoglenoid is gone. A type B3 glenoid may be very difficult to distinguish from a type C glenoid, looking only at axial cuts.

Shoulder (Glenoid) Dysplasia

Dysplasia may affect the shoulder joint either in very obvious or far more subtle manners (5–7). Patients with multiple epiphyseal dysplasia and other forms of dysplasia will exhibit substantial abnormalities of the humerus and glenoid (Figure 9.6A and B) (8). The humerus may be bowed abnormally, the greater tuberosity may be seen riding higher than the humeral head, and, more importantly (as in hip dysplasia), humeral version may be very abnormal and difficult to assess prior to surgery.

Glenoid dysplasia may be seen in the setting of dysmorphic dysplasia or it may manifest as a subtle, isolated condition (Figure 9.6C and D) (5,7). The hallmarks of glenoid dysplasia on the anteroposterior view include a flat, elongated glenoid face and a short (or absent) glenoid neck. On axillary radiography or axial views on CT, the glenoid often has excessive posterior retroversion, and the posterior corner of the glenoid may be rounded (type C glenoid in the Walch classification) (4). Cartilage degeneration in shoulder dysplasia may lead to moderate to severe pain before complete obliteration of the articular joint line is appreciated on radiography.

The main challenge when performing shoulder arthroplasty in patients with dysplasia is to determine the ideal spatial orientation of the components. In dysmorphic dysplasia, it is probably best to replicate the native version of the humerus and correct glenoid version just enough to safely fit the component. In patients with milder degrees of glenoid dysplasia, it is unclear whether it is best to place the glenoid component in the native retroversion or if glenoid version should be corrected to some extent (7).

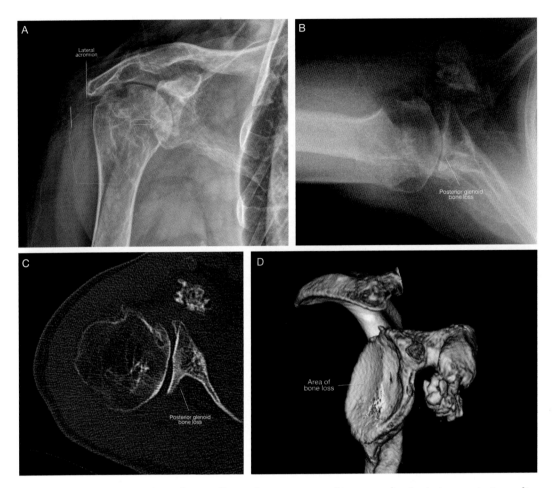

Figure 9.3 *Bone loss may be assessed on plain radiographs or computed tomography.* **A,** *Anteroposterior radiograph shows loss of offset; in a normal shoulder, the lateral aspect of the tuberosity (green line) is lateral to the acromion, whereas in this shoulder with substantial glenoid bone loss, it is medial (red line).* **B,** *Axillary radiograph demonstrates posterior bone loss.* **C and D,** *Computed tomography.*

Cuff Tear Arthropathy

The term *cuff tear arthropathy* was coined by Neer to describe those shoulders that develop progressive degeneration of the glenohumeral joint and secondary bone loss as a consequence of longstanding large rotator cuff tears (Figure 9.7) (9). The sequence of events leading to cuff tear arthropathy probably involves a combination of biomechanical and biochemical changes. Severe cuff insufficiency typically leads to superior humeral head migration; eccentric point loading of the articular cartilage on the superior glenoid and humeral head likely contributes to joint degeneration. Cuff deficiency also leads to an uncontained articular space; synovial fluid leakage may alter the nutrition of the articular cartilage, further contributing to joint degeneration.

Radiographically, cuff tear arthropathy is characterized by obliteration of the glenohumeral joint space, superior humeral head migration, and various degrees of bone loss. Typically, glenoid bone loss is superior. Humeral bone loss may lead to humeral head collapse and erosion of the medial humerus just below the surgical neck, where it contacts the inferior glenoid rim. There may be thinning of bone or even a stress fracture involving the acromion or distal end of the clavicle. Magnetic resonance imaging (MRI) confirms all these changes and shows a large, retracted rotator cuff tear with atrophy and fatty infiltration (see chapter 6, The Rotator Cuff and Biceps Tendon). Occasionally, large ganglion cysts develop on the superior aspect of the acromioclavicular joint.

Inflammatory Arthritis

Rheumatoid arthritis is the most common inflammatory arthropathy involving the shoulder joint. Other inflammatory conditions (e.g., lupus or psoriatic arthropathy) may affect the glenohumeral joint as well. Shoulder symptoms in patients with inflammatory arthritis may be due to a number of conditions, including glenohumeral joint synovitis, loss of the articular cartilage at the glenohumeral

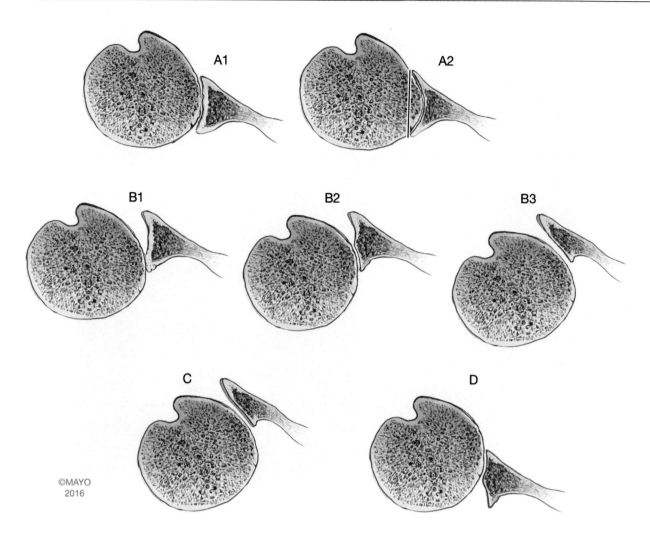

Figure 9.4 *Glenoid classification (Walch) in primary osteoarthritis.*

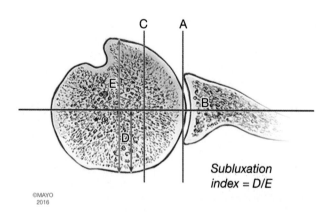

Subluxation index = D/E

©MAYO 2016

Figure 9.5 *Calculating posterior subluxation: the amount of humeral head posterior to the centerline of the glenoid as measured at the medial third of the humeral head on the axillary radiograph (D) is divided by the diameter of the humeral head at the same level.*

joint, subacromial bursitis, acromioclavicular joint arthritis, sternoclavicular joint arthritis, or a rotator cuff tear. These disorders may coexist and contribute to symptoms in a given patient (10).

When synovitis is the only source of symptoms, plain radiographs may appear normal or, at most, show mild osteopenia. Later on, inflammatory conditions lead to obliteration of the joint line space and progressive medial glenoid erosion with little hypertrophic osteophyte formation (Figure 9.8). As the disease involves the rotator cuff, various degrees of proximal humeral head migration may occur, and, in extreme cases, the humeral head may contact the acromion and thin the coracoacromial arch and distal clavicle.

Avascular Necrosis

The humeral head is one classic location of AVN. Bone infarction typically involves a segmental portion of the

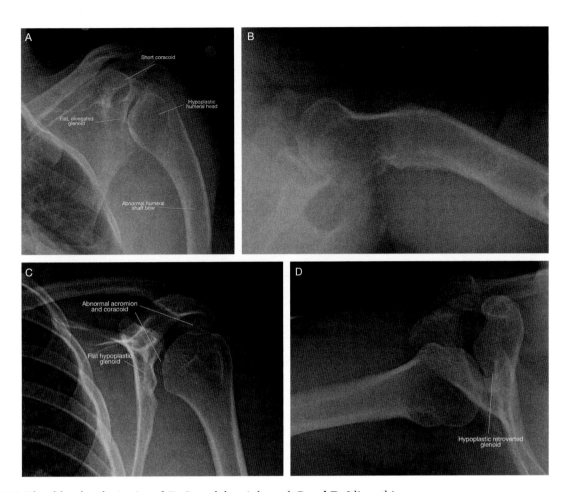

Figure 9.6 *Shoulder dysplasia.* **A and B,** *Spondyloepiphyseal.* **C and D,** *Idiopathic.*

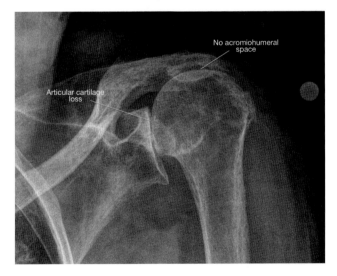

Figure 9.7 *Cuff tear arthropathy. Note proximal humeral head migration, with the head contacting the acromion.*

subchondral bone on the superior and central aspects of the humeral head. As in other locations, plain radiographs are negative in the early stages of AVN. Progressive radiographic changes are usually categorized using the Cruess classification (Figure 9.9) (11). The main turning points in terms of surgical evaluation and treatment are the development of subchondral collapse with interruption of the humeral head outline and, later, secondary degenerative changes on the glenoid side (Figure 9.10).

Posttraumatic Conditions

Proximal humerus fractures may lead to a number of problems, including posttraumatic AVN, nonunion, malunion, posttraumatic osteoarthritis, locked anterior dislocation, locked posterior dislocation, or a combination of one or more of these. Each of these conditions presents a particular set of challenges (12). These challenges may be complicated further by the presence of failed hardware

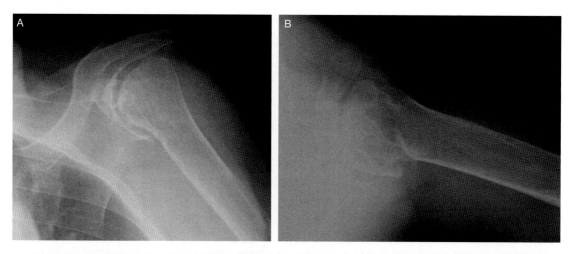

Figure 9.8 *Rheumatoid arthritis. Note central glenoid bone loss (erosion), loss of offset, and marked osteopenia.*

in those patients who have previously undergone surgery (Figure 9.11).

Posttraumatic AVN

Avascular changes may develop after a proximal humerus fracture as a consequence of the initial fracture pattern (i.e., traumatic devascularization of the humeral head) and/or iatrogenic damage to the vasculature of the humeral head at the time of internal fixation. A number of individuals develop changes consistent with AVN on radiography but complain of minimal symptoms (Figure 9.11A). Other patients may complain of pain and poor function when AVN develops despite otherwise perfect restoration of the proximal humerus geometry and complete fracture union. When patients with posttraumatic AVN develop symptoms, it is important to understand whether symptoms are associated with the area of AVN only or if they are at least partly related to associated nonunion, malunion, or retained hardware.

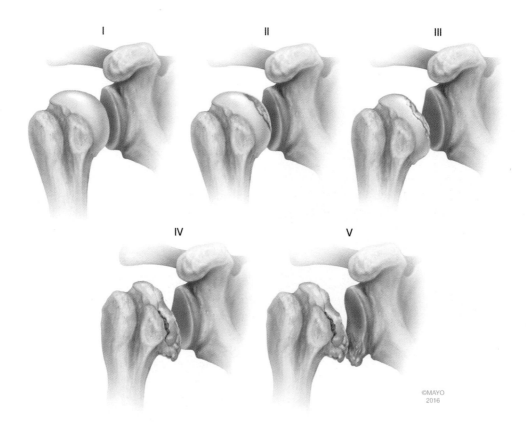

Figure 9.9 *Cruess classification for avascular necrosis. Stage I, normal radiographs; stage II, segmental humeral head condensation; stage III, subchondral fracture and collapse; stage IV, severe head collapse without glenoid changes; stage V, glenoid involvement.*

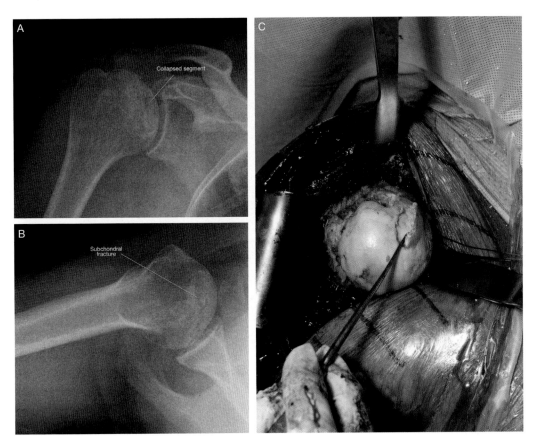

Figure 9.10 *Avascular necrosis.* **A and B,** *In earlier stages, the humeral head shows subchondral collapse but the glenoid is well preserved.* **C,** *Intraoperative aspect of the area of subchondral failure.*

Proximal Humerus Nonunion

Most nonunions affect the surgical neck of the humerus. Nonunion of the greater or lesser tuberosity may also occur either as an isolated condition or associated with nonunion at the head-shaft junction. The nonunited proximal fragment is oftentimes in varus, and the severity of bone loss and disuse osteopenia are often underestimated on plain radiographs (Figure 9.11B and C). Retained hardware may further contribute to poor bone stock. Secondary contracture of the capsule and rotator cuff is not uncommon.

Proximal Humerus Malunion

A certain degree of malunion is well tolerated in the absence of associated AVN or cartilage degeneration. Some patients with a proximal humerus malunion may complain most of loss of motion with minor pain. Severe pain is almost always secondary to a combination of malunion and posttraumatic arthrosis (Figure 9.11D).

Locked Dislocations

Locked posterior dislocation may be discovered after an initial incorrect diagnosis. Most locked posterior dislocations present as substantial impaction fractures of the humeral head where it collides with the posterior rim of the glenoid (see chapter 7, Shoulder Instability and the Labrum). Over time, the defect may increase in size as a result of toggling with attempted movement of the arm. In addition, disuse osteopenia and secondary contractures develop, making reduction of the dislocated shoulder more and more difficult as time goes by.

Missed anterior dislocations are much more rare but occasionally are seen, mostly in elderly patients with dementia. Although some dislocations may be impacted on the anterior glenoid rim with a substantial head defect, it is not uncommon for the whole humeral head to be dislocated anteriorly with disuse osteopenia but no structural deficiency. On the contrary, most shoulders develop progressive wear of the anterior glenoid rim over time. The dislocated humeral head and adjacent soft tissues may become adherent to the brachial plexus and subclavian vessels, which should be taken into consideration at the time of surgery.

Posttraumatic Osteoarthritis and Complicating Hardware

Rarely, isolated cartilage degeneration may develop as a consequence of trauma in patients with no other sequelae. More commonly, progressive settling of the head segment, AVN, or secondary fracture displacement may lead

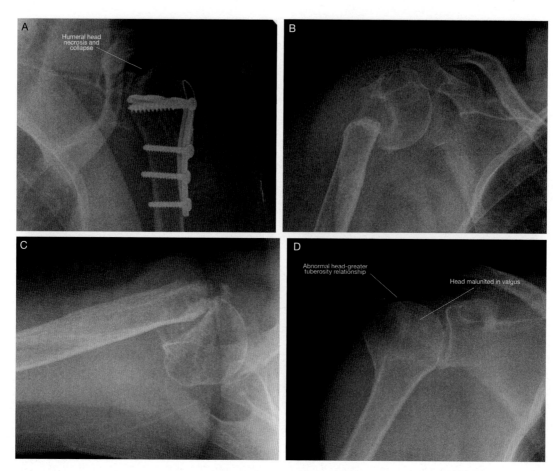

Figure 9.11 *Posttraumatic glenohumeral disorders.* **A,** *Posttraumatic avascular necrosis.* **B and C,** *Posttraumatic nonunion.* **D,** *Posttraumatic malunion.*

to hardware penetration past the humeral head. Once prominent hardware (most commonly, locked screws) is in contact with the glenoid, rapid destruction of the glenoid cartilage, and, possibly, progressive glenoid bone damage may ensue.

Instability and Capsulorraphy Arthritis (Arthropathy)

Anterior and posterior shoulder instability have been associated with late arthrosis. The relative contribution of multiple episodes of dislocation and the resultant shear damage on the articular cartilage versus excessive tightening of the soft tissues or adverse effects of devices used for shoulder stabilization varies from patient to patient.

Radiographic arthrosis has been documented in most studies that have investigated the natural history of recurrent anterior instability (13). The term *capsulorraphy arthropathy* is used when patients develop arthritis after prior anterior stabilization surgery (Figure 9.12). Theoretically, this condition can be caused by iatrogenic damage to the cartilage at the time of surgery, intra-articular migration or damage of anchors or alternative fixation devices, abnormal

mechanics after bone augmentation procedures (Latarjet coracoid transfer and other), or excessive tightness of the anterior soft-tissue structures (capsule and/or subscapularis) leading to increased joint reaction forces over time. When arthroplasty is performed in these patients, shortening of the anterior soft tissues may create challenges for both exposure and soft-tissue balance, as detailed later.

Patients with progressive arthritis after recurrent posterior instability most often have existing cartilage damage at the posterior junction between the glenoid cartilage and the posterior labrum at the time of their index surgery. Persistent posterior laxity combined with progressive wear of the posterior glenoid rim makes these patients prone to residual posterior instability after arthroplasty.

Chondrolysis

The term *chondrolysis* is used when patients develop relatively rapid joint degeneration (a few months to a couple of years) after arthroscopic shoulder surgery (14). Unfortunately, this condition has been reported most in very young patients after arthroscopic instability surgery or repair of superior labral tears (Figure 9.13). Accelerated destruction

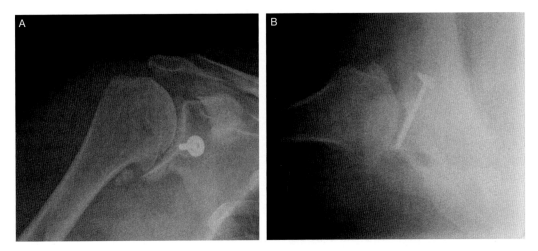

Figure 9.12 Capsulorraphy arthropathy.

of the articular cartilage has been linked to a number of possible culprits, including arthroscopic thermal devices, prominent anchors or suture material (especially knots on the articular side of the labrum), biochemical adverse effects of biodegradable material, prolonged (24–48 hours) intra-articular infusion of local anesthetics for postoperative pain relief using a pump, or low-grade infection. In these patients, cartilage damage on the glenoid side is oftentimes as bad as on the humeral side.

Infection

Joint degeneration may be a consequence of septic arthritis with or without osteomyelitis. In some individuals, the diagnosis is pretty clear based on their history (e.g., prolonged drainage after surgery or fistulas), especially when there are confirmatory positive cultures. However, infection may be extremely difficult to identify in some individuals, especially when the causative microorganism is

Cutibacterium acnes (formerly, *Propionibacterium acnes*), a slow-growing bacterium (15). Low-grade postoperative infections will lead to joint destruction and constant deep-seated pain, but patients often have no systemic symptoms (i.e., no fever, chills, or excessive sweating) and blood markers (i.e., cell count, sedimentation rate, C-reactive protein) are normal; cultures of aspirated joint fluid take longer than 2 to 3 weeks to grow and many may be negative (16,17). When patients undergo arthroplasty in the face of possible lingering infection, intraoperative pathology will be oftentimes appear negative for acute inflammation, although it may be positive for chronic inflammation.

Charcot (Neurotrophic or Neuropathic) Arthropathy

Charcot (or neurotrophic) arthropathy should be suspected in patients presenting with severe destructive bone changes involving the glenohumeral joint in the absence of an alternative explanation (e.g., no trauma, infection, or

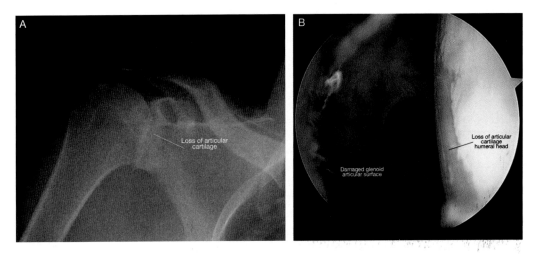

Figure 9.13 Chondrolysis. **A,** *Radiographic aspect.* **B,** *Arthroscopic findings.*

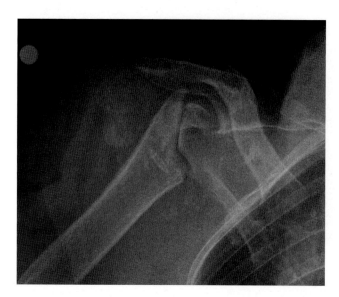

Figure 9.14 *Charcot arthropathy (neurotrophic arthropathy).*

inflammatory arthropathy) (18,19). The proposed mechanisms leading to progressive joint destruction include decreased peripheral sensation, compromised proprioception, and poor fine motor control. The 2 most common conditions responsible for neuropathic arthropathy are diabetes mellitus and syringomyelia. Other central and peripheral neurologic conditions that may lead to Charcot arthropathy include spinal cord disorders (e.g., spinal cord injury, myelitis) and peripheral neuropathies that are either acquired (e.g., alcoholic neuropathy, syphilis, leprosy) or congenital (i.e., congenital insensitivity to pain).

Pain severity varies among patients, but most individuals do complain of pain to some extent. Progressive destruction of the articulating bony ends, rotator cuff, and capsule lead to poor motion, decreased strength, and joint instability. Occasionally, neurotrophic arthropathy will lead to acute inflammatory symptoms (e.g., redness, warmth, and swelling) either as part of the pathologic process or secondary to a bacterial superinfection. Joint destruction usually affects the humeral head, glenoid, and, in severe cases, the coracoid, acromion, and distal clavicle (Figure 9.14).

Evaluation

Basic Concepts

Most patients presenting with shoulder pain and dysfunction can be assessed properly with a good history, physical examination, and plain radiographs. As detailed in chapter 1 (Evaluation of the Shoulder), glenohumeral joint pain is typically felt over the deltoid region. Pain along the posterior glenohumeral joint line is considered somewhat specific to glenohumeral joint pain. The articular shear test (described in chapter 1) also aims to identify

glenohumeral joint degeneration as a cause of pain. Some patients may have additional sources of pain, such as the acromioclavicular joint, the biceps tendon, or, rarely, the sternoclavicular joint.

Other goals of the evaluation of the arthritic joint are to identify and grade stiffness and to assess strength as a surrogate of cuff integrity. Active motion may be more limited than passive motion secondary to pain. Passive motion in elevation, external rotation, and internal rotation should be assessed and recorded in order to plan certain surgical details (e.g., soft-tissue releases and head sizing) if arthroplasty is performed, to evaluate progression of disease, and to assess the outcome of treatment. Strength assessment can also be confounded by pain. In patients with glenohumeral arthritis, strength testing should be gentle: the examiner should use short lever arms (force is applied at the elbow, not the wrist) and add force progressively while trying to keep the patient from moving the shoulder; movement generates pain and can lead to giveaway "pseudoweakness." For patients with suspected associated cuff insufficiency, lag signs are extremely useful (see chapter 1, Evaluation of the Shoulder). Plain radiographs are the main imaging study used in the evaluation of patients with glenohumeral arthritis. Other tests discussed later are used selectively (Table 9.1).

Specific Arthritic Conditions

Glenohumeral Osteoarthritis and Dysplasia

Patients with glenohumeral osteoarthritis may report a family history of arthritis and oftentimes will have arthritis in other joints. A history of heavy lifting for a prolonged period of time is not uncommon, either for work (e.g., farmers and construction workers) or sport (e.g., weight training). Typically, patients present to the office with various degrees of stiffness; in most, strength testing suggests an intact rotator cuff.

Classic radiographic findings include a narrow glenohumeral joint line space and osteophyte formation (Figure 9.1). In the early stages of disease, cartilage loss may only be inferred from an axillary radiograph; a small osteophyte at the head-neck junction on the anteroposterior view may also tip off the surgeon to osteoarthritis. As the disease progresses, subluxation and bone loss may be appreciated on radiography. The space between the proximal humerus and the acromion may look narrow secondary to osteophyte formation in the tuberosity region and acromion; this should not prompt a conclusion that the supraspinatus tendon is torn. Posterior subluxation may project on anteroposterior views as proximal humeral head migration, but most often the so-called gothic arch, or Shenton line, of the shoulder (shape formed by the medial aspect of the humeral shaft and the lateral aspect of the scapular body) is maintained.

Underlying dysplasia may be easy to identify in patients with a glenoid that looks flat and tall in the anteroposterior

Table 9.1 • Arthritic Conditions of the Glenohumeral Joint

Condition	History	Physical Examination	Complementary Studies
Glenohumeral osteoarthritis	Family history Weight lifting	Pain Stiffness Crepitus Good strength	Radiographic narrowing of the joint line space, osteophytes Posterior glenoid bone loss is common Underlying dysplasia may be identified
Cuff tear arthropathy	Injury in the past Prior rotator cuff surgery	Pain Worse active than passive motion May present with pseudoparalysis Evaluate incision and deltoid integrity in patients with prior surgery	Proximal humeral head migration Joint line narrowing, superior glenoid bone loss May develop humeral head collapse and bone loss at the acromion, distal clavicle, and coracoid
Inflammatory arthritis	Polyarticular involvement	Pain Various degrees of stiffness and weakness Involvement of other joints	Positive blood markers for rheumatoid arthritis and others Synovitis, osteopenia, joint line narrowing, minimal osteophyte formation Medial glenoid bone loss Superior migration when cuff affected
Avascular necrosis	Risk factors	Pain Motion and strength can be very well preserved	Early avascular necrosis can only be identified on magnetic resonance imaging Evolves through progressive stages, most importantly subchondral collapse and glenoid involvement
Posttraumatic conditions	Index injury	Most will have a combination of pain, stiffness, and weakness Carefully assess the axillary nerve, deltoid integrity, skin condition	Radiographs identify malunion, nonunion, posttraumatic arthritis, posttraumatic avascular necrosis, and/or locked dislocations Computed tomography is very helpful in the decision-making process Assess the need for hardware removal Rule out infection
Instability and capsulorraphy arthropathy	Prior dislocations and instability surgery	Pain, crepitus, markedly limited external rotation Carefully assess the axillary nerve, deltoid integrity, skin condition	Joint line narrowing, osteophytes, bone loss Radiographs may show prior hardware (screws, staples) and transferred bone blocks
Chondrolysis	Prior arthroscopic shoulder surgery	Pain and stiffness Good strength Question patient regarding use of intra-articular thermal devices, absorbable anchors, intra-articular pain pumps	Joint line space narrowing (rapid progression) Rule out infection
Infection	Debilitated elderly patients with acute onset of shoulder pain Lingering pain after surgery	Pain with various degrees of stiffness Good strength May present with redness and swelling or not	Plain radiographs may be negative or show prior surgical procedures Cultures of fluid or tissue are required to confirm the diagnosis The diagnostic yield of classic tests for infection may be low when caused by *Cutibacterium acnes*
Neuropathic arthropathy	Associated conditions	Pain is present but less than expected Very poor function	Marked bony destruction involving the proximal humerus, glenoid, and occasionally other portions of the scapula For patients with unexplained neuropathic arthropathy, investigate for diabetes and cervical syrinx

view and very steeply retroverted (Walch type C) in the axillary view (Figure 9.6) (4). Minor degrees of dysplasia may be more difficult to recognize (6). A short glenoid neck, excessive glenoid retroversion, and a rounded posterior glenoid rim may indicate subtle underlying dysplasia and should prompt careful analysis of humeral and glenoid geometry if surgery is performed.

Cuff Tear Arthropathy

Patients with cuff tear arthropathy may present with various degrees of pain and dysfunction (9). The classic patient with advanced cuff tear arthropathy will complain of severe pain and lack of active elevation ("pseudoparalysis" in elevation; Figure 9.15). However, surprisingly, some individuals with concerning radiographic findings will have little pain and/or good active motion. The lack of correlation between radiographic findings and symptoms continues to be one of the most confusing aspects of shoulder surgery.

It is important to know whether these patients have undergone previous surgery (attempted rotator cuff repair, débridement, biceps tenotomy or tenodesis, or even attempted tendon transfers). The presence of previous incisions and surgical alterations of anatomy need to be considered when further surgery is planned. Special attention should be paid to the condition of the deltoid muscle in patients with prior surgery. The deltoid may be compromised as a result of prior surgical exposures for open rotator cuff repair or, rarely, iatrogenic injury to the axillary nerve. As in other patients with failed surgery, the possibility of a deep infection should be thoroughly investigated, as detailed later.

The extent of cuff damage should be assessed using physical examination tests and, occasionally, advanced imaging studies. With the advent of reverse shoulder arthroplasty, the importance of the posterior rotator cuff as it relates to functional outcomes after arthroplasty is now better understood. Special attention should be paid to assessing the function of the infraspinatus and teres minor (i.e., active external rotation, strength in external rotation, and external rotation lag and drop signs). The ability to perform active external rotation with the shoulder in abduction is considered a good indicator of the integrity of the teres minor (see chapter 1, Evaluation of the Shoulder) (20).

Cuff tear arthropathy can occasionally lead to substantial synovitis, joint effusion, and even recurrent hemarthrosis. These conditions may manifest as substantial swelling on physical examination. As mentioned before, some patients may also develop large subcutaneous ganglion cysts over the acromioclavicular joint.

Inflammatory Arthritis

Most patients with inflammatory arthritis consult an orthopedic surgeon with a diagnosis already established. When a rheumatoid patient is referred to the orthopedic surgeon for a surgical consultation regarding the shoulder joint, the evaluation should not only assess the affected glenohumeral joint in detail but also determine involvement of other joints in the upper extremity (e.g., sternoclavicular joint, acromioclavicular joint, elbow, wrist, or hand), as well as the cervical spine (which may impact anesthesia techniques), and the lower extremities (the use of assistive devices may increase load across the shoulder joint) (10).

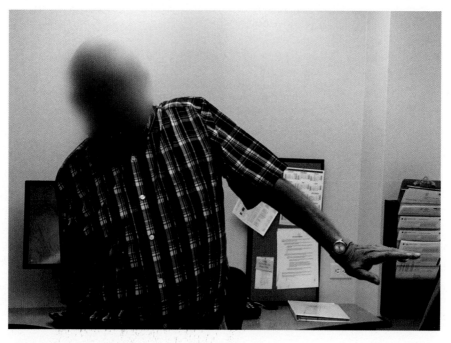

Figure 9.15 *Poor active motion in a patient with pseudoparalysis.*

Efforts should be made to learn the pharmacological treatment each patient is receiving (21). Many patients referred to the orthopedic surgeon will be receiving a combination of a traditional disease-modifying antirheumatic drug (DMARD)—such as methotrexate—and a biologic DMARD (anti-tumor necrosis factor, interleukin [IL]-1 and IL-6 receptor antagonists, T-cell blockers, or B-lymphocyte modulators). Currently, corticosteroids are used to control symptoms when DMARDs are first introduced, while the DMARDs are becoming effective (typically 4–6 weeks), as well as for episodes of flare-up; rarely, they are used long term for patients who have not responded to anything else.

There are multiple reasons for a thorough understanding of pharmacological treatment for these patients. First, it is important to make sure that the pharmacological treatment of inflammatory conditions has been optimized before surgery is recommended. Second, DMARDs may interfere with healing (e.g., methotrexate) and facilitate infection (biologic DMARDs), and most surgeons would agree that they should be discontinued around the time of surgery (22). The specific time off DMARDs needs to be discussed carefully with the patient, since oftentimes other joints flare up as DMARDs are stopped, complicating recovery after surgery. The ideal time off DMARDs depends on the pharmacokinetics of each specific medication (Table 9.2) (21).

Depending on the chronicity and severity of synovitis, inflammatory arthritis will present with various degrees of cuff deficiency and bone loss. The rotator cuff may be completely normal in some patients, but oftentimes it is attenuated. A number of patients have developed a full-thickness tear by the time they present for surgery (23). Cuff function needs to be evaluated carefully using physical examination and imaging studies. Sometimes, the status of the rotator cuff will be documented in previous surgery (e.g., synovectomy). As mentioned previously, glenoid bone loss translates most often into progressive medial glenoid erosion. Severe cases may also develop bone loss at the acromion, distal clavicle, or proximal humerus.

Avascular Necrosis

When patients present early in their course of the disease, AVN may be difficult to diagnose because radiographic changes have not yet occurred (11). AVN should be suspected in patients presenting with deep-seated glenohumeral pain at rest and at night, good motion and strength, and otherwise negative radiographic results, especially when risk factors are identified (Table 9.3). Some patients may report a history of AVN in other locations, most commonly the hip. MRI helps confirm the diagnosis when radiographs are negative (Figure 9.16). As mentioned before, AVN tends to progress in stages, described in the Cruess classification (Figure 9.9) (11). Identification of modifiable risk factors (e.g., corticosteroid treatment or excessive alcohol intake) is important when formulating a treatment plan.

Posttraumatic Conditions and Arthritis Complicating Shoulder Instability

A key element in the evaluation of patients with progressive joint degeneration after trauma is understanding the nature of the index injury and all treatment attempts prior to presentation. Special attention should be paid to ruling out associated neurovascular injuries and evaluating the shoulder for joint infection. Information should also be collected regarding hardware used in previous surgeries.

Table 9.2 ∘ Recommendations for Perioperative Medication Management of Pharmacologic Agents in Inflammatory Arthritis

Agent	Dosing	Withhold
Methotrexate	Weekly	No
Hydroxychloroquine	Daily	No
Azathioprine	Daily	No
Sulfasalazine	Daily	No
Leflunomide	Daily	Yes (1 week)
Etanercept	Weekly	Yes (2 weeks)
Golimumab	Monthly	Yes (6 weeks)
Adalimumab	2 weeks	Yes (3 weeks)
Infliximab	4–8 weeks	Yes (6 weeks)
Certolizumab pegol	4 weeks	Yes (6 weeks)
Tocilizumab	SC 1–2 weeks, IV 4 weeks	Yes (3 weeks SC, 4 weeks IV)
Rituximab	16–24 weeks	No
Abatacept	SC 1 week, IV 4 weeks	Yes (2 weeks SC, 4 weeks IV)

Abbreviations: IV, intravenous administration; SC, Subcutaneous administration.
Adapted from Goodman (21). Used with permission.

Table 9.3 ∘ Main Risk Factors for Nontraumatic Avascular Necrosis

Treatment with corticosteroids

Excessive alcohol intake

Systemic lupus erythematosus

Antiphospholipid antibodies

Sickle cell hemiglobinopathies

Gaucher disease

Decompression disease

Transplantation (e.g., kidney, hematopoietic stem cell)

Radiation therapy

Inherited thrombophilia or hypofibrinolysis

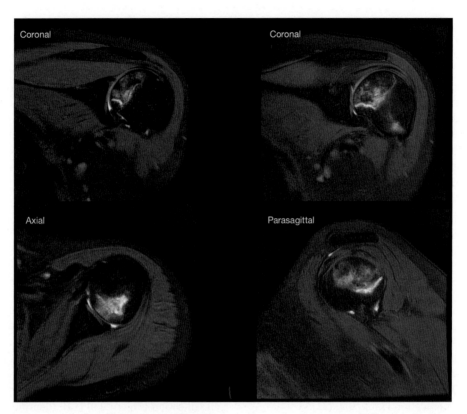

Figure 9.16 *Magnetic resonance imaging shows avascular necrosis results in a segmental increase in bone marrow signal in the humeral head.*

Injuries to the axillary nerve, brachial plexus, and musculocutaneous nerve may occur as a consequence of the initial injury or as a complication of previous surgical procedures. Sensory and motor deficits can usually be noted at the time of physical examination. Further testing using electromyography (EMG) and nerve conduction studies (NCS) may help confirm the diagnosis and grade the extent and severity of nerve involvement. Patients present having had an associated vascular injury needing surgery in rare cases; extreme care should be taken if further surgery is contemplated in the future.

The possibility of an associated infection should be considered in any patient presenting with a poor outcome after previous surgery. Patients should be asked whether they developed drainage, fever, or redness after previous surgeries; if the word "infection" was mentioned previously; or if they were placed on antibiotics (even a few days of oral antibiotics) for some time after surgery. Unfortunately, the diagnostic yield of various tests for infection has proven to be low for the shoulder joint, as detailed later.

Imaging studies in patients with a complicated course after trauma should be evaluated not only for posttraumatic arthritis but also for nonunion, malunion, and hardware issues. Special attention should be placed on evaluating glenoid bone stock because hardware protruding through the humeral head into the joint may create a fair amount of glenoid bone destruction. CT is particularly useful for evaluation of the posttraumatic shoulder (Figure 9.17).

Infection and Chondrolysis

Glenohumeral infection most commonly results from surgery; however, hematogenous glenohumeral joint septic arthritis and osteomyelitis can also occur in unoperated shoulders of elderly, frail patients with substantial comorbidities (15). In some patients, infection can be suspected on the basis of their presentation (e.g., prolonged drainage or fever), but in many the presentation is less obvious and the diagnosis of infection may be overlooked. As noted later, the diagnosis of infection may be difficult to prove with diagnostic tests.

Radiographically, infection typically leads to a decreased joint line space and various degrees of bone destruction, most often with little reactive bone osteophyte formation. These changes can also be the result of chondrolysis. In fact, some patients' initial diagnosis of chondrolysis (based on their history of arthroscopic surgery and rapid joint destruction) ends up being chondrolytic changes developed due to infection (14).

Charcot Arthropathy

Charcot (or neurotrophic) arthropathy should be suspected in patients with severe bone destruction for no apparent

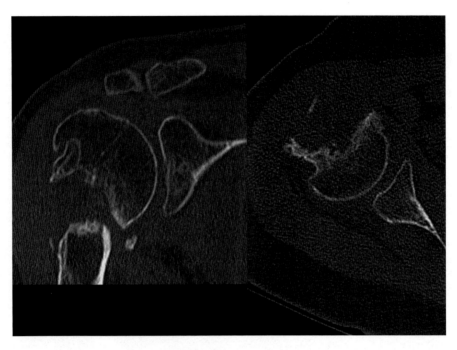

Figure 9.17 *Computed tomogram in a patient with a proximal humerus nonunion.*

reason (Figure 9.14). Other conditions—such as cuff tear arthropathy, advanced inflammatory arthritis, infection, advanced AVN, and severe trauma—may lead to similar radiographic changes and should be excluded (19).

When Charcot arthropathy is suspected, efforts should be made to identify the underlying condition responsible for the neurotrophic changes. Peripheral neuropathy secondary to diabetes mellitus is one of the most common conditions. In patients with no obvious explanation for their joint changes, a consultation with a neurologist and an MRI of the cervical spine should be considered to exclude an underlying syrinx.

Neuropathic arthropathy may occasionally lead to episodes of substantial inflammation, with increased pain, redness, and warmth. Although these symptoms may be part of the disease process, superinfection should be suspected and excluded.

Additional Studies

Computed Tomography

There are 2 main indications for CT in the evaluation of the conditions reviewed in this chapter: evaluation of certain traumatic conditions and preoperative planning for shoulder arthroplasty.

CT in Posttraumatic Conditions

CT is extremely helpful in the evaluation of posttraumatic conditions of the shoulder that lead to glenohumeral joint degeneration. It is particularly useful in assessing bone loss in the humeral head segment and when deciding between internal fixation and arthroplasty. CT is also useful in the

assessment of deformity in malunions, the condition of the tuberosities, and any secondary joint penetration and glenoid damage that may be caused by hardware.

CT in Preoperative Planning for Arthroplasty

Many surgeons obtain a CT scan for every patient undergoing shoulder arthroplasty in order to better understand the morphology of the glenoid. Although a good axillary radiograph can provide enough information to understand glenoid version and bone loss, CT is much more helpful, especially in patients with more severe abnormalities (Figure 9.18). The condition of the rotator cuff can also be assessed using CT, not only for tendon ruptures but also for grading muscle quality (see chapter 6, The Rotator Cuff and Biceps Tendon, Goutallier classification).

The information provided by CT can be visually analyzed by the surgeon and can also be imported into software packages. These packages create accurate 3-dimensional models of the scapula, provide accurate measurements of various parameters (e.g., version, inclination), allow virtual placement of prosthetic components, and can be used to create intraoperative guides used to replicate the position that was planned virtually (Figure 9.19) (24,25).

Magnetic Resonance Imaging

MRI can be of value in some of the conditions reviewed in this chapter. MRI can identify synovitis and areas of cartilage damage in the early stages of inflammatory conditions or chondrolysis. It also helps confirm the diagnosis of AVN in patients presenting before changes become apparent on radiography. MRI also helps identify areas of osteomyelitis.

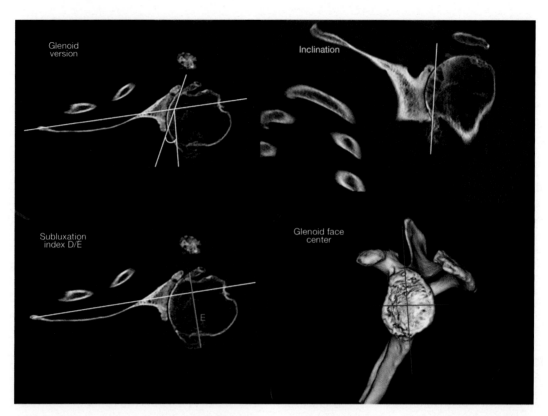

Figure 9.18 *Computed tomogram provides useful information for surgical planning of shoulder arthroplasty.*

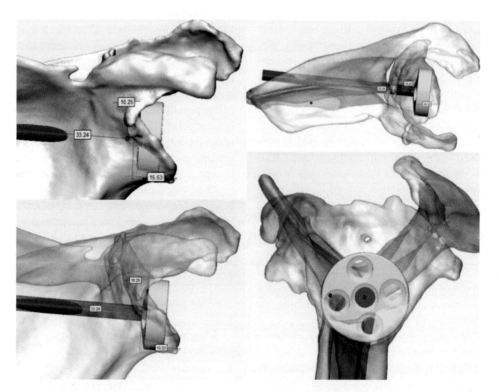

Figure 9.19 *Screenshot of one of the available software packages that uses computed tomography data to create 3-dimensional models of the shoulder skeleton for accurate measuring, virtual implantation, and creation of surgical guides.*

Although MRI is one of the best imaging studies to assess the rotator cuff, it is not necessary for the evaluation of most patients with cuff tear arthropathy or neuropathic arthropathy. Cuff evaluation with MRI can be more helpful in patients with primary osteoarthritis or inflammatory arthritis when physical examination maneuvers suggest associated cuff insufficiency. As mentioned before, the rotator cuff can also be evaluated with CT obtained for other reasons.

Infection Workup

Infection should be considered in patients presenting with a worrisome history and those presenting with fever, drainage, redness, or unexpected severe joint destruction. Infection can also be a complicating factor for patients with previous surgery resulting in chondrolysis, capsulorraphy arthropathy, failed surgery for trauma, or a recurrent cuff tear leading to arthropathy. Infection should be investigated in all patients with overt signs and symptoms; some surgeons order an infection workup in every patient with previous failed surgery.

The microbiology of shoulder infection has a certain impact on the diagnostic yield of infection tests (16). *Cutibacterium acnes* (formerly *Propionibacterium acnes*) is particularly common in glenohumeral infections after surgery (17). This microorganism generates a chronic inflammatory response that oftentimes will not be detected by acute phase reactants (e.g., erythrocyte sedimentation rate and C-reactive protein [CRP]); in addition, *C acnes* grows slowly in culture media, so that samples after a few days will appear falsely negative. For these reasons, it is important to prolong the culture time to 2 to 3 weeks. Shoulder infections can also be caused by other common bacteria, such as *Staphylococcus aureus* or *epidermidis, Corynebacteria* spp, and others. The diagnostic yield of infection tests for these microorganisms is typically higher.

Peripheral blood tests useful in the evaluation of shoulder infection include total leukocyte count (WBC), neutrophil count, erythrocyte sedimentation rate, and CRP; blood cultures are obtained in patients with a high fever or symptoms and signs of sepsis. In addition, articular joint fluid is obtained by aspiration either blindly or under imaging guidance, most commonly ultrasonography. Articular fluid is analyzed for cell count and differential, and it is also sent for culture. The cutoff values considered having good sensitivity, specificity, and predictive values are different for patients with and without joint replacement. In the absence of joint replacement, synovial fluid WBC counts over 50,000/mm³ with more than 90% neutrophils are accepted by most as predictive of infection. However, infections in patients with associated peripheral leukopenia or sepsis and *C acnes* infections can be associated with lower values. Current research is underway to clarify the diagnostic value of measuring ILs (specifically IL-1 and IL-6), α-defensin, and other molecules in aspirated synovial fluid (26,27).

When the clinical suspicion of infection is very high and all indicated tests are negative or joint fluid cannot be aspirated, consideration should be given to obtaining surgical biopsies for culture. Biopsies can be obtained arthroscopically with relatively little morbidity (28). Bone scan, using either technetium or indium-labeled WBCs, may provide additional information but is considered to have poor specificity and predictive value.

Other Tests

As mentioned before, EMG with NCS is used to assess patients with motor or sensory deficits. Vascular studies (i.e., angiography, CT angiography, or magnetic resonance angiography) should be ordered in the rare patient with a history of vascular injury after prior trauma or surgery; they should also be considered in chronic anterior dislocations. For patients with unexplained Charcot arthropathy, an MRI of the cervical spine is commonly ordered to look for a spinal cord syrinx.

Nonoperative Treatment

Shoulder arthroplasty is often the best option for patients with advanced glenohumeral joint degeneration. However, some patients feel that their symptoms are not severe enough to justify surgery, and in those circumstances nonoperative treatment may help (29).

Activity Modifications and Physical Therapy

Pain secondary to glenohumeral joint degeneration is aggravated by motion under loading conditions. Patients should be instructed to avoid lifting heavy objects with their shoulders and educated about the difference between lifting and carrying. Carrying an object, such as a heavy suitcase, with the arm at the side has little detrimental effect on symptoms, whereas lifting that same suitcase to a high shelf, by elevating the shoulder, can be very painful.

Formal physical therapy is of some value in patients with shoulder arthritis in order to maintain motion and for patient education on activity modifications such as those just described. Gentle stretching exercises can help slow progression of stiffness, but these exercises can become painful in the presence of large osteophytes, especially if the osteophytes fracture. Patients interested in weight training to maintain their strength are advised to avoid weight-lifting exercises that require glenohumeral motion (i.e., military press, flies, and similar exercises should be avoided). Patients can strengthen their shoulder muscles using either isometrics or elastic bands instead (see chapter 12, Rehabilitation and Injections). Weight training for the biceps and triceps is typically well tolerated.

Pharmacologic Treatment

Arthritic pain responds, to some extent, to a combination of acetaminophen and nonsteroidal anti-inflammatory drugs. Patients should be advised to combine both families of medications (multimodal analgesia seems to be more effective than the plain sum of 2 medications) and to maximize the dose of each (for example, up to 1 g acetaminophen every 6 hours and up to 600 mg ibuprofen every 8 hours). Narcotic pain medication is not recommended. If the pain level is severe enough to require narcotics, surgery should be considered instead. Patients on long-term treatment with pharmacologic agents should be monitored for adverse effects, especially liver toxicity, gastric ulceration, and kidney toxicity.

Patients who develop AVN as a complication of corticosteroid treatment should be counseled to discontinue corticosteroids if at all possible; hopefully this step will not only halt shoulder AVN but also (more importantly) decrease the chance of AVN developing in the other shoulder, hips, or ankles. As mentioned earlier, patients with inflammatory arthritis should maximize pharmacologic treatment with DMARDs under the supervision of a rheumatologist. Pharmacologic management of glenohumeral joint infection is discussed later.

Intra-articular Injections

Injection of a corticosteroid solution into the glenohumeral joint can be extremely helpful in alleviating pain during flare-up episodes of shoulder arthritis (see chapter 12, Rehabilitation and Injections) (30,31). Inserting a needle-tip into an arthritic glenohumeral joint can be difficult, especially in the presence of a very narrow joint line space, large osteophytes, thick capsular fibrosis, or deformity. For these reasons, my preference is to perform intra-articular injections under imaging guidance (typically ultrasonography) although some studies do demonstrate good success with "blind" injections.

As discussed in chapter 12, there are very little objective data to help understand the ideal dose, frequency, and expected outcome of intra-articular glenohumeral corticosteroid injections for arthritis. Most surgeons use a relatively high dose, and recommend no more than 3 injections per year. Patients with relative contraindications to corticosteroid use (e.g., diabetes mellitus or possible allergy) may be considered for injection with other agents, such as ketorolac or hyaluronic acid. Most patients do experience improvement in pain levels, and the improvement typically last weeks to months.

A number of recent studies seem to indicate that the rate of deep infection after arthroplasty is increased when surgery is performed soon after an intra-articular injection with corticosteroids; this is clearly the case for the knee joint and likely applied to the shoulder joint as well (32). The number

of weeks after which this increased risk no longer exists is unknown. My current practice is to avoid surgery within the 2 to 3 months following a corticosteroid injection.

Shoulder Arthroplasty

General Principles

Shoulder arthroplasty is the procedure of choice for most patients with advanced glenohumeral arthritis when symptoms interfere substantially with the patient's quality of life and do not respond to nonoperative treatment (1). When patients are undecided about surgery based on their symptoms, I do recommend replacement in 2 circumstances: confirmed progression of glenoid bone loss and progressive stiffness. Progression of glenoid bone loss may make the procedure technically more challenging and increase the chance of complications (33). In addition, there seems to be some correlation between preoperative motion and motion after recovery from replacement surgery; therefore, when patients are getting more and more stiff, surgery should probably be performed sooner rather than later.

Like any other implant replacement surgery, shoulder arthroplasty carries the risk of mechanical failure (e.g., loosening and wear). Mechanical failure rates are probably influenced by activity level. Most patients are advised to comply with certain postoperative restrictions in hopes of prolonging the durability of implants, although specific data to guide patients about restrictions are largely lacking. Patients unwilling to comply with restrictions can be considered for alternative surgical procedures (e.g., arthroscopic débridement). Shoulder arthroplasty should be avoided in patients with active infection, severe neuromuscular deficits, or extremely compromised bone stock.

The field of shoulder arthroplasty is in constant evolution. Implants currently used belong to 1 of 2 major categories: anatomic and reverse (Figure 9.20) (1). Anatomic components replicate, to some extent, the morphology of the articulating ends: the humeral component has an articulating round hemispherical component, whereas the glenoid component—when used—has a concave articulating surface. The terms *anatomic hemiarthroplasty, partial shoulder arthroplasty*, or *humeral head replacement* are used when the humeral component articulates with the native glenoid and a glenoid component is not used. The term *total shoulder arthroplasty* is used when both a humeral and a glenoid anatomic component are implanted. In a reverse shoulder arthroplasty, the natural ball and socket structure is reversed; the glenoid component has a convex hemispherical articular surface, whereas the humeral component has a concave humeral bearing articulating surface. A detailed description of shoulder arthroplasty using a hemiarthroplasty or a reverse shoulder arthroplasty for acute proximal

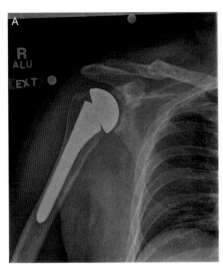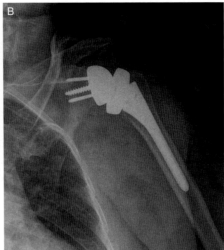

Figure 9.20 Postoperative radiographs after anatomic (A) and reverse (B) shoulder arthroplasty.

humerus fractures is found in chapter 4, Proximal Humerus Fractures.

Anatomic Arthroplasty (Total Shoulder Arthroplasty and Hemiarthroplasty)

Historical Background, Anatomical and Biomechanical Considerations, and Implant Design

Dr. Charles S. Neer is credited with the development of modern anatomical arthroplasty in the United States. The very first modern component was a monoblock hemiarthroplasty manufactured in only 3 sizes and intended for fixation with polymethylmethacrylate. A glenoid component made of polyethylene with a keel for cemented fixation into the glenoid vault was developed later. A number of design modifications were introduced over time, some more successful than others. Dr. Robert H. Cofield is credited with the introduction of modularity and ingrowth components. Dr. Gilles Walch and Dr. Pascal Boileau are credited with the introduction of third-generation components to allow for a more accurate reproduction of individual anatomy.

Humeral Component

Anatomical Considerations The anatomical dimensions of the proximal humerus have been carefully investigated (Table 9.4, Figure 9.21) (34–37). There is some variation in certain parameters, such as head diameter, head thickness, version, and medullary canal alignment and dimensions, among individuals. Some surgeons believe that every attempt should be made to reproduce the humeral anatomy of each individual accurately; this requires adapting resection angles and head to stem positioning in every single case (38). Other surgeons aim for a reasonable average position for most patients, and deviate from these general parameters only in the presence of extreme anatomical abnormalities (i.e., dysplasia).

Table 9.4 • Anatomical Considerations: Humerus and Glenoid

Consideration	Measurement, Mean (SD); Range
Humerus	
Head diameter/curvature	46.2 (5.4) mm; 37–57 mm
Articular surface diameter/curvature	43.3 (4.3) mm; 36–51 mm
Articular surface thickness	15.2 (1.6) mm; 12–18 mm
Head-to-tuberosity relationship	6 (2) mm; 3–8 mm
Head retroversion	21.5° (15.1°); -6°–48°
Glenoid	
Retroversion	5° (6°); -9°–13°
Superior vertical inclination	15.7° (5.1°)
Height	39 (3.5) mm; 30–48 mm
Width	29 (3.2) mm; 21–35 mm
Radius of curvature	2.3; 0.2 mm greater than humeral head

There are 3 commonly accepted parameters for positioning: 30° of retroversion of the humeral component as referenced from the forearm, positioning of the humeral head to restore the anatomical height relative to the greater tuberosity (head 5–10 mm proud), and thickness selection relative to both the resected humeral head and secondary changes in the soft tissues. Most currently available systems provide multiple head-diameter options. For each head-diameter option, there are several options for thickness. In addition, head eccentricity allows for selection of the ideal canal (or stem) to head positioning.

Fixation and Bearing Material Classically, humeral components for shoulder arthroplasty were designed with a relatively long stem designed for cement fixation. Over

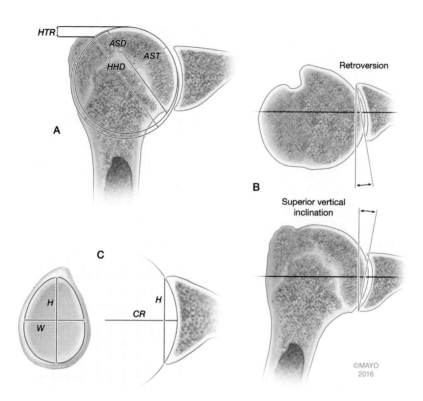

Figure 9.21 *Dimensions of the humeral head and the glenoid. Calculation of glenoid version and inclination. ASD indicates articular surface diameter; AST, articular surface thickness; CR, curvature radius; H, height; HHD, humeral head diameter; HTR, head-to-tuberosity relationship; W, width.*

the past few years, as with the hip joint, fixation without cement has become the standard. In addition, there is growing interest in the use of components with shorter stems, components with no stems, and resurfacing components (Figure 9.22). Most humeral head components are manufactured using a cobalt and chrome alloy. There is also interest in using alternative materials for the joint surface, including ceramic for total shoulder arthroplasty (e.g., ceramic

against polyethylene shows favorable wear characteristics) and pyrocarbon for hemiarthroplasty (e.g., pyrocarbon has a very low coefficient of friction against bone).

Glenoid Component
Anatomical Considerations The anatomical dimensions of the human glenoid have also been investigated carefully (Table 9.4, Figure 9.21) (34,39). The most important

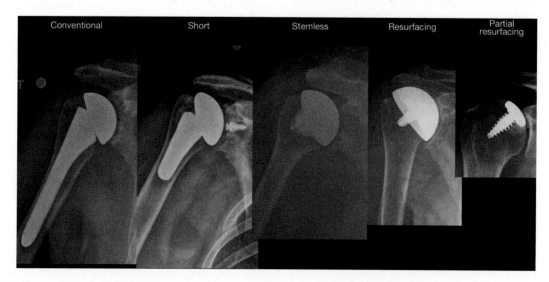

Figure 9.22 *Conventional, short, stemless, resurfacing, and partial resurfacing humeral components.*

parameters for surgical planning are version and vertical inclination. It is important to realize that most of the studies on the anatomy of the glenoid have not taken into account articular cartilage. It is also important to remember that 3 points can define any geometrical plane.

Version is typically calculated on CT as the angle between the plane of the glenoid bony articular surface and the vertical plane of the scapula (defined by the os trigonum medially, the center of the glenoid articular surface, and the inferior scapular angle). Interestingly, the ideal target version when implanting an anatomical glenoid component has not been fully defined. Most surgeons aim for 0° to 10° of retroversion (Figure 9.18) (40). Vertical inclination is typically calculated on CT as the angle between the plane of the glenoid bony articular surface and the horizontal plane of the scapula (defined by the os trigonum medially, the midpoint of the anterior glenoid rim, and the midpoint of the posterior glenoid rim). Again, the ideal target vertical inclination for anatomical total shoulder arthroplasty has not been defined, but most surgeons aim for 0° to 10° of inferior inclination.

Fixation and Bone Loss Cemented, all-polyethylene glenoid components, first introduced by Neer, continue to be considered the gold standard in anatomic shoulder arthroplasty (41). As detailed later, this type of component has been associated with a relatively high rate of mechanical failure (loosening and wear), although reported revision rates are lower (42,43). To date, attempts to improve glenoid component performance have included switching from keels to pegs and using cement-free fixation or hybrid fixation (Figure 9.23).

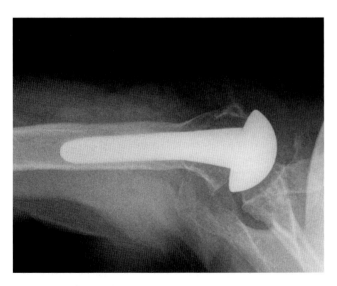

Figure 9.23 *Axillary radiograph after implantation of a modern, cemented, bone-preserving, self-pressurizing component.*

The portion of all-polyethylene glenoid components that is inserted into the glenoid vault typically consists of either a triangular keel or multiple pegs. In our experience, triangular keels and components with 3 pegs in line have performed similarly (44). In theory, components where some pegs are not in line (typically the inferior pegs are anterior and posterior to the midline) are thought to provide more resistance to rocking forces, which should translate to better long-term performance (Figure 9.24).

Three factors related to surgical technique have been noted to have some influence in long-term fixation of all-polyethylene glenoid components: maintaining cancellous bone in the glenoid vault, providing good support to the back side of the glenoid component, and absence of radiolucent lines in the immediate postoperative radiograph.

In the past, it was thought that having a larger amount of cement in the glenoid vault would contribute to macro interlock and provide better fixation. We now know that cement interdigitation with cancellous bone provides the best fixation. *Efforts should be made at the time of surgery to avoid excessively removing cancellous bone* (45).

Some studies have also demonstrated that component subsidence is more likely to happen when a fair amount of bone is removed at the time of reaming, leaving the glenoid component resting in relatively poor cancellous bone (39,45). *Minimal reaming* is now emphasized to preserve stronger subchondral bone. However, the glenoid component is also more stable if fully supported by bone and thus less likely to subside or deform. *Curved-backed components* (as opposed to flat-backed components) allow more bone preservation with better support from the underlying concave glenoid bone.

Goals of glenoid component implantation conflict with each other in the presence of asymmetric bone loss, which is problematic. If substantial posterior bone loss develops (think about a B2 glenoid), it is not possible to implant a component in 0° to 10° of retroversion and provide complete support of the back of the component with minimal reaming; either the posterior aspect of the component will not rest on bone or so much reaming is required that the component will rest in very poor cancellous bone (Figure 9.25). Options to deal with asymmetric bone loss include using a bone graft (most commonly from the resected humeral head) or implanting a component with a built-up portion (hemiwedge, full wedge, or hemiblock) (46–48). In cases of severe bone loss, many surgeons currently opt for a reverse arthroplasty instead of an anatomic shoulder arthroplasty (49).

Radiolucent lines seen in immediate postoperative radiographs are thought to represent areas of poor bonding between cement and cancellous bone at the time of surgery. New radiolucent lines that develop during follow-up are thought to represent progressive loss of cement bond and fixation. Some studies seem to indicate that the presence of radiolucent lines right after surgery increases the risk of loosening seen as progression of radiolucent lines (50).

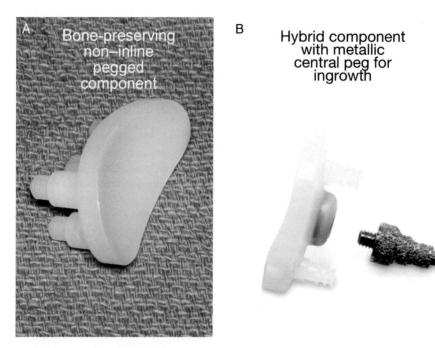

Figure 9.24 *Contemporary glenoid components:* **A,** *All polyethylene, bone preserving, with non–inline pegs.* **B,** *Component designed for hybrid fixation.*

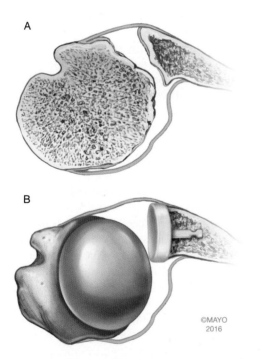

Figure 9.25 *Problems with anatomical TSA and B2 glenoid implantation.* **A,** *Preoperative combination of glenoid bone loss and stretching of the posterior soft-tissues.* **B,** *After surgery, medial reaming in neutral version will aggravate soft-tissue imbalance and leave the glenoid component supported by poor cancellous bone. B2 indicates Walch classification (see Figure 9.4); TSA, total shoulder arthroplasty.*

Every effort should be made to avoid or decrease the presence of radiolucent lines in immediate postoperative radiographs. Most likely these lines are due to blood and bone marrow accumulation at the cement–bone interface. They can be reduced with accurate bone preparation, complete suctioning of fluids at the time of implantation, and mechanical cement pressurization. Some modern components have design features in their pegs that self-pressurize the cement at the time of insertion, which prevents early lucent lines (Figure 9.24A).

Several attempts have been made to use completely cement-free, metal-backed anatomic glenoid components. Unfortunately, they have been associated with a high failure rate secondary to catastrophic polyethylene wear (51,52). This has been due to the fact that, since the lateral offset of the shoulder joint cannot be increased beyond the limits imposed by the rotator cuff tension, most components were designed with a very thin polyethylene liner. Currently, several of the implant components aim for hybrid fixation (the central peg is typically cement-free but cement is still used for fixation of the peripheral pegs and/or the back of the component (Figure 9.24B). There is also interest in developing a completely new generation of cement-free components using fixation strategies borrowed from reverse arthroplasty implants and possibly hard bearing surfaces.

The Concept of Mismatch When the shoulder moves, the humeral head rotates and translates on the glenoid surface. After anatomic joint replacement, as the prosthetic humeral head translates on the glenoid surface, it will tend to tilt

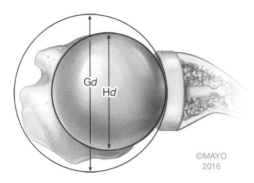

Figure 9.26 *The concept of mismatch. Gd indicates diameter of curvature of the prosthetic glenoid articular surface; Hd, diameter of curvature of the prosthetic humeral head articular surface.*

or rock the glenoid component on the edges, which could potentially contribute to glenoid component loosening. To minimize this stress on the glenoid component, some designs include a certain amount of mismatch between the radius of curvature of the humeral head and that of the glenoid (Figure 9.26); the arc of the humeral head is smaller than the arc of the articular surface of the glenoid, typically between 2 mm and 10 mm, depending on the design and sizing. Biomechanical and clinical studies seem to demonstrate that some degree of mismatch is beneficial (53,54). The ideal diametrical mismatch seems to be between 6 mm and 10 mm. Our preference is to use a design system that provides mismatch and to implant head and glenoid sizes that maintain this mismatch.

Indications

Anatomic shoulder arthroplasty currently is considered for patients with glenohumeral joint degeneration and a functional rotator cuff. The most common indications include primary glenohumeral osteoarthritis (with or without underlying dysplasia), inflammatory arthritis, AVN, certain posttraumatic conditions, capsulorraphy arthropathy, and chondrolysis (1). However, the indications for reverse shoulder arthroplasty have continued to expand to include patients with severe glenoid bone loss or marked soft-tissue imbalance that occurs in many of these conditions.

When anatomic components are deemed ideal for shoulder arthroplasty, the question then becomes whether to use a hemiarthroplasty or total shoulder arthroplasty. The decision to implant a glenoid component rests on 2 questions: Is glenoid resurfacing necessary to achieve a successful outcome? Are risk factors present that may make glenoid component failure likely?

Hemiarthroplasty versus Total Shoulder Arthroplasty for Arthritic Conditions

The outcome of hemiarthroplasty versus total shoulder arthroplasty has been investigated most in primary glenohumeral osteoarthritis. Hemiarthroplasty is associated with an approximate 20% chance of persistent shoulder pain (55).

Total shoulder arthroplasty provides pain relief in the vast majority of patients and also seems to provide better motion. Based on these data, most surgeons favor total shoulder arthroplasty over hemiarthroplasty whenever the glenoid surface is involved by the primary disease (e.g., osteoarthritis, inflammatory arthritis, capsulorraphy arthropathy, and chondrolysis), provided that the glenoid bone stock is sufficient, the rotator cuff is intact, and there is no major soft-tissue imbalance. Conversely, hemiarthroplasty is favored by many in patients with AVN or sequelae of trauma without glenoid involvement at the time of arthroplasty.

Risk Factors for Glenoid Component Failure

Some technical risk factors increase the likelihood of glenoid component wear or loosening (e.g., excessive reaming, incomplete glenoid support on bone). Other factors are likely associated with a higher risk of anatomic glenoid component failure (e.g., compromised bone stock, associated rotator cuff tearing, and marked soft-tissue imbalance). Prior to the advent of reverse shoulder arthroplasty, patients with osteoarthritis and inflammatory arthritis were advised to consider hemiarthroplasty instead of a total shoulder arthroplasty if any of these 2 sets of factors were present. Additionally, hemiarthroplasty was the procedure of choice for cuff tear arthropathy. Currently, many of these patients are advised to consider reverse arthroplasty.

Activity level has a role in the long-term performance of anatomic total shoulder arthroplasty (56). This factor comes into play most often in younger patients with physically demanding jobs or sports participation. Classically, these patients have been considered at very high risk of glenoid failure, and hemiarthroplasty is recommended by most surgeons for patients who desire absolutely no restrictions after surgery. The disadvantage of hemiarthroplasty for these patients is that some will not experience pain relief (57). The relative benefits and risks of implantation of a glenoid component should be assessed for, and discussed with, each patient individually.

Fear of glenoid component failure in young, active patients has led to investigating other alternatives—namely, using hemiarthroplasty (with a metallic implant) in combination with resurfacing the glenoid with various soft-tissue materials (e.g., Achilles tendon allograft, meniscus, and synthetic patches). Studies from multiple institutions have demonstrated high failure rates, sometimes higher than those reported in plain hemiarthroplasty (58). I do not currently consider this alternative approach in my surgical treatment armamentarium.

Preoperative Planning

Preoperative planning is extremely important (Figure 9.27). Plain radiographs and CT may be used to estimate the size of the humeral head, size of the humeral canal, head-to-tuberosity distance, size of the glenoid vault, and assess glenoid version and inclination, and bone loss. As

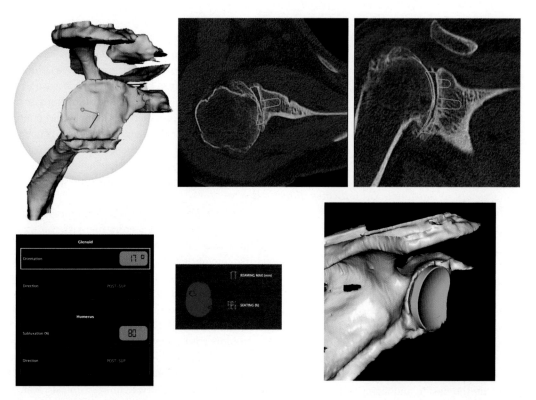

Figure 9.27 *Preoperative planning for anatomical total shoulder arthroplasty on computed tomography.*

mentioned earlier, there is commercially available software that creates tridimensional models of the shoulder skeleton based on CT imaging, allows for virtual planning, and facilitates creation of patient-specific guides (24,25). Special attention should be paid to abnormalities in glenoid version (to plan for the possibility of augmented components or bone graft), and to the location of osteophytes at the glenoid periphery, which oftentimes will result in poor alignment of the glenoid face with the glenoid vault.

Surgical Technique

My preference is to perform this procedure with the patient in the beach chair position using a long deltopectoral approach (chapter 3, Surgical Exposures). There are a number of technical aspects important to the successful performance of shoulder arthroplasty; however, some are not yet universally accepted. An acknowledged key element for the successful performance of total shoulder arthroplasty is good glenoid exposure (⬤ Video 9.1, Table 9.5).

Subscapularis Management

Although some surgeons have described cuff-sparing approaches for shoulder arthroplasty (most commonly insertion of a hemiarthroplasty through the rotator cuff interval), most expose the joint through some sort of subscapularis mobilization. My preference is to perform anatomic shoulder arthroplasty through a subscapularis tenotomy. Others prefer to detach the subscapularis with a

Table 9.5 • Top 10 Recommendations for Good Glenoid Exposure

Lateral skin incision

Truly long deltopectoral approach

Selective pectoralis major release

Selective biceps tenotomy or tenodesis

Large inferior capsular release

Low humeral head cut

Medial humeral osteophyte removal and metaphyseal trimming

Good (multiple) glenoid retractors

Use of arm holder/Mayo stand

Selective paralysis

portion of the lesser tuberosity (i.e., lesser tuberosity osteotomy) or to detach the subscapularis off bone (i.e., subscapularis peel) (Figure 9.28).

Advocates of the lesser tuberosity osteotomy state that bone-to-bone healing is more reliable than tendon-to-tendon or tendon-to-bone healing; in addition, osteotomizing the lesser tuberosity debulks the proximal humerus, which facilitates glenoid exposure. However, osteotomy of the lesser tuberosity has some disadvantages. It is difficult to ensure consistent fragment size; it is more time consuming; and, finally, weakening of the proximal humeral

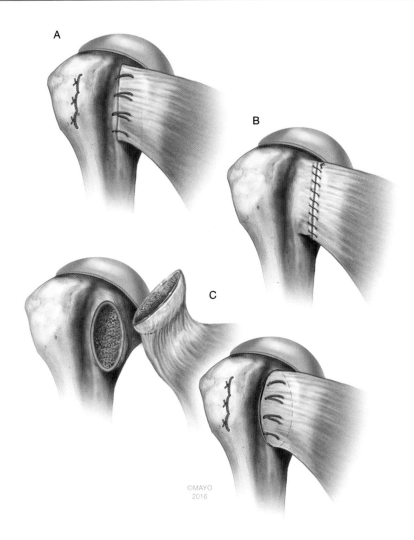

Figure 9.28 *Tenotomy* **(A)**, *osteotomy* **(B)**, *and peel* **(C)**.

cortex may lead to severe damage to metaphyseal bone at the time of posterior retraction of the humerus for glenoid exposure; this damage may compromise fixation with proximally coated, cementless implants (59). Osteotomy of the lesser tuberosity can be particularly worrisome when implanting stemless humeral components. Most cadaver studies comparing osteotomy, tenotomy, and peel have not replicated clinical practice. I tend to use multiple sutures for repair of the tenotomy, whereas the cadaver experiments have used a limited number of sutures. Some comparative studies suggest lower subscapularis failure rates with lesser tuberosity osteotomy, but the best evidence to date shows no difference between subscapularis peel and osteotomy (59–61).

Regardless of the method of subscapularis detachment, a meticulous repair is mandatory (Figure 9.29). Most surgeons repair tenotomies with tendon-to-tendon suture. Osteotomies and peels are repaired with transosseous sutures, oftentimes passing the sutures around the stem of the prosthesis

for additional fixation. As described later, protection after surgery is mandatory to avoid subscapularis insufficiency, which can lead to poor function and anterior instability that may be difficult to overcome with a second attempted repair.

Management of the Long Head of the Biceps
Tenotomy of the long head of the biceps (with or without soft tissue tenodesis) currently is performed commonly at the time of shoulder arthroplasty (62,63). Most advocates state that removing the intra-articular portion of the long head of the biceps facilitates exposure and addresses a potential pain generator. On the other hand, if the tenodesis fails to heal or a tenotomy is performed, some patients experience deformity and cramping (see chapter 6, The Rotator Cuff and Biceps Tendon). In theory, if patients were to develop a late cuff tear (years after their index arthroplasty), an intact long head of the biceps would be the last barrier preventing anterosuperior escape of the prosthesis. In patients with either pain around the biceps tendon area or gross

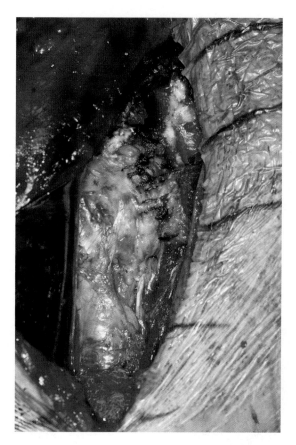

Figure 9.29 Subscapularis repair.

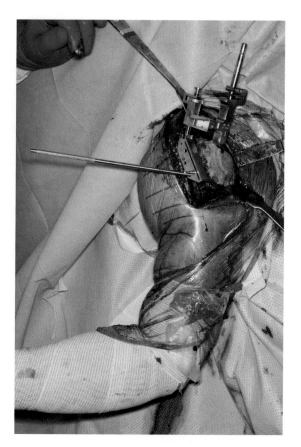

Figure 9.30 Humeral resection guide.

tenosynovitis at the time of surgery, my preference is to perform a tenodesis by suturing the biceps to the pectoralis or conjoined tendon.

Humeral Preparation

The key elements of humeral preparation include performing a humeral head cut at the right height and version and preparing the canal for fixation of the humeral component. Details regarding humeral preparation for resurfacing, partial resurfacing, and stemless components are outside the scope of this book.

The version and inclination of the humeral head cut either can be matched to each individual by performing a free-hand resection at the anatomical neck level after osteophyte removal or, except in severe anatomical abnormalities, a reasonable average cut may be made, depending on the system used and surgeon preference. Free-hand osteotomies with visual estimation require some level of expertise, and I have evaluated patients referred to our practice for failed surgery where the surgeon clearly performed the wrong cut. For those reasons, my preference is to use an accurate intramedullary guide and resect the humeral head flush with the posterosuperior cuff and in approximately 30° of retroversion in reference to the forearm. The component I currently use has

135° of head inclination (Figure 9.30). A relatively low humeral head cut (flush with the cuff) avoids humeral overlengthening, which is detrimental to motion and can facilitate late cuff attrition. In addition, a lower cut facilitates glenoid exposure.

Cementless fixation of the humeral component is favored in most cases. In many patients, adequate primary stability can be achieved by combining distal line-to-line fit, proximal underbroaching, and 3-point fixation. In patients with severe osteopenia, morselized bone graft from the osteotomized humeral head can be packed proximally to enhance fixation and promote ingrowth (64). Rarely, adequate primary stability cannot be obtained with cementless, proximally coated components, and components designed for distal or cemented fixation must be considered. The ideal length of the stem is largely unknown and likely depends on bone quality and other design features. The current trend is to use shorter stems.

Once the humeral osteotomy, reaming, and broaching are finalized, it is wise to leave the broach in the medullary canal to protect the humeral bone stock. Some systems provide a proximal humerus plate protector to prevent inadvertent crushing of the proximal humerus bone with retractors.

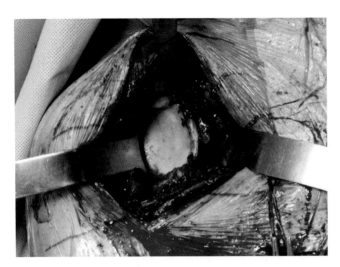

Figure 9.31 Adequate glenoid exposure is critical for successful glenoid preparation and implantation.

Glenoid Preparation

Next, the glenoid is inspected for cartilage damage. In patients with AVN or sequelae of trauma, a glenoid component is not implanted if the cartilage looks pristine; the hemiarthroplasty is finalized with head selection and soft-tissue balance. If an anatomical glenoid component is to be used, adequate exposure is obtained and all soft tissues around the glenoid are removed to identify the outline of the face of the glenoid (Figure 9.31). It is then a good time to pause; take a look at radiographs, CT images, and preoperative planning; and understand the goals for version, inclination, and reaming depth. Next, the humeral head is measured so that glenoid size selection can be performed to ensure some mismatch.

Reaming is best performed with cannulated reamers. Insertion of the guide pin in the correct orientation is critical because it will determine version and inclination. The position of the guide pin may be estimated visually (using internal landmarks) or using a 3D-printed guide. Accurate preparation and minimal reaming are emphasized. The trial component should be used to confirm adequate contact and support with no rocking. Most current components are fixed with bone cement (Figure 9.32). I add vancomycin and methylene blue to polymethylmetacrylate. Some components are very stable once implanted, but care must be taken not to change the position of the glenoid component while the cement is curing.

Head Selection and Soft-Tissue Balance

My preference is to select the diameter of the humeral head to match the diameter of the resected humeral head, discounting osteophytes. Once the diameter of the humeral head is selected, eccentricity can be used to ensure adequate coverage of the neck osteotomy and adequate restoration of the head-to-greater tuberosity distance.

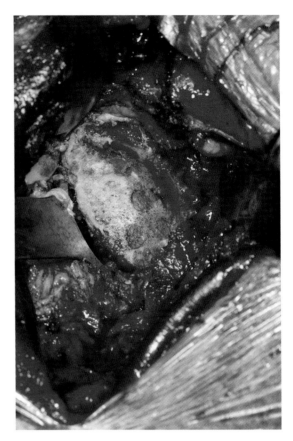

Figure 9.32 Glenoid prepared for implantation of a cemented glenoid component.

Once the appropriate diameter and eccentricity are selected, various thicknesses are trialed to determine the ideal lateral offset and soft-tissue tension. The most common soft-tissue imbalances in primary osteoarthritis include inferior capsular contracture, leading to limited elevation; anterior capsular contracture, leading to limited external rotation; and elongation of the posterior capsule or cuff, leading to posterior subluxation.

Inferior Capsular Contracture Release of the inferior capsule is critical to restoring good overhead motion (Figure 9.33). A large inferior capsular release is performed during exposure; right after the subscapularis is mobilized, the inferior capsule is released around the neck of the humerus past the 6-o'clock position. The inferior capsule is also detensioned (released) by removing medial humeral neck osteophytes and some medial metaphyseal bone (i.e., metaphyseal trimming). Additionally, a flap of the inferior capsule can be removed at the time of glenoid preparation.

Anterior Capsular Contracture The anterior capsule is thick and short and tethers the subscapularis, limiting external rotation (Figure 9.34). My preference is to release

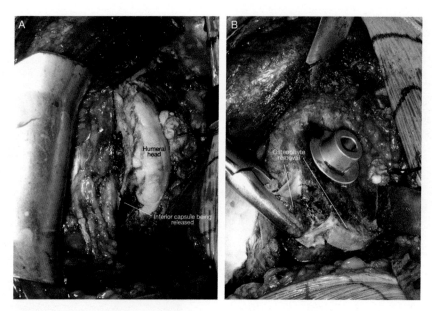

Figure 9.33 *Subperiosteal release of the inferior capsule* **(A)** *and removal of medial humeral osteophytes and bone* **(B)** *contribute to better elevation after surgery.*

the anterior capsule once the glenoid is exposed. The capsule is released along 3 anatomical locations: the superior aspect of the subscapularis tendon (coracohumeral and superior glenohumeral ligaments); along the inferior aspect of the subscapularis (at the 7-o'clock position for the left shoulder or the 5-o'clock for the right shoulder); and the capsule-labrum junction. Traction sutures are used to confirm unrestricted lateral subscapularis excursion. Leaving a free rectangle of capsule on the posterior aspect of the subscapularis tendon provides a better anchor for sutures at the time of closure.

Head Thickness (Offset) and Anteroposterior Balancing
Once the glenoid component is implanted and the humeral broach is in place, head thickness is selected so that the humeral head will translate approximately 50% of its diameter posteriorly (to the rim of the glenoid) and bounce back to a perfectly centered position when stress is released. A thinner head is selected if there is less translation or the subscapularis will not accommodate the distance. A thicker head is selected if there is more than 50% translation. As thickness is increased, tension on the posterior capsule and cuff increases and the tendency for

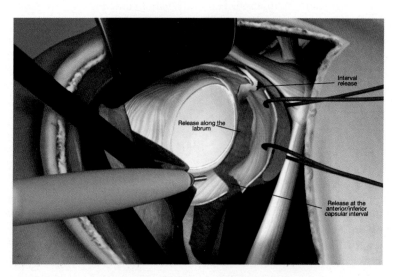

Figure 9.34 *Release of the anterior capsule to free up the subscapularis provides better external rotation and decreases the chance of subscapularis failure with external rotation exercises.*

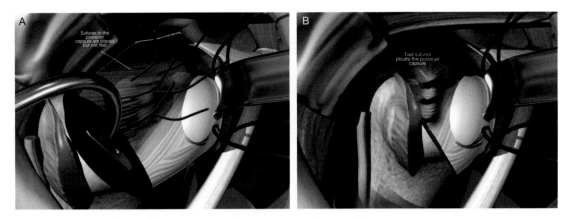

Figure 9.35 *Posterior capsular plication.* **A,** *All sutures are placed.* **B,** *Tied sutures shorten the posterior capsule and cuff.*

posterior subluxation decreases. Once the ideal thickness is selected, the surgeon must confirm full elevation, and external and internal rotation or adjust the head size and soft-tissue balance accordingly.

In cases of marked soft tissue imbalance, even the thickest head likely will not prevent excessive posterior translation, or if it does prevent excessive posterior translation, it will not allow subscapularis closure. Options at that point include plicating the posterior capsule and cuff or converting to a reverse shoulder arthroplasty in these circumstances. The outcome of capsular plication is largely unknown. The capsule and cuff are plicated by placing vertical sutures medially and laterally through the joint and into the tissue (Figure 9.35). Sutures are tied once all sutures have been passed, and the shoulder must be immobilized in external rotation for 6 weeks. Currently, most surgeons convert to a reverse arthroplasty in cases such as these.

Postoperative Management

For the standard, uncomplicated, anatomic total shoulder arthroplasty or hemiarthroplasty, I recommend use of a shoulder immobilizer for 6 weeks. Passive shoulder motion is begun on postoperative day 1 within the safe limits determined intraoperatively based on tension on the subscapularis repair and overall motion and tracking. Active elbow range-of-motion exercises are also started right away to prevent elbow stiffness and irritation of the ulnar nerve. Patients then progress to active assisted range-of-motion exercises with stretching at week 6, adding isometric strengthening at week 10, and elastic band strengthening at week 12 (see chapter 12, Rehabilitation and Injections). As mentioned earlier, patients with a tendency for intraoperative posterior subluxation are immobilized in external rotation for the first 6 weeks, especially if capsular plication is performed. Motion may be delayed for patients with frail soft tissues (subscapularis).

Outcomes

Anatomical shoulder arthroplasty is very successful in terms of pain relief. Unless complications arise, most patients experience complete pain relief. Average range of motion after recovery is at least two-thirds normal, and many patients recover almost complete motion, although stiffness can occur.

Worse functional outcomes should be expected in patients with rheumatoid arthritis with severe loss of offset or in posttraumatic conditions. Restoration of a good arc of motion is also more difficult to obtain in arthritis of instability and chondrolysis, as well as in patients with severe preoperative stiffness. Some patients with AVN are also predisposed to postoperative stiffness.

Complications

The most common complications of anatomic total shoulder arthroplasty include instability, infection, periprosthetic fractures, implant loosening or wear, and late cuff failure. Hemiarthroplasties can also be complicated with progressive painful glenoid erosion.

Instability

Shoulder subluxation or dislocation after anatomic total shoulder arthroplasty or hemiarthroplasty can be secondary to insufficiency of the soft tissues, component malposition, or a combination of the 2 (Figure 9.36) (65). Excessive anteversion or retroversion of either the humeral or the glenoid component (or both) facilitates instability. Anterior instability is almost always associated with subscapularis disruption. Elongation of the posterior capsule and cuff is almost always present in posterior instability.

Subluxation and dislocation do not respond to nonoperative treatment. If a patient presents with subscapularis disruption in the first few weeks after surgery leading to anterior instability, repair or reconstruction of the subscapularis should be attempted soon (although the success rate is moderate). For patients with chronic instability, revision for component exchange and soft-tissue repair has a very high failure rate; allograft augmentation and tendon transfers have not been successful in the setting of an unstable arthroplasty (65). For these reasons, most patients with a

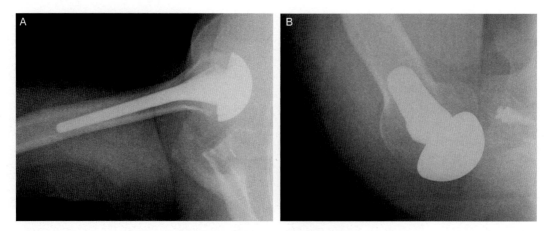

Figure 9.36 *Dislocated anatomical shoulder arthroplasty.* **A,** *Anterior dislocation.* **B,** *Posterior dislocation.*

chronic, symptomatic, unstable shoulder arthroplasty are advised to proceed with revision to a reverse prosthesis (66).

Infection

Deep infection is relatively uncommon after primary anatomic shoulder arthroplasty. It should be suspected in patients with pain present from the time of surgery that cannot otherwise be explained, as well as patients with overt signs of infection. Humeral component loosening is very uncommon in the absence of infection; radiographic evidence of humeral loosening should prompt initiation of an infection work-up (Figure 9.37A). As mentioned earlier, the bacteriology of periprosthetic shoulder infection is such that the diagnosis is difficult to establish (see Infection Workup). Prevention of infection with *C acnes* (formerly *P acnes*) may be particularly difficult because there are high counts of bacteria in the dermal sebaceous

glands and superficial skin preparation may not be effective in reaching deeper structures (17).

Once a deep infection is confirmed, options include oral antibiotic suppression, irrigation and débridement with component retention, 1-stage or 2-stage reimplantation, arthrodesis, and resection arthroplasty (67,68). Irrigation and débridement is attempted in patients presenting within the first few days of symptoms of acute infection, which is uncommon. Most patients with deep infection are advised to undergo 2-stage reimplantation with use of an antibiotic-loaded cement spacer in between the resection procedure and the reimplantation procedure (Figure 9.37B).

Deep infection not only compromises implant fixation but also can lead to damage to the capsular structures and the rotator cuff. Even if the deep infection is eradicated, patients may have poor functional outcomes with pain,

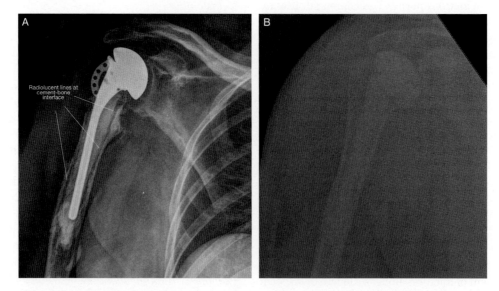

Figure 9.37 *Radiographs showing* **(A)** *loose humeral component in the setting of infection and* **(B)** *cement spacer loaded with antibiotics.*

stiffness, or instability; therefore, use of a reverse design at the time of reimplantation is a growing trend since better outcomes may be obtained even if the rotator cuff is compromised (69). In fact, since reverse arthroplasty provides the opportunity for a more aggressive soft-tissue débridement, 1-stage reimplantation may be considered if the microorganism is susceptible to antibiotics.

Periprosthetic Fractures
Intraoperative Fractures Both the humerus and the glenoid can be fractured at the time of replacement, although this is uncommon (70). Fractures of the humerus can occur at the tuberosity region or in the midshaft. Greater tuberosity fractures can occur during manipulation of the shoulder or trialing in patients with severe osteopenia. A stiff rotator cuff can lead to fracture, especially after broaching, leaving a relatively fragile shell of bone in the tuberosity region. Fractures of the midshaft may occur at the time of dislocation if the humerus is torqued in rotation and the soft tissues have not been released sufficiently, especially in patients with rheumatoid arthritis. Fracture can also occur at the time of implantation of the humeral component if distal reaming was too tight. Greater tuberosity fractures may be handled with suture fixation (as in acute proximal humerus fractures) or may require intraoperative conversion to a reverse prosthesis. Fractures of the shaft may be managed with a longer stem and/or cerclage or plate fixation. My preference is to use a standard-length stem and plate the humeral shaft. Intraoperative fractures of the glenoid almost always occur at the time of reaming; care must be taken to activate the reamer prior to fully seating it in bone. If the reamer is initiated when caught in a bone irregularity, it may fracture the glenoid.

Postoperative Fractures Postoperative fractures of the glenoid are almost always the consequence of glenoid loosening, wear, and osteolysis. Postoperative fractures of the humeral shaft are more commonly traumatic (71,72). As a general rule, periprosthetic fractures of the humeral shaft require a much longer healing time than conventional humeral shaft fractures. Periprosthetic humeral fractures are classified and managed with criteria identical to those of the Vancouver classification of periprosthetic fractures of the femur (Figure 9.38).

Fracture of the Greater Tuberosity A spontaneous fracture of the greater tuberosity can occur secondary to proximal humerus osteolysis, but this is not common. Most cases are associated with mechanical failure that would require revision surgery, regardless of the fracture itself.

Fracture of the Humeral Shaft Along the Length of the Stem Management of fractures along the length of the stem will differ, depending on if the stem is well fixed or loose. If the stem is well fixed and the fracture is not displaced,

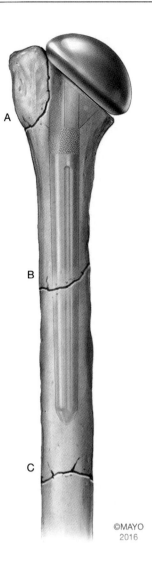

Figure 9.38 *Classification of periprosthetic humeral fractures* **A,** *Tuberosity fractures.* **B,** *Fractures at the level of the humeral stem.* **C,** *Fractures distal to the humeral stem.*

nonoperative treatment may lead to successful fracture healing. Otherwise, plate fixation is recommended. If the stem is loose, humeral component revision surgery is necessary. Bone management in these circumstances is discussed later in this chapter.

Fracture of the Humeral Shaft Distal to the Stem Oftentimes, these fractures can be managed nonoperatively, as if they had occurred in a patient without a prosthesis. Internal fixation is considered for severe fracture displacement or when union is not progressing after a trial of nonoperative treatment.

Glenoid Complications
Glenoid Erosion in Hemiarthroplasty Replacement of the humeral head with a metal prosthesis may lead to progressive loss of glenoid cartilage and bone. This type of

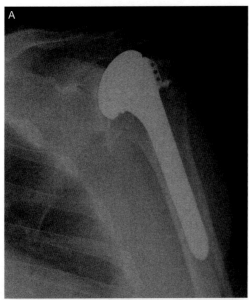

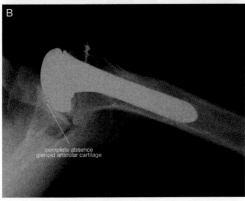

Figure 9.39 Progressive glenoid erosion after hemiarthroplasty. **A,** *Anteroposterior.* **B,** *Axillary.*

loss is particularly likely to occur if the glenoid cartilage is already compromised at the time of hemiarthroplasty (such as in primary osteoarthritis or after years of heavy use of the shoulder joint). Glenoid erosion is oftentimes seen on radiography, but does not always lead to symptoms (Figure 9.39). However, in a number of individuals with good initial pain relief after hemiarthroplasty, pain may recur secondary to progressive glenoid erosion. If the severity of pain justifies revision surgery, these patients can be considered for implantation of a glenoid component (i.e., revision to a total shoulder arthroplasty). Several studies have documented that the outcome of the revised hemiarthroplasty to a total shoulder arthroplasty may be inferior to the outcome of a primary total shoulder arthroplasty (73,74).

Glenoid Loosening in Total Shoulder Arthroplasty A common type of failure of total shoulder arthroplasty is wear and loosening of all-polyethylene, cemented glenoid components. As in progressive glenoid erosion,

glenoid component loosening does not always lead to symptoms.

Glenoid loosening is best identified by comparison of sequential radiographs (Figure 9.40A and B). Small changes in the projection of the beam may result in radiographs that are difficult to compare or to assess for radiolucent lines. For this reason, my preference is to use fluoroscopically guided radiographs (Figure 9.40C). Glenoid loosening is most often diagnosed when there is a tilt or shift in component position on sequential radiographs. A complete radiolucent line around the whole periphery of the component is also considered diagnostic of loosening. Incomplete radiolucent lines are worrisome when they are progressive. Radiographs may also reveal wear and osteolysis. When radiographs are inconclusive, a CT with intra-articular contrast may demonstrate leakage of contrast at the component-cement-bone interface (Figure 9.40D).

The rate of radiographic loosening is substantially disproportionate to the rate of revision for glenoid loosening. Several studies seem to indicate that radiographic loosening may occur in up to 50% of total shoulder arthroplasties with a minimum of 10 years of follow-up. However, reported revision rates for glenoid failure are approximately 5% to 10% (42). This discrepancy is due partly to the fact that glenoid loosening may remain minimally symptomatic for quite some time and partly to the fact that by the time patients may consider revision surgery, they may be considered too old or may have decreased their functional demands substantially.

Symptomatic glenoid loosening may be treated surgically by either removing the glenoid component (i.e., revision to a hemiarthroplasty) or by exchanging the glenoid component for a new one (i.e., revision total shoulder arthroplasty) (75).

Classically, revision to a hemiarthroplasty was performed when the remaining bone stock would not allow safe implantation of a new glenoid component. The goals of the revision hemiarthroplasty are removal of the glenoid component, bone grafting of any glenoid defects, and adjustment of soft-tissue tension, which oftentimes requires using a different humeral head prosthesis size. More recently, techniques for arthroscopic removal of the glenoid component have been developed; major benefits of this approach include less morbidity and better subscapularis preservation. However, when arthroscopic component removal is performed, bone grafting is difficult to accomplish (many surgeons do not even attempt it) and the soft tissues cannot be properly rebalanced by exchanging the humeral head to a different size.

In shoulders with enough remaining glenoid bone stock, revision of the failed total shoulder arthroplasty with implantation of a new component is performed. Comparative studies have shown that implantation of a new glenoid component provides better outcomes

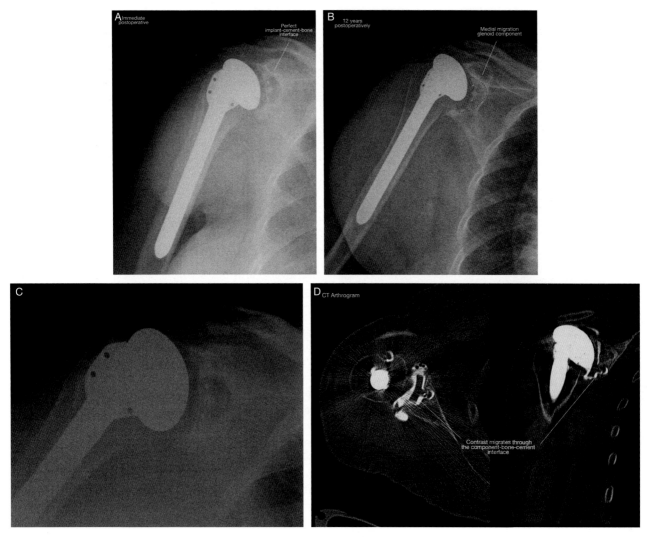

Figure 9.40 *Glenoid loosening.* **A and B,** *Progressive migration.* **C,** *Fluoroscopically positioned radiographs provide a perfect view of the component-cement-bone interface.* **D,** *Contrast migration on computed tomographic arthrogram.*

than revision to a hemiarthroplasty. However, the long-term outcome of cementing a polyethylene component in the revision setting are not very well understood. Currently, there is a growing trend to consider revision to a reverse arthroplasty in these circumstances; reverse glenoid components are believed to provide better fixation in compromised bone, and reverse arthroplasty is also more forgiving in terms of soft-tissue imbalance or insufficiency.

Patients need to be counseled carefully regarding all these treatment options. Many patients with low physical demands, who are looking for pain relief but could tolerate absence of functional improvement, may prefer arthroscopic component removal. On the other hand, if revision surgery is to be performed, it may be best to go "all in" and revise the failed total shoulder arthroplasty to a reverse arthroplasty. Comparative studies are required to further delineate the relative indications of all these options.

Late Cuff Failure

Replacement of the humeral head and resurfacing of the glenoid does not change the fact that progressive cuff degeneration related to age and other factors may still occur (3). In the section on instability, we discussed how early failure of subscapularis healing can occur in some patients, contributing to anterior instability. Progressive cuff attrition can also occur late in patients who had a normal rotator cuff after arthroplasty. The rate of late rotator cuff tears after arthroplasty is difficult to assess; most studies use progressive proximal humeral head migration as a surrogate (Figure 9.41).

Risk factors for late cuff failure include length of follow-up, placement of the glenoid component with superior tilt, placement of the humeral component proud, preoperative fatty infiltration of the cuff, rheumatoid arthritis, and advanced age. In one study, the likelihood of not developing cuff tearing after anatomic total shoulder arthroplasty

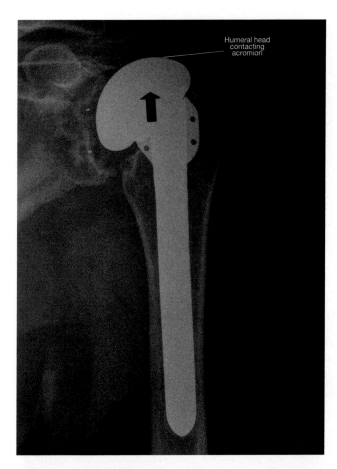

Humeral head contacting acromion

Figure 9.41 Progressive proximal humeral head migration after arthroplasty typically is secondary to late cuff failure.

was 100% at 5 years, 85% at 10 years, and 45% at 15 years. Cuff tearing leads to worsening pain and function. It also facilitates glenoid component loosening, possibly through edge loading.

The management of cuff tears after arthroplasty has evolved over time. Prior to the advent of reverse arthroplasty, rotator cuff repair was performed with poor success rates. Currently, most surgeons favor revision to a reverse arthroplasty, especially when the glenoid component is also loose (2,76,77).

Other

Other complications reported after anatomic total shoulder arthroplasty and hemiarthroplasty include humeral loosening, vascular injuries, infection, and nerve injuries. Axillary nerve injury is uncommon in the primary setting, but inadvertent damage to the axillary nerve during glenoid exposure can lead to catastrophic consequences. The occurrence of brachial plexopathy has diminished over time because the procedure is now more streamlined, requiring less time spent with the arm in abduction and external rotation. After anatomic shoulder arthroplasty, most brachial plexopathies recover spontaneously over a few months.

Reverse Shoulder Arthroplasty

Historical Background, Anatomical and Biomechanical Considerations, and Implant Design

As mentioned earlier, components used in reverse arthroplasty are nonanatomical prostheses that combine a cementless glenoid component with a convex hemisphere and a humeral component with a concave articulating surface (78,79). The rationale and essential design features of reverse prostheses were developed by Dr. Paul M. Grammont; this design provides a fixed fulcrum and increases the resting length of the deltoid so that active elevation is restored in the absence of a functional rotator cuff (Figure 9.42A) (80). The reverse prosthesis was initially developed to provide a better solution for patients with cuff-tear arthropathy. As noted later, the indications for reverse arthroplasty have been expanded substantially over the last 10 years.

Reverse Glenoid Component

Reverse glenoid components are modular. A baseplate with variable ingrowth features is fixed to the glenoid with screws (typically locking screws). The so-called "glenosphere" is then fixed to the baseplate using a morse taper or a screw or both. Baseplates are made of titanium to facilitate ingrowth. Glenospheres are typically made of a cobalt-chrome alloy, although there are alternative designs with ceramic or polyethylene glenospheres.

In the final iteration of the design efforts introduced by Grammont (i.e., Delta III), the glenosphere was a third of a sphere with a 19-mm offset. The center of rotation of the prosthesis is thus medial to the baseplate-bone interface; this design feature was incorporated so that (with use of the shoulder) forces across the joint would translate into compression at the interface vs. shear in order to minimize mechanical failure. This defines the so-called "medial center of rotation" style of reverse arthroplasty (Figure 9.42B) (80). A reverse arthroplasty with a medial center of rotation is theoretically less prone to the high failure rate historically reported with constrained shoulder arthroplasties. In addition, it changes the vector of the deltoid fibers, recruiting more fibers for elevation.

However, a medial center of rotation also has a number of potential disadvantages (81). First, the humeral component is closer to the scapula; in adduction (especially when rotation or extension is added), there is impingement between the humeral component and the glenoid bone, leading to scapular bone resorption known as "notching." Second, any intact posterior cuff and the posterior deltoid are detensioned, which can contribute to less strength in external rotation. Third, the shoulder loses offset, which translates in cosmetic changes and, if extreme, can turn the deltoid moment arm into a dislocating force. An alternative style of reverse was designed by Dr. Mark A. Frankle with

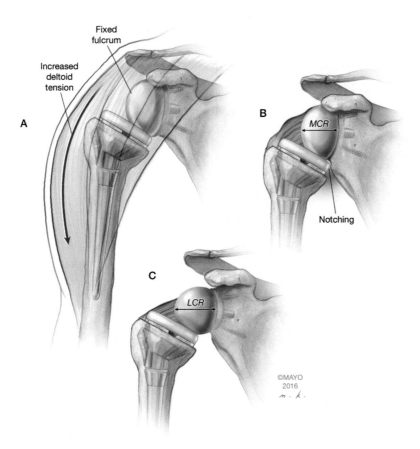

Figure 9.42 *Reverse rationale.* **A,** *Fixed fulcrum with deltoid tensioning.* **B,** *Medial center of rotation (MCR).* **C,** *Lateral center of rotation (LCR).*

a more "lateralized center of rotation," with thicker glenospheres for all of these reasons (Figure 9.42C). The first generation of lateralized reverse arthroplasties had a relatively high mechanical failure rate, but once baseplate fixation was optimized the rate of loosening decreased substantially.

Controversy continues regarding which of these 2 design philosophies is best. Some implants offer only a medial center of rotation; others offer a lateral center of rotation, and some offer both options. My preference is to select the center of rotation best for each individual patient. As mentioned later in this chapter, some designs achieve more overall shoulder offset by lateralizing on the humeral size, which also needs to be taken into consideration. Some surgeons propose an intermediate solution: use of a design with a medial center of rotation design, adding structural bone graft (from the humeral head) underneath the baseplate to create a more lateralized bony glenoid neck (bio-RSA) (82). This approach will lateralize the shoulder; however, once the graft is healed the center of rotation will still be medial to the component-bone interface.

Most designs offer the possibility of various glenosphere diameters (32 mm, 36–38 mm, 40–42 mm). Theoretically, larger glenospheres provide a greater arc of motion before

impingement, which should translate in more motion, less notching, and more stability. Clinical differences between glenosphere sizes, however, have not been investigated in depth. A prosthesis with a large glenosphere diameter may be difficult to implant in a very small patient.

Much has been learned regarding the ideal position of the baseplate on the glenoid in terms of superior to inferior positioning, version, inclination, and rotation (78,79,83) (Figure 9.43).

Superior to Inferior Positioning In order to avoid impingement between the medial humerus and the glenoid neck, reverse baseplates are typically placed flush with the inferior rim of the glenoid. When adequate fixation requires more superior positioning (typically in the revision setting), glenospheres with inferior eccentricity may be used to minimize notching (Figure 9.43A and B).

Version Reverse arthroplasty is more forgiving than anatomic arthroplasty in terms of glenoid version; a sphere allows good prosthetic articulation in various degrees of version better than a flat surface. Most surgeons aim for neutral version or slight retroversion in shoulders with minimal bone loss (Figure 9.43C). In patients with

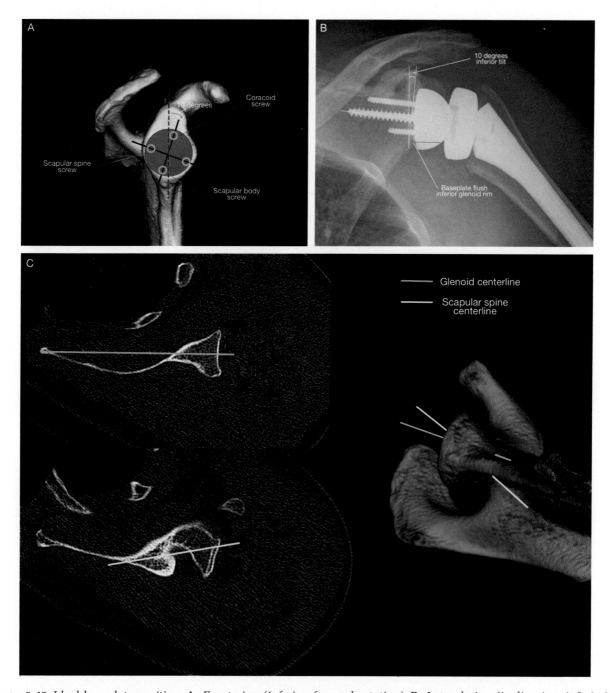

Figure 9.43 *Ideal baseplate position.* **A,** *Front view (inferior, forward rotation).* **B,** *Lateral view (inclination, inferior).* **C,** *Superior view of the glenoid centerline and the alternative scapular spine centerline.*

severe bone loss at the glenoid vault, the central fixation mechanism (i.e., screw or post) of the baseplate can be fixed to the spine of the scapula; this requires placing the component in a fair amount of anteversion, perpendicular to the so-called "alternative scapular spine centerline."

Inclination Most surgeons aim for some (5°–10°) inferior tilt when implanting the baseplate (Figure 9.43B). Various studies seem to indicate that inferior tilt results in compressive rather than shear force, and depending on the design, inferior inclination or tilt may also decrease notching.

Rotation The superior and inferior screws get good purchase along the base of the coracoid (superiorly) and the body of the scapula (inferiorly). Rotating the baseplate forward (to the 1-o'clock position for the right shoulder or the 11-o'clock position for the left shoulder) places the superior and inferior screw holes in the best trajectory for most individuals (Figure 9.43A).

Reverse Humeral Component

The humeral component of the Grammont Delta III reverse prosthesis was designed as a modular component and combines a stem and a humeral bearing segment. The humeral bearing portion is inset into the proximal humerus and has a concave polyethylene design available in 2 sizes (36 mm and 42 mm) to match the 2 glenosphere diameters initially offered. In addition, the neck-shaft angle is 155° (more flat on top of the humerus). Once articulating with the glenosphere, the humerus is displaced distally, which increases the resting length of the deltoid, providing more power for elevation. A flatter neck-shaft angle helps prevent superolateral dislocation in a medialized reverse arthroplasty, but (unfortunately) it also facilitates medial impingement and notching. Initially, implanting the humeral component in 0° to 10° of retroversion was recommended to facilitate internal rotation (see later) and prevent dislocation (2,79,80).

Currently, some of the available implants replicate the design principles of the Delta III humeral component. However, a number of changes have been introduced in many other reverse prosthesis designs, in part to provide the possibility of easy conversion between anatomic and reverse arthroplasties using the same humeral stem and in part to decrease notching (Figure 9.44) (81).

An anatomic humeral component implanted in less than 20° to 30° of anteversion with a 155° neck-shaft angle creates a number of issues, including anterior instability. Most surgeons prefer to select a design where the same stem can be used for either anatomic or reverse arthroplasty; hopefully, this allows for an easier revision by not needing to

exchange the stem and also decreases inventory. For these reasons, many current reverse arthroplasties have an "anatomic" neck-shaft angle around 135° and the humeral component is implanted in approximately 30° of retroversion. There is also a trend to implant shorter and shorter stems uncemented and some interest in stemless reverse designs.

Another recent design modification is related to the introduction of "onset" as opposed to "inset" humeral bearings. In many current designs, the humeral bearing rests on the cut surface of the humeral neck, which translates to a more lateral position of the humerus for the same position of the glenoid component. Lateralizing on the humeral side has the potential benefit of maintaining good tension on the external rotators while allowing a medial center of rotation. However, the line of pull of the deltoid is less vertical, which could result in less strength in elevation.

Internal and External Rotation After Reverse Arthroplasty

In patients with an insufficient rotator cuff, reverse arthroplasty restores active elevation thanks to its fixed fulcrum and changes in the tension and line of action of the deltoid. However, reverse arthroplasty oftentimes leads to decreased internal rotation and may also be associated with poor external rotation.

Internal Rotation Decreased internal rotation after reverse arthroplasty is due mostly to impingement: the semiconstrained nature of the prosthesis blocks internal rotation

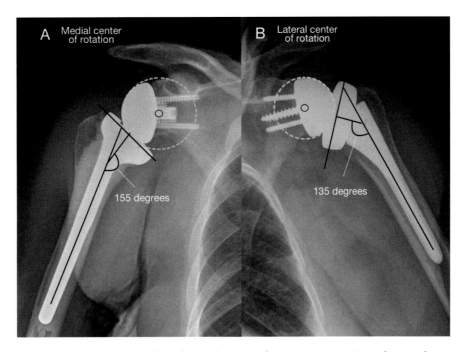

Figure 9.44 A, *Inset humeral component with a relative horizontal orientation.* **B,** *Onset humeral component with a more anatomic orientation.*

at the point of impingement. In addition, if the design medializes the shoulder offset, the internal rotators are less tensioned and will have a more vertical vector. Internal rotation also will largely depend on the flexibility of the scapulothoracic joint. Patients able to protract the scapula may still be able to get their hand behind their backs even though glenohumeral rotation is limited.

Placing the humeral component in less retroversion provides a little extra internal rotation. However, since the trend is now to implant reverse stems in 30° of retroversion, limited internal rotation still remains problematic in some patients. For these reasons, it is important to inform patients prior to surgery that loss of internal rotation is likely. This loss can be especially concerning for patients requiring reverse arthroplasty bilaterally, since neither hand could be placed behind the back for personal hygiene. However, most patients with bilateral reverse arthroplasty seem to find a way to adjust.

External Rotation Poor external rotation is particularly likely when a prosthesis with a medial center of rotation is placed in neutral version. The posterior deltoid and rotator cuff are detensioned, and the humerus version places the hand in a starting point with relatively internal rotation. Several studies have demonstrated that lack of active external rotation after reverse arthroplasty leads to worse function. This lack of active external rotation is especially likely to occur when both the infraspinatus and the teres minor are affected; a positive hornblower sign, lack of active external rotation with the arm in abduction, and confirmation of teres minor rupture and fatty infiltration on imaging are predictors of poor external rotation after reverse arthroplasty (84).

Better resting tension on the posterior external rotators can be achieved by restoring a more lateral shoulder offset on the glenoid side, the humeral side, or both (78). Placing the humeral component in more retroversion may also provide more active external rotation; however, in the complete absence of the posterior rotator cuff, it may not be enough. That is why emphasis has been placed on achieving greater tuberosity healing when reverse is used for proximal humerus fractures and nonunions (see chapter 4, Proximal Humerus Fractures). In patients with combined loss of active elevation and external rotation (Figure 9.45), some surgeons advocate transferring the latissimus dorsi (with or without the teres major) at the time of reverse arthroplasty (20,85). The details of this combined procedure are described later. (See also chapter 6, The Rotator Cuff and Biceps Tendon.)

Indications

The prime indication for reverse shoulder arthroplasty is cuff tear arthropathy; however, over time the indications have expanded substantially (Table 9.6) (1,79). Reverse arthroplasty is very attractive for patients with pain and pseudoparalysis. The recommendation of reverse arthroplasty should be discussed cautiously for 2 groups of patients: those with pseudoparalysis and no pain and those with a painful irreparable cuff tear but good active motion (86).

The use of reverse arthroplasty to restore active motion in the absence of pain is a departure from traditional theory on shoulder arthroplasty; for most joints, arthroplasty is recommended to relieve pain. Patients electing to undergo reverse arthroplasty for only functional improvements need to be aware of the possibility that they could have increased pain after surgery. At the other end of the spectrum, patients

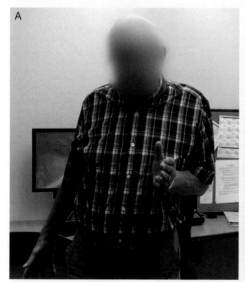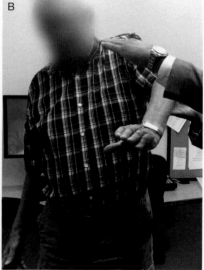

*Figure 9.45 Combined loss of elevation and external rotation. Pseudoparalysis in elevation is shown in Figure 9.15. This same patient has pseudoparalysis in external rotation **(A)** and inability to actively externally rotate in abduction **(B)**.*

Table 9.6 • Indications for Reverse Shoulder Arthroplasty

Cuff tear arthropathy

Massive irreparable cuff tear

Rheumatoid arthritis with cuff insufficiency

Primary osteoarthritis or dysplasia with either
Large associated cuff tear
Severe posterior subluxation (over 80%)
Severe bone loss (typically posterior)

Certain posttraumatic conditions
Nonunion
Malunion
Locked dislocation

Certain acute proximal humerus fractures (see chapter 4, Proximal Humerus Fractures)

Two-stage reimplantation for infection (selectively)

Neuropathic arthropathy (selectively)

Revision surgery (selectively)

Shoulder reconstruction after tumor resection

with a painful irreparable cuff tear but great motion (e.g., those with well-compensated cuff tear arthropathy, or even in the absence of arthropathy) may be disappointed with outcome after surgery, even if their pain goes away, since they may lose some motion (e.g., worse elevation and/or rotation after reverse arthroplasty).

Preoperative Planning

Plain radiographs may provide enough information to plan in patients with severe cuff insufficiency but almost no glenoid abnormalities. However, CT is used commonly for preoperative planning, especially for patients with glenoid abnormalities or after trauma. As mentioned in the section on anatomic arthroplasty, an added benefit of CT is the use of software to perform virtual surgery and even create custom-made guides. Some patients will come to the shoulder surgeon with an MRI and, if the MRI is of good quality, it may provide enough information to plan the bony part of the operation. Special attention should be paid to assessment of the posterior cuff during the planning phase. As mentioned earlier, in the absence of functional infraspinatus and teres minor, consideration should be given to a combined tendon transfer at the time of arthroplasty.

Surgical Technique

Exposure

Reverse arthroplasty is performed in the beach chair position (🔘 Video 9.2). Some surgeons favor a deltopectoral approach; others prefer a superior approach (see chapter 3, Surgical Exposures). Table 9.7 summarizes the relative benefits of these 2 exposures for reverse arthroplasty. Since the arm is elongated with reverse arthroplasty, most surgeons recommend biceps tenotomy or tenodesis. The subscapularis is not always present at the time of arthroplasty; when intact, it can be completely preserved when a superior approach is used. When reverse arthroplasty is performed through a deltopectoral approach, the subscapularis can be mobilized through a tenotomy, peel, or lesser tuberosity osteotomy, as detailed in the section on anatomic shoulder arthroplasty. As with anatomic shoulder arthroplasty, it is essential to achieve good glenoid exposure (Table 9.5). When reverse arthroplasty is performed for a proximal humerus fracture, nonunion, or malunion, the tuberosities are mobilized or osteotomized for exposure.

Humeral Preparation

With current platform systems, many surgeons use the exact same stem for anatomic and reverse arthroplasty. Preparation of the humerus is identical to that described

Table 9.7 • Deltopectoral Versus Superior Approach for Reverse Shoulder Arthroplasty

Relative To	Deltopectoral	Superior
Deltoid	Deltoid preserving	Of benefit in patients with prior deltoid weakening secondary to open cuff repair attempts
Subscapularis	Needs to be mobilized	Can be preserved
Access to the greater tuberosity	More difficult	Easier (helpful in fractures and sequels of trauma)
Inferior humeral capsular release/ osteophytes	Easier	More difficult
Extensile to the humeral shaft	Yes (important for revision cases)	No
Access to the inferior glenoid rim	Easier	More difficult (except in shoulders with a fracture, nonunion, or severe humeral bone loss)
Combined latissimus dorsi/teres major transfer	Easier	More difficult

for anatomic shoulder arthroplasty, although the neck oste-otomy is oftentimes performed a few millimeters lower in order to be able to relocate the prosthesis. Care must be taken to preserve any intact posterior cuff.

Glenoid Preparation

Most surgeons favor placing the baseplate flush with the inferior glenoid rim, with approximately 10° of inferior tilt. Reaming is performed to the point where there is good-quality cancellous bone for ingrowth. Most compo-nents are designed with a post or a large screw for fixation at the center of the baseplate; my preference is to use a component with a screw in the primary setting as opposed to a post in order to preserve more bone (Figure 9.46). Fixation is then supplemented with multiple locking screws. Glenosphere selection is based on all the parame-ters described before, and is largely based on patient size, surgeon's preference, underlying structural changes, and trialing.

Humeral Bearing Selection

Once the glenoid component is implanted, the ideal soft-tissue tension is determined by trialing several humeral bearing thicknesses. To date, there are few objective data to use for selecting the thickness of the humeral bearing intra-operatively, and selection is most often based on the sub-jective feeling of soft-tissue tension. Most surgeons select the bearing that will make it difficult (but not impossible) to relocate the shoulder so that if the trials are relocated, they are difficult to dislocate.

The main risks of under sizing humeral bearing thick-ness are postoperative dislocation and poor deltoid tension. However, overlengthening the arm by using too thick a humeral bearing can lead to other complications (e.g., brachial plexus injuries, stress fractures of the acro-mion or spine, and muscular pain secondary to excessive tension).

When the shoulder feels too loose with a given humeral bearing, the thickness can be increased until the soft-tissue tension is felt to be optimal; sometimes, more lateral offset is required to obtain the right tension. Use of a more lateral-ized glenoid may be required. If the shoulder is still loose with a lateralized construct and the thickest possible bear-ing, a glenosphere with inferior offset may be used or the stem may be cemented proud.

When the shoulder feels too tight with the thinnest pos-sible bearing, better soft-tissue tension can be achieved by releasing any remaining supraspinatus, releasing the biceps tendon if still intact, lowering the humeral cut, or using a more medialized glenosphere.

It is important to check for range of motion and impinge-ment. In some circumstances, the greater tuberosity may impinge on the acromion and should be trimmed down. More rarely, the lesser tuberosity may impinge on the cor-acoid; this can be addressed by using a glenosphere with posterior offset or by trimming down the lesser tuberosity. Inferior impingement should be avoided if at all possible to minimize notching.

Latissimus Dorsi and Teres Major Transfer It is estimated that combined tendon transfer is required in 1% to 10% of the cases; this rate varies depending on the combina-tion of diagnoses, design features of the implant, and surgeon preference. I consider tendon transfers (in the

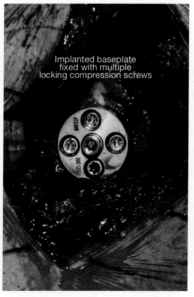
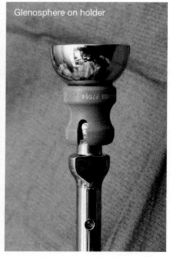

Figure 9.46 Glenoid component of a reverse prosthesis design.

setting of reverse shoulder arthroplasty) for patients with combined pseudoparalysis in elevation and external rotation (i.e., preoperative active external rotation not even to neutral and extension of cuff insufficiency to the teres minor) (⬤ Video 9.3) (84).

The tendons of the latissimus dorsi and teres major blend together as they attach to the humeral shaft. They can be harvested easily with a deltopectoral approach by dividing the majority of the pectoralis, which is repaired at the end of the procedure (Figure 9.47). Alternatively, the latissimus dorsi may be harvested individually under the intact pectoralis major. Once the combined tendon is harvested, the muscles are mobilized and transferred around the humeral shaft. Some surgeons favor reattachment to the greater tuberosity; others favor reattachment to the humeral shaft (20,85). It is important to reattach the tendons not too anteriorly in order to avoid severe restriction of internal rotation. My preference is to reattach the tendons to the shaft just below the greater tuberosity using intramedullary sutures around the stem. As detailed later, tendon transfer requires a different program of rehabilitation.

Closure The main controversy regarding closure after reverse arthroplasty involves the subscapularis. If the subscapularis is intact at the beginning of the procedure, I favor repairing it at the end (if at all possible). Subscapularis repair has been noted to decrease the rate of dislocation when a medial center of rotation reverse

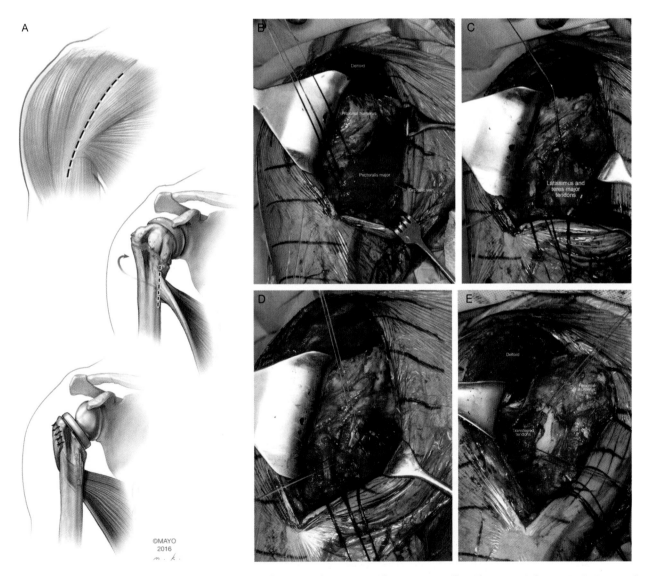

Figure 9.47 *Latissimus dorsi and teres major transfer in combination with a reverse arthroplasty.* **A,** *Schematic.* **B,** *Pectoralis major elevated.* **C,** *Latissimus dorsi and teres major tendons harvested.* **D,** *Nonabsorbable sutures placed in the tendons to be transferred in a locking running fashion.* **E,** *The tendons have been transferred around the humeral shaft and are ready to be attached.*

is implanted through a deltopectoral approach (87,88). Subscapularis repair may be less critical for stability when an implant with a lateral center of rotation is used. If the repair is too tight, external rotation could be limited further. On the other hand, if the repair is performed optimally, it may provide more strength in internal rotation. Some surgeons never repair the subscapularis, and others repair the subscapularis when they can. There is no general consensus on optimal treatment.

Postoperative Management

The inherently semiconstrained nature of reverse arthroplasty is more protective for the soft tissues; there is not much to protect unless the subscapularis is intact and repaired. On the other hand, the absence of a rotator cuff does not allow sealing the joint, and postoperative hematomas can easily migrate through the deltopectoral interval and collect under the skin. The absence of a rotator cuff also makes subacromial scarring less likely to limit motion. Reverse arthroplasty is also used commonly for older patients who benefit from a simplified program of rehabilitation and faster return to use of their arm to avoid dependence. For all these reasons, my preferred protocol is to delay motion for the first 2 to 3 weeks only, and allow active assisted motion and discontinue use of an immobilizer much earlier than would be typical in anatomic shoulder arthroplasty.

After surgery, I favor use of a shoulder immobilizer with a small abduction pillow for the first 2 to 3 weeks. During that time patients perform no shoulder physical therapy (to decrease the chance of a subcutaneous hematoma) but are instructed to exercise their elbow, wrist, and hand. At 2 to 3 weeks after surgery, the immobilizer is removed and patients start on a program of passive and active assisted motion exercises. Strength training typically starts 6 weeks after surgery, first using isometrics and later, elastic bands. Strength training focuses on the deltoid and the posterior rotator cuff.

Postoperative management is different for patients who undergo a combined latissimus dorsi-teres major transfer; the shoulder is immobilized in external rotation for 6 weeks to protect the transfer, and internal rotation is incorporated carefully to avoid stretching of the transferred tendons.

Outcomes

The outcomes of reverse shoulder arthroplasty are difficult to summarize. Reported outcomes are influenced largely by the surgeon's and the orthopedic community's learning curves, the type of implant used, and the underlying diagnosis (89). The best results have been published using modern implants in cuff tear arthropathy. Pain relief is very predictable after reverse arthroplasty for any of the indications summarized in Table 9.6. However, gains in motion and function are very good in patients with cuff tear arthropathy, primary osteoarthritis, and rheumatoid arthritis, and less predictable in patients with an acute fracture, sequelae of trauma, previous infection, tumors, and revision surgery.

Complications

Reverse arthroplasty shares some complications with anatomic arthroplasty, including loosening glenoid or humeral component loosening, periprosthetic fractures, and infection. A few complications are particularly relevant to reverse arthroplasty, including dislocation, notching, brachial plexopathy, and stress fractures of the scapula.

Dislocation

When instability occurs, the constrained nature of reverse arthroplasty results in a substantial event. Dislocation of a reverse arthroplasty is typically felt as a painful episode followed by deformity and loss of motion, as opposed to the progressive development of subluxation and dislocation after anatomical arthroplasty. The diagnosis of dislocation is also quite evident on plain radiographs (Figure 9.48).

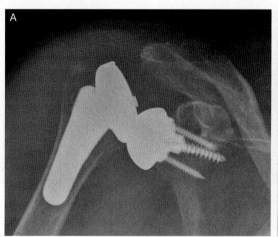
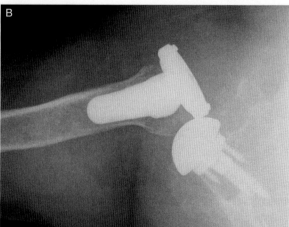

Figure 9.48 *Plain radiographs show dislocated reverse arthroplasty.* **A,** *Anteroposterior.* **B,** *Axillary.*

The most common causes for dislocation in reverse arthroplasty include lack of restoration of sufficient arm length, impingement, extreme medialization, and loss of proximal humerus bone stock. Dislocation is common in revision surgery and in patients with sequelae of trauma. All factors possibly contributing to instability should be assessed when formulating a treatment plan.

Some authors have reported successful treatment of early dislocations with closed reduction; approximately 50% to 60% of the patients did not experience further dislocation episodes (90). When closed reduction is unsuccessful, recurrence occurs, or gross problems can be identified, revision surgery is recommended (91). Radiographs of both arms with magnifier markers are useful to measure arm length. At the time of revision surgery, sources of impingement are identified and eliminated. Stability may be increased by using a large-diameter glenosphere, increasing lateral offset of the shoulder, and adding length on the humeral side (by using thicker bearings or revising the component). More constrained liners with deeper polyethylene are available, but their walls are thin and may be predisposed to catastrophic wear; I use them only when everything else has been tried and the implant is still unstable. For patients with a large segment of proximal humerus missing, reconstruction using a humeral allograft-prosthetic composite should be considered (see later in the chapter).

Notching

As discussed previously, the term notching refers to progressive loss of bone on the inferior aspect of the glenoid caused by repetitive impingement. Retrieval studies show that notching is associated with medial polyethylene wear. The incidence of radiographic notching is reported to be very high when using reverse designs with a medial center of rotation (Figure 9.49) (92). A number of patients with radiographic notching do not seem to experience adverse clinical effects; however, long-term studies have reported worse results in patients with severe notching. Although not every patient with notching does poorly, I prefer to do everything I can during preoperative planning and surgery to minimize medial impingement.

Brachial Plexopathy

As mentioned in the section on anatomic arthroplasty, the brachial plexus can be transiently stretched at the time of surgery, leading to sensory and motor dysfunction that typically resolves over time. Brachial plexopathy complicating a reverse arthroplasty may not resolve when it is secondary to permanent arm lengthening (as opposed to transient stretch during surgery). Care must be taken to avoid excessive arm overlengthening because, if symptoms of brachial plexopathy do not resolve over time, revision surgery to a shorter reverse construct may be needed. By then the soft tissues may be so stretched that instability may occur. Over time, surgeons have tended to implant reverse arthroplasties slightly looser, which (hopefully) will translate into a lower rate of permanent brachial plexopathy.

Stress Fractures of the Acromion and Spine of the Scapula

The increased tension on the deltoid after reverse shoulder arthroplasty can also lead to a stress fracture of either the acromion or the spine of the scapula (93). Multiple cycles of motion are required for stress fractures to occur; therefore, most patients develop this complication a few months into their recovery. Risk factors for stress fracture include a very thin acromion, substantial arm overlengthening, rheumatoid arthritis, and osteopenia.

Typically, patients report that after having recovered a good, pain-free arc motion, they suddenly experience pain and decrease in active elevation. Physical examination reveals pain on palpation along the acromion, or spine, of the scapula in addition to loss of active elevation. These fractures may be extremely difficult to identify on plain radiographs, but can be confirmed with CT (Figure 9.50). Conservative treatment of stress fracture of the acromion leads to resolution of pain in many patients, but active elevation seldom returns to the level that was achieved shortly after surgery. Occasionally, surgery is considered to fix the fracture or remove the fractured fragment. Fractures of the spine of the scapula are much more problematic, and plate fixation of the spine should be considered when symptoms continue.

Other Complications

As with anatomic shoulder arthroplasty, reverse arthroplasty can be complicated by deep infection, axillary nerve injury, vascular injuries, and mechanical failure. Humeral loosening is uncommon. Glenoid loosening has been found to be less common than initially expected. There are also reports of other modes of mechanical failure (e.g.,

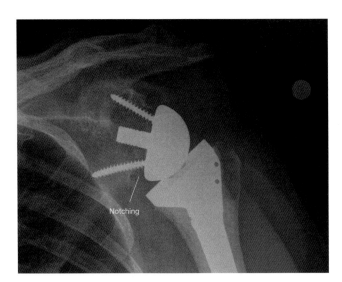

Figure 9.49 *Radiograph showing notching.*

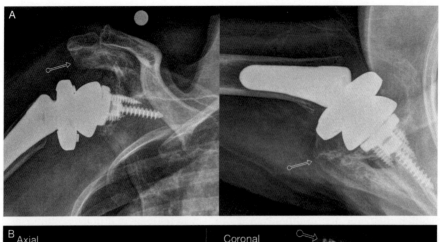

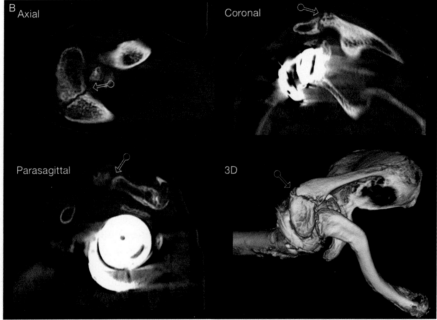

Figure 9.50 *Most commonly, stress fractures of the acromion are not seen on plain radiographs* **(A)**. *Typically, they can be diagnosed on computed tomography* **(B)**.

disassociation of components on either the glenoid side or the humeral side) and metal fracture at the base of the humeral bearing in certain designs.

Surgical Alternatives to Arthroplasty

Surgical alternatives to arthroplasty may be of some benefit in selected patients with glenohumeral arthritis.

Débridement

Arthroscopic débridement may benefit patients who have milder forms of joint degeneration and do not want to face the recovery time, rehabilitation, restrictions, and potential complications of shoulder arthroplasty. Débridement is most commonly considered for patients with early

rheumatoid arthritis, osteoarthritis, chondrolysis, cuff tear arthropathy with well-preserved motion, and septic arthritis (94–96).

The goals and extent of the procedure differ depending on the indication. Synovectomy is the main goal of arthroscopic débridement for inflammatory arthritis. In osteoarthritis and chondrolysis, débridement involves removal of loose pieces of articular cartilage, capsular release for stiff shoulders, and (when present) removal of osteophytes (Figure 9.51) (94). Biceps tenotomy or tenodesis is commonly associated with débridement, and some surgeons reshape the glenoid in patients with asymmetric bone loss. In cuff tear arthropathy with well-preserved motion, pain may improve with débridement of cartilage, frayed tendon edges, and biceps tenotomy or tenodesis. Débridement for septic arthritis may be successful in the absence of osteomyelitis (15).

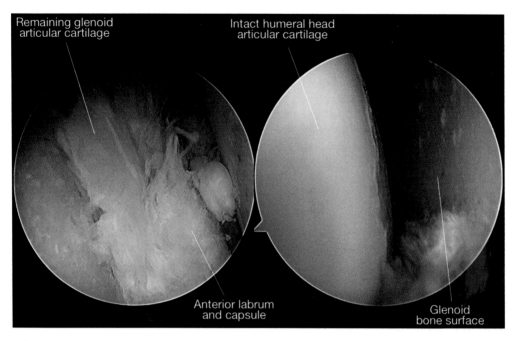

Figure 9.51 *Arthroscopic débridement for glenohumeral osteoarthritis.*

After surgery, protection of repaired structures is not required, so patients can initiate active use of the shoulder as soon as their pain subsides. Patients with preoperative stiffness released at the time of arthroscopy may benefit from a program of stretching.

Arthrodesis and Resection Arthroplasty

These 2 options are discussed in detail in chapter 11, Salvage Procedures. They are seldom indicated in patients with glenohumeral joint degeneration unless patients present with deep infection unresponsive to any other treatment, complete absence of deltoid function, paralysis secondary to axillary nerve or brachial plexus palsy, or severe unreconstructable bone loss.

Surgical Management of Specific Conditions

Glenohumeral Osteoarthritis, Posttraumatic Arthritis, Chondrolysis, and Arthritis of Dislocation

Anatomic total shoulder arthroplasty is the procedure of choice for most patients with these conditions (1). As mentioned before, arthroscopic débridement may be considered for individuals with milder forms of disease and unwilling to deal with the recovery, restrictions, and potential complications of shoulder arthroplasty (94).

Patients with chondrolysis are typically younger than most arthroplasty candidates, and their underlying inflammatory process may still be active at the time of surgery,

making them more prone to stiffness (14). Patients with arthritis of dislocation and capsulorrhaphy arthropathy present 2 particular challenges: 1) exposure may be difficult secondary to previous surgery (especially when the local anatomy was markedly distorted, such as after a previous coracoid transfer procedure), and 2) the anterior soft tissues are most often extremely shortened and scarred, making it difficult to balance the shoulder and to obtain a functional arc of motion (13). In my practice, retained hardware is removed from the glenoid only if it interferes with glenoid preparation and implantation; otherwise it is left in place to avoid further compromising any remaining glenoid bone stock.

Primary glenohumeral osteoarthritis is an ideal condition for treatment with anatomic total shoulder arthroplasty; however, reverse arthroplasty is considered for patients with 1) an associated medium to large cuff tear, 2) severe posterior humeral subluxation (>80%), and/or 3) severe posterior glenoid bone loss (49,97). In these circumstances, surgeons commonly will obtain patient consent for both anatomic and reverse arthroplasty and make the final decision intraoperatively.

Cuff Tear Arthropathy

Reverse shoulder arthroplasty has become the procedure of choice for patients with cuff tear arthropathy (97). Arthroscopic débridement may be considered for selected patients with preserved active motion and severe pain, especially if the long head of the biceps is intact. Hemiarthroplasty may also be considered for this subgroup of patients, but pain relief and motion are much less predictable. As mentioned before, combined tendon transfer may be considered for patients with cuff tear arthropathy and loss of active external rotation. Arthrodesis rarely is considered for patients who have no deltoid function (as a consequence of previous surgery) or younger patients with conditions requiring use of the upper extremities to transfer (e.g., paraplegia, amputation, or severe poliomyelitis). The safety of hemiarthroplasty and reverse arthroplasty in patients who use their upper extremities to transfer has not been defined, but some surgeons do not consider this an absolute contraindication.

Inflammatory Arthritis

Arthroscopic synovectomy is the procedure of choice for most patients with early-stage rheumatoid arthritis. Improvement of symptoms is common, although pain and loss of function eventually return. Synovectomy has not been shown to alter the course of inflammatory arthritis (10).

For more advanced inflammatory disease, anatomical total shoulder arthroplasty is the procedure of choice (98). Currently, reverse arthroplasty is considered more often for inflammatory arthritis with associated cuff insufficiency and for those patients with severe bone loss (23,99). However, reverse arthroplasty has to be considered more cautiously in patients with inflammatory arthropathy because osteopenia is more common in that condition (possibly leading to a higher rate of mechanical failure of the glenoid component) and the risk of fracture of the acromion and scapular spine is high. Hemiarthroplasty is a good option for patients with cuff dysfunction or compromised bone stock who are willing to accept less functional improvement in order to avoid the potential complications of reverse arthroplasty.

Patients with rheumatoid arthritis are also more prone to intraoperative fractures of the humeral shaft during exposure; care must be taken to avoid forced rotational manipulation of the shoulder in these patients, giving consideration to the so-called "anteromedial approach" (chapter 3, Surgical Exposures) to facilitate dislocation and avoid fracture. Cemented fixation of the humeral component may also be required in patients with severe osteopenia.

Avascular Necrosis

Hemiarthroplasty is the procedure of choice for patients with no glenoid involvement. Most patients give consent for both hemiarthroplasty and total shoulder arthroplasty prior to surgery, in case glenoid damage assessed at the time of surgery is worse than expected. A subset of patients with AVN develops a marked inflammatory response after shoulder arthroplasty with a tendency for stiffness. Since the rotator cuff is typically very well preserved in patients

with AVN, most surgeons tend to downsize the humeral head slightly to guarantee motion (100).

Posttraumatic Conditions

Posttraumatic AVN and posttraumatic osteoarthritis have already been discussed. As a general rule, for patients with retained humeral hardware and complications after trauma, it is only wise to remove hardware that is in the way. The development of shorter stems, stemless prostheses, and resurfacing arthroplasty allow the surgeon to leave some hardware in place, removing only those screws that are in the way (Figure 9.52). When hardware needs to be removed at the time of arthroplasty, another important consideration is to fully dislocate the joint prior to removing the hardware. Otherwise, stress risers (left after hardware removal) can facilitate intraoperative fracture when the shoulder is being rotated externally during exposure and dislocation.

Nonunion

Isolated nonunions of the surgical neck or the greater tuberosity may be considered for internal fixation with bone grafting, provided that the articular cartilage is

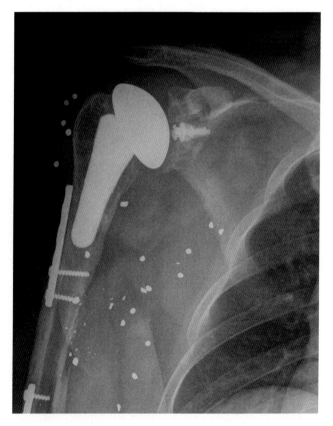

Figure 9.52 *Short stems allow joint replacement with only partial removal of hardware.*

well preserved and the remaining bone stock is reasonable enough to allow fixation. Hemiarthroplasty has been associated with a relatively high rate of unsatisfactory results secondary to tuberosity or cuff dysfunction (101). This is especially true when the tuberosities are osteotomized and then fixed around the hemiarthroplasty. Currently, most surgeons prefer reverse shoulder arthroplasty for those nonunions not amenable to internal fixation for these reasons (102). As in acute fractures, reconstruction of the tuberosities should still be attempted when reverse arthroplasty is performed for nonunion. In cases with severe bone loss, consideration should be given to reconstruction with an allograft-prosthetic composite or a tumor prosthesis; otherwise, the functional results and dislocation rate may be unacceptable (103).

Malunion

Isolated malunions of the greater tuberosity can be treated with osteotomy or tuberoplasty and cuff repair. More complex malunions involving the head segment can also be considered for osteotomy, but the rate of complications is high. When the articular cartilage also is compromised, anatomic and reverse arthroplasties are oftentimes considered.

Hemiarthroplasty can be successful if the humeral head replacement can be positioned in such a way that it restores the head-greater tuberosity distance without a tuberosity osteotomy. If the glenoid cartilage is relatively well preserved, a hemiarthroplasty may be all that is required. On the other hand, it may be impossible to reconstruct severe distortion of the anatomy of the proximal humerus properly with anatomic components, and many surgeons currently favor reverse arthroplasty, especially for older patients (102,104).

Locked Dislocations

Most chronic anterior and posterior shoulder dislocations are associated with an impaction fracture of the humeral head (see chapter 4, Proximal Humerus Fractures) (12). Once reduction is achieved, smaller nonengaging defects may be ignored; larger defects may require filling the defect with soft tissue (subscapularis anteriorly and infraspinatus posteriorly [so-called "McLaughlin procedure"] and remplissage [see chapter 7, Shoulder Instability and the Labrum]) or bone. When defects involve more than 40% to 50% of the head segment, or for long-standing dislocations with damaged articular cartilage, arthroplasty is favored.

Arthroplasty for locked dislocations can be difficult to perform. Exposure can be a challenge, and (after some time) the proximal humerus and the glenoid develop disuse osteopenia. In addition, the glenoid rim may be worn anteriorly (anterior dislocations) or posteriorly (posterior dislocations), leaving less bone stock for support of the glenoid component and making hemiarthroplasty more prone to instability. In anterior dislocations, detachment of the conjoined tendon (with or without the tip of the coracoid) may aid in exposure and avoid injury to the brachial plexus or brachial vessels. In posterior dislocations, it is critical to perform an extensive release of the inferior capsule and use a bone hook to displace the proximal humerus laterally before rotating the humerus into the reduced position. Hemiarthroplasty can be a successful option, but patients should give consent for a total shoulder arthroplasty (in case the glenoid cartilage is worse than expected) and for a reverse arthroplasty (in case the soft tissues cannot be balanced properly or intraoperative tuberosity fractures occur).

Infection

Spontaneous acute septic arthritis of the glenohumeral joint is relatively uncommon and tends to affect elderly individuals with substantial comorbidities. Arthroscopic débridement and lavage followed by antibiotic treatment can be successful in a large number of patients, although the concern always remains about the possibility of dormant osteomyelitis that could be reactivated at any time (15).

Patients with more chronic infections, especially those complicating surgery and leading to marked destruction of the articular cartilage, are oftentimes considered for 2-stage joint replacement surgery (67–69). In the first surgery, the humeral head is resected, the glenoid is reamed (if needed), an antibiotic-loaded cement spacer is placed, and a program of intravenous antibiotic therapy is initiated based on the results of cultures and sensitivities (⊙ Video 9.4). After 6 weeks of intravenous antibiotic therapy, antibiotics are discontinued for 2 to 4 additional weeks and implantation of shoulder arthroplasty components is then performed as a second surgery, provided all indicators show that the infection is resolved. Reverse arthroplasty has become increasingly popular in the second stage, since the previous infection commonly compromises the integrity of the rotator cuff to some extent.

Single-stage joint replacement for glenohumeral infections remains controversial in the United States. The introduction of reverse arthroplasty has made it more attractive because reverse replacement allows for more aggressive soft-tissue débridement.

Extremely frail patients may be considered for a permanent resection arthroplasty, which typically solves the infection clinically but is associated with mediocre pain relief and function. Arthrodesis may be considered for the very young patient, those with compromised deltoid function, or those unwilling to consider the potential for recurrence of infection.

Neuropathic Arthropathy

Classically, neuropathic arthropathy has been considered a contraindication for reconstructive orthopedic surgery (19). The nature of this condition makes any attempt to reconstruct the shoulder joint more likely to fail. Every effort should be made to treat these patients nonoperatively, with activity modifications and pain management modalities. Underlying conditions (e.g., uncontrolled diabetes mellitus) also should be identified and addressed accordingly.

For patients with severe pain and dysfunction despite control of their underlying disease and pain management modalities, I have considered shoulder arthroplasty selectively with reasonable outcomes. In addition, arthrodesis and resection arthroplasty are always considered in the decision-making process, although the rate of successful arthrodesis is likely decreased in patients with neuropathic arthropathy. Most patients are not candidates for anatomic total shoulder arthroplasty, based not only on their bone abnormalities but also on their soft-tissue insufficiencies. Hemiarthroplasty and reverse arthroplasty have been somewhat successful in the management of these patients, although the mechanical failure rate is expected to be higher than for other conditions.

When arthroplasty is considered, every effort is made to determine whether the underlying condition is stable and neuropathic damage is no longer progressive. Special attention needs to be paid to those individuals presenting with an inflammatory component since (as discussed before) it could be due to the nature of Charcot arthropathy; but it could also represent superinfection. Workup for infection in these circumstances is mandatory prior to considering any type of surgical intervention.

Complex Surgery and Revision Surgery

Revision shoulder arthroplasty and complex reconstructive surgery represent a major portion of my practice. All principles regarding arthritic conditions and shoulder arthroplasty discussed throughout this chapter need to be applied when complex surgery and revision surgery are considered. Most of the time, management of bone loss on the humeral side, the glenoid side, or both is paramount for the successful surgical management of these patients.

Revision Shoulder Arthroplasty: General Principles

The evaluation of patients with persistent pain and poor function after shoulder arthroplasty requires a systematic approach in order to identify the reason or reasons for a poor outcome and to formulate a successful treatment plan (105). Understanding the nature of the pathologic features of each particular shoulder prior to the index arthroplasty is paramount. If possible, imaging studies

---

Table 9.8 • Evaluation Checklist for Patient With Failed Shoulder Arthroplasty

Pain and dysfunction
Pain score
Subjective shoulder value
Pain plotted over time

Previous skin incision(s)

Motion and strength testing

Assessment of stability

Plain radiographs
Sequential radiographs
Fluoroscopically positioned radiographs
Radiographs of both humeri with magnifier markers (reverse TSA)

CT with intra-articular contrast (arthro-CT)
Cuff tears, atrophy and fatty infiltration
Component fixation (glenoid)
Bone loss

MRI with metal suppression
Soft tissue integrity
Component version

Ultrasonography

Bone scan

EMG

Arthroscopic evaluation
Biopsies for culture (infection)
Cuff integrity
Component fixation

The question of infection
Symptoms and signs (drainage, redness, fever, chills)
Did your surgeon treat you with antibiotics after surgery?
Pain at rest, severe unexplained pain
Radiographic findings (humeral loosening)
Blood markers (CBC, ESR, CRP)
Aspiration
   Cell count
   Culture
   Other markers (interlekukins, α-defensin)
Arthroscopy for biopsies
Cultures and pathology at the time of surgery

Abbreviations: CBC, complete blood count; CRP, C-reactive protein; CT, computed tomography; EMG, electromyography; ESR, erythrocyte sedimentation rate; MRI, magnetic resonance imaging; TSA, total shoulder arthroplasty.

(i.e., radiographs, CT, and MRI) obtained before the primary procedure should be reviewed. In addition, the operative report and all clinical notes should be reviewed. Table 9.8 summarizes the evaluation of patients with a failed shoulder arthroplasty.

Patients should be questioned carefully about pain, function, and their postoperative course. What is their average pain level? What is their subjective shoulder value? Is pain present all the time and at night, or is it mostly related to activity? Was there a short or long period of time when pain was much better or absent, or has pain been present ever since the time of the index arthroplasty? Were there any complications identified by the referring physician after surgery? Was there drainage, redness, fever, or chills after surgery? Were antibiotics prescribed? Have there been any injuries after surgery?

Physical examination should assess the location and status of the previous skin incision(s), areas of muscular atrophy (deltoid, rotator cuff), active and passive motion, strength, skin sensation (especially in the territory of the axillary nerve), and evidence of gross instability or subscapularis failure (excessive passive external rotation, positive belly press, and bear hug tests).

Plain radiographs are extremely helpful in the evaluation of the failed shoulder arthroplasty. It is useful to review the clinical evaluation, preoperative imaging studies, and operative report of the index procedure. Radiographs obtained after surgery should be assessed for component position and fixation. Sequential radiographs are especially helpful to assess component migration and oftentimes are the only indicator of glenoid failure after anatomical shoulder arthroplasty. As mentioned previously, fluoroscopically positioned radiographs are necessary to assess the shoulder after arthroplasty for radiolucent lines. Radiographs should also be evaluated for component version, especially in patients with prosthetic instability. Fluoroscopy can be extremely useful in evaluating humeral component version. What position of the forearm is necessary to obtain a perfectly perpendicular view of the humeral head-neck interface? Radiographs of both humeri with magnifier markers are particularly useful in the assessment of the unstable reverse shoulder arthroplasty.

Advanced imaging studies may be necessary in the evaluation of failed shoulder arthroplasty. CT is frequently obtained to assess bone loss and remaining bone stock in preparation for revision shoulder arthroplasty. Intra-articular contrast is useful when cuff tears or component loosening are suspected, but they are not required routinely. MRI with metal suppression may help in assessment of cuff integrity and component version. Ultrasonography may also be useful in assessment of cuff integrity. Bone scan is considered for patients with unexplained pain despite a thorough workup, whereas EMG with NCS is considered for patients with evidence of associated nerve dysfunction on physical examination.

In my practice, all patients referred for revision surgery undergo a basic workup for infection, including complete blood count, erythrocyte sedimentation rate, CRP, and aspiration of joint fluid for cultures and cell count. I realize that the yield of these tests for deep periprosthetic shoulder infections is low; however, it is not nonexistent. If an infection is identified and sensitivities are obtained preoperatively, that information is priceless for patient management (106).

When the index of suspicion for infection is high and all preoperative studies for infection are negative, I discuss the possibility of diagnostic arthroscopy with my patients (Figure 9.53) (28). The diagnostic yield of culturing biopsies obtained arthroscopically is much better, and arthroscopy allows direct visual assessment of the rotator cuff, the biceps tendon if still present, and fixation of the glenoid component. In addition, I favor sending tissue samples for pathologic assessment and culture in all patients undergoing revision shoulder arthroplasty at the time of the revision procedure (106).

Table 9.9 summarizes treatment options for the most common failure mechanisms after anatomic arthroplasty

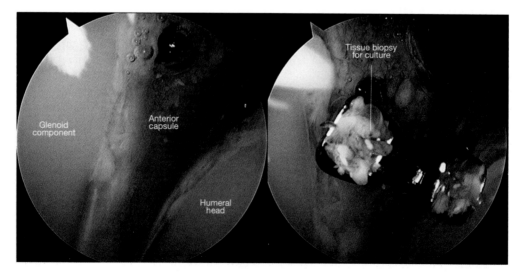

Figure 9.53 *Diagnostic arthroscopy to obtain tissue samples for cultures in a patient with a high index of suspicion for infection after shoulder arthroplasty.*

Table 9.9 • Surgical Management of the Failed Shoulder Arthroplasty

Failure Mechanism	Surgical Management Options
Symptomatic glenoid erosion in hemiarthroplasty	Revision to an anatomic or reverse shoulder arthroplasty

Glenoid loosening	Revision surgery
	Conversion to hemiarthroplasty
	  Arthroscopic
	  Open
	Revision using an anatomic or reverse prosthesis

Humeral loosening	Revision
Instability and cuff failure after anatomical arthroplasty	Revision to a reverse Rarely, cuff repair ± component revision
Instability after reverse arthroplasty	Closed reduction Revision surgery
Periprosthetic fractures	Conservative treatment, ORIF, or revision surgery depending on fracture location and component fixation
Deep infection	One-stage reimplantation Two-stage reimplantation Arthrodesis Permanent resection
Fractures of the acromion and spine of the scapula after reverse arthroplasty	Nonoperative treatment vs excision vs. ORIF
Stiffness	Arthroscopic capsular release Component revision with open contracture release

Abbreviation: ORIF, open reduction internal fixation.

and reverse shoulder arthroplasty. Most of these mechanisms and treatment options have been reviewed in my description of complications of anatomic and reverse shoulder arthroplasty. Techniques to remove components safely, implant revision components, and manage bone loss are common themes in revision shoulder arthroplasty.

Component Removal, Humeral Revision, and Management of Humeral Bone Loss

Humeral Component Removal

Grossly loose humeral components are removed easily. Removal of retained cement is more difficult with failed cemented components, and I attempt complete removal of all retained cement only in the presence of infection. Removal of well-fixed humeral components is very different depending on the extent of the fixation. Proximally fixed, cementless prostheses can be removed relatively easily with minimal bone loss, whereas removal of well-fixed cemented stems or fully textured cementless stems oftentimes require special maneuvers and may lead to substantial bone loss. Care must be taken to avoid an uncontrolled fracture of the greater tuberosity or the humeral shaft at the time of component removal.

I proceed with component removal in a stepwise fashion (Figure 9.54). Once the humeral head prosthesis is removed, access to the component interface is gained and a thin bur (pencil tip or router bur) is used circumferentially to free up the proximal interface; osteotomes may be used when fixation extends distally. Once reasonable release has been achieved, use of slap-hammer extractors or a square-tip impactor are oftentimes successful.

If the aforementioned strategy is unsuccessful, a corticotomy is my next step. Longitudinal division of the anterior cortex of the humeral diaphysis (along part or the whole length of the prosthesis) has to be performed, bearing in mind that it may need to be converted to a window. Corticotomies are particularly useful for removal of well-fixed cemented humeral components. A microsagittal saw is used to divide both bone and cement along the whole extent of the prosthesis; the split is carefully dilated with osteotomes and, often, the stem can then be removed, though most of the cement remains in place. When corticotomies are unsuccessful, a medial or anterior window is the next step to provide better access to the component interface. Care must be taken during component removal and arm manipulation once a corticotomy or window has been performed because both act as stress risers and can facilitate an uncontrolled catastrophic humeral shaft fracture.

Humeral Revision Options

Once the humeral component is removed, implantation of the revision humeral component should be planned (⊙ Video 9.5). Long-stemmed, cemented components

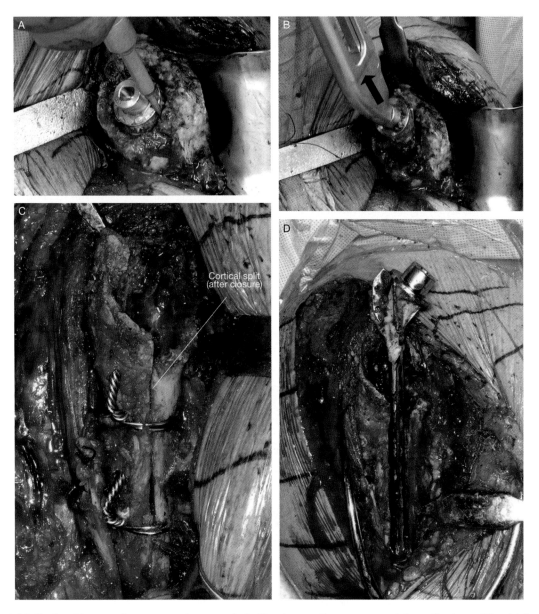

Figure 9.54 *Methods of humeral component removal.* **A,** *Freeing up the component from the top with a high-speed bur.* **B,** *Extractor/impactor.* **C,** *Cortical split.* **D,** *Cortical window.*

have commonly been used in the revision setting, a concept borrowed from hip arthroplasty, trying to obtain fixation in new bone. My preference is to avoid this revision strategy whenever possible because removal of cement from the whole humeral shaft is so difficult, should it become necessary. When the humeral bone stock is reasonable, I try to implant a regular-length, proximally coated, cementless humeral component. Fixation is usually achieved by a combination of distal diaphyseal fit and a wider implant proximally, oftentimes combined with impacted cancellous allograft chips. When fixation with a cementless, regular-length component is not anticipated to work or in patients with retained bone cement, I favor cementing a regular-length component in the patient's

native bone or on the layer of retained cement (i.e., cement within cement fixation).

Management of Bone Loss

Marked proximal humerus bone loss may be faced in revision surgery, after segmental resection of tumors, or in certain posttraumatic conditions. An insufficient proximal humerus creates a number of problems: the area of metaphyseal fixation—best for fixation of modern humeral components—is compromised; the attachment sites of the rotator cuff are gone; and the lack of proximal humerus results in loss of offset and deltoid detensioning (107). It is tempting to place the humeral component deeper into the humeral canal in these cases, which would detension the deltoid further (Figure 9.55A). In these circumstances, consideration should be given to allograft reconstruction of the proximal humerus or implantation of a tumor prosthesis with a relatively bulky proximal humeral body (▣ Video 9.6). Since the attachment sites of the rotator cuff are compromised, reverse prostheses are favored.

Allograft-Prosthetic Composites
In this type of reconstruction, a prosthesis is cemented into a structural humeral allograft, and this composite is fixed to the patient's remaining humerus (Figure 9.55B, C) (108). My preference is to bypass the host-graft junction with the cemented stem only when the length of the allograft is shorter than the stem of the prosthesis. Compression plating across the host-graft junction is paramount to achieve a stable construct, promote union, and decrease bone resorption. An allograft-prosthetic composite offers a number of benefits: 1) length is restored, 2) the component gains vertical and rotational stability in good quality allograft, 3) the deltoid is tensioned properly, and 4) repair of the patient's

cuff to the allograft cuff provides additional stability and the potential for active external rotation.

Tumor Prostheses
In this type of reconstruction, the prostheses are fixed to the remaining diaphysis and have proximal metal bodies to restore length and offset (Figure 9.56). This reconstruction is technically much less demanding than allograft-prosthetic composites; however, the bodies of current tumor prostheses do not tension the deltoid laterally as much as an allograft. In addition, the chances of component loosening are increased due to cantilever bending; the length of unsupported prosthesis can be equal to or longer than the portion fixed into bone. Some tumor prostheses offer areas of porous metal to serve as attachment sites for soft tissues, but the rate of successful tendon-to-metal healing is largely unknown. At this point, comparative studies between allograft-prosthetic composites and tumor prostheses are missing in the field of shoulder arthroplasty.

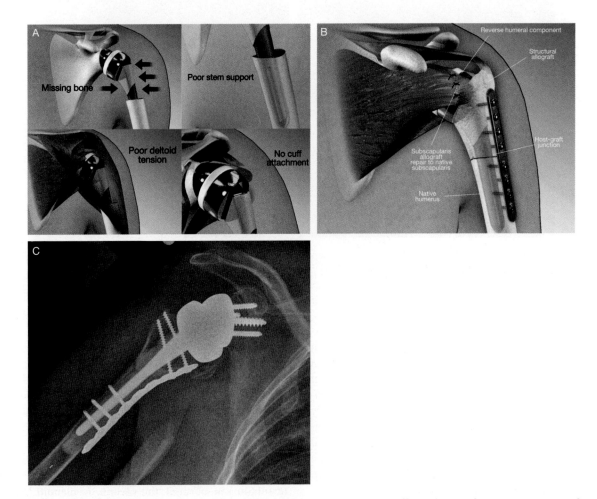

Figure 9.55 **A,** *Adverse consequences of proximal humerus bone loss.* **B,** *Allograft prosthetic composite schematic.* **C,** *Allograft prosthetic composite radiograph.*

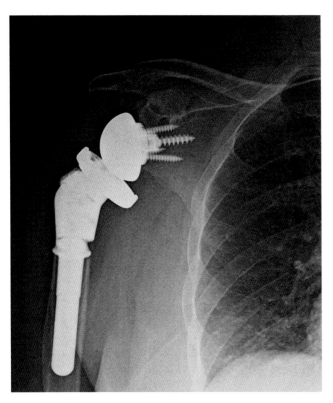

Figure 9.56 Revision reverse arthroplasty using a compo-nent with metal replacement of the proximal humerus.

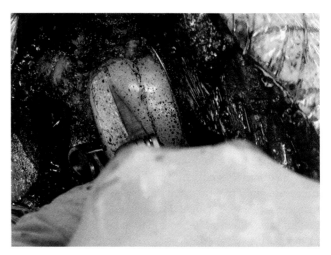

Figure 9.57 Well-fixed glenoid components are best removed in separate segments using a microsaggital saw to divide the face of the component.

Glenoid Component Removal, Glenoid Revision, and Management of Glenoid Bone Loss

Component Removal

Loose glenoid components are removed easily. If cement was used for fixation in these circumstances, often it is fragmented and easy to remove; burs can be used to remove any retained, well-fixed cement.

Removal of a well-fixed, cemented, all polyethylene gle-noid component is best performed by cutting the compo-nent in situ with a microsagittal saw (Figure 9.57). Prying the component out with an osteotome is tempting, but often-times the component does not come out and, on the contrary, the soft glenoid bone underneath gets crushed. A microsagit-tal saw can be used to divide the polyethylene component in segments that can be removed separately. Modern hybrid components can be removed in a similar way, but the central ingrowth portion needs to be removed using a trephine.

Removal of well-fixed, cementless, anatomic or reverse components may be more cumbersome and could lead to substantial bone loss. The modular polyethylene or gleno-sphere are removed first. All screws are removed next. If possible, dedicated extractors are used to back out the base-plate. When that maneuver is unsuccessful, use of curved osteotomes, a 90° angled microsagittal saw, or a pencil tip bur can be considered.

Not uncommonly, glenoid bone loss is not contained at least in portions of the anterior and posterior wall. Thick fibrous tissue, however, surrounds the glenoid vault; it should be preserved to provide some containment for bone grafting procedures when performed.

Glenoid Revision Options

Implantation of a new, cemented, all-polyethylene glenoid component was the only available revision option until the reverse prosthesis was popularized (75). Oftentimes, there is a substantial central defect after removal of the failed component and fibrous tissue, and keeled components tend to fit best in this situation; however, the long-term results of cemented fixation of polyethylene components in the revision setting have not been very successful. Implantation of an anatomic glenoid component may also cause concern in the setting of associated cuff insufficiency or marked tissue imbalance that could lead to edge load-ing, wear, and loosening.

Reverse arthroplasty is more and more commonly considered in the revision setting not so much to com-pensate for the rotator cuff but mostly to provide better glenoid fixation (105). The use of multiple locking com-pression screws at different angles can provide very good implant stability in the face of compromised glenoid bone stock. It also facilitates bone grafting under compression. It is important to achieve a minimum amount of contact between the ingrowth surfaces of the component and native bone; the threshold value has not been defined com-pletely, but I aim for at least 50% contact with native bone. Components with longer central ingrowth posts may be useful in these circumstances.

Management of Glenoid Bone Loss

In some circumstances, the severity of glenoid bone loss and the poor quality of the remaining bone stock are such that safe implantation of another glenoid component is not feasible. In these circumstances, the failed total shoulder arthroplasty is converted to a hemiarthroplasty by packing morselized cancellous bone graft tightly, sometimes using a reamer in a reverse direction. Over time, some of this bone incorporates and some resorbs. Pain relief seems to be less predictable with revision to a hemiarthroplasty as opposed to anatomic or reverse total shoulder arthroplasty, and there are reports of patients treated operatively once the bone graft on the glenoid has incorporated in order to implant a glenoid component.

Cancellous allograft chips are used mostly to deal with contained defects. Structural autograft or allograft may be required in larger segmental defects that are contained or uncontained. Bone grafts seem to incorporate more reliably in the setting of reverse arthroplasty (109). For very large defects, autograft (typically from the iliac crest) is needed to avoid having most of the reverse baseplate sitting on allograft (⊙ Video 9.7). In some circumstances, it may be best to stage the surgery: in the first procedure the bone graft and baseplate implantation are performed. The rest of the arthroplasty is not completed in order to allow for graft incorporation under no stress. Once the graft is thought to have healed (typically 3 months), the glenosphere and humeral component are implanted in a second procedure.

KEY POINTS

✓ Multiple conditions can lead to progressive glenohumeral joint degeneration; each presents with specific pathologic abnormalities that need to be taken into account at the time of surgical management.

✓ Most arthritic conditions can be evaluated properly with a careful physical examination and plain radiographs; however, CT has become extremely useful when shoulder arthroplasty is considered, and its value increases further with computer planning.

✓ Many arthritic conditions can be managed initially with activity modifications, pharmacologic agents, and occasional intra-articular corticosteroid injections; arthroplasty should be avoided for 2 to 3 months after an intra-articular corticosteroid injection to decrease the risk of periprosthetic infection.

✓ The main limiting factor for the long-term survival of anatomic shoulder arthroplasty is glenoid component failure. Careful implant selection, surgical technique, and postoperative protection all translate into longer lasting arthroplasties.

✓ Patterns of soft-tissue imbalance and glenoid bone loss are now recognized as critical in the evaluation of shoulders considered for arthroplasty and the decision-making process between anatomic and reverse arthroplasties.

✓ Reverse arthroplasty provides a fixed fulcrum and improved deltoid function. Available implants provide various options regarding the center of rotation (medial or lateral) and sizing of the glenoid component as well as humeral component opening angle, lateralization, and version. Initially introduced for the management of cuff tear arthropathy, the indications of reverse arthroplasty have expanded substantially.

✓ Reverse arthroplasty may lead to decreased internal rotation. Improvements in external rotation may require adding tendon transfers to the procedure in patients with no intact posterior cuff.

✓ Surgical management of arthritic shoulder conditions may include arthroscopic débridement or synovectomy, hemiarthroplasty, anatomic total shoulder arthroplasty, reverse shoulder arthroplasty. and rarely salvage with arthrodesis or permanent resection.

✓ *Cutibacterium acnes* (formerly, *Propionibacterium acnes*) is particularly common in periprosthetic shoulder infections. Since these bacteria generate a low-grade infection, the diagnosis may be elusive and sometimes can be confirmed only with cultures of tissue samples obtained at the time of revision surgery or arthroscopy.

✓ Revision of failed shoulder arthroplasty components requires dedicated techniques for safe component removal and reconstruction of missing bone on the humeral or glenoid side.

Acknowledgment

Portions previously published in Sanchez-Sotelo J. Elbow rheumatoid elbow: surgical treatment options. Curr Rev Musculoskelet Med. 2016 Jun;9(2):224–31. Used with permission.

REFERENCES

1. Sanchez-Sotelo J. Shoulder arthroplasty. Rosemont (IL): American Academy of Orthopedic Surgeons; c2012. 122 p.
2. Sanchez-Sotelo J. Total shoulder arthroplasty. Open Orthop J. 2011 Mar 16;5:106–14.
3. Young AA, Walch G, Pape G, Gohlke F, Favard L. Secondary rotator cuff dysfunction following total shoulder arthroplasty for primary glenohumeral osteoarthritis: results of a multicenter study with more than five years of follow-up. J Bone Joint Surg Am. 2012 Apr 18;94(8):685–93.
4. Walch G, Badet R, Boulahia A, Khoury A. Morphologic study of the glenoid in primary glenohumeral osteoarthritis. J Arthroplasty. 1999 Sep;14(6):756–60.
5. Wirth MA, Lyons FR, Rockwood CA Jr. Hypoplasia of the glenoid: a review of sixteen patients. J Bone Joint Surg Am. 1993 Aug;75(8):1175–84.
6. Smith SP, Bunker TD. Primary glenoid dysplasia: a review of 12 patients. J Bone Joint Surg Br. 2001 Aug;83(6):868–72.
7. Sperling JW, Cofield RH, Steinmann SP. Shoulder arthroplasty for osteoarthritis secondary to glenoid dysplasia. J Bone Joint Surg Am. 2002 Apr;84-A(4):541–6.

8. Anthony S, Munk R, Skakun W, Masini M. Multiple epiphyseal dysplasia. J Am Acad Orthop Surg. 2015 Mar;23(3):164–72. Epub 2015 Feb 9. Erratum in: J Am Acad Orthop Surg. 2015 Apr;23(4):266.

9. Neer CS 2nd, Craig EV, Fukuda H. Cuff-tear arthropathy. J Bone Joint Surg Am. 1983 Dec;65(9):1232–44.

10. Chen AL, Joseph TN, Zuckerman JD. Rheumatoid arthritis of the shoulder. J Am Acad Orthop Surg. 2003 Jan-Feb;11(1):12–24.

11. Hattrup SJ, Cofield RH. Osteonecrosis of the humeral head: relationship of disease stage, extent, and cause to natural history. J Shoulder Elbow Surg. 1999 Nov-Dec;8(6):559–64.

12. Boileau P, Trojani C, Walch G, Krishnan SG, Romeo A, Sinnerton R. Shoulder arthroplasty for the treatment of the sequelae of fractures of the proximal humerus. J Shoulder Elbow Surg. 2001 Jul-Aug;10(4):299–308.

13. Plath JE, Aboalata M, Seppel G, Juretzko J, Waldt S, Vogt S, et al. Prevalence of and risk factors for dislocation arthropathy: radiological long-term outcome of arthroscopic bankart repair in 100 shoulders at an average 13-year follow-up. Am J Sports Med. 2015 May;43(5):1084–90. Epub 2015 Mar 2.

14. Scheffel PT, Clinton J, Lynch JR, Warme WJ, Bertelsen AL, Matsen FA 3rd. Glenohumeral chondrolysis: a systematic review of 100 cases from the English language literature. J Shoulder Elbow Surg. 2010 Sep;19(6):944–9. Epub 2010 Apr 24.

15. Abdel MP, Perry KI, Morrey ME, Steinmann SP, Sperling JW, Cass JR. Arthroscopic management of native shoulder septic arthritis. J Shoulder Elbow Surg. 2013 Mar;22(3):418–21. Epub 2012 Jun 27.

16. Warme WJ, Hsu JE. Definition of a "true" periprosthetic shoulder infection still eludes us. J Bone Joint Surg Am. 2015 Jul 15;97(14):e56.

17. Horneff JG, Hsu JE, Huffman GR. Propionibacterium acnes infections in shoulder surgery. Orthop Clin North Am. 2014 Oct;45(4):515–21. Epub 2014 Jul 11.

18. Edison J, Finger DR. Neuropathic osteoarthropathy of the shoulder. J Clin Rheumatol. 2005 Dec;11(6):333–4.

19. Hatzis N, Kaar TK, Wirth MA, Toro F, Rockwood CA Jr. Neuropathic arthropathy of the shoulder. J Bone Joint Surg Am. 1998 Sep;80(9):1314–9.

20. Boileau P, Chuinard C, Roussanne Y, Bicknell RT, Rochet N, Trojani C. Reverse shoulder arthroplasty combined with a modified latissimus dorsi and teres major tendon transfer for shoulder pseudoparalysis associated with dropping arm. Clin Orthop Relat Res. 2008 Mar;466(3):584–93. Epub 2008 Jan 25.

21. Goodman SM. Rheumatoid arthritis: perioperative management of biologics and DMARDs. Semin Arthritis Rheum. 2015 Jun;44(6):627–32. Epub 2015 Jan 30.

22. Wright J, Potts C, Smyth MP, Ferrara L, Sperling JW, Throckmorton TW. A quantitative analysis of the effect of baseplate and glenosphere position on deltoid lengthening in reverse total shoulder arthroplasty. Int J Shoulder Surg. 2015 Apr-Jun;9(2):33–7.

23. Hattrup SJ, Sanchez-Sotelo J, Sperling JW, Cofield RH. Reverse shoulder replacement for patients with inflammatory arthritis. J Hand Surg Am. 2012 Sep;37(9):1888–94. Epub 2012 Jun 30.

24. Iannotti JP, Weiner S, Rodriguez E, Subhas N, Patterson TE, Jun BJ, et al. Three-dimensional imaging and templating improve glenoid implant positioning. J Bone Joint Surg Am. 2015 Apr 15;97(8):651–8.

25. Walch G, Vezeridis PS, Boileau P, Deransart P, Chaoui J. Three-dimensional planning and use of patient-specific guides improve glenoid component position: an in vitro study. J Shoulder Elbow Surg. 2015 Feb;24(2):302–9. Epub 2014 Aug 31.

26. Frangiamore SJ, Saleh A, Kovac MF, Grosso MJ, Zhang X, Bauer TW, et al. Synovial fluid interleukin-6 as a predictor of periprosthetic shoulder infection. J Bone Joint Surg Am. 2015 Jan 7;97(1):63–70.

27. Frangiamore SJ, Saleh A, Grosso MJ, Kovac MF, Higuera CA, Iannotti JP, et al. α-Defensin as a predictor of periprosthetic shoulder infection. J Shoulder Elbow Surg. 2015 Jul;24(7):1021–7. Epub 2015 Feb 8.

28. Dilisio MF, Miller LR, Warner JJ, Higgins LD. Arthroscopic tissue culture for the evaluation of periprosthetic shoulder infection. J Bone Joint Surg Am. 2014 Dec 3;96(23):1952–8.

29. Millett PJ, Gobezie R, Boykin RE. Shoulder osteoarthritis: diagnosis and management. Am Fam Physician. 2008 Sep 1;78(5):605–11.

30. Kwon YW, Eisenberg G, Zuckerman JD. Sodium hyaluronate for the treatment of chronic shoulder pain associated with glenohumeral osteoarthritis: a multicenter, randomized, double-blind, placebo-controlled trial. J Shoulder Elbow Surg. 2013 May;22(5):584–94. Epub 2013 Jan 16.

31. Cunnington J, Marshall N, Hide G, Bracewell C, Isaacs J, Platt P, et al. A randomized, double-blind, controlled study of ultrasound-guided corticosteroid injection into the joint of patients with inflammatory arthritis. Arthritis Rheum. 2010 Jul;62(7):1862–9.

32. Amin NH, Omiyi D, Kuczynski B, Cushner FD, Scuderi GR. The risk of a deep infection associated with intraarticular injections before a total knee arthroplasty. J Arthroplasty. 2016 Jan;31(1):240–4. Epub 2015 Aug 20.

33. Denard PJ, Walch G. Current concepts in the surgical management of primary glenohumeral arthritis with a biconcave glenoid. J Shoulder Elbow Surg. 2013 Nov;22(11):1589–98. Epub 2013 Sep 3.

34. Iannotti JP, Gabriel JP, Schneck SL, Evans BG, Misra S. The normal glenohumeral relationships: an anatomical study of one hundred and forty shoulders. J Bone Joint Surg Am. 1992 Apr;74(4):491–500.

35. Pearl ML, Volk AG. Coronal plane geometry of the proximal humerus relevant to prosthetic arthroplasty. J Shoulder Elbow Surg. 1996 Jul-Aug;5(4):320–6.

36. Boileau P, Walch G. The three-dimensional geometry of the proximal humerus. Implications for surgical technique and prosthetic design. J Bone Joint Surg Br. 1997 Sep;79(5):857–65.

37. Robertson DD, Yuan J, Bigliani LU, Flatow EL, Yamaguchi K. Three-dimensional analysis of the proximal part of the humerus: relevance to arthroplasty. J Bone Joint Surg Am. 2000 Nov;82-A(11):1594–602.

38. Walch G, Boileau P. Prosthetic adaptability: a new concept for shoulder arthroplasty. J Shoulder Elbow Surg. 1999 Sep-Oct;8(5):443–51.

39. Walch G, Mesiha M, Boileau P, Edwards TB, Levigne C, Moineau G, et al. Three-dimensional assessment of the dimensions of the osteoarthritic glenoid. Bone Joint J. 2013 Oct;95-B(10):1377–82.

40. Ho JC, Sabesan VJ, Iannotti JP. Glenoid component retroversion is associated with osteolysis. J Bone Joint Surg Am. 2013 Jun 19;95(12):e82.

41. Pinkas D, Wiater B, Wiater JM. The glenoid component in anatomic shoulder arthroplasty. J Am Acad Orthop Surg. 2015 May;23(5):317–26. Epub 2015 Mar 31.

42. Papadonikolakis A, Neradilek MB, Matsen FA 3rd. Failure of the glenoid component in anatomic total shoulder arthroplasty: a systematic review of the English-language literature between 2006 and 2012. J Bone Joint Surg Am. 2013 Dec 18;95(24):2205–12.

43. Vavken P, Sadoghi P, von Keudell A, Rosso C, Valderrabano V, Muller AM. Rates of radiolucency and loosening after total shoulder arthroplasty with pegged or keeled glenoid components. J Bone Joint Surg Am. 2013 Feb 6;95(3):215–21.

44. Fox TJ, Cil A, Sperling JW, Sanchez-Sotelo J, Schleck CD, Cofield RH. Survival of the glenoid component in shoulder arthroplasty. J Shoulder Elbow Surg. 2009 Nov-Dec;18(6):859–63. Epub 2009 Mar 17.

45. Walch G, Young AA, Boileau P, Loew M, Gazielly D, Mole D. Patterns of loosening of polyethylene keeled glenoid components after shoulder arthroplasty for primary osteoarthritis: results of a multicenter study with more than five years of follow-up. J Bone Joint Surg Am. 2012 Jan 18;94(2):145–50.

46. Wang T, Abrams GD, Behn AW, Lindsey D, Giori N, Cheung EV. Posterior glenoid wear in total shoulder arthroplasty: eccentric anterior reaming is superior to posterior augment. Clin Orthop Relat Res. 2015 Dec;473(12):3928–36. Epub 2015 Aug 5.

47. Sabesan V, Callanan M, Sharma V, Iannotti JP. Correction of acquired glenoid bone loss in osteoarthritis with a standard versus an augmented glenoid component. J Shoulder Elbow Surg. 2014 Jul;23(7):964–73. Epub 2014 Jan 7.

48. Sabesan V, Callanan M, Ho J, Iannotti JP. Clinical and radiographic outcomes of total shoulder arthroplasty with bone graft for osteoarthritis with severe glenoid bone loss. J Bone Joint Surg Am. 2013 Jul 17;95(14):1290–6.

49. Mizuno N, Denard PJ, Raiss P, Walch G. Reverse total shoulder arthroplasty for primary glenohumeral osteoarthritis in patients with a biconcave glenoid. J Bone Joint Surg Am. 2013 Jul 17;95(14):1297–304.

50. Choi T, Horodyski M, Struk AM, Sahajpal DT, Wright TW. Incidence of early radiolucent lines after glenoid component insertion for total shoulder arthroplasty: a radiographic study comparing pressurized and unpressurized cementing techniques. J Shoulder Elbow Surg. 2013 Mar;22(3):403–8. Epub 2012 Sep 7.

51. Tammachote N, Sperling JW, Vathana T, Cofield RH, Harmsen WS, Schleck CD. Long-term results of cemented metal-backed glenoid components for osteoarthritis of the shoulder. J Bone Joint Surg Am. 2009 Jan;91(1):160–6.

52. Boileau P, Moineau G, Morin-Salvo N, Avidor C, Godeneche A, Levigne C, et al. Metal-backed glenoid implant with polyethylene insert is not a viable long-term therapeutic option. J Shoulder Elbow Surg. 2015 Oct;24(10):1534–43. Epub 2015 Jul 27.

53. Sabesan VJ, Ackerman J, Sharma V, Baker KC, Kurdziel MD, Wiater JM. Glenohumeral mismatch affects micromotion of cemented glenoid components in total shoulder arthroplasty. J Shoulder Elbow Surg. 2015 May;24(5):814–22. Epub 2014 Dec 2.

54. Walch G, Edwards TB, Boulahia A, Boileau P, Mole D, Adeleine P. The influence of glenohumeral prosthetic mismatch on glenoid radiolucent lines: results of a multicenter study. J Bone Joint Surg Am. 2002 Dec;84-A(12):2186–91.

55. van den Bekerom MP, Geervliet PC, Somford MP, van den Borne MP, Boer R. Total shoulder arthroplasty versus hemiarthroplasty for glenohumeral arthritis: a systematic review of the literature at long-term follow-up. Int J Shoulder Surg. 2013 Jul;7(3):110–5.

56. Zarkadas PC, Throckmorton TQ, Dahm DL, Sperling J, Schleck CD, Cofield R. Patient reported activities after shoulder replacement: total and hemiarthroplasty. J Shoulder Elbow Surg. 2011 Mar;20(2):273–80. Epub 2010 Oct 15.

57. Schoch B, Schleck C, Cofield RH, Sperling JW. Shoulder arthroplasty in patients younger than 50 years: minimum 20-year follow-up. J Shoulder Elbow Surg. 2015 May;24(5):705–10. Epub 2014 Oct 8.

58. Puskas GJ, Meyer DC, Lebschi JA, Gerber C. Unacceptable failure of hemiarthroplasty combined with biological glenoid resurfacing in the treatment of glenohumeral arthritis in the young. J Shoulder Elbow Surg. 2015 Dec;24(12):1900–7. Epub 2015 Jul 15.

59. Lapner PL, Sabri E, Rakhra K, Bell K, Athwal GS. Comparison of lesser tuberosity osteotomy to subscapularis peel in shoulder arthroplasty: a randomized controlled trial. J Bone Joint Surg Am. 2012 Dec 19;94(24):2239–46.

60. Shi LL, Jiang JJ, Ek ET, Higgins LD. Failure of the lesser tuberosity osteotomy after total shoulder arthroplasty. J Shoulder Elbow Surg. 2015 Feb;24(2):203–9. Epub 2014 Aug 5.

61. Small KM, Siegel EJ, Miller LR, Higgins LD. Imaging characteristics of lesser tuberosity osteotomy after total shoulder replacement: a study of 220 patients. J Shoulder Elbow Surg. 2014 Sep;23(9):1318–26. Epub 2014 Mar 4.

62. Simmen BR, Bachmann LM, Drerup S, Schwyzer HK, Burkhart A, Flury MP, et al. Usefulness of concomitant biceps tenodesis in total shoulder arthroplasty: a prospective cohort study. J Shoulder Elbow Surg. 2008 Nov-Dec;17(6):921–4. Epub 2008 Sep 24.

63. Fama G, Edwards TB, Boulahia A, Kempf JF, Boileau P, Nemoz C, et al. The role of concomitant biceps tenodesis in shoulder arthroplasty for primary osteoarthritis: results of a multicentric study. Orthopedics. 2004 Apr;27(4):401–5.

64. Wirth MA, Lim MS, Southworth C, Loredo R, Kaar TK, Rockwood CA Jr. Compaction bone-grafting in prosthetic shoulder arthroplasty. J Bone Joint Surg Am. 2007 Jan;89(1):49–57.

65. Sanchez-Sotelo J, Sperling JW, Rowland CM, Cofield RH. Instability after shoulder arthroplasty: results of surgical treatment. J Bone Joint Surg Am. 2003 Apr;85-A(4):622–31.

66. Abdel MP, Hattrup SJ, Sperling JW, Cofield RH, Kreofsky CR, Sanchez-Sotelo J. Revision of an unstable hemiarthroplasty or anatomical total shoulder replacement using a reverse design prosthesis. Bone Joint J. 2013 May;95-B(5):668–72.

67. Singh JA, Sperling JW, Schleck C, Harmsen WS, Cofield RH. Periprosthetic infections after total shoulder arthroplasty: a 33-year perspective. J Shoulder Elbow Surg. 2012 Nov;21(11):1534–41. Epub 2012 Apr 18.

68. Sperling JW, Kozak TK, Hanssen AD, Cofield RH. Infection after shoulder arthroplasty. Clin Orthop Relat Res. 2001 Jan;(382):206–16.

69. Cuff DJ, Virani NA, Levy J, Frankle MA, Derasari A, Hines B, et al. The treatment of deep shoulder infection and glenohumeral instability with debridement, reverse shoulder arthroplasty and postoperative antibiotics. J Bone Joint Surg Br. 2008 Mar;90(3):336–42.

70. Athwal GS, Sperling JW, Rispoli DM, Cofield RH. Periprosthetic humeral fractures during shoulder arthroplasty. J Bone Joint Surg Am. 2009 Mar 1;91(3):594–603.

71. Singh JA, Sperling J, Schleck C, Harmsen W, Cofield R. Periprosthetic fractures associated with primary total shoulder arthroplasty and primary humeral head replacement: a thirty-three-year study. J Bone Joint Surg Am. 2012 Oct 3;94(19):1777–85.

72. Steinmann SP, Cheung EV. Treatment of periprosthetic humerus fractures associated with shoulder arthroplasty. J Am Acad Orthop Surg. 2008 Apr;16(4):199–207.

73. Sassoon AA, Rhee PC, Schleck CD, Harmsen WS, Sperling JW, Cofield RH. Revision total shoulder arthroplasty for painful glenoid arthrosis after humeral head replacement: the nontraumatic shoulder. J Shoulder Elbow Surg. 2012 Nov;21(11):1484–91. Epub 2012 Mar 23.

74. Carroll RM, Izquierdo R, Vazquez M, Blaine TA, Levine WN, Bigliani LU. Conversion of painful hemiarthroplasty to total shoulder arthroplasty: long-term results. J Shoulder Elbow Surg. 2004 Nov-Dec;13(6):599–603.

75. Cheung EV, Sperling JW, Cofield RH. Revision shoulder arthroplasty for glenoid component loosening. J Shoulder Elbow Surg. 2008 May-Jun;17(3):371–5. Epub 2008 Feb 20.

76. Patel DN, Young B, Onyekwelu I, Zuckerman JD, Kwon YW. Reverse total shoulder arthroplasty for failed shoulder arthroplasty. J Shoulder Elbow Surg. 2012 Nov;21(11):1478–83. Epub 2012 Feb 22.

77. Melis B, Bonnevialle N, Neyton L, Levigne C, Favard L, Walch G, et al. Glenoid loosening and failure in anatomical total shoulder arthroplasty: is revision with a reverse shoulder arthroplasty a reliable option? J Shoulder Elbow Surg. 2012 Mar;21(3):342–9. Epub 2011 Nov 1.

78. Berliner JL, Regalado-Magdos A, Ma CB, Feeley BT. Biomechanics of reverse total shoulder arthroplasty. J Shoulder Elbow Surg. 2015 Jan;24(1):150–60. Epub 2014 Oct 29.

79. Sanchez-Sotelo J. Reverse total shoulder arthroplasty. Clin Anat. 2009 Mar;22(2):172–82.

80. Boileau P, Watkinson DJ, Hatzidakis AM, Balg F. Grammont reverse prosthesis: design, rationale, and biomechanics. J Shoulder Elbow Surg. 2005 Jan-Feb;14(1 Suppl S):147S-161S.

81. Walker M, Brooks J, Willis M, Frankle M. How reverse shoulder arthroplasty works. Clin Orthop Relat Res. 2011 Sep;469(9):2440–51.

82. Boileau P, Moineau G, Roussanne Y, O'Shea K. Bony increased-offset reversed shoulder arthroplasty: minimizing scapular impingement while maximizing glenoid fixation. Clin Orthop Relat Res. 2011 Sep;469(9):2558–67.

83. Sabesan V, Callanan M, Sharma V, Wiater JM. Assessment of scapular morphology and surgical technique as predictors of notching in reverse shoulder arthroplasty. Am J Orthop (Belle Mead NJ). 2015 May;44(5):E148–52.

84. Simovitch RW, Helmy N, Zumstein MA, Gerber C. Impact of fatty infiltration of the teres minor muscle on the outcome of reverse total shoulder arthroplasty. J Bone Joint Surg Am. 2007 May;89(5):934–9.

85. Favre P, Loeb MD, Helmy N, Gerber C. Latissimus dorsi transfer to restore external rotation with reverse shoulder arthroplasty: a biomechanical study. J Shoulder Elbow Surg. 2008 Jul-Aug;17(4):650–8. Epub 2008 Apr 21.

86. Hartzler RU, Steen BM, Hussey MM, Cusick MC, Cottrell BJ, Clark RE, et al. Reverse shoulder arthroplasty for massive rotator cuff tear: risk factors for poor functional improvement. J Shoulder Elbow Surg. 2015 Nov;24(11):1698–706. Epub 2015 Jul 11.

87. Edwards TB, Williams MD, Labriola JE, Elkousy HA, Gartsman GM, O'Connor DP. Subscapularis insufficiency and the risk of shoulder dislocation after reverse shoulder arthroplasty. J Shoulder Elbow Surg. 2009 Nov-Dec;18(6):892–6. Epub 2009 Mar 17.

88. Clark JC, Ritchie J, Song FS, Kissenberth MJ, Tolan SJ, Hart ND, et al. Complication rates, dislocation, pain, and postoperative range of motion after reverse shoulder arthroplasty in patients with and without repair of the subscapularis. J Shoulder Elbow Surg. 2012 Jan;21(1):36–41. Epub 2011 Jul 31.

89. Boileau P, Watkinson D, Hatzidakis AM, Hovorka I. Neer Award 2005: the Grammont reverse shoulder prosthesis: results in cuff tear arthritis, fracture sequelae, and revision arthroplasty. J Shoulder Elbow Surg. 2006 Sep-Oct;15(5):527–40.

90. Teusink MJ, Pappou IP, Schwartz DG, Cottrell BJ, Frankle MA. Results of closed management of acute dislocation after reverse shoulder arthroplasty. J Shoulder Elbow Surg. 2015 Apr;24(4):621–7. Epub 2014 Oct 25.

91. Chalmers PN, Rahman Z, Romeo AA, Nicholson GP. Early dislocation after reverse total shoulder arthroplasty. J Shoulder Elbow Surg. 2014 May;23(5):737–44. Epub 2013 Nov 1.

92. Nicholson GP, Strauss EJ, Sherman SL. Scapular notching: Recognition and strategies to minimize clinical impact. Clin Orthop Relat Res. 2011 Sep;469(9):2521–30.

93. Levy JC, Anderson C, Samson A. Classification of postoperative acromial fractures following reverse shoulder arthroplasty. J Bone Joint Surg Am. 2013 Aug 7;95(15):e104.

94. Skelley NW, Namdari S, Chamberlain AM, Keener JD, Galatz LM, Yamaguchi K. Arthroscopic debridement and capsular release for the treatment of shoulder osteoarthritis. Arthroscopy. 2015 Mar;31(3):494–500. Epub 2014 Nov 8.

95. Sayegh ET, Mascarenhas R, Chalmers PN, Cole BJ, Romeo AA, Verma NN. Surgical treatment options for glenohumeral arthritis in young patients: a systematic review and meta-analysis. Arthroscopy. 2015 Jun;31(6):1156–1166.e8. Epub 2014 Dec 25.

96. Spiegl UJ, Faucett SC, Horan MP, Warth RJ, Millett PJ. The role of arthroscopy in the management of glenohumeral osteoarthritis: a Markov decision model. Arthroscopy. 2014 Nov;30(11):1392–9. Epub 2014 Aug 14.

97. Leung B, Horodyski M, Struk AM, Wright TW. Functional outcome of hemiarthroplasty compared with reverse total shoulder arthroplasty in the treatment of rotator cuff tear arthropathy. J Shoulder Elbow Surg. 2012 Mar;21(3):319–23. Epub 2011 Aug 26.

98. Sperling JW, Cofield RH, Schleck CD, Harmsen WS. Total shoulder arthroplasty versus hemiarthroplasty for rheumatoid arthritis of the shoulder: results of 303 consecutive cases. J Shoulder Elbow Surg. 2007 Nov-Dec;16(6):683–90. Epub 2007 Oct 29.

99. Young AA, Smith MM, Bacle G, Moraga C, Walch G. Early results of reverse shoulder arthroplasty in patients with rheumatoid arthritis. J Bone Joint Surg Am. 2011 Oct 19;93(20):1915–23.

100. Schoch BS, Barlow JD, Schleck C, Cofield RH, Sperling JW. Shoulder arthroplasty for post-traumatic osteonecrosis of the humeral head. J Shoulder Elbow Surg. 2016 Mar;25(3):406–12. Epub 2015 Nov 14.

101. Duquin TR, Jacobson JA, Sanchez-Sotelo J, Sperling JW, Cofield RH. Unconstrained shoulder arthroplasty for treatment of proximal humeral nonunions. J Bone Joint Surg Am. 2012 Sep 5;94(17):1610–7.

102. Hattrup SJ, Waldrop R, Sanchez-Sotelo J. Reverse total shoulder arthroplasty for posttraumatic sequelae. J Orthop Trauma. 2016 Feb;30(2):e41–7.

103. Raiss P, Edwards TB, da Silva MR, Bruckner T, Loew M, Walch G. Reverse shoulder arthroplasty for the treatment of nonunions of the surgical neck of the proximal part of the humerus (type-3 fracture sequelae). J Bone Joint Surg Am. 2014 Dec 17;96(24):2070–6.

104. Jacobson JA, Duquin TR, Sanchez-Sotelo J, Schleck CD, Sperling JW, Cofield RH. Anatomic shoulder arthroplasty for treatment of proximal humerus malunions. J Shoulder Elbow Surg. 2014 Aug;23(8):1232–9. Epub 2014 Jan 15.

105. Favard L. Revision of total shoulder arthroplasty. Orthop Traumatol Surg Res. 2013 Feb;99(1 Suppl):S12–21. Epub 2013 Jan 16.

106. Updegrove GF, Armstrong AD, Kim HM. Preoperative and intraoperative infection workup in apparently aseptic revision shoulder arthroplasty. J Shoulder Elbow Surg. 2015 Mar;24(3):491–500. Epub 2014 Dec 2.

107. Stephens SP, Paisley KC, Giveans MR, Wirth MA. The effect of proximal humeral bone loss on revision reverse total shoulder arthroplasty. J Shoulder Elbow Surg. 2015 Oct;24(10):1519–26. Epub 2015 Apr 7.

108. Chacon A, Virani N, Shannon R, Levy JC, Pupello D, Frankle M. Revision arthroplasty with use of a reverse shoulder prosthesis-allograft composite. J Bone Joint Surg Am. 2009 Jan;91(1):119–27.

109. Wagner E, Houdek MT, Griffith T, Elhassan BT, Sanchez-Sotelo J, Sperling JW, et al. Glenoid bone-grafting in revision to a reverse total shoulder arthroplasty. J Bone Joint Surg Am. 2015 Oct 21;97(20):1653–60.

10 The Scapula

Most orthopedic surgeons, and even many shoulder experts, are a little intimidated by the evaluation and management of patients with conditions affecting primarily the scapula, periscapular muscles, and scapulothoracic joint. A number of reasons explain these feelings, including relative unfamiliarity with the anatomy, function, physical examination, and diagnostic categories related to the scapula, as well as the fact that surgical procedures around the scapula are less commonly performed and sometimes not completely understood.

As mentioned in previous chapters of this book, dysfunction of the scapulothoracic joint may play a major role in patients with diverse shoulder conditions (disorders of the clavicle and the acromioclavicular joint, shoulder instability, rotator cuff disease, and others). In addition, the scapulothoracic joint and periscapular muscles may be affected by specific disorders (traumatic muscle avulsions, injuries to various nerves responsible for the function of periscapular muscles, fractures of the scapula and the glenoid cavity, bursitis, osteochondromas, congenital abnormalities, and others). Finally, some patients will present with pain and dysfunction secondary to poor control of the periscapular muscles in the absence of specific structural pathology.

In chapter 1, Evaluation of the Shoulder, we introduced a few basic concepts related to the scapula, including muscles and planes of motion, and observations derived from physical examination, including winging, snapping, scapular dyskinesis, and the evaluation of individual muscle groups involved in the function of the scapulothoracic joint. Consider reviewing the section on the scapula and periscapular muscles in chapter 1, Evaluation of the Shoulder, before diving into the content of this chapter. Table 10.1 summarizes the physical examination of the scapula as described in chapter 1.

There are 3 major impediments for proper assessment of the scapula: patient examination without uncovering the shoulder, examination of the shoulder from the front aspect

Table 10.1 • Physical Examination of the Scapula

Resting position of the scapula
Winging (trapezius and serratus anterior dysfunction most common)
Subtle malpositioning
  Prominence of the inferomedial border
  Coracoid malpositioning
  Tape measurements (compare with opposite side)
    Medial, superior, and inferior scapula to midline
    Coracoid to wall distance (measures pectoralis minor contracture)

Scapular motion
Scapular dyskinesis unmasked by repetitive active arm elevation
Crepitus
Snapping

Specific muscle testing
Serratus
  Winging aggravated by
    Push-ups on a wall
    Low grades of resisted arm elevation
  Weakness in the boxing punch position
Trapezius
  Winging accentuated with resisted abduction or external rotation
  Assess superior (shrug) and middle trapezius (resisted scapular retraction) separately
Rhomboids
  Subtle winging in a patient with no trapezius atrophy and a strong shrug

Scapular repositioning maneuvers
Scapular assistance test (elevation improves)
Scapular retraction test (secondary impingement disappears)

alone, and lack of knowledge regarding scapular conditions. These aspects of the examination are easy to address: get used to examining your patients with their shoulders and scapulae uncovered from the front *and* back. The goal of this chapter is to address the final impediment, insufficient knowledge of scapular conditions.

Brief Focused Review of the Scapulothoracic Musculature

The scapula floats suspended over the chest wall. It is connected to the trunk by the clavicle anteriorly, and by some of the periscapular muscles all around. Smooth adaptations of the relative position of the scapula in space provide a mobile platform for the glenohumeral joint and the rest of the upper extremity. In addition, the scapula provides the take-off point for a number of extremely important muscles for the glenohumeral joint, especially the deltoid and the rotator cuff.

How would you build this adaptable, mobile platform if you were to design it from scratch? You would need strong ligamentous connections between the scapula and the anterior clavicular struts. You would then need muscles to fine tune the position of the scapula in space in all directions. These muscles were summarized in chapter 1, Evaluation of the Shoulder, Table 1.7. They can be conceptually divided in 2 groups: anterior and posterior.

The anterior group includes the serratus anterior and the pectoralis minor (Figure 10.1, left). The serratus anterior keeps the scapula apposed to the chest wall and moves the scapular body around the chest wall in 3 planes: abduction (forward around the chest wall), extension (the inferior pole is closer to the chest wall), and upward rotation (the glenoid face is oriented up). Some call the serratus anterior the muscle of boxing: it positions the scapula for punching. With serratus insufficiency, the medial border of the scapula cannot be apposed to the chest wall and wings posteriorly. Elevation of the arm is compromised, since the glenoid cannot be positioned anteriorly and facing upwards. Abnormal anterior tilt of the scapula can lead to secondary impingement.

The pectoralis minor is the second muscle of the anterior group. Think of the pectoralis minor as a hand controlling the scapular position through a joystick: the coracoid. If you grasped the coracoid process with your fingertips and moved the coracoid in the line of pull of the pectoralis minor, it would abduct, depress, and downward rotate

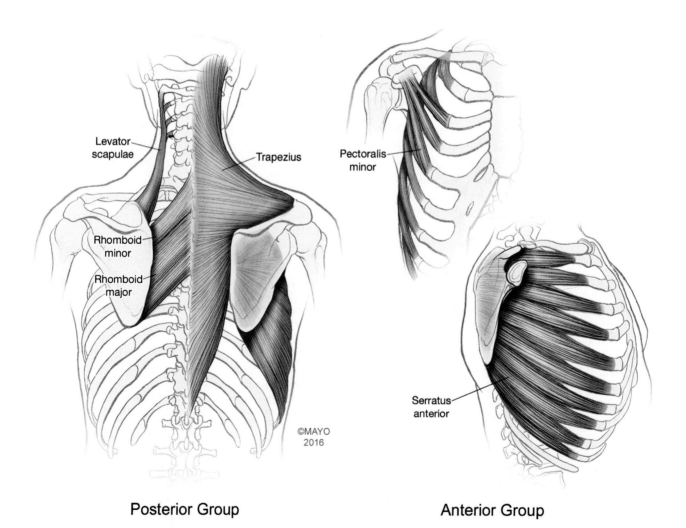

Posterior Group

Anterior Group

Figure 10.1 *Main periscapular muscles.*

the scapula. More importantly, it results in anterior tilt. The most common pathologic condition affecting the pectoralis minor seems to be contracture with fibrosis and shortening. This results in a scapula that is permanently tilted anteriorly, generating secondary impingement and a certain degree of stiffness. In addition, it can lead to compressive brachial plexopathy, oftentimes difficult to diagnose, where thoracic outlet syndrome symptoms are aggravated by direct pressure medial and inferior to the coracoid.

The posterior group includes a deeper group of 3 muscles (rhomboid minor, rhomboid major, and levator scapulae) and a large superficial muscle, the trapezius (Figure 10.1). All 3 muscles of the deep layer move the scapular body superiorly (shrug) and rotate the scapula inferiorly (the glenoid faces down); in addition, the rhomboid muscles bring the scapular body closer to the midline (adduction). Rhomboid insufficiency is difficult to detect, since the larger, more superficial middle and superior trapezius have similar functions. Since the trapezius would need to work harder after losing the help of the rhomboids, it may become achy (trapezius hypercontracture and tenderness) and eventually fatigue and allow winging to some extent.

The trapezius is a very large muscle, and like the deltoid, different portions serve different functions. The superior trapezius elevates, whereas the inferior trapezius depresses the scapula; they both result in upward rotation (glenoid facing up) by controlling the superior and inferior poles of the medial scapula. The middle trapezius moves the scapula closer to the midline and tilts the scapula posteriorly. Trapezius insufficiency results in visible atrophy (most evident at the sides of the neck). The weight of the arm takes the scapula laterally and distally (winging). Active elevation is compromised by weakness in upward rotation. Anterior tilt results in secondary subacromial impingement.

Functional Scapular Dyskinesis

As mentioned in chapter 1, Evaluation of the Shoulder, and at the beginning of this chapter, some patients will present with symptoms secondary to poor muscular control of the scapula in the absence of specific structural pathology in the scapulothoracic joint or surrounding neuromuscular structures. The term *scapular dyskinesis* is often used to refer to this situation (1). Most studies seem to suggest that functional scapular dyskinesis is associated with decreased activity in the serratus anterior and middle and inferior trapezius, and increased activity in the upper trapezius (2).

In some patients, scapular dyskinesis develops as a primary problem: for reasons that oftentimes are not completely clear, patients lose control of the periscapular musculature and develop discomfort in the periscapular region.

The abnormal position of the scapula can then lead to symptoms of cuff impingement (secondary to anterior tilt of the acromion) or instability (secondary to poor positioning of the glenoid).

In other patients, scapular dyskinesis develops secondarily, as a poor adaptation to a painful shoulder, or after an injury or surgery. For example, a patient may have undergone surgery, and as a consequence of the immobilization time or postural changes to deal with pain, adequate control of the periscapular musculature is lost. Classic examples of conditions leading to secondary functional scapular dyskinesis include certain acromioclavicular joint separations (3,4) and clavicle fractures leading to malunion or nonunion.

Evaluation

The goals of patient evaluation for suspected functional scapular dyskinesis are as follows: rule out any *structural* conditions to confirm that the dyskinesis is *functional*, identify any associated pathology outside of the periscapular region (e.g., cuff disease, biceps pathology, glenohumeral instability), reassure the patient, and formulate a specific physical therapy plan.

The most common patient complaints in functional scapular dyskinesis include pain in the trapezius, neck, and periscapular region; difficulties with use of the arm overhead; and a sense of lack of control of the upper extremity. Some patients with scapular dyskinesis are referred to the shoulder specialist with symptoms attributed to impingement, a superior labral tear, or glenohumeral instability. If proper examination of the scapula is not performed, and the underlying scapular dyskinesis not managed accordingly, treatment directed to these secondary problems will fail. It has also been my observation, although not well documented in the literature, that patients with collagen abnormalities leading to hypermobility (e.g., Ehlers-Danlos syndrome and Marfan syndrome) also have a tendency to present with scapular dyskinesis. Criteria for diagnosing hypermobility conditions are summarized in chapter 7, Shoulder Instability and the Labrum (see Table 7.12 for Beighton criteria).

On inspection, patients with functional scapular dyskinesis may have a normal resting position of the scapula; however, subtle malpositioning is common: the inferomedial border or the whole medial border of the scapula is prominent in the back and the coracoid is prominent in the front. A measuring tape or ruler may be used to measure the distance between the medial, superior, and inferior scapula to the midline as compared with the opposite side. The distance between the tip of the coracoid and the examining table or a wall can be used to assess pectoralis minor shortening (5). As mentioned in chapter 1, Evaluation of the Shoulder, the term *SICK* scapula has been coined as a mnemonic to remember the combination of *Scapular* malposition at rest, prominence of the *I*nferior medial border of the scapula, *C*oracoid malpositioning with pain, and scapular dys*K*inesis (6).

The next step of the physical examination is to compare the motion of both scapulae in space with active elevation and lowering of the upper extremities (7). Most of the time, there are obvious differences in motion in terms of rotation and prominence. Crepitus and snapping may be noted. The scapular assistance and retraction tests can then be used to confirm improvement of symptoms in the office with better support and positioning of the scapula. Specific testing of individual muscles is then performed as detailed in chapter 1, Evaluation of the Shoulder, and Table 10.1.

Some patients with scapular dyskinesis may complain of distal sensory changes. These symptoms are likely secondary to brachial plexus compression underneath the clavicle or, more commonly, behind the pectoralis minor. In addition, do not forget to examine for a possible associated suprascapular neuropathy, since the suprascapular nerve tethered under the suprascapular ligament may become stretched secondary to chronic scapular malpositioning (see chapter 6, Suprascapular Nerve section).

Plain radiographs are typically obtained in patients with suspected functional scapular dyskinesis. Most of the time they are negative; occasionally, malposition of the scapula may be noted on radiographs. Magnetic resonance imaging of the shoulder can be misleading, since signal changes in the labrum or rotator cuff may be interpreted as pathologic. In patients with severe scapular dyskinesis and physical examination findings consistent with structural neuromuscular pathology, consideration should be given to electromyography and nerve conduction studies. As detailed later, evaluation of the periscapular muscles requires ordering magnetic resonance imaging of the chest, not the shoulder. Patients suspected of having collagen abnormalities can be referred for genetic testing.

Management

Management of functional scapular dyskinesis can be extremely challenging. Although physical therapy represents the ideal treatment modality, improvement is neither quick nor predictable. Many of these patients may have already tried physical therapy unsuccessfully, and they feel frustrated when the only additional recommendation is *more physical therapy!* It is important to educate and reassure these patients, and also to understand the details of the programs attempted so far, since a good program of periscapular rehabilitation commonly has not been followed (8).

As mentioned before, most of these patients have relative weakness of the serratus anterior and the middle and inferior trapezius. In addition, some may have contracture of the pectoralis minor. Strengthening of the serratus anterior and middle and inferior trapezius is essential; details on

exercises recommended in patients with functional scapular dyskinesis are covered in chapter 12. Rehabilitation and Injections.

Long-standing, functional scapular dyskinesis in active sport players (especially throwers) can lead to secondary structural pathology such as rotator cuff impingement or cuff tears, labral tears, or instability (7,9). Surgery may be needed to deal with these secondary problems, but the outcome of surgery will be poor if the scapular dyskinesis is not corrected as well.

If a clearly symptomatic nerve entrapment is also detected, it should be managed accordingly. Corticosteroid injections around the location of the suprascapular nerve may be of benefit for patients with associated suprascapular neuropathy; if they are successful only on a temporary basis, arthroscopic suprascapular nerve release may be considered. Patients with marked contracture of the pectoralis minor and compressive brachial plexopathy may rarely require surgical release of the pectoralis minor.

Periscapular Neuromuscular Conditions

Dysfunction of one or more of the muscles governing the scapulothoracic joint may be secondary to either an injury of the brachial plexus or any of its proximal branches (10), a traumatic muscular rupture or avulsion (11), or inherited dystrophic conditions (12).

Injuries to the Brachial Plexus and Its Branches
Injury to the Spinal Accessory Nerve
Etiology
The spinal accessory nerve (cranial nerve XI) innervates the sternocleidomastoid and trapezius muscles. Since the proximal aspect of the nerve is protected by the sternocleidomastoid, the spinal accessory nerve typically is injured distal to it, resulting in isolated trapezius palsy. Occasionally, both muscles are affected. The most common etiology for injuries to the spinal accessory nerve is iatrogenic damage during surgical procedures in the lateral aspect of the neck (posterior triangle): cervical lymph node biopsy, cervical lymphadenectomy, radical neck dissection, and so on. However, it can also be the result of blunt or penetrating trauma, or residual after Parsonage-Turner syndrome. Finally, spontaneous idiopathic spinal accessory mononeuropathy has also been reported (13–15).

Evaluation
The diagnosis of injury to the spinal accessory nerve and trapezius palsy may be missed initially. Patients complain of shoulder pain and poor active elevation. Occasionally, they will present after having undergone an unsuccessful arthroscopic subacromial decompression, labral repair, or biceps tenodesis for the wrong diagnosis. The hallmarks of trapezius palsy include atrophy (best appreciated

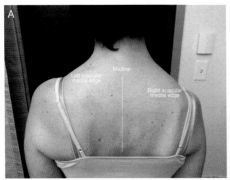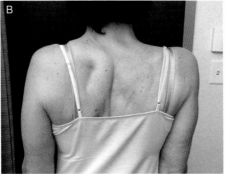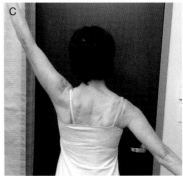

Figure 10.2 Clinical aspect of a patient with long-standing trapezius palsy (right side). **A,** *Lateralized scapula in the resting position.* **B,** *Inability to perform a shoulder shrug.* **C,** *Limited active elevation with winging and atrophy; the muscle bellies of the levator scapulae and rhomboids can be seen on the right side.*

comparing the shape of the neck to back transition and the muscle bulk medial to the scapula); drooping of the shoulder laterally and inferiorly; winging; and weakness when performing active elevation, a shrug, or scapular retraction to the midline (Figure 10.2). Winging and improvement of elevation with the scapular assistance test are less marked than in patients with serratus anterior dysfunction. If the sternocleidomastoid muscle is also affected, the patient will have weakness when turning the chin to the opposite side of the injury.

Management
Some patients with a nonpenetrating injury to the spinal accessory nerve may recover spontaneously. Iatrogenic injuries are best treated with neurolysis, direct nerve repair, or repair with intervening grafting if surgery is performed within the first 6 months to a year after the injury; improvement rates over 85% have been reported, especially when the nerve is found in continuity and neurolysis is performed (14,16). Risk factors for incomplete recovery after nerve repair or grafting include age over 50, duration of the palsy over 20 months, spontaneous palsy, penetrating injuries, and radical neck dissection (14).

For long-standing symptomatic trapezius palsy, tendon transfers are the treatment of choice. The most popular choice is to transfer the levator scapulae, rhomboid minor, and rhomboid major to a different location. In the so-called Eden-Lange procedure, the levator scapulae is transferred from the superomedial border of the scapula to the lateral spine or acromion, and the rhomboids are transferred to the infraspinatus fossa, typically under the infraspinatus (Figure 10.3A) (14,17). The current trend is to transfer the rhomboids to the spine of the scapula instead, just medial to the transferred levator scapule, to better replicate the line of pull of the trapezius and facilitate upward rotation (Figure 10.3B) (13). Care must be taken to protect the dorsal scapular nerve when performing these procedures. Brace immobilization in abduction and external rotation is recommended for 6 to 8 weeks. Reported improvement

rates have ranged from 60% to over 90%, depending on the study (13,14,17).

Patients with relative contraindications for tendon transfer (collagen disorders, issues with compliance) and those with failed tendon transfer surgery can be considered for scapulothoracic arthrodesis, a salvage procedure described in chapter 11, Salvage Procedures.

Injury to the Long Thoracic Nerve
Etiology
The long thoracic nerve (C5–C7) crosses over the lateral aspect of the rib cage for 10 to 20 centimeters to innervate the serratus anterior. A number of studies have tried to analyze various reasons and mechanisms leading to long thoracic neuropathy (Table 10.2) (18–23). Although a clear inciting event can be identified in some cases (chest wall trauma or surgery), in some individuals the etiology and mechanism of dysfunction are never identified.

Evaluation
Most patients complain of posterior periscapular pain, difficulty with arm elevation (especially after prolonged activity), and occasional periscapular crepitus or snapping. Classic physical examination findings include winging (the scapular medial border lifts off the chest wall, Figure 10.4), limited active arm elevation, a positive boxer punch sign, and worsening of the winging with resisted arm elevation or when performing push-ups on the wall. The scapular assistance test clearly improves active elevation in the majority of these cases.

Plain radiographs are usually obtained to rule out other reasons for scapular winging, but imaging studies are usually normal. Magnetic resonance imaging of the chest may show atrophy of the serratus anterior, but this test is seldom necessary to confirm the diagnosis. Electromyography with nerve conduction studies usually confirm the diagnosis, but these studies are also negative in a number of patients with clear dysfunction of the long thoracic nerve (24).

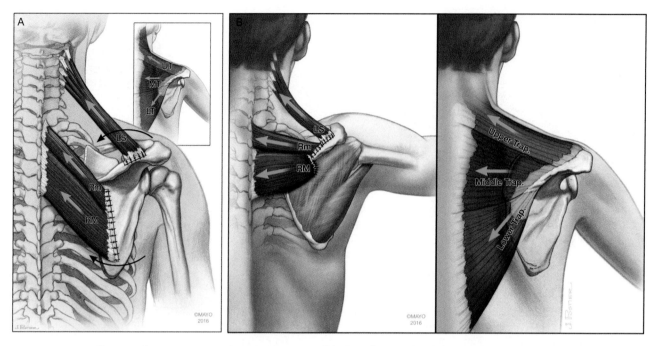

Figure 10.3 A, *Classic Eden-Lange procedure.* **B,** *Mayo-modified triple transfer (left) more accurately reproduces the lines of action of the 3 portions of the trapezius. LS indicates levator scapulae; LT, lower trapezius; MT, middle trapezius; Rm, rhomboid minor; RM, rhomboid major; Trap., trapezius; UT, upper trapezius.*

Table 10.2 • Causes of Injury to the Long Thoracic Nerve

Cause	Examples
Iatrogenic injury in surgery	Resection of the first rib for thoracic outlet syndrome Mastectomy Thoracotomy Other
Traumatic injuries to the lateral aspect of the chest wall	Motor vehicle accident Multiple rib fractures
Inflammatory neuropathies	Viral Parsonage-Turner syndrome After vaccination Idiopathic
Prolonged compression due to incorrect positioning during general anesthesia	Lateral decubitus position
Sports-related injury	Traction injury Overexertion

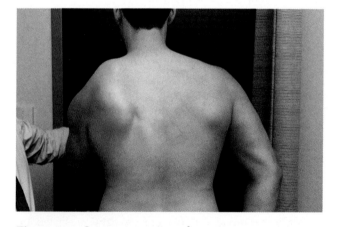

Figure 10.4 *Serratus anterior palsy.*

Management

Many patients with serratus anterior palsy recover spontaneously, although the interval time to complete resolution may range between 6 months and 2 years. A trial of conservative treatment is thus warranted, and focused on preventing secondary contracture (especially of the pectoralis minor), scapular stabilizing exercises, and the occasional use of braces or orthesis.

Patients without evidence of improvement despite an adequate program of nonoperative treatment and those with long-standing, debilitating serratus anterior palsies may be considered for surgery. Similar to what has been discussed regarding the spinal accessory nerve, surgical options include nerve decompression, repair, or grafting; tendon transfers; or scapulothoracic arthrodesis as a salvage (Chapter 11, Salvage Procedures).

A number of studies have reported relatively good outcomes with surgical release of the long thoracic nerve (18,19). In a recent study on surgical release of the long thoracic nerve performed on 52 consecutive patients, complete correction of winging occurred in 60% of the cases and 85% of the patients had satisfactory results. Release was particularly effective when performed within 1 year of the onset of symptoms.

For patients with long-standing, symptomatic serratus anterior palsy, the tendon transfer of choice involves transferring the tendon of the sternal head of the pectoralis major to the inferior angle of the scapula (21,24). Preservation of the clavicular portion of the pectoralis major aids with cosmesis and strength in internal rotation. The transfer may be performed directly or indirectly. Direct transfers involve attachment of the end of the pectoralis tendon to the scapula, whereas indirect transfers use some kind of interposed material for anchoring, most commonly an Achilles tendon allograft extension of the pectoralis tendon (25). Theoretically, direct transfers should be associated with more predictable healing, but might lead to excessive tension, with either inability of the pectoralis to reach the scapula, or a stretch injury to the pectoralis nerves. A recent study from our institution

reported on the outcome of 51 shoulders treated with direct transfer harvesting the pectoralis tendon with a segment of bone (Figure 10.5). Complete resolution of winging was noted in almost 90% of the patients, with substantial improvements in pain and function (24).

Brachial Plexus Dysfunction

Although isolated dysfunction of the dorsal scapular nerve has been described (26), most patients presenting with a neurogenic scapula will have isolated trapezius palsy, isolated serratus anterior palsy, or combined dysfunction of several components of the brachial plexus (27). Brachial plexus dysfunction leading to periscapular problems can be the result of trauma or inflammatory neuropathy (Parsonage-Turner syndrome). Details regarding the evaluation and management of brachial plexus injuries exceed the scope of this book.

Commonly, patients with brachial plexopathy will eventually present with patchy involvement secondary to

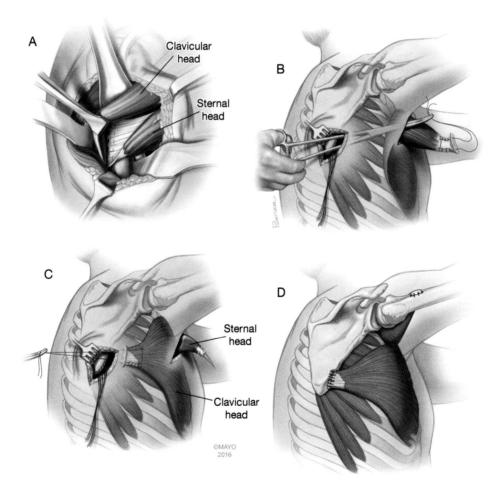

Figure 10.5 *Direct pectoralis major transfer for the surgical management of serratus anterior palsy.* **A,** *Harvesting the sternal head under the clavicular head.* **B and C,** *Transfer of the sternal head.* **D,** *Reattachment of the clavicular head.*

the nature of the injury or various states of recovery. These patients may be referred for shoulder surgery when further recovery is not expected and nerve repair, grafting, or neurotization are not reliable. Glenohumeral arthrodesis is commonly considered as a salvage procedure for patients with sequelae of brachial plexus injuries and paralysis of the deltoid and the rotator cuff, but it requires that the trapezius and serratus anterior (and ideally the levator scapulae and rhomboids) are intact (28). In patients with combined involvement of the rotator cuff, deltoid, and periscapular musculature, tendon transfers are preferred (27,29).

Currently, transfer of the lower trapezius to the infraspinatus (similar to the technique described for management of rotator cuff tears in chapter 6, The Rotator Cuff and Biceps Tendon) is preferred for restoration of external rotation (30). In patients with a paralyzed trapezius, the contralateral trapezius may be considered for transfer (31). Additional transfers are performed depending on the functional status of the remaining muscles, and may include transfers of the levator scapulae to the supraspinatus, the upper portion of the serratus anterior to the subscapularis, the teres major (if available) to the teres minor, the latissimus dorsi (if available) to the anterior portion of the deltoid, and the upper and middle portions of the trapezius to the deltoid (27).

Dystrophic Conditions

Progressive bilateral scapular winging is one of the hallmarks of facioscapulohumeral muscular dystrophy (FSHD) (32). This condition is one of the most prevalent adult muscular dystrophies (1:15,000 to 1:20,000), and it is characterized by asymmetric and often descending weakness affecting the face, shoulder, and arms, followed by weakness of the distal lower extremities and pelvic girdle. Severe cases may present extramuscular manifestations, such as symptomatic retinal vascular disease and hearing loss. Approximately 20% of these patients over the age of 50 require use of a wheelchair. Ninety-five percent of these patients inherit the disease in an autosomal dominant fashion linked to chromosome 4 (FSHD type 1). The remaining 5% demonstrate a variable inherited pattern. Both result in hyperactivation of the retrogene DUX4.

Regarding the shoulder region, studies performed using whole-body magnetic resonance imaging have demonstrated that muscular changes commonly affect the serratus anterior (80%), latissimus dorsi (80%), trapezius (50%), pectoralis major (50%), teres major (50%), rhomboids (40%), and pectoralis minor (30%), among others (33). This translates into the typical shoulder manifestations of FSHD: shoulder ache, limited active elevation over 90°, and unsightly winging. With attempted elevation, the scapula wings posteriorly and superiorly (Figure 10.6). Winging is oftentimes bilateral, although asymmetric. Commonly, patients are aware of other family members with the diagnosis. FSHD can be confirmed by genetic testing.

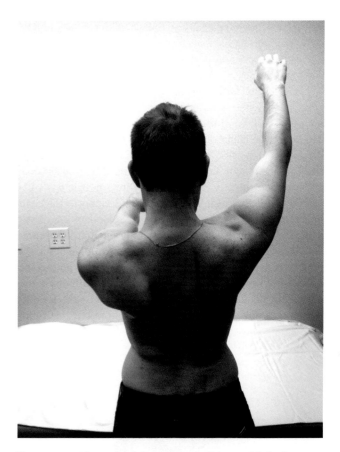

Figure 10.6 *Scapular winging in a patient with facioscapulohumeral dystrophy. On the left side, active elevation is limited and there is marked winging. On the right side, scapulothoracic arthrodesis has resulted in correction of winging and improved active elevation.*

Physical therapy may be tried to maintain conditioning and strength, but the progressive nature of the disease makes it less successful over time. Scapulothoracic arthrodesis is the surgical procedure of choice to correct scapular winging in FSHD (34). Typically, the procedure needs to be performed on both sides, but patients seem to tolerate the effect of bilateral restriction of rib excursion well (see chapter 11, Salvage Procedures). A number of pharmacologic treatments (corticosteroids, anabolic agents, creatine, myostatin inhibitors) have been tested without much success (12).

Traumatic Periscapular Muscle Detachment

Scapular winging can also occur after injuries resulting in traumatic detachment of the periscapular muscles (11,35). This type of injury may be more common than previously acknowledged. These patients report acute onset of periscapular pain after either a direct (collision with an object posteriorly) or tensile injury; seat-belted motor vehicle accidents are particularly common.

Typically, these patients complain of moderate to severe pain along the medial border of the scapula. Not uncommonly, they have been seen by one or more health care providers, diagnosed with functional scapular dyskinesis, and managed with physical therapy without success. Some are dependent on chronic narcotic pain medication. They express difficulty or inability to perform overhead activities or maintain the arm in elevation. Physical examination is consistent with dysfunction of the trapezius and/or rhomboids: winging, atrophy, and weakness in scapular retraction to the midline. Occasionally, a defect may be palpated just medial to the scapular border. Elevation improves with the scapular assistance test. Some patients may complain of secondary impingement. Plain radiographs are essentially negative. Electromyography and nerve conduction studies may be used to exclude an injury to the long thoracic, spinal accessory, or dorsal scapular nerves. Magnetic resonance imaging of the chest may be used to compare the attachment sites of the trapezius and rhomboids on the medial scapular body with the opposite, nonaffected side.

Although conservative management (physical therapy) may be tried, patients with a substantial muscular avulsion seem to improve only with surgical management. Substantial improvements in pain and function have been reported in a study on 72 patients treated with surgical repair of the trapezius and rhomboids, although functional scores in this study did not return to normal (11). The procedure involves resecting the interposed stretched scar tissue and primary repair to the body (rhomboids) or spine (trapezius) through bone tunnels. The surgeon should be ready to convert intraoperatively to a triple tendon transfer if needed (13). Scapulothoracic arthrodesis should only be considered in the very rare patient with a massive irreparable avulsion.

Scapular Snapping and Crepitus

The term *scapular snapping syndrome* is used to define a group of patients that develop sounds of crepitus or snapping as the scapula glides over the posterior aspect of the thorax with active motion of the upper extremity (36–40). While some patients have minimal or no pain, others complain of severe pain and dysfunction even with common activities of daily living. These symptoms may be the result of specific structural pathology, such as a space-occupying skeletal lesion (Table 10.3), but in some individuals it can only be attributed to scapulothoracic bursitis.

Evaluation

Patients with scapular snapping syndrome usually complain of pain and noise around the scapula with use of the arm, especially overhead use. Each of these symptoms may vary in intensity: pain may be minor to excruciating, and snapping and crepitus may be audible or only palpable. It is important to recognize that scapular noises may be asymptomatic, with some potential for secondary gain in worker's compensation and litigation cases. On the other hand, some patients are truly disabled and respond beautifully to surgery.

Physical examination is conducted along the lines summarized in Table 10.1, assessing the resting position of the scapula, abnormal scapular motion, testing of individual muscles, and changes in symptoms with scapular repositioning maneuvers. Patients with scapular snapping syndrome may have a normal position of the scapula at rest or they may present with winging or pseudowinging (prominence of the scapula posteriorly due to a space-occupying abnormality or scapular malunion). Most of the time, patients can reproduce their symptoms and noise with active use of the arm, and the examiner may be able to better detect snapping or crepitus by placing the hand on the posteromedial aspect of the scapula while the patient elevates the arm. The examiner may unmask

---

Table 10.3 • Scapular Snapping Syndrome: Possible Underlying Abnormalities

Type of Abnormality	Examples
Osseous	**Scapular osseous topography** Thick inferomedial or superomedial (Luschke tubercle) angle Deep, undulating costal surfaces Scapular malunion or exuberant callus after fracture Other
	Rib cage osseous topography Sequelae of rib fractures After surgery (e.g., rib resection, thoracotomy) Scoliosis or kyphosis with secondary rib cage deformity
Inflamed or fibrotic bursae (see Figure 10.6)	Acute trauma Chronic overuse (e.g., swimming, pitching, gymnastics, weight training)
Subscapularis or serratus anterior atrophy	
Elastofibroma dorsi	
Functional scapular dyskinesis	Underlying collagen abnormalities (e.g., Ehlers-Danlos syndrome, Marfan syndrome) Idiopathic

crepitus and snapping by applying an anteriorly directed force to the scapula during active motion. The shoulder region should be assessed for pectoralis minor contracture or weakness of individual periscapular muscles. Traumatic muscle avulsion needs to be excluded in those patients with a clear history of injury. Patients should also be assessed for associated glenohumeral pathology (labral tearing, cuff impingement, instability), especially overhead athletes. Finally, it is important to assess the vertebral spine for scoliosis of kyphosis, and to determine if the patient has a primary collagen disorder.

Plain radiographs are routinely obtained and will sometimes reveal certain abnormalities, such as scapular malunion or an osteochondroma. However, osseous abnormalities of the scapulothoracic joint are best assessed using computed tomography with 3-dimensional reconstruction. Magenetic resonance imaging is useful for the evaluation of mass-occupying lesions (elastofibroma dorsi), and may occasionally show excessive bursal thickening, cysts, or selective muscle atrophy. Electromyography with nerve conduction studies is ordered in patients suspected to have a primary neurologic dysfunction. Although still investigational, 4-dimensional computed tomography looks very promising in the evaluation of the scapular snapping syndrome (41).

Management

Patients with scapular snapping syndrome should undergo a good program of conservative management as a first line of treatment unless structural pathology can be clearly identified (space occupying lesions, scapular malunion, exhuberant callus). Nonoperative management includes activity modifications, nonsteroidal anti-inflammatory drugs, physical therapy, and the occasional use of corticosteroid injections. These injections may be performed under ultrasonography, but they can also be performed in the office with the patient prone and the wrist resting on the small of the back ("chicken-wing" position).

Surgical management is considered for patients with structural pathology as well as those not responding to a good program of nonoperative treatment for 3 to 6 months. The most common procedure performed for patients with snapping scapula syndrome and no space-occupying lesions is bursectomy with or without partial resection of the superomedial border of the scapula. Although this procedure was initially described and may be performed

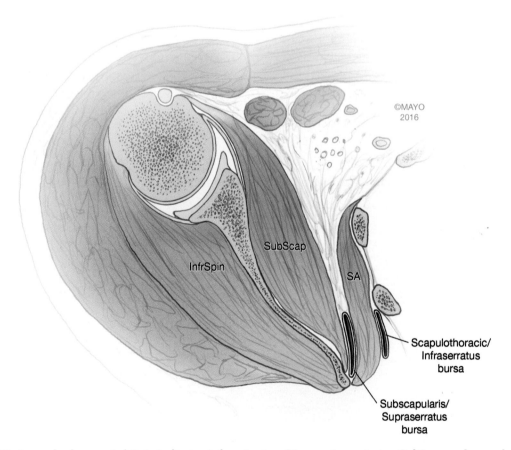

Figure 10.7 *Periscapular bursae. InfrSpin indicates infraspinatus; SA, serratus anterior; SubScap, subscapularis.*

through an open approach, currently it is most commonly performed endoscopically.

Endoscopic Bursectomy and
Partial Scapular Resection

Performing this procedure endoscopically has a number of benefits in my opinion, especially avoidance of ample muscular periscapular detachment and improved cosmesis. However, the procedure carries some risk of injury to various neurovascular structures, and some authors argue that it is difficult to perform an adequate resection arthroscopically. Most of the time pathology is centered around the supraserratus bursa (⏺ Video 10.1, Figure 10.7).

The patient is placed prone and the arm is draped free. Placing the wrist of the patient over the low thoracic spine ("chicken-wing" position) raises the medial border of the scapula and facilitates the procedure (Figure 10.8). Portal

placement is critical to avoid iatrogenic neurovascular injuries (Figure 10.9). The spinal accessory nerve may be damaged by portals placed proximal to the level of the scapular spine. The dorsal scapular nerve and artery are located approximately 1 to 2 centimeters medial to the medial border of the scapula. For these reasons, all portals should be placed distal to the location of the spine of the scapula and at least 3 centimeters medial to the medial border.

My preference is to place my viewing portal distally, proximal to the inferomedial border of the scapula and 3 cm medial to the medial border. The main working portal is established proximally, again about 3 cm medial to the medial border, and not proximal to the level to the spine of the scapula. Removal of inflamed bursal tissue is performed first. The superomedial border of the scapula is then skeletonized using a radiofrequency ablation device. The outlines of the scapula may be marked with spinal needles.

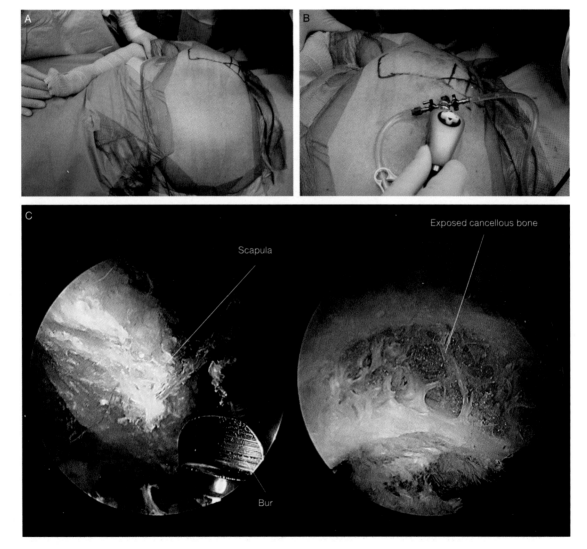

Figure 10.8 *Endoscopic resection of the superomedial border of the scapula.* **A,** *Patient positioning (prone, arm behind lower back).* **B,** *Portal for visualization.* **C,** *Superomedial angle exposed and bone removal.*

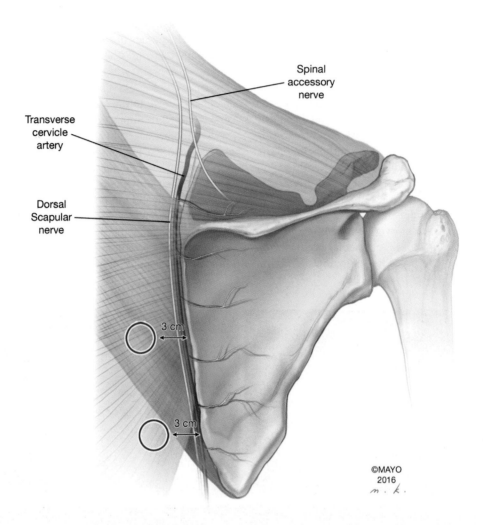

Figure 10.9 Neurovascular structures at risk when performing endoscopic procedures in the scapulothoracic space.

Bone is then removed with an arthroscopic bur. Some authors have reported performing the bursectomy endoscopically and completing the bone removal through a miniopen approach. After surgery, a sling is used for comfort and patients are recommended a well-structured program of scapular isometrics followed by strengthening once the inflammatory postsurgical response subsides.

Outcome of Bursectomy and Partial Scapular Resection

Most studies on the outcome of surgical management for snapping scapula syndrome have included a relatively small number of patients (36,38–40,42). Nickolson and Duckworth (40) reported on 17 patients treated with open bursectomy; 5 patients (30%) also underwent bone resection to some extent. At a mean follow-up of 2 years, pain and function improved in all but 1 patient (40). In a large series of 23 shoulders with a minimum 2-year follow-up, Millett et al. (38) demonstrated measurable improvement

in pain and function after arthroscopic bursectomy with or without scapuloplasty. However, despite these improvements, median patient satisfaction was only 6 of 10 in this series. Multiple other authors have reported a relatively high rate of satisfactory results (36).

Congenital Abnormalities

A few congenital abnormalities may result in scapular dysfunction. These include congenital absence of one or more periscapular muscles, congenital pseudoarthrosis of the clavicle, and the uncommon, but well known, congenital undescended scapula (Sprengel deformity).

Sprengel deformity is characterized by a hypoplastic scapula with decreased vertical length that is superiorly placed and medially rotated on the posterior thorax compared with normal, with the glenoid abnormally tilted (Figure 10.10) (43–46). It is more common in females and typically unilateral. The shoulder musculature is hypotrophic, fibrotic,

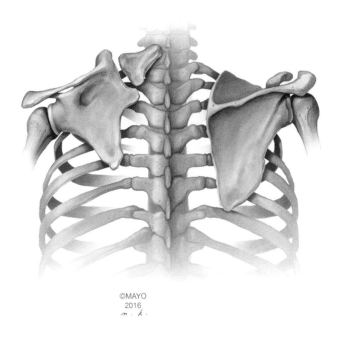

©MAYO
2016
m. k.

Figure 10.10 *Sprengel deformity (hypoplastic undescended scapula).*

or even absent, and many patients present with winging of the hypoplastic scapula. In one-third of the patients there is a bony or cartilaginous connection between the superior angle of the scapula and the spinous processes of the cervical vertebrae (omovertebral bone).

A congenital undescended scapula results in asymmetry of the shoulder and thorax and, in severe cases, a webbed neck appearance. Most patients do not complain of pain, but elevation is restricted, typically to less than 90°. Associated abnormalities, such as scoliosis and Klippel-Feil syndrome, are common. Plain radiographs demonstrate the small size and abnormal location of the scapula.

Surgical management is indicated for those patients with substantial dysfunction or marked cosmetic abnormalities. Surgery is typically considered when the patient is between 5 and 10 years of age. Surgical options include partial scapulectomy or positioning of the scapula in a more typical anatomic location. Repositioning of the scapula requires detachment of the trapezius, levator scapulae, and rhomboids from either the vertebral spine (i.e., Woodward procedure) or the scapula (i.e., Green procedure); translation of the scapula; and muscle reattachment in the more anatomic location.

Since the scapula is hypoplastic, it should not be brought down to the level of the inferior angle of the opposite side, but aligned at the level of the spine of the opposite scapula. Care must be taken to derotate the scapula in order to superiorly orient the glenoid, and the scapula is typically secured to the ribs in the new position with sutures or tapes. Osteotomy of the clavicle may be necessary in severe cases to avoid iatrogenic compression of the brachial plexus as

the scapula and clavicle are translated inferiorly. If there is an associated omovertebral bone, it needs to be removed as well. Satisfactory studies have been reported using variations of these surgical techniques (43–46). Elevation seems to improve by 30° to 60°.

Fractures of the Scapula

The anatomic location of the scapula behind the thorax, and the fact that the scapula is surrounded by layers of muscles, have a number of implications. On one hand, being protected by the thorax and muscles, fractures of the scapula are relatively uncommon (approximately 1% of all fractures and 3% of all injuries of the shoulder region). By the same token, and for the same exact reasons, for the scapula to fracture, high-energy trauma is required (except for glenoid rim fractures in the setting of a glenohumeral dislocation), which means that not uncommonly fractures of the scapular body are associated with substantial chest injuries.

The layers of muscles around the scapula may function as an external splint after a fracture and provide lots of vascularity, leading to uneventful healing of many fractures without surgery. Exposure of fractures of the scapula for surgical management may obviously require a fair amount of muscle detachment (see chapter 3, Surgical Exposures). All these reasons add up to explain why surgical management of scapular fractures has not been very common in the past. However, certain fractures involving the glenoid do require surgery to avoid glenohumeral instability or incongruity. Similarly, scapular malunion beyond a certain threshold can lead to substantial pseudowinging, painful snapping, and scapular dyskinesis. Some fractures of the scapula definitely do better with surgery.

Classification and Displacement

Classifying fractures of the scapula is not easy (47–52). There are many different patterns of fracture that may involve a segment of the scapula in isolation or may be associated with fractures in other areas. The *international scapula fracture classification* represents a very good starting point to understand the potential complexity of these fractures (Figure 10.11, Table 10.4) (51). The scapula is divided into 4 areas: glenoid fossa, coracoid, acromion, and body. The glenoid fossa is defined as the portion of the scapula lateral to the plane parallel to the glenoid face through the suprascapular notch, not extending proximal to the superior articular rim.

Although this classification system has been shown to have better agreement than others (48,51), it does not fully serve the purpose of orienting toward nonoperative or operative treatment. The indications for surgery will obviously vary depending on not only the location of the fracture but also the amount of displacement, the consequences

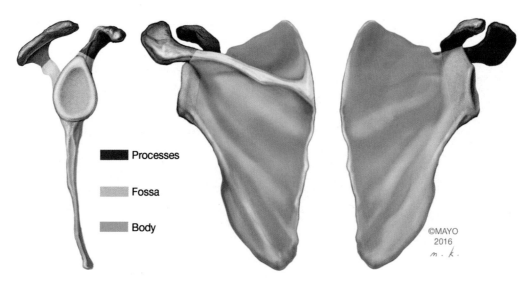

Figure 10.11 *Segments considered in the international scapula fracture classification.*

Table 10.4 • International Scapula Fracture Classification

F: Glenoid fossa fractures
F0: Extra-articular fracture (no part of the fossa is attached to the body)
F1: Intra-articular, simple (rim, transverse, oblique)
F2: Intra-articular, multifragmentary

B: Body fractures
B1: Fracture lines exit at 1 or 2 spots
B2: Fracture line exits at 3 or more spots

P: Process fractures
P1: Coracoid fracture
P2: Acromion fracture
P3: Fracture of both processes

Data from Harvey et al. (51).

on the glenohumeral joint for those fractures involving the glenoid fossa, and associated injuries both within the scapula and outside of the scapula (associated fractures of the clavicle, injuries to the sternoclavicular joint or acromioclavicular joint, rib fractures). The term *superior shoulder suspensory complex* was coined to emphasize that the glenoid, coracoid, clavicle, and acromion form a ringlike structure along with the connecting ligaments and other soft tissues between these structures (Figure 10.12) (53). Disruption of 2 or more structures in this ring results in a complete interruption of the suspension between the upper extremity and the trunk.

Evaluation

Fractures involving the scapula may be secondary to a high-energy injury (e.g., motor vehicle accident or fall from a height), resulting in a fracture of the body with or without extension into the glenoid and its processes; a sports-related injury or fall from a standing height, resulting in an intra-articular fracture of the glenoid; or repetitive stress, resulting in a fracture of the coracoid, acromion, or spine of the scapula (Figure 10.13).

Complex Fractures in the Setting of High-Energy Trauma

Scapular fractures in the setting of high-energy trauma are commonly associated with other injuries. This fact has 2 implications: (1) active search for associated injuries is important in order to identify life-threatening or severe injuries, and (2) scapular fractures may be missed in the midst of evaluating a patient with many other substantial injuries. The most commonly associated injuries involve the thorax (80%), ipsilateral extremity (50%), head (50%), and spine (25%).

The evaluation of these patients should include radiographs of the chest and shoulder (trauma series, see chapter 4, Proximal Humerus Fractures). In patients with fracture extension into the glenoid or marked displacement of the body segments possibly meeting surgical indications, computed tomography with 3-dimensional reconstruction should be obtained for accurate measurements of displacement and angular deformity.

Intra-articular Fractures of the Glenoid

A fall on the outstretched hand or similar type of injury may result in a fracture of the glenoid rim or a more substantial fracture with variable extension into the glenoid vault. Some of these fractures occur as a consequence of a glenohumeral joint dislocation (see chapter 7, Shoulder Instability and the Labrum). Although plain radiographs may be all that is needed for evaluation of very small rim fractures, most of the time accurate evaluation of size and displacement requires use of computed tomography.

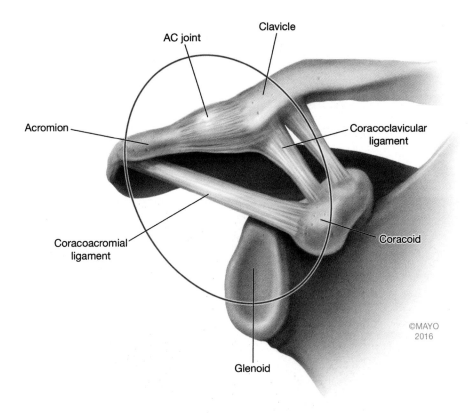

Figure 10.12 *Suspensory complex of the shoulder. AC indicates acromioclavicular.*

Stress Fractures

The acromion and spine of the scapula may develop stress fractures in patients with substantial osteopenia and bone thinning. This was typically seen in the past in patients with either cuff tear arthropathy or rheumatoid arthritis. Interestingly, the rate of stress fractures of both the acromion and spine of the scapula has increased substantially with the introduction of reverse arthroplasty. Fractures complicating reverse arthroplasty are discussed in detail in chapter 9, Shoulder Arthritis and Arthroplasty. Occasionally, stress fractures of the acromion and coracoid may also be the result of repetitive stress during the practice of sports. Stress fractures may be extremely difficult to identify on radiographs. Computed tomography, magnetic resonance imaging, or bone scanning may be required to confirm the diagnosis.

Management

Intra-articular Fractures of the Glenoid Fossa

As with other intra-articular fractures, philosophically, fractures of the glenoid should be treated with anatomic internal fixation if they are associated with incongruity or instability. The problem is that clear criteria for size and displacement values considered to be excessive are lacking (52,54,55). I consider internal fixation for fractures involving more than 20% of the glenoid articular surface

if they are displaced more than 2 to 5 mm, or if they are associated with static subluxation or recurrent instability. Some authors have recommended use of the Ideberg classification, more useful to describe fracture patterns than to determine indications for surgery (Figure 10.14) (56).

Stable fixation of intra-articular simple glenoid fractures can usually be obtained with interfragmentary compression using screws; larger fractures with comminution may benefit from additional plate neutralization. Anterior fractures are approached through a low deltopectoral approach, whereas posterior fractures are exposed through a direct or extensile posterior approach, as described in chapter 3, Surgical Exposures. Arthroscopically assisted reduction and percutaneous screw fixation is commonly attempted currently (Figure 10.15) (57). The outcome of both open and arthroscopic fixation for intra-articular fractures of the glenoid has been successful in the absence of complications (54,55,57–59). The management of these fractures in the setting of glenohumeral instability is discussed in chapter 7, Shoulder Instability and the Labrum.

Extra-articular Fractures Involving the Scapular Body or Neck

Management of this fracture category remains controversial (52,60,61). Union usually occurs reliably, and the shoulder region has a tremendous capability for compensatory

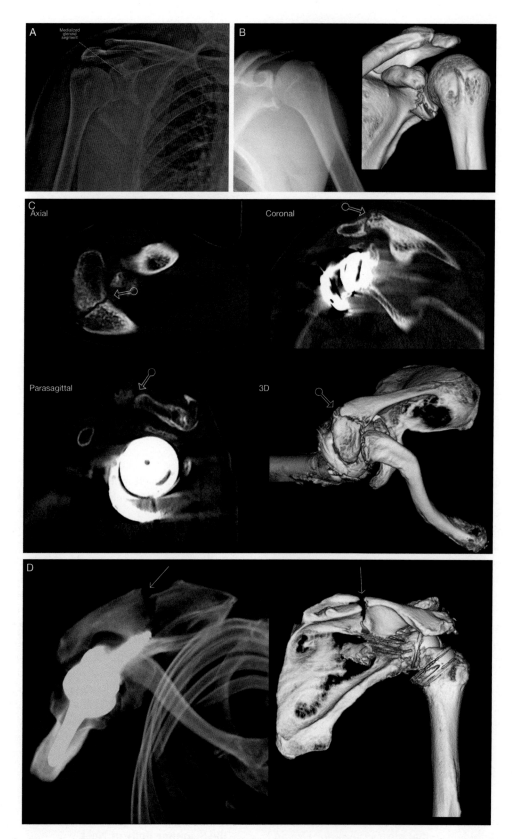

Figure 10.13 A, *Complex fracture of the scapula sustained in a motor-vehicle accident.* **B,** *Intra-articular glenoid fracture.* **C,** *Stress fracture of the acromion in a patient with a prior reverse arthroplasty. Arrows indicate the stress fracture location.* **D,** *Fracture of the spine of the scapula in a patient with a prior reverse arthroplasty. Arrows indicate the stress fracture location.*

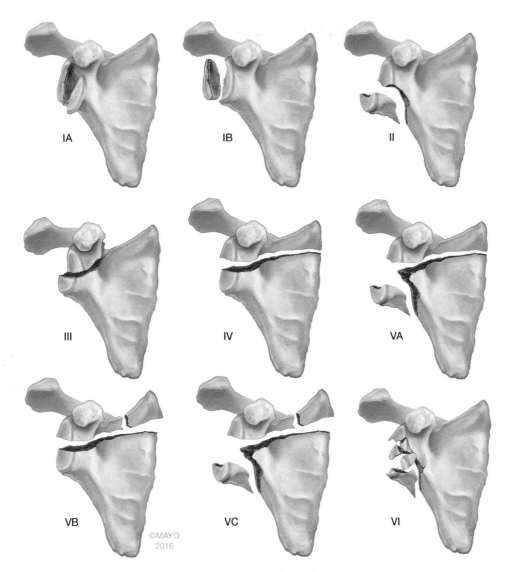

Figure 10.14 Ideberg classification for intra-articular fractures of the glenoid.

motion. Nonoperative treatment is thus considered for most of these fractures, but in some patients residual malunion will lead to either snapping scapula syndrome or symptomatic scapular dyskinesis. The question is, can we predict when?

In an attempt to assess displacement accurately and eventually correlate displacement and outcome, a number of measurements can be performed on computed tomography (Figure 10.16), including the glenopolar angle, the angulation of the scapular body, and mediolateral displacement. Some authors recommend open reduction and internal fixation when medial displacement is greater than 25 mm, angular deformity is greater than 45°, or the glenopolar angle is less than 20° to 30° (52).

Most extra-articular fractures of the scapula managed surgically are exposed through a direct or extensile posterior approach, depending on their complexity. Precontoured scapular plates are extremely useful for the management of

these injuries. Modern studies have reported satisfactory outcomes after internal fixation of displaced fractures of the body or neck (61–64). When compared with nonoperative treatment, the outcome of surgery seems to be favorable, and the reported complication rate is approximately 10% (60).

Coracoid, Acromion, and Spine

Isolated fractures of the coracoid and acromion are uncommon when stress fractures (in the setting of cuff-tear arthropathy, rheumatoid arthritis, or reverse arthroplasty) are excluded. For traumatic fractures of these processes, internal fixation may be considered if an associated fracture of the glenoid or scapular body requires surgery, the fracture of the coracoid or acromion is part of a double injury to the suspensory complex, or there is displacement over 1 centimeter. A few studies have reported specifically on the outcome of surgical management of these fractures with good overall results (65).

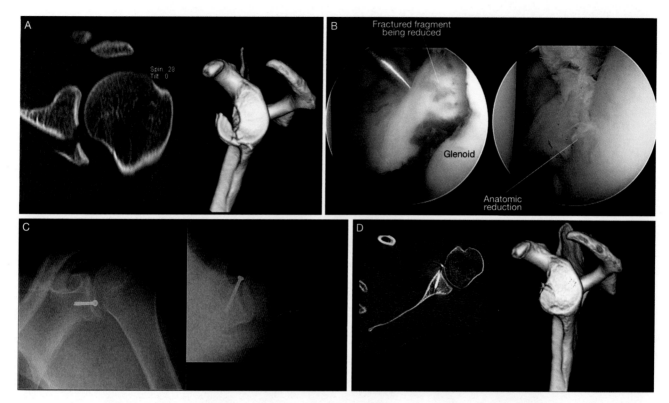

Figure 10.15 *Simple intra-articular fracture of the glenoid rim managed with arthroscopically assisted internal fixation.* **A,** *Preoperative CT scan.* **B,** *Arthroscopic pictures.* **C,** *Postoperative radiographs.* **D,** *Postoperative CT scan. CT indicates computed tomography.*

Double Injuries to the Suspensory Complex

These injuries, also referred to as *floating shoulder*, translate in a complete disconnection between the upper extremity and the trunk, leading to poor outcomes unless one or both of the ring interruptions are stabilized surgically (53).

Examples include the combinations of fracture of the scapular neck and clavicle, or a grade III or greater acromioclavicular joint injury combined with a coracoid fracture (52). Some authors have reported very good outcome with surgical stabilization of both sides of the ring (66), but surgical

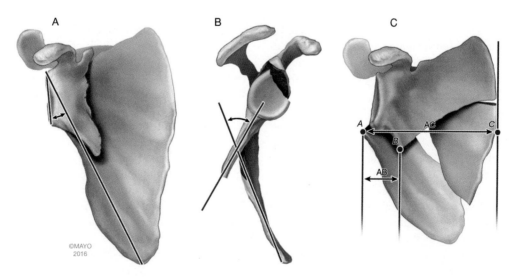

Figure 10.16 *Tomographic measurements of displacement.* **A,** *Glenopolar angle.* **B,** *Scapular body angulation.* **C,** *Mediolateral displacement.*

stabilization of one of the two points of disruption may be enough (67), and nondisplaced double injuries do well without surgery (68). My preference is to address only one of the two points of disruption (clavicle fracture or acromioclavicular joint injury) and add fixation to the second ring injury if it merits surgery on its own.

Scapulothoracic Dissociation

This injury is characterized by severe lateral displacement of the scapula with traumatic avulsion of multiple periscapular muscles (69). This injury is uncommon, but important and not to be missed, since it is commonly associated with injuries to the subclavian vessels and/or brachial plexus. Because of the violent forces involved, any of the three bones in the shoulder complex (clavicle, scapula, and proximal humerus) may be fractured, and any of the remaining three articulations (glenohumeral, acromioclavicular, and sternoclavicular) may be dislocated.

Clinically, these patients present with severe swelling after high-energy trauma, and there is commonly evidence of an associated brachial plexus injury; the vascularity of the upper extremity may be compromised. Plain radiographs show a very lateralized scapula in reference to the chest wall, as well as associated traumatic injuries.

Initially, management is aimed at dealing with associated neurovascular injuries. Injuries to the sternoclavicular or acromioclavicular joint and clavicle fractures need to be stabilized surgically in the acute phase, whereas muscle disruptions around the scapula are typically addressed later with repair or tendon transfers if needed (69).

KEY POINTS

✓ The main periscapular muscles can be divided into an anterior group (serratus anterior and pectoralis minor) and a posterior group (levator scapulae, rhomboids, and trapezius).

✓ Functional scapular dyskinesis is the clinical expression of poor muscular control of the scapula. Provided true structural abnormalities are ruled out, a tailored program of physical therapy helps overcome symptoms in many patients.

✓ Injuries to the spinal accessory nerve can be iatrogenic, the result of trauma or idiopathic. Trapezius paralysis leads to pain, atrophy, limited elevation, and winging. Direct nerve repair may be successful when performed early (within 6 months). Older patients and long-standing injuries are indications for transfer of the levator and rhomboids. The condition may be salvaged with a scapulothoracic fusion.

✓ Injuries to the long thoracic nerve are multifactorial. Spontaneous neuropathy may recover without treatment. Serratus anterior paralysis results in pain, limited elevation, and winging. Neurolysis or repair

may be considered in the first year. Long-standing palsy is best managed with transfer of the sternal head of the pectoralis major.

✓ FSHD is typically inherited as an autosomal dominant disease linked to chromosome 4. Patients develop progressive periscapular weakness with pain, limited active elevation, and winging. The diagnosis may be confirmed by genetic testing. Scapulothoracic arthrodesis is the treatment of choice.

✓ Traumatic injuries may result in avulsion of the periscapular muscles. Surgical repair or tendon transfers are required in many of these patients to decrease pain and improve function.

✓ The scapular snapping syndrome may be secondary to space-occupying lesions, bursitis, or osseous abnormalities of the scapulothoracic joint. Surgical removal of space-occupying lesions solves the problem. In the rest of the cases, bursectomy with selective removal of bone from the superomedial angle of the scapula may be considered when nonoperative treatment fails.

✓ Sprengel deformity is the result of a congenital undescended, hypoplastic scapulae. Omovertebral bones are identified in one-third of patients. Severe cases are treated surgically between the ages of 5 and 10, most commonly with scapular repositioning and transfer of the spinal origin of the medial periscapular muscles. Clavicle osteotomy may be needed to prevent brachial plexopathy at the time of surgery.

✓ Intra-articular fractures of the glenoid require surgery in the presence of instability or incongruity. This is typically the case with fragments larger than 20% of the articular surface displaced more than 2 to 5 mm. Internal fixation may be performed with open or arthroscopically assisted techniques.

✓ Extra-articular fractures of the scapular body and glenoid neck typically are associated with injuries to the chest, head, spine, and ipsilateral upper extremity. Most do well with nonoperative treatment. Surgery is considered for fractures with more than 25 mm of mediolateral displacement, a glenopolar angle under 20° to 30°, or angulation of the body over 45°.

✓ Double lesions to the superior shoulder suspensory complex require surgery only when displaced. Controversy persists regarding the need to stabilize one or both points of ring disruption.

✓ Scapulothoracic dissociation is a rare injury commonly associated with neurovascular disruption. Associated injuries to the clavicle or its joints should be stabilized surgically in the acute phase.

REFERENCES

1. Kibler WB, Sciascia A. Current concepts: scapular dyskinesis. Br J Sports Med. 2010 Apr;44(5):300–5. Epub 2009 Dec 8.
2. Huang TS, Ou HL, Huang CY, Lin JJ. Specific kinematics and associated muscle activation in individuals

with scapular dyskinesis. J Shoulder Elbow Surg. 2015 Aug;24(8):1227–34.

3. Carbone S, Postacchini R, Gumina S. Scapular dyskinesis and SICK syndrome in patients with a chronic type III acromioclavicular dislocation: results of rehabilitation. Knee Surg Sports Traumatol Arthrosc. 2015 May;23(5):1473–80. Epub 2014 Jan 24.

4. Murena L, Canton G, Vulcano E, Cherubino P. Scapular dyskinesis and SICK scapula syndrome following surgical treatment of type III acute acromioclavicular dislocations. Knee Surg Sports Traumatol Arthrosc. 2013 May;21(5):1146–50. Epub 2012 Mar 30.

5. Struyf F, Nijs J, Mottram S, Roussel NA, Cools AM, Meeusen R. Clinical assessment of the scapula: a review of the literature. Br J Sports Med. 2014 Jun;48(11):883–90. Epub 2012 Jul 21.

6. Burkhart SS, Morgan CD, Kibler WB. The disabled throwing shoulder: spectrum of pathology Part III: the SICK scapula, scapular dyskinesis, the kinetic chain, and rehabilitation. Arthroscopy. 2003 Jul-Aug;19(6):641–61.

7. Kibler WB, Sciascia A, Wilkes T. Scapular dyskinesis and its relation to shoulder injury. J Am Acad Orthop Surg. 2012 Jun;20(6):364–72.

8. McClure P, Greenberg E, Kareha S. Evaluation and management of scapular dysfunction. Sports Med Arthrosc. 2012 Mar;20(1):39–48.

9. Provencher CM, Makani A, McNeil JW, Pomerantz ML, Golijanin P, Gross D. The role of the scapula in throwing disorders. Sports Med Arthrosc. 2014 Jun;22(2):80–7.

10. Lee S, Savin DD, Shah NR, Bronsnick D, Goldberg B. Scapular winging: evaluation and treatment: AAOS exhibit selection. J Bone Joint Surg Am. 2015 Oct 21;97(20):1708–16.

11. Kibler WB, Sciascia A, Uhl T. Medial scapular muscle detachment: clinical presentation and surgical treatment. J Shoulder Elbow Surg. 2014 Jan;23(1):58–67.

12. Statland J, Tawil R. Facioscapulohumeral muscular dystrophy. Neurol Clin. 2014 Aug;32(3):721–8. Epub 2014 May 15.

13. Elhassan BT, Wagner ER. Outcome of triple-tendon transfer, an Eden-Lange variant, to reconstruct trapezius paralysis. J Shoulder Elbow Surg. 2015 Aug;24(8):1307–13.

14. Teboul F, Bizot P, Kakkar R, Sedel L. Surgical management of trapezius palsy. J Bone Joint Surg Am. 2004 Sep;86-A(9):1884–90.

15. Wiater JM, Bigliani LU. Spinal accessory nerve injury. Clin Orthop Relat Res. 1999 Nov;(368):5–16.

16. Park SH, Esquenazi Y, Kline DG, Kim DH. Surgical outcomes of 156 spinal accessory nerve injuries caused by lymph node biopsy procedures. J Neurosurg Spine. 2015 Oct;23(4):518–25. Epub 2015 Jun 26.

17. Romero J, Gerber C. Levator scapulae and rhomboid transfer for paralysis of trapezius: the Eden-Lange procedure. J Bone Joint Surg Br. 2003 Nov;85(8):1141–5.

18. Le Nail LR, Bacle G, Marteau E, Corcia P, Favard L, Laulan J. Isolated paralysis of the serratus anterior muscle: surgical release of the distal segment of the long thoracic nerve in 52 patients. Orthop Traumatol Surg Res. 2014 Jun;100(4 Suppl):S243–8. Epub 2014 Apr 3.

19. Schippert DW, Li Z. Supraclavicular long thoracic nerve decompression for traumatic scapular winging. J Surg Orthop Adv. 2013 Fall;22(3):219–23.

20. Maire N, Abane L, Kempf JF, Clavert P; French Society for Shoulder and Elbow SOFEC. Long thoracic nerve release for scapular winging: clinical study of a continuous series of eight patients. Orthop Traumatol Surg Res. 2013 Oct;99(6 Suppl):S329–35. Epub 2013 Aug 20.

21. Streit JJ, Lenarz CJ, Shishani Y, McCrum C, Wanner JP, Nowinski RJ, et al. Pectoralis major tendon transfer for the treatment of scapular winging due to long thoracic nerve palsy. J Shoulder Elbow Surg. 2012 May;21(5):685–90.

22. Nath RK, Lyons AB, Bietz G. Microneurolysis and decompression of long thoracic nerve injury are effective in reversing scapular winging: long-term results in 50 cases. BMC Musculoskelet Disord. 2007 Mar 7;8:25.

23. Wiater JM, Flatow EL. Long thoracic nerve injury. Clin Orthop Relat Res. 1999 Nov;(368):17–27.

24. Elhassan BT, Wagner ER. Outcome of transfer of the sternal head of the pectoralis major with its bone insertion to the scapula to manage scapular winging. J Shoulder Elbow Surg. 2015 May;24(5):733–40.

25. Chalmers PN, Saltzman BM, Feldheim TF, Mascarenhas R, Mellano C, Cole BJ, et al. A comprehensive analysis of pectoralis major transfer for long thoracic nerve palsy. J Shoulder Elbow Surg. 2015 Jul;24(7):1028–35.

26. Argyriou AA, Karanasios P, Makridou A, Makris N. Dorsal scapular neuropathy causing rhomboids palsy and scapular winging. J Back Musculoskelet Rehabil. 2015;28(4):883–5.

27. Elhassan B, Bishop AT, Hartzler RU, Shin AY, Spinner RJ. Tendon transfer options about the shoulder in patients with brachial plexus injury. J Bone Joint Surg Am. 2012 Aug 1;94(15):1391–8.

28. Atlan F, Durand S, Fox M, Levy P, Belkheyar Z, Oberlin C. Functional outcome of glenohumeral fusion in brachial plexus palsy: a report of 54 cases. J Hand Surg Am. 2012 Apr;37(4):683–8.

29. Carlsen BT, Bishop AT, Shin AY. Late reconstruction for brachial plexus injury. Neurosurg Clin N Am. 2009 Jan;20(1):51–64.

30. Crowe MM, Elhassan BT. Scapular and shoulder girdle muscular anatomy: its role in periscapular tendon transfers. J Hand Surg Am. 2016 Feb;41(2):306–14. Epub 2016 Jan 1.

31. Elhassan BT, Wagner ER, Spinner RJ, Bishop AT, Shin AY. Contralateral trapezius transfer to restore shoulder external rotation following adult brachial plexus injury. J Hand Surg Am. 2016 Apr;41(4):e45–51. Epub 2016 Jan 16.

32. Goel DP, Romanowski JR, Shi LL, Warner JJ. Scapulothoracic fusion: outcomes and complications. J Shoulder Elbow Surg. 2014 Apr;23(4):542–7.

33. Leung DG, Carrino JA, Wagner KR, Jacobs MA. Whole-body magnetic resonance imaging evaluation of facioscapulohumeral muscular dystrophy. Muscle Nerve. 2015 Oct;52(4):512–20. Epub 2015 Mar 31.

34. Diab M, Darras BT, Shapiro F. Scapulothoracic fusion for facioscapulohumeral muscular dystrophy. J Bone Joint Surg Am. 2005 Oct;87(10):2267–75.

35. Hayes JM, Zehr DJ. Traumatic muscle avulsion causing winging of the scapula: a case report. J Bone Joint Surg Am. 1981 Mar;63(3):495–7.

36. Warth RJ, Spiegl UJ, Millett PJ. Scapulothoracic bursitis and snapping scapula syndrome: a critical review of current evidence. Am J Sports Med. 2015 Jan;43(1):236–45. Epub 2014 Mar 24.

37. Frank RM, Ramirez J, Chalmers PN, McCormick FM, Romeo AA. Scapulothoracic anatomy and snapping scapula syndrome. Anat Res Int. 2013;2013:635628. Epub 2013 Nov 28.

38. Millett PJ, Gaskill TR, Horan MP, van der Meijden OA. Technique and outcomes of arthroscopic scapulothoracic bursectomy and partial scapulectomy. Arthroscopy. 2012 Dec;28(12):1776–83. Epub 2012 Oct 16.

39. Lehtinen JT, Macy JC, Cassinelli E, Warner JJ. The painful scapulothoracic articulation: surgical management. Clin Orthop Relat Res. 2004 Jun;(423):99–105.

40. Nicholson GP, Duckworth MA. Scapulothoracic bursectomy for snapping scapula syndrome. J Shoulder Elbow Surg. 2002 Jan-Feb;11(1):80–5.

41. Bell SN, Troupis JM, Miller D, Alta TD, Coghlan JA, Wijeratna MD. Four-dimensional computed tomography scans facilitate preoperative planning in snapping scapula syndrome. J Shoulder Elbow Surg. 2015 Apr;24(4):e83–90.

42. Conduah AH, Baker CL 3rd, Baker CL Jr. Clinical management of scapulothoracic bursitis and the snapping scapula. Sports Health. 2010 Mar;2(2):147–55.

43. Wada A, Nakamura T, Fujii T, Takamura K, Yanagida H, Yamaguchi T, et al. Sprengel deformity: morphometric assessment and surgical treatment by the modified green procedure. J Pediatr Orthop. 2014 Jan;34(1):55–62.

44. Walstra FE, Alta TD, van der Eijken JW, Willems WJ, Ham SJ. Long-term follow-up of Sprengel's deformity treated with the Woodward procedure. J Shoulder Elbow Surg. 2013 Jun;22(6):752–9.

45. Harvey EJ, Bernstein M, Desy NM, Saran N, Ouellet JA. Sprengel deformity: pathogenesis and management. J Am Acad Orthop Surg. 2012 Mar;20(3):177–86.

46. Di Gennaro GL, Fosco M, Spina M, Donzelli O. Surgical treatment of Sprengel's shoulder: experience at the Rizzoli Orthopaedic Institute 1975-2010. J Bone Joint Surg Br. 2012 May;94(5):709–12.

47. van Oostveen DP, Temmerman OP, Burger BJ, van Noort A, Robinson M. Glenoid fractures: a review of pathology, classification, treatment and results. Acta Orthop Belg. 2014 Mar;80(1):88–98.

48. Neuhaus V, Bot AG, Guitton TG, Ring DC, et al; Science of Variation Group. Scapula fractures: interobserver reliability of classification and treatment. J Orthop Trauma. 2014 Mar;28(3):124–9.

49. Bartonicek J, Tucek M, Fric V, Obruba P. Fractures of the scapular neck: diagnosis, classifications and treatment. Int Orthop. 2014 Oct;38(10):2163–73. Epub 2014 Jul 5.

50. Zuckerman SL, Song Y, Obremskey WT. Understanding the concept of medialization in scapula fractures. J Orthop Trauma. 2012 Jun;26(6):350–7.

51. Harvey E, Audige L, Herscovici D Jr, Agel J, Madsen JE, Babst R, et al. Development and validation of the new international classification for scapula fractures. J Orthop Trauma. 2012 Jun;26(6):364–9.

52. Cole PA, Gauger EM, Schroder LK. Management of scapular fractures. J Am Acad Orthop Surg. 2012 Mar;20(3):130–41.

53. Goss TP. Double disruptions of the superior shoulder suspensory complex. J Orthop Trauma. 1993;7(2):99–106.

54. Schandelmaier P, Blauth M, Schneider C, Krettek C. Fractures of the glenoid treated by operation: a 5- to 23-year follow-up of 22 cases. J Bone Joint Surg Br. 2002 Mar;84(2):173–7.

55. Kavanagh BF, Bradway JK, Cofield RH. Open reduction and internal fixation of displaced intra-articular fractures of the glenoid fossa. J Bone Joint Surg Am. 1993 Apr;75(4):479–84.

56. Ideberg R, Grevsten S, Larsson S. Epidemiology of scapular fractures. Incidence and classification of 338 fractures. Acta Orthop Scand. 1995 Oct;66(5):395–7.

57. Scheibel M, Hug K, Gerhardt C, Krueger D. Arthroscopic reduction and fixation of large solitary and multifragmented anterior glenoid rim fractures. J Shoulder Elbow Surg. 2016 May;25(5):781–90.

58. Hu C, Zhang W, Qin H, Shen Y, Xue Z, Ding H, et al. Open reduction and internal fixation of Ideberg IV and V glenoid intra-articular fractures through a Judet approach: a retrospective analysis of 11 cases. Arch Orthop Trauma Surg. 2015 Feb;135(2):193–9. Epub 2014 Dec 11.

59. Anavian J, Gauger EM, Schroder LK, Wijdicks CA, Cole PA. Surgical and functional outcomes after operative management of complex and displaced intra-articular glenoid fractures. J Bone Joint Surg Am. 2012 Apr 4;94(7):645–53.

60. Dienstknecht T, Horst K, Pishnamaz M, Sellei RM, Kobbe P, Berner A. A meta-analysis of operative versus nonoperative treatment in 463 scapular neck fractures. Scand J Surg. 2013;102(2):69–76.

61. Cole PA, Gauger EM, Herrera DA, Anavian J, Tarkin IS. Radiographic follow-up of 84 operatively treated scapula neck and body fractures. Injury. 2012 Mar;43(3):327–33. Epub 2011 Oct 27.

62. Jones CB, Cornelius JP, Sietsema DL, Ringler JR, Endres TJ. Modified Judet approach and minifragment fixation of scapular body and glenoid neck fractures. J Orthop Trauma. 2009 Sep;23(8):558–64.

63. Herrera DA, Anavian J, Tarkin IS, Armitage BA, Schroder LK, Cole PA. Delayed operative management of fractures of the scapula. J Bone Joint Surg Br. 2009 May;91(5):619–26.

64. Pizanis A, Tosounidis G, Braun C, Pohlemann T, Wirbel RJ. The posterior two-portal approach for reconstruction of scapula fractures: results of 39 patients. Injury. 2013 Nov;44(11):1630–5. Epub 2013 Aug 6.

65. Anavian J, Wijdicks CA, Schroder LK, Vang S, Cole PA. Surgery for scapula process fractures: good outcome in 26 patients. Acta Orthop. 2009 Jun;80(3):344–50.

66. Leung KS, Lam TP. Open reduction and internal fixation of ipsilateral fractures of the scapular neck and clavicle. J Bone Joint Surg Am. 1993 Jul;75(7):1015–8.

67. Herscovici D Jr, Fiennes AG, Allgower M, Ruedi TP. The floating shoulder: ipsilateral clavicle and scapular neck fractures. J Bone Joint Surg Br. 1992 May;74(3):362–4.

68. Edwards SG, Whittle AP, Wood GW 2nd. Nonoperative treatment of ipsilateral fractures of the scapula and clavicle. J Bone Joint Surg Am. 2000 Jun;82(6):774–80.

69. Flanagin BA, Leslie MP. Scapulothoracic dissociation. Orthop Clin North Am. 2013 Jan;44(1):1–7.

11 Salvage Procedures

If you have read this book up to this chapter, you already realize that the field of shoulder surgery has advanced tremendously. The many surgical procedures summarized in previous chapters allow successful management of most shoulder conditions and result in improved pain, motion, and function. However, salvage procedures that sacrifice the glenohumeral joint or the scapulothoracic joint represent the best surgical option for a few patients. These salvage procedures are uncommon, but shoulder surgeons need to be familiar with their indications, surgical technique, and reported outcomes.

Glenohumeral Arthrodesis

This procedure involves achieving solid union between the proximal humerus and the scapula (Figure 11.1). Shoulder fusion was a relatively common procedure in the early years of shoulder surgery. Mobility at the scapulothoracic joint allows a surprising range of motion of the upper extremity despite absence of motion at the glenohumeral joint (Figure 11.2). There is some controversy regarding the ideal position of the arthrodesis, fixation modalities, and modes of postoperative immobilization.

Indications

The indications of glenohumeral osteoarthritis have continued to evolve over time. Table 11.1 summarizes my current indications for shoulder fusion. Arthrodesis has been traditionally considered for patients with lack of motor function (paralysis), tuberculosis and other refractory deep infections, after resection of a tumor, and for the sequels of shoulder trauma with deltoid insufficiency (primary muscular damage, axillary nerve injury, or brachial plexus injuries).

Reverse shoulder arthroplasty is currently considered for conditions where arthrodesis used to be commonly indicated. Reverse shoulder arthroplasty is considered after tumor resection provided the function of the deltoid can be preserved or restored by combining the arthroplasty with a muscle transfer (typically pectoralis major transfer). Reverse arthroplasty has also become the procedure of choice for

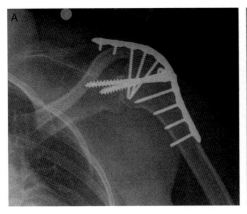
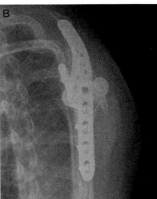
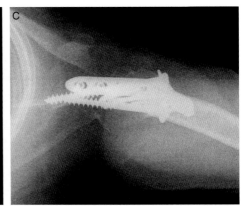

Figure 11.1 *Postoperative radiographs after shoulder arthrodesis.* **A**, *Anteroposterior.* **B**, *Lateral,* **C**, *Axillary.*

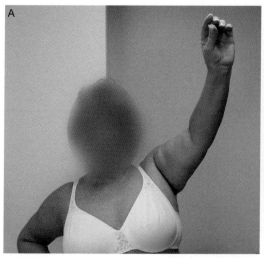
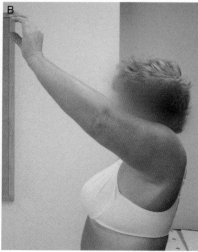
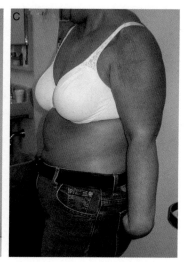

Figure 11.2 *Motion after glenohumeral arthrodesis.* **A,** *Flexion.* **B,** *Elevation.* **C,** *Internal rotation.*

Table 11.1 • Current Indications for Shoulder Arthrodesis

Shoulder paralysis (i.e., brachial plexus injuries, severe poliomyelitis)

Glenohumeral osteoarthritis in the presence of complete deltoid dysfunction (most commonly after trauma)

Refractory deep infection (i.e., tuberculosis, refractory osteomyelitis)

Resection of a tumor

Recurrent instability after multiple failed procedures in young patients with marked soft-tissue or bony deficiencies

Massive irreparable rotator cuff tear with pseudoparalysis when reverse arthroplasty is contraindicated (ultrayoung age, use of upper extremities for transfer in patients with paralysis of the lower extremities)

Failed shoulder arthroplasty not amenable to revision arthroplasty

---

patients with massive irreparable rotator cuff tearing and pseudoparalysis; however, arthrodesis is still considered for the ultrayoung patient in these circumstances due to concerns with implant longevity.

Persistent instability after multiple failed stabilizing procedures is a relatively common indication for shoulder arthrodesis. These patients typically present at a young age with substantial soft-tissue and bone deficiencies, sometimes with an underlying collagen disorder such as Ehlers-Danlos syndrome. Some may have developed cartilage damage secondary to dislocation arthropathy or chondrolysis.

Failed shoulder arthroplasty is oftentimes salvageable with implant revision. However, a subset of patients may present with catastrophic bone loss or severe deltoid dysfunction, making them better candidates for arthrodesis than revision arthroplasty.

Surgical Technique

There is controversy regarding a number of details related to the surgical technique for shoulder arthrodesis (Table 11.2, Figure 11.3). Several of these technical details are interrelated. The procedure involves preparation of the bone surfaces of the proximal humerus and scapula to eliminate all residual cartilage and contour the bones to maximize

---

Table 11.2 • Controversies Regarding the Surgical Technique for Glenohumeral Arthrodesis

Exposure
Deltopectoral
Anteromedial
Arthroscopically assisted

Position of the arm in space
Degree of flexion, abduction, and internal rotation

Relative position of the proximal humerus and scapula
Humeral head positioned superiorly against upper glenoid and acromion
Humeral head positioned directly across the glenoid
Bone graft interposed between top of the humeral head and acromion
Acromion osteotomy to tip the acromion inferiorly

Fixation
Screw fixation
Screw fixation + plate neutralization
External fixation

Need for bone graft
None
Autograft
Allograft

Postoperative immobilization
Shoulder spica cast
Dedicated shoulder brace
Shoulder immobilizer with abduction pillow

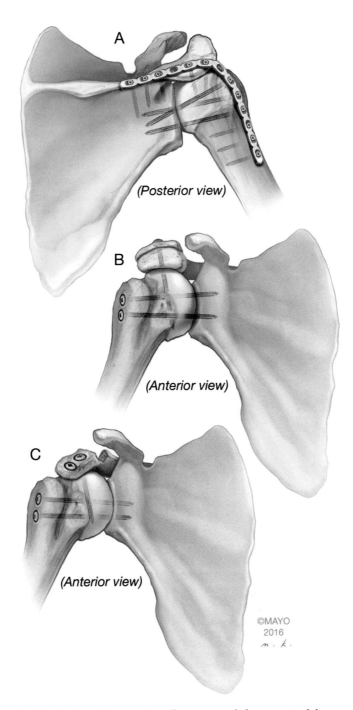

Figure 11.3 A, *Glenohumeral arthrodesis with superior placement of the proximal humerus and plate neutralization.* **B,** *Glenohumeral arthrodesis placing the humeral head across the glenoid, with intercalary subacromial bone graft and multiple screw fixation.* **C,** *Glenohumeral arthrodesis placing the humeral head across the glenoid, with acromion osteotomy and screw fixation.*

contact and compression. The posterosuperior cuff is oftentimes resected to allow union between the superior aspect of the humeral head and the acromion as well. Bone graft may be used. The arm is then positioned and fixed in the desired position. Protection of the shoulder until solid union is achieved is extremely important (▶ Video 11.1).

Position of Arthrodesis

In order to provide the best position of the hand in space, the glenohumeral joint needs to be fused so that the humerus rests in some degree of flexion, abduction, and internal rotation relative to the trunk. Most surgeons aim for a position that will allow easily reaching the center of the face with the hand as the elbow is flexed. Angles of approximately 20° of flexion and 45° of internal rotation are commonly recommended and reported in most studies (Figure 11.4A).

There is less agreement in the angle of abduction: higher angles will allow better active elevation at the expense of overuse of the periscapular musculature in the resting position, which may result in fatigue and periscapular pain. It is probably best to discuss this particular aspect with the patient and individualize the angle of abduction to each patient's needs. Patients interested in as much elevation as possible are fused in abduction angles of 40° or higher, whereas patients interested in minimizing periscapular pain are fused in abduction angles around 20° (Figures 11.4B and C). Higher abduction angles are also selected for overweight patients.

Regarding the relative position of the proximal humerus and the scapula, my preference is to place the prepared humeral head high, so that it contacts both the glenoid and the acromion (Figure 11.3A). This provides a much larger area of bone contact: The humeral head will be fused to both the acromion superiorly and the glenoid medially without the need for bone graft. However, some prefer to fuse the humeral head directly across the glenoid and either leave a space between the humeral head and the acromion, or place an intercalary bone graft in the subacromial space, or osteotomize the acromion to angle it inferiorly.

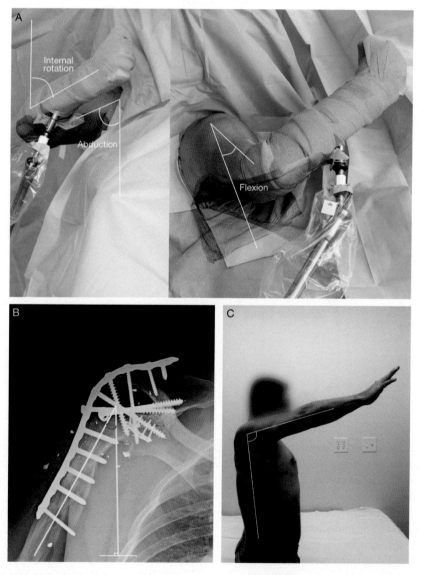

Figure 11.4 **A,** *Intraoperative photographs show positioning of the arm for glenohumeral arthrodesis in flexion, abduction, and internal rotation.* **B,** *Radiographic measurement of the abduction angle after arthrodesis.* **C,** *Range of motion in elevation.*

Fixation

My preference is to use interfragmentary screw fixation combined with plate neutralization (Figure 11.5). This fixation modality provides the strongest possible construct and may be particularly useful in less compliant patients or those with risk factors for nonunion. However, contouring the plate to place it properly across the spine of the scapula, acromion, and proximal humerus is time consuming and somewhat difficult. In addition, the plate may become prominent and bothersome in thinner patients or those with poor muscle coverage secondary to muscle atrophy (paralysis). Finally, adequate screw fixation of the plate may be difficult in patients with severe osteopenia or hypoplastic bones after a longstanding brachial plexus injury. Alternatively, fixation may be obtained with screw fixation only; this is particularly attractive when performed percutaneously in the setting of arthroscopically assisted arthrodesis. Use of an external fixator for arthrodesis can be considered for patients with persistent osteomyelitis, but was much more commonly used in the past and is currently largely abandoned.

Exposure

When glenohumeral arthrodesis is performed so that the humeral head will contact both the glenoid and the

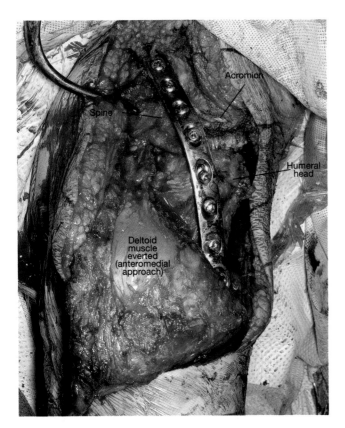

Figure 11.5 *Intraoperative photograph shows plate fixation across the arthrodesis site.*

acromion, and plate neutralization will be used for fixation, the anteromedial approach is ideal (see chapter 3, Surgical Exposures). Detachment of the deltoid from the clavicle, acromion, and the spine of the scapula provides great exposure to resect the posterosuperior cuff; prepares the humeral head, glenoid, and acromion surfaces; and places the neutralization plate across the spine of the scapula and proximal humerus. Alternatively, shoulder arthrodesis may be performed through a standard deltopectoral approach when more limited fixation is considered. As mentioned before, arthroscopically assisted arthrodesis has been described as well, with removal of cartilage from the humeral head and the glenoid with an arthroscopic bur followed by percutaneous or mini-open internal fixation.

Other Technical Details

Solid union across the arthrodesis site is more likely to occur if there is perfect preparation of the bone surfaces, adequate contact and compression, and stable fixation. During bone preparation, efforts are made to remove all remaining cartilage and to contour the bone surfaces so that they will have the best possible contact. My preference is to use a combination of a saw blade and a high-speed bur to accomplish these 2 goals.

Substantial bone loss may compromise the ability to achieve union. Small areas of bone deficiency may be addressed with allograft, but my preference is to use iliac crest autograft for larger defects. Occasionally, substantial bone defects after resection of a tumor or catastrophic implant failure require use of a vascularized autograft, typically from the fibula (1).

Postoperative Management

The shoulder region should be protected until union is confirmed. The modality and length of immobilization depend on bone quality, the fixation method used, and patient compliance and comorbidities. The upper extremity is heavy, and lack of support can really endanger the success of the fixation. My preference has been to use a shoulder spica cast for most patients (Figure 11.6A). Having the upper extremity perfectly supported by a cast seems to help control pain in the immediate postoperative period. In addition, it does not rely on compliance or adjustments as much as brace immobilization. However, when adequate compression and stable fixation have been achieved, brace immobilization may suffice to achieve union, and some patients find it more comfortable (Figure 11.6B). When a shoulder spica cast is used, patients are typically transitioned to a brace at week 8. Some sort of immobilization is used for 3 to 4 months for most patients. Care must be taken with cast management in patients with compromised sensation secondary to brachial plexus injuries, since they can develop painless full-thickness skin erosions secondary to pressure.

During the immobilization time, patients cannot be allowed to perform shoulder range of motion exercises.

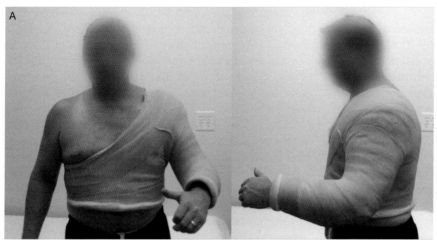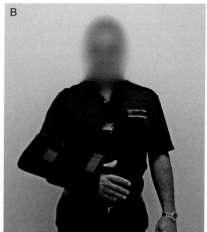

Figure 11.6 **A,** *Shoulder spica cast.* **B,** *Shoulder immobilizer.*

However, isometric strengthening of the scapular stabilizers should be initiated as soon as pain allows. In addition, all factors that may possibly interfere with union need to be addressed. The 2 most common are smoking and infection. As a general rule, I delay surgery on smokers until cessation of tobacco use is confirmed. Patients undergoing an arthrodesis in the setting of infection require adequate antibiotic treatment and may need to be considered for staged surgery.

Outcome and Complications

A number of studies have reported on the outcome of glenohumeral arthrodesis (Table 11.3) (2–10). Some studies with larger numbers of patients include several diagnoses, whereas others have included only 1 specific condition. Reported union rates have approximated 100%, although secondary bone grafting is required in some patients. Union may be more difficult to achieve when arthrodesis is attempted for failed shoulder arthroplasty (7), likely due to a combination of substantial bone loss and devitalized bone surfaces. Shoulder arthrodesis has been reported to improve pain reliably in 75% to 90% of the patients. Scapulothoracic motion allows some degree of elevation; in Cofield and Brigg's study (2), 75% of the patients could easily reach the trunk level, 50% reached the head level, and 25% reached overhead.

The main complication of shoulder arthrodesis is fracture of the humeral shaft distal to the fusion site (Figure 11.7). Reported fracture rates have ranged from 2% to 15% (2–10). Most fractures are the consequence of a fall: The arthrodesed shoulder cannot be easily protected from impact, and the long lever arm distal to the fusion facilitates fracture. Osteopenia may also play a role in selected patients, such as those with long-standing brachial plexus palsy. Other complications include nonunion requiring bone grafting and infection. Some patients will complain of periscapular pain, likely secondary to excessive muscle loads after fusion. Finally, some individuals are bothered by their hardware, and in some studies the rate of hardware removal has been as high as 25% to 50%.

Scapulothoracic Arthrodesis

Surgical stabilization of the scapula to the chest wall was developed at the beginning of the last century for patients with severe muscular dystrophy resulting in painful scapular winging (see chapter 10, The Scapula, for an in-depth review of scapular disorders). Over time, 2 main procedures evolved: scapulopexy and scapulothoracic arthrodesis. *Scapulopexy* involves stabilizing the scapula to the chest wall by using fascial slings or synthetic material (11). *Scapulothoracic arthrodesis* (also known as *scapulodesis* or *scapulothoracic fusion*) involves achieving solid bony union between the body of the scapula and several ribs. The results of scapulopexy tend to deteriorate over time due to stretching of the material used to suspend the scapula off the ribs. Scapulothoracic arthrodesis has thus become the procedure of choice.

Rationale and Indications

Isolated dysfunction of certain periscapular muscles can be successfully managed with tendon transfers or surgery on the involved peripheral nerve (see chapter 10, The Scapula). However, when multiple or most periscapular muscles are either detached (as occurs in scapulothoracic dissociation) or dysfunctional (as in extensive injuries to the brachial plexus or dystrophic muscular conditions), scapulothoracic arthrodesis typically is a better solution. These patients with extensive damage to the periscapular musculature complain of periscapular and shoulder pain, limited active elevation, and winging.

Table 11.3 • Outcome of Glenohumeral Arthrodesis as Reported in Selected Studies

Study	No. of Patients	Indications	Follow-up, y	Union, %	Pain	Function	Complications	Comments
Cofield and Briggs (2)	71	Paralysis Cuff tear Osteoarthritis Infection Instability Rheumatoid arthritis	9.5	96	75% no or mild pain	Trunk level 75% Head level 50% Overhead 25%	Postoperative fracture 14% Infection 1.5% Hardware removal 24%	Subjective satisfaction 82% Results did not deteriorate over time
Rybka et al (3)	41	Rheumatoid arthritis	6	90	90% no or mild pain	Good or excellent results in 68%	Postoperative fracture 2.5% Hardware removal 10%	Subjective satisfaction 95%
Richards et al (4)	14	Brachial plexus injury	2.6	100	78% no or mild pain	Minimum abduction 60°	Hardware removal 50%	All patients felt function had improved
Diaz et al (5)	8	Instability	2.9	100	Mean VAS 3.1	Mean VAS 4.7	Hardware removal 62% ACJ resection 25%	Subjective satisfaction 100%
Fuchs et al (6)	21	Tumor resection	11	N/A	N/A	81% Toronto score	Overall complication rate 43%	8 primary and 13 salvage arthrodesis
Scalise and Iannotti (7)	7	Failed arthroplasty	4	42 (71 after secondary bone grafting)	Pain score 26/30	Function score 26/30	Secondary bone grafting 57% Hardware removal 28%	4 cases required vascularized fibular autograft
Atlan et al (8)	54	Brachial plexus injury	3	76 (94 after additional surgery)	N/A	Abduction >45° in 75%, rotation >45° in 65%	Secondary bone grafting 24% Infection 3.7%	Graft used between acromion and humeral head Only 12% of patients were immobilized
Porcellini et al (9)	12	Instability Deep infection Cuff deficiency Brachial plexus palsy	2	83 (100 after additional bone grafting)	N/A	Spadi score improved 60 points	Secondary bone grafting 17%	Arthroscopically assisted arthrodesis
Thangarajah et al (10)	6	Epilepsy-associated instability	3	100	N/A	SSV 42%, Oxford instability score 24	Hardware removal 16% Postoperative fracture 16%	Cast immobilization 3 months

Abbreviations: ACJ, acromioclavicular joint; N/A, not available; SSV, Subjective Shoulder Value; VAS, Visual Analog Scale; y, years.

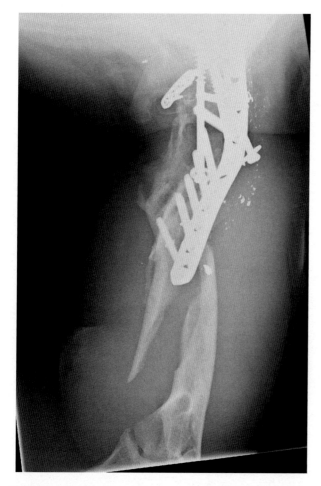

Figure 11.7 Late fracture in a patient injured after undergoing successful glenohumeral arthrodesis.

Table 11.4 • Indications for Scapulothoracic Arthrodesis
Muscular dystrophy
Facioscapulohumeral dystrophy and others
Congenital abnormalities
Sprengel deformity
Congenital absence of multiple periscapular muscles
Injuries to the brachial plexus or its branches not amenable to successful nerve repair or tendon transfer
Widespread involvement
Salvage of previous transfer
Associated collagen disease (i.e., Ehlers-Danlos syndrome)
Severe traumatic disruption of periscapular musculature not amenable to repair or reconstruction
Scapulothoracic dissociation with persistent symptoms despite adequate stabilization of the clavicle
Severe clavicular insufficiency
Congenital (cleidocranial dysostosis)
Traumatic
After surgical resection (tumor, uncontrolled osteomyelitis, trauma)

Permanent fusion of the scapula to the chest wall typically results in improvement of all 3 symptoms. Improvements in active elevation after scapulothoracic arthrodesis may be predicted to some extent with the scapular assistance test (see chapter 1, Evaluation of the Shoulder).

Table 11.4 summarizes the most common current indications for scapulothoracic arthrodesis. After scapulothoracic arthrodesis, active shoulder motion depends on the deltoid and the rotator cuff; this procedure should thus be avoided in patients with dysfunction of the axillary or suprascapular nerves or other reasons for poor deltoid or cuff function (12).

Surgical Technique

Basic Principles

Bone union between the body of the scapula and the ribs requires adequate contact between well-prepared bone surfaces, compression, and stable fixation until a solid fusion mass develops. There are a number of practical problems that make it difficult to achieve these goals at the scapulothoracic joint: Muscles between the scapula and the ribs need to be widely mobilized or partially resected, fixation needs to be achieved between bone structures that do not provide a whole lot of bone stock (the ribs are relatively narrow cylinders with the pleura and lungs underneath, and the body of the scapula can be paper thin), and the whole upper extremity hangs off the scapula creating a large weight to support during healing.

Various techniques have been described to perform this procedure. My preference is to use cables around the ribs and through the body of the scapula for fixation (Figure 11.8) (13). Others have reported use of wires or screws (14,15), but modern cables are very strong and can be adequately tensioned (13,16). Since the body of the scapula is so thin, cables or wires can easily break it; this is avoided by using a plate on the dorsal aspect of the scapula, so that cables go through the body of the scapula and then through the plate. The plate protects the scapular body from fracture as the cables are tensioned. Wires are favored when arthrodesis is performed in children with dystrophy, for example, fascioscapulohumeral dystrophy (17).

Bone graft is commonly added at the interface between the body of the scapula and the ribs to promote successful union. Good results have been reported using both autograft and allograft (13–16,18). My preference is to use autograft obtained from the posterior iliac crest. The fixation must be protected to some extent until fusion

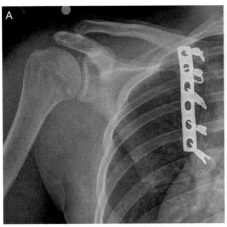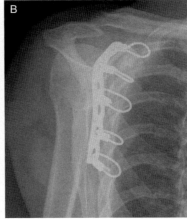

Figure 11.8 *Postoperative radiographs (**A,** anteroposterior; **B,** lateral Y) after scapulothoracic arthrodesis.*

occurs. I favor use of a shoulder spica cast, but other authors have reported use of custom-made or commercial braces (13).

Since several ribs are used to secure the scapula, chest excursion is somewhat restricted after surgery permanently. This is particularly relevant in patients with associated thoracic pathology or those with dystrophy possibly requiring bilateral scapulothoracic arthrodesis (19–21). However, clinically relevant pulmonary insufficiency seems to be uncommon, even after bilateral arthrodesis (21).

Surgical Procedure

The patient is placed prone (Figure 11.9). The opposite upper extremity is placed on an arm board with the shoulder in approximately 140° of abduction; the scapula on the noninvolved side can then be used as a reference to determine in which position to fuse the involved scapula. The affected upper extremity is draped free and can be rested in a Mayo stand in the same position of 140° of abduction at the time of fusion, but can also be moved freely for other portions of the procedure (⬤ Video 11.2).

The medial edge of the scapula is exposed using a vertical skin incision. The trapezius and rhomboids are detached from the scapular body. The serratus anterior and paraspinal musculature are mobilized as needed or partially resected to expose the inferior aspect of the body of the scapula and the ribs. The origins of the supraspinatus and infraspinatus are mobilized laterally to expose the dorsal aspect of the body of the scapula. Changes in position of the arm help expose the inferior aspect of the scapula and the ribs.

The spine of the scapula can be palpated on the noninvolved side and the spine of the scapula on the affected side can be positioned symmetrically to select the rib that will be fixed to the scapula at the level of the spine. Additional ribs are exposed proximally and distally. Most of the time the scapula is fixed to 4 or 5 ribs, depending on the size of

the patient. Most commonly the scapula is fixed to ribs 3 to 7 or 4 to 8. A high-speed bur is used to lightly decorticate the dorsal aspect of the ribs and the inferior aspect of the body of the scapula. A large fragment 5- or 6-hole plate is then contoured to fit the dorsal aspect of the scapula over the spine. This requires removing a small amount of bone from the scapular spine for the plate to sit flat.

The posterior iliac crest is then exposed and corticocancellous struts are obtained with a microsagittal saw and osteotomes. Additional cancellous chips are harvested as well, and the iliac crest donor site is closed, typically leaving a drain underneath.

The most delicate part of the procedure involves passing the cables around the ribs. Anesthesia can help with use of smaller end-tidal lung volumes or selective hypoventilation of the lung on the operative side. Dedicated small curved instruments are used to pass the cables as close to the ribs as possible. After each cable is passed, the surgical field is irrigated, avoiding suction for a few seconds to confirm that no bubbles are coming out of the chest wall. If bubbles are seen, the pleura is likely perforated, and the patient will probably require placement of a chest tube at the end of the procedure to manage the resultant pneumothorax.

Once all cables are passed under the ribs, the plate is placed over the dorsal aspect of the scapula and the scapular body is drilled in line with the plate holes to pass the cables. All harvested iliac crest is placed as a sandwich between the body of the scapula and the ribs, and the cables are tensioned simultaneously with mechanical tensioners and secured with crimp connectors. The rhomboids and trapezius are then repaired to the supraspinatus and infraspinatus to cover the plate. The rest of the closure is routine.

Postoperative Management

A chest radiograph with the patient sitting up should be obtained after surgery to identify pneumothorax and place

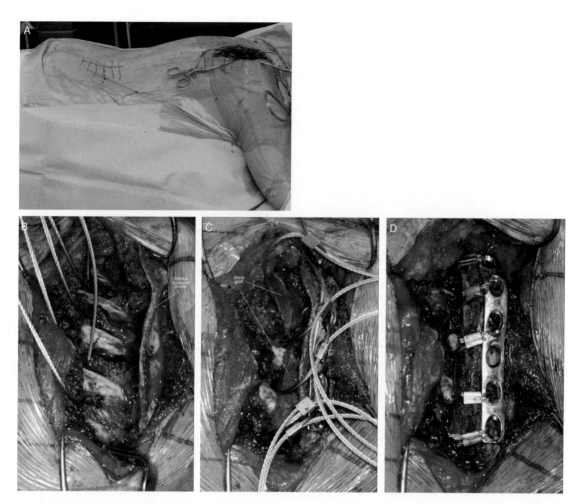

Figure 11.9 *Scapulothoracic arthrodesis.* **A,** *Positioning.* **B,** *Exposure.* **C,** *Bone grafting and cable placement.* **D,** *Final reconstruction.*

a chest tube if needed. My preference is to use a shoulder spica cast to protect the arthrodesis site by immobilizing the shoulder and supporting the weight of the upper extremity. The cast is removed between week 6 and 8, and a commercial shoulder immobilizer is used for the following 6 weeks but removed for physical therapy exercises. Radiographs are interpreted as consistent with arthrodesis when there is no change in the position of the scapula on sequential radiographs and all hardware remains intact. However, if there is any question about the arthrodesis, such as in patients with persistent pain, computed tomography is necessary to confirm successful fusion.

Outcome and Complications

Most published studies on scapulothoracic arthrodesis have reported the results in patients with fascioscapulo-humeral dystrophy (13,14,17–23) or a mixed group of diagnoses (15,16). A few studies have reported the outcome specifically in nondystrophic conditions (24–26). In most studies, scapulothoracic arthrodesis has been reported to provide satisfactory pain relief, improved active elevation,

and satisfactory cosmesis (Table 11.5). Most studies have reported improvements in active flexion or elevation from below the horizontal to over the horizontal. However, some studies have reported late deterioration of motion over time in patients with facioscapulohumeral muscular dystrophy as their underlying condition deteriorates (17) (Figure 11.10).

The main complications of scapulothoracic arthrodesis include pulmonary complications (pneumothorax, pleural effusion, atelectasis), nonunion, fractures of the ribs or the scapula, and intercostal neuralgia. The rate of union has ranged between 70% and 100%; 1 study correlated nonunion with a number of risk factors, including smoking, age over 35 years, and prior shoulder surgery (16). An uncommon complication of scapulothoracic fusion is compression of the brachial plexus and the subclavian vessels (27). Brachial plexopathy after scapulothoracic arthrodesis may recover spontaneously, but sometimes may require removing the fixation construct and allowing the scapula and clavicle to return to the preoperative position.

Table 11.5 • Reported Outcomes After Scapulothoracic Arthrodesis

Author	No.	Indications	Follow-up, y	Union, %	Elevation/Flexion, Degrees		Complications, No.
					Pre	Final	
Letournel et al (19)	Patients, 9 Shoulders, 16	FSHD	5.7	93	75	108	Reduced pulmonary function, 1 Pneumothorax, 3 Pleural effusion, 1 Atelectasis, 1 Rib fracture or nonunion, 2 Scapula fracture, 2
Bunch and Siegel (23)	Patients, 12 Shoulders, 17	FSHD	3–21	100	30	125	Transient brachial plexus compression, 1 Frozen shoulder, 1
Bizot et al (26)	Patients, 10	Serratus anterior palsy (isolated in 5, combined in 5)	6.3 (range, 1–15)	70	83	101	Pleural effusion, 2 Nonunion, 3 Postoperative arthrodesis fracture, 1 Frozen shoulder, 1
Diab et al (17)	Patients, 8 Shoulders, 11	FSHD	6.5	100	75	145	Hardware removal, 2
Jeon et al (25)	Shoulders, 6	Trapezius palsy, 3 Brachial plexus injury, 2 Sprengel deformity, 1	4	83	80	98	Hardware discomfort, 6 Nonunion, 1
Rhee and Ha (22)	Patients, 6 Shoulders, 9	FSHD	4	100	71	109	Pleural effusion, 1
Demirhan et al (13)	Patients, 13 Shoulders, 18	FSHD	3	89	55	126	Nonunion, 2 Hardware failure and removal, 1
Sewell et al (16)	Patients, 34 Shoulders, 42	Dystrophic conditions (e.g., FSHD and others), 15 Nondystrophic conditions (e.g., nerve palsies and others), 19	5	86	59	97	Nonunion, 6 Rib fracture, 2 Pneumothorax, 2 Pleural effusion, 3
Van Tongel et al (14)	Patients, 24 Shoulders, 35	FSHD	2	86	65	119	Pneumothorax, 1 Nonunion, 5 Fracture, 1
Cooney et al (18)	Patients, 11 Shoulders, 14	FSHD	2.4	93	70	115	Pneumonia, 1 Pleural effusion, 1 Nonunion, 1 Hardware removal, 5 Transient brachial plexus injury, 1
Goel et al (15)	Patients, 10 Shoulders, 12	FSHD, 3 Clavicular insufficiency, 2 Trapezius palsy, 5	3.4	83	90	117	Pleural effusion, 1 Pneumothorax, 1 Infection, 1 Pulmonary embolism, 1 Nonunion, 2 Hardware removal, 6

Abbreviations: FSHD, facioscapulohumeral muscular dystrophy; y, years.

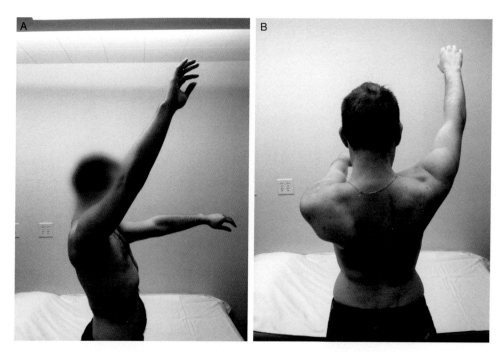

Figure 11.10 Range of motion in a patient with facioscapulohumeral muscular dystrophy. **A,** *Lateral view.* **B,** *Posterior view. The left shoulder has not undergone surgery and displays limited active elevation and winging. The right shoulder has undergone scapulothoracic arthrodesis resulting in improved elevation and absence of winging.*

Glenohumeral Resection Arthroplasty

Resection procedures involve removing a variable portion of the proximal humerus, and occasionally a portion of the scapula as well, leaving a space at the old location of the glenohumeral joint. Fibrous tissue eventually fills this space and can provide some degree of stability (Figure 11.11).

Indications

Permanent resection arthroplasty with no intention of further reconstructing the glenohumeral joint is indicated

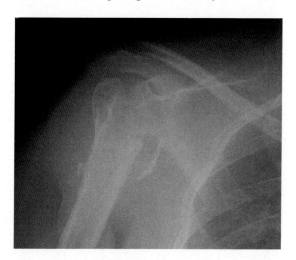

Figure 11.11 Postoperative radiograph after permanent resection of the glenohumeral joint.

as a salvage procedure only in the following situations: in frail patients, those with multiple failed procedures with persistence of infection, or those with deep infection (periprosthetic joint infection or osteomyelitis); in cases of catastrophic failure of arthroplasty with severely compromised bone stock not amenable to arthroplasty or arthrodesis; and in frail patients with locally aggressive or malignant tumors, short anticipated survival, or disinterest in arthroplasty or arthrodesis.

As discussed in chapter 9, Shoulder Arthritis and Arthroplasty, a 2-stage reimplantation is the most common treatment strategy offered to patients with deep infection after arthroplasty, as well as to patients with osteomyelitis of the native glenohumeral joint. At the time of resection, most surgeons implant a cement spacer, planning to remove it and replace it with a prosthesis at the second stage reimplantation. However, some patients experience good pain relief and reasonable function with their temporary spacer, and choose to avoid the second stage and maintain it permanently.

Surgical Technique

Nononcologic Resection Arthroplasties

Most resection arthroplasties are performed through a deltopectoral approach; occasionally, extension into an anteromedial approach is necessary (see chapter 3, Surgical Exposures). Even when resection is expected to be permanent, the soft tissues and bone stock at the shoulder should be preserved as best as possible, in case further reconstruction is contemplated in the future. On the other hand, when resection is performed for infection, all infected-looking tissue and most, if not all, foreign material should be removed. The exception may be areas of extremely well bonded cement when the risk of fracture, catastrophic bone loss, or nerve injury is too high to justify cement removal at all costs.

In patients with a native septic joint, if possible only the humeral head is resected at the anatomical neck level. However, additional bone removal may be required based on the gross aspect of bone and tissues. If there is any glenoid cartilage left, consideration should be given to reaming the glenoid, since bacteria may potentially survive in the avascular cartilage. When performing a permanent resection for a failed or infected shoulder arthroplasty, careful removal of the components should be attempted following the principles and techniques outlined in the section on revision arthroplasty in chapter 9, Shoulder Arthritis and Arthroplasty. Again, an attempt should be made to preserve bone stock and soft tissues without retaining infected tissue or foreign materials.

The goal of postoperative management is to let the joint "stiffen up" so that the resected joint is somewhat stable, which is perceived to lead to better pain relief and function. Most authors have reported use of a shoulder immobilizer for 6 to 12 weeks, gentle motion afterwards, and delayed strengthening for up to 6 months (28). Obviously, infected shoulders do require appropriate antibiotic treatment, typically 6 weeks of intravenous antibiotics followed by a variable course of oral antibiotics.

Oncologic Resections

Resections performed for the surgical management of malignancy follow general oncologic principles and may require surgical removal of not only various segments of bone but also the rotator cuff, some or part of the deltoid, and occasionally the axillary and/or radial nerves. An in-depth discussion of shoulder oncology exceeds the scope of this book, but a few concepts are useful to the shoulder surgeon. Most patients will be offered, and elect, reconstruction of the resected shoulder with an arthrodesis or an arthroplasty. Frail patients with an expected low life expectancy may be better served with a permanent resection (1).

The Musculoskeletal Tumor Society classification is most commonly used to describe the extent of the resection (Figure 11.12). The skeleton of the scapula is divided in 2 segments, and the proximal humerus in 3. The letter A is used when the deltoid or rotator cuff can be preserved or reconstructed, whereas the letter B indicates sacrifice of the deltoid or cuff. For example, S234B means that the body of the scapula and humeral shaft are preserved, but the glenoid fossa and the upper third of the proximal humerus are resected with poor integrity of the deltoid or cuff. The Tikhoff-Linberg procedure is an S1234B resection (1).

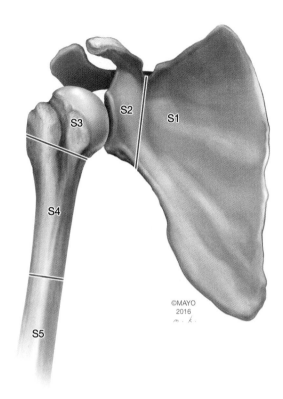

Figure 11.12 *Musculoskeletal Tumor Society classification of resections of the shoulder girdle. S denotes bone segment. The number of skeletal segments resected is expressed numerically and qualified as A if the deltoid and rotator cuff are either preserved or reconstructed and as B if the deltoid or rotator cuff needs to be resected and cannot be reconstructed.*

Outcome

Few studies have reported the outcome of resection arthroplasty in detail. Braman et al (29) reported on 7 resection arthroplasties performed for the management of deep periprosthetic infection. Pain was rated as none or mild in 5, and moderate with activity in 2 shoulders. Motion was extremely limited (mean elevation to 30° and mean external rotation to 10°), but all patients were able to use the hand on the affected side to feed themselves and reach the perineum. There were no recurrences of infection and no complications. Rispoli et al (28) reported a total of 18 resections: 13 performed for periprosthetic joint infection, 4 performed for catastrophic implant failure, and 1 performed for osteomyelitis. Pain level decreased, but 5 patients continued to complain of moderate to severe pain. Mean motion included elevation to 70°, with minimal active rotation. Most patients were unable to perform the majority of the activities included in shoulder outcome tools. Other studies have reported similar results (30–32). As expected, in oncologic patients the outcome of permanent resection is worse than the outcome obtained with arthrodesis, arthroplasty, or osteoarticular allografts (1).

Based on all the available data, it seems fair to conclude that resection arthroplasty will eradicate deep infection when present. Pain tends to improve, but not to zero, and some patients will have continued pain. Function is poor for the most part, but a number of patients are subjectively satisfied taking into account their starting point. At the present time, alternatives to resection arthroplasty are considered when possible in order to provide the opportunity for a better functional result, but the potential for improvement in pain and eradication of infection should be discussed with patients facing a permanent resection as an alternative.

KEY POINTS

✓ Glenohumeral arthrodesis, scapulothoracic arthrodesis, and permanent glenohumeral resection are 3 salvage procedures occasionally performed for selected patients with no other good surgical solution.

✓ The main indications for glenohumeral arthrodesis are shoulder paralysis, glenohumeral arthritis in the presence of complete deltoid dysfunction, refractory deep infection, tumor resection, and selected cases of failed arthroplasty, cuff-tear arthropathy, and instability when other alternatives are contraindicated.

✓ Most surgeons agree with fusing the glenohumeral joint in 20° of flexion and 45° of internal rotation; abduction is typically set between 20° and 40°.

✓ There are various techniques described to perform glenohumeral arthrodesis. I tend to prefer use of an anteromedial approach, placement of the humeral head against both the glenoid and the acromion, and use a combination of interfragmentary screw compression and plate neutralization.

✓ Several studies have reported satisfactory pain relief in most patients and very high union rates after glenohumeral arthrodesis. Scapulothoracic motion does allow some degree of elevation for many patients.

✓ The main complications of glenohumeral arthrodesis are fracture of the humeral shaft, nonunion, infection, periscapular pain, and symptomatic hardware requiring removal.

✓ The main indications of scapulothoracic arthrodesis include facioscapulohumeral dystrophy, Sprengel deformity, multiple severe neuromuscular injuries not amenable to repair or transfer, and severe clavicular insufficiency.

✓ There are multiple techniques described to perform scapulothoracic arthrodesis. My preference is to fuse the scapula to ribs 3 to 7 using cables through a plate to avoid fracture of the scapular body, and adding iliac crest bone autograft.

✓ Most studies on scapulothoracic arthrodesis have reported satisfactory rates of pain relief and improvements in active elevation.

✓ The main complications of scapulothoracic arthrodesis include pneumothorax, pleural effusion, atelectasis, nonunion, fractures of the ribs or scapula, and intercostal neuralgia.

✓ Permanent resection of the glenohumeral joint is uncommonly performed for frail patients with recalcitrant deep infection, catastrophic implant failure, or resection of malignant tumors.

✓ Postoperatively, patients are immobilized for a number of weeks to let the resection "stiffen up" and hopefully provide some stability and the potential for some motion.

✓ Permanent resection tends to provide some pain relief, but function is extremely limited.

REFERENCES

1. O'Connor MI, Sim FH, Chao EY. Limb salvage for neoplasms of the shoulder girdle: intermediate reconstructive and functional results. J Bone Joint Surg Am. 1996 Dec;78(12):1872–88.
2. Cofield RH, Briggs BT. Glenohumeral arthrodesis. Operative and long-term functional results. J Bone Joint Surg Am. 1979 Jul;61(5):668–77.
3. Rybka V, Raunio P, Vainio K. Arthrodesis of the shoulder in rheumatoid arthritis: a review of forty-one cases. J Bone Joint Surg Br. 1979 May;61-B(2):155–8.
4. Richards RR, Waddell JP, Hudson AR. Shoulder arthrodesis for the treatment of brachial plexus palsy. Clin Orthop Relat Res. 1985 Sep;(198):250–8.
5. Diaz JA, Cohen SB, Warren RF, Craig EV, Allen AA. Arthrodesis as a salvage procedure for recurrent instability of the shoulder. J Shoulder Elbow Surg. 2003 May-Jun;12(3):237–41.
6. Fuchs B, O'Connor MI, Padgett DJ, Kaufman KR, Sim FH. Arthrodesis of the shoulder after tumor resection. Clin Orthop Relat Res. 2005 Jul;(436):202–7.
7. Scalise JJ, Iannotti JP. Glenohumeral arthrodesis after failed prosthetic shoulder arthroplasty. J Bone Joint Surg Am. 2008 Jan;90(1):70–7.
8. Atlan F, Durand S, Fox M, Levy P, Belkheyar Z, Oberlin C. Functional outcome of glenohumeral fusion in brachial plexus palsy: a report of 54 cases. J Hand Surg Am. 2012 Apr;37(4):683–8.
9. Porcellini G, Savoie FH 3rd, Campi F, Merolla G, Paladini P. Arthroscopically assisted shoulder arthrodesis: is it an effective technique? Arthroscopy. 2014 Dec;30(12):1550–6. Epub 2014 Aug 29.
10. Thangarajah T, Alexander S, Bayley I, Lambert SM. Glenohumeral arthrodesis for the treatment of recurrent shoulder instability in epileptic patients. Bone Joint J. 2014 Nov;96-B(11):1525–9.
11. Ketenjian AY. Scapulocostal stabilization for scapular winging in facioscapulohumeral muscular dystrophy. J Bone Joint Surg Am. 1978 Jun;60(4):476–80.
12. DeFranco MJ, Nho S, Romeo AA. scapulothoracic fusion. J Am Acad Orthop Surg. 2010 Apr;18(4):236–42.
13. Demirhan M, Uysal O, Atalar AC, Kilicoglu O, Serdaroglu P. Scapulothoracic arthrodesis in facioscapulohumeral dystrophy with multifilament cable. Clin Orthop Relat Res. 2009 Aug;467(8):2090–7. Epub 2009 Mar 31.

14. Van Tongel A, Atoun E, Narvani A, Sforza G, Copeland S, Levy O. Medium to long-term outcome of thoracoscapular arthrodesis with screw fixation for facioscapulohumeral muscular dystrophy. J Bone Joint Surg Am. 2013 Aug 7;95(15):1404–8.

15. Goel DP, Romanowski JR, Shi LL, Warner JJ. scapulothoracic fusion: outcomes and complications. J Shoulder Elbow Surg. 2014 Apr;23(4):542–7.

16. Sewell MD, Higgs DS, Al-Hadithy N, Falworth M, Bayley I, Lambert SM. The outcome of scapulothoracic fusion for painful winging of the scapula in dystrophic and non-dystrophic conditions. J Bone Joint Surg Br. 2012 Sep;94(9):1253–9.

17. Diab M, Darras BT, Shapiro F. Scapulothoracic fusion for facioscapulohumeral muscular dystrophy. J Bone Joint Surg Am. 2005 Oct;87(10):2267–75.

18. Cooney AD, Gill I, Stuart PR. The outcome of scapulothoracic arthrodesis using cerclage wires, plates, and allograft for facioscapulohumeral dystrophy. J Shoulder Elbow Surg. 2014 Jan;23(1):e8–13.

19. Letournel E, Fardeau M, Lytle JO, Serrault M, Gosselin RA. Scapulothoracic arthrodesis for patients who have fascioscapulohumeral muscular dystrophy. J Bone Joint Surg Am. 1990 Jan;72(1):78–84.

20. Andrews CT, Taylor TC, Patterson VH. Scapulothoracic arthrodesis for patients with facioscapulohumeral muscular dystrophy. Neuromuscul Disord. 1998 Dec;8(8):580–4.

21. Berne D, Laude F, Laporte C, Fardeau M, Saillant G. Scapulothoracic arthrodesis in facioscapulohumeral muscular dystrophy. Clin Orthop Relat Res. 2003 Apr;(409):106–13.

22. Rhee YG, Ha JH. Long-term results of scapulothoracic arthrodesis of facioscapulohumeral muscular dystrophy. J Shoulder Elbow Surg. 2006 Jul-Aug;15(4):445–50.

23. Bunch WH, Siegel IM. Scapulothoracic arthrodesis in facioscapulohumeral muscular dystrophy: review of seventeen procedures with three to twenty-one-year follow-up. J Bone Joint Surg Am. 1993 Mar;75(3):372–6.

24. Elhassan B, Chung ST, Ozbaydar M, Diller D, Warner JJ. Scapulothoracic fusion for clavicular insufficiency: a report of two cases. J Bone Joint Surg Am. 2008 Apr;90(4):875–80.

25. Jeon IH, Neumann L, Wallace WA. Scapulothoracic fusion for painful winging of the scapula in non-dystrophic patients. J Shoulder Elbow Surg. 2005 Jul-Aug;14(4):400–6.

26. Bizot P, Teboul F, Nizard R, Sedel L. Scapulothoracic fusion for serratus anterior paralysis. J Shoulder Elbow Surg. 2003 Nov-Dec;12(6):561–5.

27. Mackenzie WG, Riddle EC, Earley JL, Sawatzky BJ. A neurovascular complication after scapulothoracic arthrodesis. Clin Orthop Relat Res. 2003 Mar;(408):157–61.

28. Rispoli DM, Sperling JW, Athwal GS, Schleck CD, Cofield RH. Pain relief and functional results after resection arthroplasty of the shoulder. J Bone Joint Surg Br. 2007 Sep;89(9):1184–7.

29. Braman JP, Sprague M, Bishop J, Lo IK, Lee EW, Flatow EL. The outcome of resection shoulder arthroplasty for recalcitrant shoulder infections. J Shoulder Elbow Surg. 2006 Sep-Oct;15(5):549–53.

30. Verhelst L, Stuyck J, Bellemans J, Debeer P. Resection arthroplasty of the shoulder as a salvage procedure for deep shoulder infection: does the use of a cement spacer improve outcome? J Shoulder Elbow Surg. 2011 Dec;20(8):1224–33.

31. Muh SJ, Streit JJ, Lenarz CJ, McCrum C, Wanner JP, Shishani Y, et al. Resection arthroplasty for failed shoulder arthroplasty. J Shoulder Elbow Surg. 2013 Feb;22(2):247–52.

32. Stevens NM, Kim HM, Armstrong AD. Functional outcomes after shoulder resection: the patient's perspective. J Shoulder Elbow Surg. 2015 Sep;24(9):e247–54.

12 Rehabilitation and Injections

A book on the principles and fundamentals of shoulder surgery must review the basic principles of shoulder rehabilitation, as well as the role of injecting medications locally in various areas and spaces.

As mentioned multiple times in this book, *rehabilitation* modalities, mostly physical therapy, are paramount for the success of shoulder surgery, and they are also the cornerstones for most programs of nonoperative management. There are whole books dedicated to the fields of physical medicine, rehabilitation, and physical therapy. In this chapter, I will review only a few essential concepts that every shoulder surgeon should know.

Regarding *injections*, most commonly performed using a combination of a local anesthetic and corticosteroids, the shoulder was among the first anatomic areas where cortisone injections were used (guess where, at Mayo Clinic for a patient with calcifying tendinitis!). Injections around the shoulder may be used for both diagnosis and treatment. They can be extremely effective, but also somewhat deleterious when abused.

Shoulder Rehabilitation

Several rehabilitation treatment modalities may be used for the shoulder. These include assistive devices (slings, immobilizers, braces), physical modalities (heat and cold, massage, electrotherapy, ultrasonography, laser, extracorporeal shock wave therapy), and exercises to improve motion, strength, and neuromuscular reeducation. Immobilization and exercises are most commonly used for the majority of shoulder conditions before or after surgery.

The importance of *patient education* cannot be overemphasized. When patients understand what is going on, they are much more likely to protect their shoulders during healing and when they return to work or sports, and also more likely to feel motivated to complete and comply with their rehabilitation program. In addition, working with a physical therapist several times a day can be afforded by only some; most patients will need to exercise on their own (or with the help of a friend or family member) in between sessions with a professional physical therapist, which typically happens 1 to 3 times a week.

A few general principles should be reviewed before discussing some details of shoulder rehabilitation (Table 12.1). No one wants to go through a rehabilitation program in pain; in fact, most people can't, which means that pain management is paramount for shoulder rehabilitation. Shoulder rehabilitation goes beyond the glenohumeral joint: the elbow, wrist, hand, scapulothoracic joint, and the rest of the kinetic chain are extremely important, too. In general, motion should be re-established before strengthening starts. This is partly due to timing (motion can be introduced at earlier stages of healing than strengthening), and partly due to difficulties getting stronger when patients still feel painful and stiff. Finally, proper return to certain jobs or sports may require rehabilitation beyond what is generally recommended for most patients.

Table 12.1 • A Few Principles of Shoulder Rehabilitation

Pain control
Rest, immobilization, pharmacologic agents, physical modalities
Avoid positions or exercises that may irritate the shoulder

Protection
Early after injury or surgery to not compromise healing
Later on to prevent reinjury/recurrence

Recover motion, then strength

Include the scapulothoracic joint and its muscles

Do not forget the elbow, wrist, and hand

Integrate the kinetic chain in your program

Specific planning to return to
Work
Sports and weight training

Regarding planes of motion for physical therapy, as a general rule I prefer to avoid exercises in abduction for both motion and strength (see chapter 1, Evaluation of the Shoulder, for planes of motion). Direct lateral abduction leads to tuberosity-acromion impingement and also generates a fair amount of strain on the supraspinatus. Elevation or flexion are better planes for shoulder rehabilitation. In general, flexion and elevation exercises are best performed with the shoulder in external rotation (thumbs-up position), since there is more impingement and strain in internal rotation (thumbs-down position).

Principles of Shoulder Immobilization

Shoulder immobilization is necessary for a period of time after recent injuries or surgery. Most patients use any of the many commercially available slings or shoulder immobilizers. Patient education is important for the proper use of all these devices, and they are often applied poorly, especially at the end of surgery when patients are still coming out of anesthesia. Surgeons, allied health staff, family members, and the patient should become knowledgeable about proper use of these devices.

Poor use of a sling or shoulder immobilizer can contribute to shoulder pain, compromise treatment outcome, and lead to poor patient compliance. Table 12.2 summarizes the most common mistakes and problems I have witnessed in my surgical practice with use of shoulder immobilizers. Occasionally, the patient is provided with a sling or immobilizer that is too large. If the strap around the neck is too long, the immobilizer does not really support the weight of the arm (Figure 12.1). The patient then feels forced to hold the weight of the arm through active muscle contraction, which leads to pain in the shoulder and periscapular regions. Also, if the elbow is positioned behind the mid-coronal plane, the shoulder falls into extension, which may

create excessive strain on anterior structures, such as the subscapularis or anterior capsule.

Remember that each patient and each condition may need a different style of sling or shoulder immobilizer. Not every shoulder should be immobilized in internal rotation. Use of immobilizers with small abduction pillows may be beneficial after cuff repair; they also provide more rotational stability of the upper extremity around the trunk. However, they are cumbersome (and should probably be avoided) in overweight patients, since their abdominal fat combined with the thickness of the abduction pillow will result in excessive abduction.

Finally, do not forget about the rest of the upper extremity during the immobilization time. The elbow, wrist, and hand are captured by the shoulder immobilizer. Hand swelling is relatively common after shoulder surgery, especially if the cephalic vein is sacrificed. Patients should be instructed in active wrist and hand exercises to minimize swelling and stiffness. The elbow can also develop some temporary stiffness after being immobilized in flexion for a while. In addition, some patients develop ulnar neuropathy after shoulder surgery (1,2), and theoretically this could be partly avoided by encouraging active motion of the elbow several times a day while the shoulder immobilizer is used (● Video 12.1).

Motion Exercises

Restoration of a functional arc of motion in all different planes represents a major goal in the management of shoulder conditions. When motion exercises are recommended or prescribed, it is important to specify the plane of motion, whether motion will be passive or active, as well as any limitations not to exceed (Table 12.3).

Passive Motion Exercises

Passive motion is advisable when musculotendinous structures, or fractured fragments connected to muscles, are at risk for healing if muscle activation occurs. Thus, passive range of motion exercises are most commonly recommended during the healing phase of cuff repairs, arthroplasty, proximal humerus fractures, and tendon transfers (Figure 12.2). These exercises require relaxation on the part of the patient and clear understanding on the part of the helper (typically a physical therapist, family member, or friend). These exercises are easier to perform with the patient lying supine and with the elbow supported by blankets or towels so that the shoulder does not fall into extension. For cuff repairs and fractures, gentle longitudinal traction along the axis of the humeral shaft may open up the subacromial space and facilitate therapy.

Arcs of passive motion are limited to safe ranges as determined based on the underlying pathology and observations at the end of the operative procedure. For example, in most anatomic arthroplasties it is safe to let patients reach 120° of passive elevation and approximately 20° to

---

Table 12.2 • Most Common Mistakes When Using a Shoulder Sling or Immobilizer

Choosing the wrong device for a given patient/procedure
Style
Size

Immobilizing every patient in internal rotation
Some external rotation is probably best for:
Proximal humerus fractures
Nonoperative management of anterior shoulder dislocations
Surgical management of posterior instability
Repair or reconstruction of a posterosuperior cuff tear
Most tendon transfers
Scapulothoracic and glenohumeral arthrodesis

Poor fitting
Neck strap excessively long
Shoulder immobilized in extension
Use of abduction pillows in overweight patients

Failure to allow/recommend elbow motion

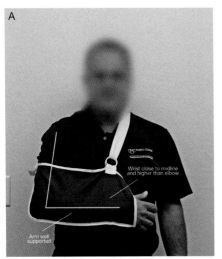
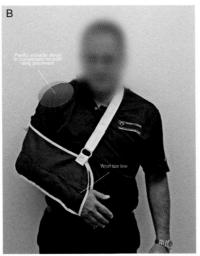
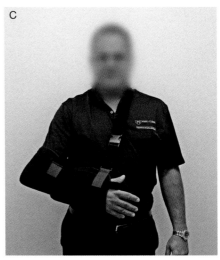

Figure 12.1 **A,** *Shoulder sling. It is important to position it correctly so that the whole upper extremity is supported, with the wrist slightly higher than the elbow and close to the midline.* **B,** *When poorly positioned, patients feel forced to shrug their shoulder to support the arm, which becomes painful.* **C,** *Shoulder immobilizer.*

Table 12.3 • Details on Shoulder Motion Exercises

Muscle use
Passive
Active-assisted
Active

Planes
Elevation, abduction, flexion
External rotation
Internal rotation

Limits (degrees of motion allowed in each plane)
Stretching allowed/recommended (yes/no)

40° of passive external rotation. However, patients with severe contracture of the anterior capsule and subscapularis may require a more restricted arc of motion during the first few weeks after surgery. Similarly, safe arcs of passive motion are determined for patients undergoing cuff repair based on observed tension on the repair at the end of the procedure.

Active Assisted Motion Exercises

This is typically the next group of exercises introduced after cuff repair, fractures, or arthroplasty, and the first group to be introduced for patients after arthroscopic instability

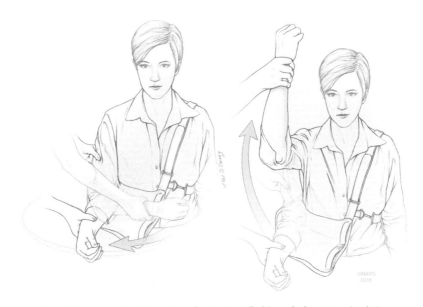

Figure 12.2 Passive range of motion exercises in external rotation (left) and elevation (right).

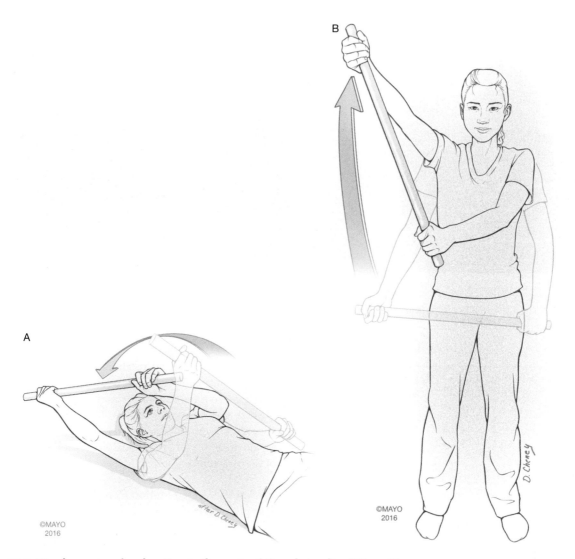

Figure 12.3 Wand exercises for elevation in the supine **(A)** and standing **(B)** positions.

surgery or bone block procedures, typically a few weeks after the index surgery. Active assisted motion exercises in elevation and external rotation are best performed with a wand, cane, or umbrella held with both hands (Figures 12.3 and 12.4). Active assisted motion exercises in internal rotation may be performed using a wand (Figure 12.5), using a towel behind the back (see Figure 12.7C), or grabbing the thumb with the opposite side and bringing it to the midline, and then superiorly.

Stretching Exercises

These exercises are directed toward improving motion in patients with stiffness secondary to either their disease process (adhesive capsulitis, arthritis) or to an injury (fractures) or surgery. In this second category of patients, stretching is not added until enough healing has occurred. Passive stretching can be performed by a physical therapist or a family member or friend. Patients can also perform their own stretching exercises (Figures 12.6 and 12.7).

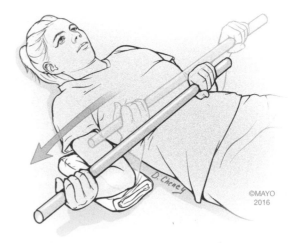

Figure 12.4 Active assisted external rotation using a wand. Note support of the arm to avoid shoulder extension.

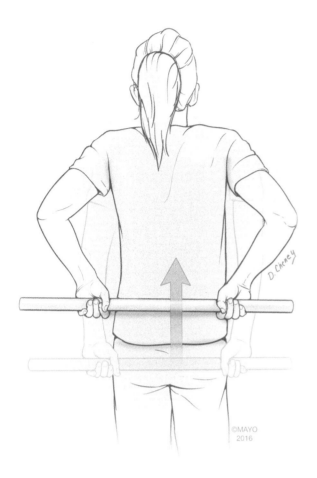

Figure 12.5 Active assisted internal rotation using a wand.

Application of heat prior to the stretching routine seems to help make it easier and maybe more effective.

Strengthening Exercises

Isometric Strengthening

Isometric exercises involve active contraction of various muscle groups without joint motion. They are typically the first strengthening exercises introduced after injuries or surgery. Isometrics are usually performed in internal rotation, external rotation, abduction, flexion, and extension depending on the condition (Figure 12.8). Most patients are recommended to perform sets of 10 sequential contractions in each direction.

Resisted Strengthening

The two most common modalities of resisted exercises involve use of elastic resistance bands or tubes or free weights. Elastic resistance bands are commonly known by the brand name of the company that makes the most popular bands, Thera-Band.

Elastic resistance bands and tubes are color coded according to their elasticity: the most elastic one is tan, and the resistance increases progressively (tan-yellow-red-green-blue-black-silver-gold). Most patients have enough strength to start with yellow bands (light resistance) and later on progress to red (medium) and green (heavy). These bands may be used for many exercises, but the ones most commonly used are shown in Figure 12.9. Most patients are recommended to perform three sets of 10 repetitions three times a day, and advance a color when they feel they can easily complete their sets with minimal difficulty.

As mentioned in chapter 6, The Rotator Cuff and Biceps Tendon, when strengthening the inferior rotator cuff with elastic resistance bands in internal and external rotation, it is helpful to place a magazine or a folded towel in the axilla and hold it actively. In theory, active adduction will result in less contraction of the deltoid, which would tend to displace the humeral head superiorly and facilitate impingement (Figure 12.10).

Free weights are used selectively. Many patients are able to achieve enough strength with isometrics and elastic bands. Weight training is obviously very effective for strengthening, but can also lead to re-injury if too much weight is used, and also with certain exercises. Weight training for internal and external rotation is best done

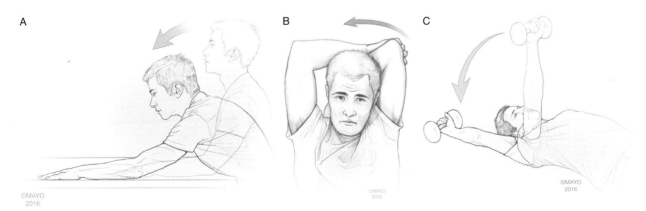

Figure 12.6 **A,** *Stretching in elevation or flexion may be performed resting the arm on a table or similar surface and leaning forward.* **B,** *Stretching in elevation can also be performed with assistance of the other hand and the affected side overhead.* **C,** *Alternatively, a weight may be used on the later phases of recovery to stretch the shoulder overhead.*

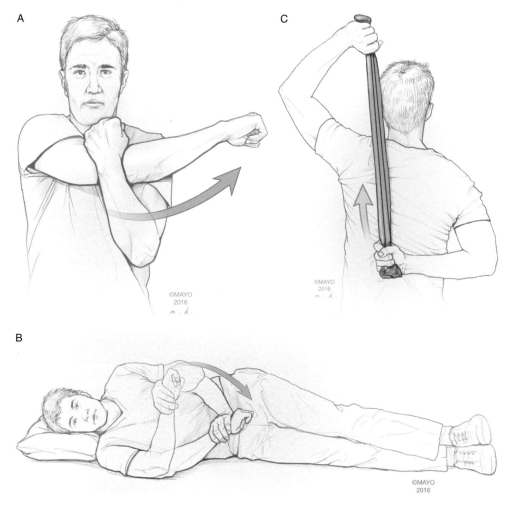

Figure 12.7 A, *Stretching in internal rotation can be performed by placing the elbow on the affected side across the body and using the opposite hand on the elbow.* **B,** *Stretching in internal rotation can also be performed lying on the side and using the opposite hand or a weight (some call this exercise "sleeper's stretch," particularly useful for glenohumeral internal rotation deficit or GIRD).* **C,** *A towel behind the back may also be used to gain internal rotation.*

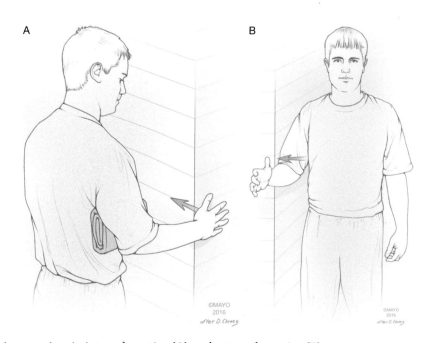

Figure 12.8 *Isometrics exercises in internal rotation* **(A)** *and external rotation* **(B).**

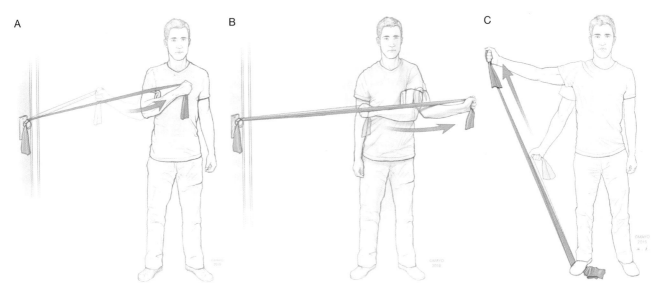

Figure 12.9 *Elastic resistance band exercises in* **(A)** *internal rotation,* **(B)** *external rotation, and* **(C)** *elevation.*

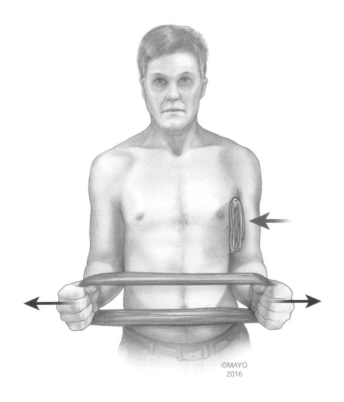

Figure 12.10 *Elastic resistance exercise in internal rotation with a magazine or folded towel under the axilla to minimize deltoid contraction.*

lying on the side (Figure 12.11). Deltoid and supraspinatus strengthening can be done lifting free weights in the plane of elevation. Advanced weight training is reserved for those individuals interested in returning to a high performance level as they are allowed to resume sports (🔴 Video 12.2).

Scapular Rehabilitation

Unfortunately, rehabilitation of the scapula is oftentimes ignored or forgotten. Scapular rehabilitation is particularly important for patients with cuff disease, instability, and primary scapular conditions.

Restoration of Scapular Motion

Stiffness at the scapulothoracic joint can really impact patient recovery in a negative way. There are two specific patterns of contracture that require attention. As detailed in chapter 10, The Scapula, some patients may present isolated contracture of the pectoralis minor leading to anterior scapular tilt. Other patients may have more generalized scapulothoracic stiffness; this can be appreciated by performing passive elevation of their shoulders while looking at them from the back and comparing the motion of both scapulae. Stretching exercises may be instituted to regain scapular flexibility when needed (Figure 12.12).

Strengthening of the Periscapular Muscles

In some individuals, selective weakness of specific scapular muscles can be detected. In those circumstances, exercises can be selected to strengthen those specific muscles. More commonly there is generalized weakness, and a comprehensive program of periscapular exercises is needed. Most of the time, patients have relative weakness of the lower trapezius and serratus anterior compared with the upper trapezius.

A useful way for patients to understand scapular strengthening is to picture how to voluntarily try to move the scapula according to the face of a clock or a compass: to 12 o'clock (north) for upper trapezius and levator scapulae, to 6 o'clock (south) for the lower trapezius, and to 9 o'clock and 3 o'clock (east and west) for serratus anterior

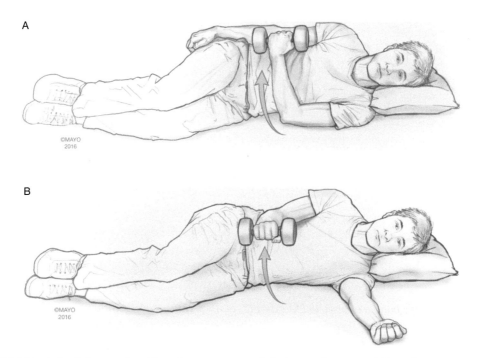

Figure 12.11 *Weight training lying on the side to increase strength in internal rotation* **(A)** *and external rotation* **(B)***.*

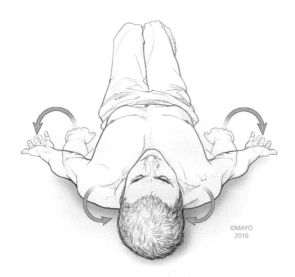

Figure 12.12 *Pectoralis minor stretch: lying on your back with your knees bent, actively pull your shoulder blades together and feel your shoulders flatten. At the same time, try to pull your shoulder blades to your feet as well. Then let your elbows fall back with your palms up to stretch further.*

and middle trapezius/rhomboids, respectively. Patients can initiate isometric exercises activating the muscles they would use for these movements, and then be advanced to some of the exercises described later. There are multiple exercises that can strengthen all these muscle groups. In this book I show only a few of my favorite exercises.

Serratus Anterior

Scapular protraction with a resistance band may be performed standing or sitting. A resistance band placed posteriorly is held with the hand at shoulder level, the shoulder extended, and the elbow flexed. The upper extremity is then moved forward as the elbow is straightened, as in a punching motion (Figure 12.13). Both shoulders can be exercised at once by placing the band around the neck and grabbing each end with one hand (dynamic hug with resistance bands, Figure 12.14). Further strengthening can be achieved punching a boxing bag.

Lower Trapezius

The lower trapezius is best strengthened lying prone with the arm hanging down the side. A dumbbell or resistance band is held with the hand and the shoulder is extended, abducted and externally rotated with the elbow straight (Figure 12.15). Alternatively the shoulder is elevated forward in the prone position.

Middle Trapezius and Rhomboids

Rowing exercises will strengthen both the middle trapezius and the rhomboids. They can be performed with resistance bands (Figure 12.16) or with a rowing machine.

Upper Trapezius

The upper trapezius rarely needs to be strengthened in patients with functional scapular dyskinesia, but it may need to be exercised in patients recovering from an injury to the spinal accessory nerve or brachial plexopathy.

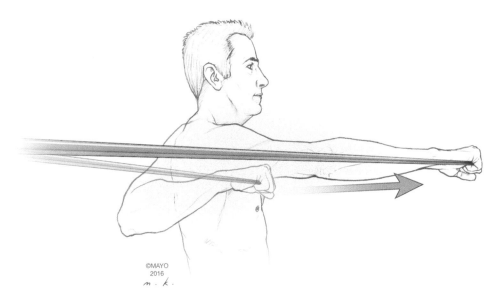

Figure 12.13 *Scapular protraction with a resistance band for serratus anterior.*

Shoulder shrugs with handheld dumbbells are very effective for the upper trapezius.

Common Programs of Rehabilitation

Physical therapy instructions may need to be individualized based on the underlying condition, the procedure performed, bone and soft-tissue quality, age, comorbidities, and personality traits that may influence compliance. However, there are some programs that can be used for many patients. Having a structured program facilitates communication with the patient, specialists in physical medicine and rehabilitation, and physical and occupational therapists (Table 12.4).

Return to Work and Sports

When to allow or advise a patient to return to work or the practice of sports obviously depends on the underlying diagnosis, the outcome of the treatment intervention, and the kind of job or sport being considered. As a general rule, most patients are allowed to return to a sedentary job between weeks 2 and 8 after the index procedure, depending on their pain level, driving needs, and ability to

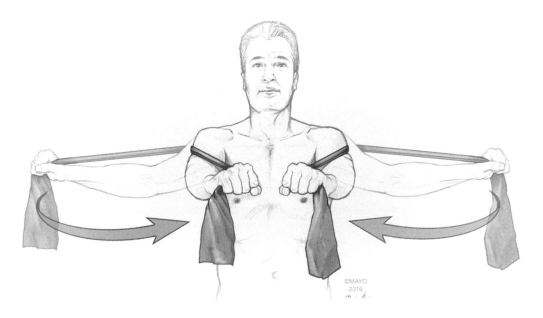

Figure 12.14 *Bilateral scapular protraction with a resistance band for serratus anterior.*

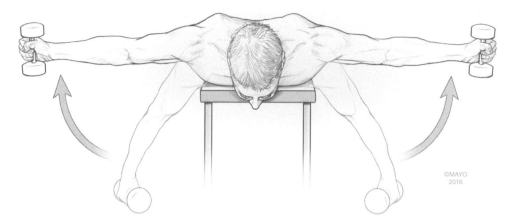

Figure 12.15 Lower trapezius strengthening. Abduction, extension, and external rotation lying prone.

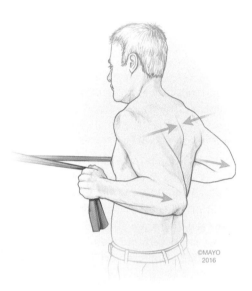

Figure 12.16 Rowing exercises with elastic bands.

free up enough time for physical therapy. Return to heavy labor cannot be initiated most of the time for at least 3 to 4 months after shoulder surgery. Return to sports involving the upper extremities are typically allowed within the same time frame, whereas contact sports are avoided for the first 6 months in most circumstances.

As mentioned before, patient education is paramount. Patients with instability need to understand how to avoid extreme positions of motion that might stress structures repaired. Patients with cuff disease need to avoid repetitive overhead activity. Patients with arthritis or after joint replacement need to understand the differences between lifting and carrying, and the potential excessive stress on the replacement components particularly when lifting heavy weights overhead. Patients interested in weight training after cuff or replacement surgery should probably avoid military press exercises and be cautious with use of excessive weight in any exercises that do involve glenohumeral motion.

Shoulder Injections

Injection of pharmacologic agents in various anatomical areas around the shoulder joint is very commonly used for both diagnosis and treatment. Classically, corticosteroids combined with a local anesthetic have been the drugs of choice for the shoulder. The deleterious effects of repeated corticosteroid injections on the soft tissues and bone (particularly the rotator cuff) and concerns regarding chondral toxicity with intra-articular administration of local anesthetics have prompted investigation of alternative pharmacologic agents, such as nonsteroidal anti-inflamatory drugs (NSAIDs), hyaluronic acid, and others. However, corticosteroid injections continue to be most commonly used in practice. As detailed later, over the last few years there has been an increased trend to use image guidance, particularly ultrasonography, to perform injections around the shoulder region.

Some Basic Principles

Pharmacologic Agents

As mentioned before, injections may be used for diagnosis, treatment, or a combination of both. When the only goal of the injection is to identify the source of pain, typically a short-acting local anesthetic is the only pharmacologic agent injected. However, commonly the needle-stick is used to also inject an anti-inflammatory agent, so that if the source of pain has been correctly identified, there is a chance for a longer lasting benefit. By the same token, corticosteroids are almost always injected in combination with a local anesthetic, so that pain relief starts even before the anti-inflamatory action is fully into effect.

Local Anesthetics

It was just mentioned that local anesthetics can be injected alone to aid with differential diagnosis, but they are also commonly combined with corticosteroids so that the diagnostic injection has the opportunity to become therapeutic

Table 12.4 • Some Common Physical Therapy Programs Used in My Practice[a]

Therapy Modality	Anterior Glenohumeral Soft-tissue Instability Surgery	Nonoperative Treatment of Cuff Disease	Cuff Repair	Anatomic Total Shoulder Arthroplasty	Reverse Total Shoulder Arthroplasty
Immobilizer	3–4 weeks	Sling for comfort	6 weeks	4–6 weeks	2–3 weeks
Passive ROM	*Not used*	*Not used*	At 2 weeks for smaller tears/stiff patients At 6 weeks otherwise	Week 1–6	*Not used*
AAROM	At 3–4 weeks	Week 1–4	At 6 weeks	At 6 weeks	At 2–3 weeks
Stretching	*Rarely (at 8 weeks)*	*Not used unless stiff*	At 12 weeks only if stiff	At 12 weeks only if stiff	*Rarely, avoid stretching in IR*
Glenohumeral isometrics	At 3–4 weeks	Week 1–4	At 10 weeks	At 10 weeks	At 8 weeks (ER and elevation)
Glenohumeral resistance bands	At 6 weeks	IR and ER at 3–4 weeks Elevation at 8 weeks	At 12 weeks	At 12 weeks	At 12 weeks (ER and elevation)
Scapular isometrics	At 3–4 weeks	Week 1–2	At 10 weeks	*Rarely, at 10 weeks*	*Rarely, at 10 weeks*
Scapular resistance exercises	At 6 weeks	At 8 weeks	At 12–14 weeks	*Rarely, at 12–14 weeks*	*Rarely, at 12 weeks*

Abbreviations: AAROM, active assisted range of motion; ER, external rotation; IR, internal rotation; ROM: range of motion.

[a] Data appearing in italics indicates that the exercise is used rarely or never for the stated indication.

as well. As detailed later, when injections are used for differential diagnosis, the most common locations targeted include the subacromial space, acromioclavicular joint, glenohumeral joint, biceps tendon sheath, sternoclavicular joint, and suprascapular nerve. Of the multiple local anesthetics available, most orthopedic surgeons choose a short-acting agent (most commonly lidocaine) when used purely for diagnosis, or a longer-acting agent (most commonly bupivacaine) when used for treatment.

There is very little information available to guide the ideal dose of a given local anesthetic to be used in various locations. Smaller spaces (acromioclavicular joint, sternoclavicular joint) may accept only 1 to 2 mL of liquid, whereas the glenohumeral joint and subacromial space will accept more. My practice is to use a larger volume (approximately 8 mL, combined with 2 to 4 mL of corticosteroids) of local anesthetic in the subacromial space, so that the medications injected reach a larger area, and use smaller volumes in the glenohumeral joint and smaller joints as detailed later.

Some studies seem to indicate that local anesthetics may be chondrotoxic (3). Thus, when intra-articular glenohumeral injections are performed, most surgeons prefer to use a lower concentration (0.25% instead of 0.50%), less volume (2–4 mL), and limit the number of injections to some extent. Worries about chondrotoxicity are less relevant in patients already presenting with end-stage glenohumeral

osteoarthritis, but are very pertinent in younger patients with pristine articular cartilage.

Corticosteroids

When the intention of the injection is therapeutic, corticosteroids continue to be the pharmacologic agents of choice. In my practice, the two corticosteroid preparations most commonly used include methylprednisolone acetate (40 mg/mL) and triamcinolone acetonide (40 mg/mL). The relative corticosteroid potency of these two pharmacologic agents seems to be about the same (4).

Interestingly, there is very little scientific data to help determine what is the ideal dose of corticosteroids to be injected in the musculoskeletal system. For larger joints like the shoulder, most recommend injecting 80 mg (2 mL) (4), but surveys of practicing surgeons, rheumatologists, and family physicians show a wide range of doses being selected, ranging from 5 mg to 200 mg (4). Different doses are selected for other anatomic areas like the subacromial space or the acromioclavicular joint, as detailed later.

Soluble NSAIDs

Since corticosteroids are known to relieve symptoms in patients with glenohumeral arthritis, subacromial impingement, and cuff disease, a few studies have investigated the possibility of using injectable NSAIDs. The 2 drugs most commonly studied are tenoxicam (20 mg) and ketorolac (60 mg) (5,6). Tenoxicam compared favorably to placebo for the management of acute painful shoulder episodes (6). Ketorolac was also found to be equal or superior to corticosteroids for the management of chronic subacromial impingement (5). NSAIDs are attractive because they can avoid the potentially detrimental effect of corticosteroids on collagen and cartilage.

Hyaluronic Acid

There are a number of commercially available injectable fluids that contain derivatives of hyaluronan, one of the major molecular components of synovial fluid. The most commonly used preparations contain hylan, sodium hyaluronate, or high-molecular-weight hyaluronan. Injection of these preparations is often referred to as viscosupplementation. Some preparations are injected 3 times, a week apart, whereas others require only 1 injection.

Since hyaluronan molecules naturally present in synovial fluid seem to facilitate joint lubrication, hyaluronan derivatives carry the potential of facilitating smoother, less painful joint function. Care should be taken to avoid hyaluronic acid injections in patients with hypersensitivity to hyaluronan products, allergies to avian proteins, women during pregnancy and lactation, as well as children.

Hyaluronic acid preparations have been approved for the treatment of knee osteoarthritis. A few studies have analyzed the outcome of hyaluronic acid injections around the shoulder for patients with glenohumeral osteoarthritis (7), subacromial impingement (8), and rotator cuff disease (9,10). Results have been mixed, with some studies showing improvement and others showing no differences. In my practice, I seldom consider use of hyaluronic acid injections except for patients with glenohumeral arthritis not responding to corticosteroid injections and unwilling to undergo surgery.

Other

Preparations of bone marrow aspirate, platelet-rich plasma, growth factors, or mesenchymal stem cells could theoretically be attractive in patients with glenohumeral arthritis and rotator cuff disease. Some of these substances have been investigated as an adjunct to surgical repair of the rotator cuff, but they are also considered by some as standalone therapeutic strategies. More evidence is needed before injection of these particular preparations can be widely recommended.

The Value of Image Guidance

Classically, orthopedic surgeons learned how to accurately inject various areas of the shoulder region based on superficial anatomy and specific landmarks. However, guidance of needle placement with imaging modalities has become very common. In the past, fluoroscopy was the main imaging study used for injections around the shoulder. Currently, ultrasound-guided injections are most common.

Ultrasonography offers various benefits, including accuracy, lack of radiation, and diagnostic abilities for soft-tissue structures. Specific details on how to perform ultrasound-guided injections exceed the scope of this book, but I will discuss how to perform injections without image guidance. Some areas like the subacromial space can be injected blindly very accurately, whereas others like the glenohumeral or acromioclavicular joints can be extremely difficult to inject without image guidance, especially in the presence of pathology: a stiff glenohumeral joint in a patient with capsulitis or an arthritic acromioclavicular joint with narrowing and osteophytes may be close to impossible to inject without imaging guidance.

Image-guided injections are particularly appealing for patients with calcifying tendinitis (see chapter 6, The Rotator Cuff and Biceps Tendon). Aspiration of the calcific material may be attempted at the time of the injection, and success in removing calcium is likely increased if the needle tip is accurately placed in the area of calcification identified with radiographs or ultrasonography. Image-guided injections are also helpful for the aspiration of paralabral cysts.

A number of studies have compared the accuracy or effectiveness of injections performed with or without image guidance. Ultrasound-guided injections are more accurate for the glenohumeral joint (11) although in some studies differences in accuracy did not reach statistical significance (12). However, surgeons with experience in shoulder arthroscopy may reach an accuracy rate of over 90% (13,14). The same seems to be true for experienced radiologists (15).

The accuracy of acromioclavicular joint injections improves using both fluoroscopy (16) and ultrasonography (17,18). Ultrasound guidance also seems to be accurate for injections into the sternoclavicular joint (19). The accuracy of injections into the subacromial space seems to be improved to a much lesser extent with ultrasound guidance (20–22).

Interestingly, for both the acromioclavicular and the glenohumeral joints, clinical improvements are sometimes experienced even if the injection is inaccurate (11,23). In fact, some studies have demonstrated equal benefits when intra-articular versus periarticular acromioclavicular joint injections are performed (24). Adhesive capsulitis has also been shown in some studies to respond to both intra-articular and subacromial injections (25).

How Many? How Often?

There is a question that comes up all the time: how many injections can be performed in a given patient, and how often? The timing of hyaluronic acid injections depends on the agent selected. Classically, 3 injections are performed 7 days apart. In order to decrease the number of procedures required, certain preparations are effective when injected only once. The timing of injections with corticosteroids and local anesthetics is related to the potential deleterious effects of the pharmacologic agents injected.

Repeated injections with corticosteroids are known to be deleterious for the soft tissues, and possibly for the bone. Thus, in patients with a full-thickness rotator cuff tear that eventually may need a tendon repair, multiple injections with corticosteroids may weaken the tendon structure as well as the bone quality at the tuberosities, leading to difficulties obtaining a sound repair. There is also a growing body of evidence that suggests the toxic side effects of local anesthetics on chondrocytes; use of lower concentrations and limited use of intra-articular injections with local anesthetics are recommended by some in order to avoid cartilage damage. Some studies suggest toxic effects on cartilage linked to corticosteroids as well. Finally, recent studies suggest a higher rate of infection when shoulder arthroplasty or cuff repair is performed in patients who recently received a corticosteroid injection (within the previous 1 to 3 months) (26).

From a practical perspective, the information just summarized leads most surgeons to avoid more than two or three injections for patients who may need soft-tissue repair (most commonly, a rotator cuff repair), space out injections at least 3 months apart, and delay surgery for several weeks (up to 3 months) if a patient has recently received a corticosteroid injection. Of course, these are no hard and fast rules; I would not hesitate injecting multiple times the glenohumeral joint of an elderly patient with severe primary glenohumeral osteoarthritis that will never be suitable for anesthesia and surgery, provided these injections are effective.

Supplies and Precautions

Although infection is extremely uncommon after a single injection, it can happen, especially if a sterile technique is not used. My preference is to decolonize the skin with a commercially available kit that combines chorhexidine and alcohol. Hand washing and use of sterile gloves are important. A larger bore needle (typically 18-gauge) is used to load the medication(s), and a smaller bore needle (22-gauge) for the injection. If the injection is performed carefully, avoiding hitting painful structures like bone prominences, there is very little value in first injecting the skin with a small amount of a local anesthetic.

Prior to the injection, the identity of the patient and the site to be injected are confirmed. Care must also be taken to confirm that the patient is not allergic to the medications to be used, and to avoid intravascular injections. After the injection is performed, the needle-stick area is covered with a small dressing or adhesive bandage. Patients are requested to wait a few minutes in the room used for the injection to confirm no adverse reactions (allergy, vasovagal syncope). Sometimes, there is value in repeating the examination of the shoulder after injections containing a local anesthetic in order to aid with the diagnosis.

Anatomic Locations

Injections around the shoulder region are targeted to a few specific locations. In most patients, only 1 of these anatomic locations is injected. Occasionally, injections are combined in patients with symptoms related to both the rotator cuff and the acromioclavicular joint (combined injection into the subacromial space and the acromioclavicular joint), or in selected patients with capsulitis that might benefit from an intra-articular glenohumeral joint injection combined with a blockade of the suprascapular nerve. There are several ways to perform injections in these various locations; I will describe only my preferred approach (Table 12.5, Figures 12.17–12.19).

Subacromial Space

Injections into the subacromial space are the most common shoulder injections performed in clinical practice. The needle may be introduced from the front, side, or back. Standard length needles are adequate for the lateral and anterior approaches, but the posterior approach may

Table 12.5 • Common Shoulder Injections

Location	Preferred Approach	Pharmacologic Agent	Volume	Most Common Indications
Subacromial	Posterior	Corticosteroids and a local anesthetic NSAIDs Hyaluronic acid (rare)	8–12 mL	Impingement Calcifying tendinitis Cuff tears
Acromioclavicular	Superior	Corticosteroids and a local anesthetic	1–2 mL	Arthritis Distal clavicle osteolysis
Biceps sheath	Anterior	Corticosteroids and a local anesthetic	2–3 mL	Tenosynovitis
Glenohumeral	Posterior Anterior	Corticosteroids and a local anesthetic NSAIDs Hyaluronic acid (rare)	4–6 mL	Arthritis Adhesive capsulitis
Suprascapular nerve	Superior	Local anesthetic +/- corticosteroids	2 mL	Diagnostic Adhesive capsulitis
Sternoclavicular	Anterior	Corticosteroids and a local anesthetic	1–2 mL	Arthritis

Abbreviation: NSAIDs, nonsteroidal anti-inflammatory drugs.

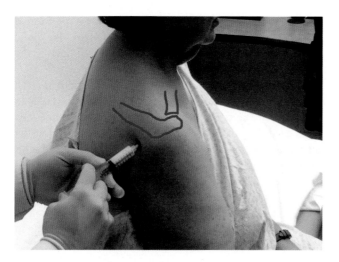

Figure 12.17 Subacromial injection from a posterior approach.

require use of a longer needle or indenting the skin and soft-tissues with the base of the needle (27). Also, some studies have noted better accuracy when the injection is performed anteriorly or laterally, particularly in women (28) (⬤Video 12.3).

For an injection using a posterior approach, the patient sits comfortably with the arm at the side (Figure 12.17). Longitudinal traction on the arm applied by an assistant may help with opening up the subacromial space. The main reference landmarks include the posterolateral and the anterior aspects of the acromion. The needle pierces the skin 1 to 2 cm distal to the posterolateral acromion and aims superiorly to the inferior aspect of the anterior acromion at approximately a 30° angle. The needle may be moved sideways as the fluid is injected. My preference is to use a larger volume of fluid in the subacromial space, so that the pharmacologic agents are distributed across the whole subacromial area. Commonly, I combine 4 mL of corticosteroid solution with 8 mL of a local anesthetic. However, this translates to a pretty high dose of corticosteroids, and repeated injections are best performed with less volume.

Acromioclavicular Joint

Injecting the acromioclavicular joint without image guidance can be a challenge. The acromioclavicular joint presents certain variability in angulation among individuals, and it is pretty small to begin with. In addition, injections are commonly performed in patients with arthritis or osteolysis, which may lead to an even narrower joint space or osteophytes that may block access to the joint. Finally, injecting too deep may place the needle tip into the subacromial space, so that the wrong target is injected.

If the acromioclavicular joint is injected without image guidance, it is important to perform the injection with shoulder radiographs available, so that the angulation of the joint, joint space, and osteophyte location can be taken into account. I prefer to visualize from superior with the patient sitting or lying supine with the torso raised 30° (Figure 12.18). The distal end of the clavicle can typically be palpated under the skin, and the injection is performed just lateral to the clavicle. The needle should be introduced

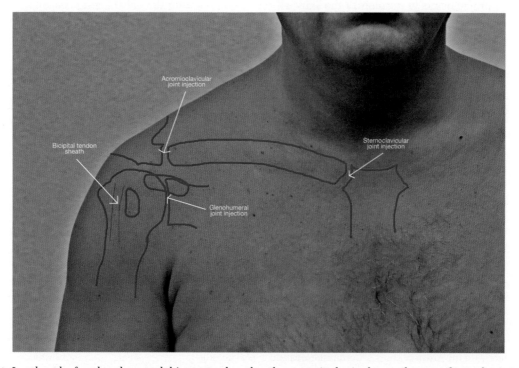

Figure 12.18 Landmarks for glenohumeral, biceps tendon sheath, acromioclavicular, and sternoclavicular injections.

just enough to pierce the superior capsule of the acromio-clavicular joint, and directed medially and inferiorly. The small capacity of this joint allows injection of only 1 to 2 mL of fluid in most patients. If the patient requires injection of both the acromioclavicular joint and the subacromial space, once the first 1 to 2 mL are injected, the needle may be advanced further into the subacromial space and the rest of the content of the syringe can be injected.

Biceps Tendon Sheath

The relationship between the long head of the biceps and the superficial landmarks will change with arm position (Figure 12.18). Localizing the injection site is facilitated by placing the arm in approximately 20° of external rotation (the long head of the biceps will face straight anteriorly) and by identifying the point of maximum tenderness. My preference is to inject anteriorly perpendicular to the skin, gently feel the bone of the humeral groove, retract the needle tip, and inject. Care must be taken to avoid injecting against resistance, which might indicate that the injection is being placed into the substance of the tendon itself.

Glenohumeral Joint

The glenohumeral joint may be injected anteriorly or posteriorly (Figure 12.18). For a posterior injection, the needle is inserted inferior and medial to the postero-lateral corner of the acromion (typically 2 cm in each direction), and the needle aimed toward the tip of the coracoid horizontally; aiming superiorly will direct the needle to the subacromial space instead. For an anterior injection, the needle is introduced in the center of a triangle formed by the coracoid, acromioclavicular joint, and lesser tuberosity (13). The needle enters the joint through the interval region. In both approaches, care must be taken to be gentle and avoid damage to the articular cartilage. Most surgeons inject between 4 and 6 mL of fluid. As mentioned before, concerns regarding chondrotoxicity make it advisable to use lower concentrations of local anesthetic (0.25%), and not to exceed 40 mg to 80 mg of corticosteroid.

Suprascapular Nerve

The suprascapular nerve is located just medial to the base of the coracoid. The needle is introduced superiorly in the triangle between the clavicle and the spine of the scapula, approximately 2 to 3 cm medial to the elbow of the scapular spine, and aiming slightly anteriorly (Figure 12.19).

Sternoclavicular Joint

The sternoclavicular joint is best injected anteriorly by feeling the prominent medial end of the clavicle and injecting just medial to it (Figure 12.18). Similar to the acromioclavicular joint, accurate injection of the sternoclavicular joint may be a challenge when the joint space is very narrow or

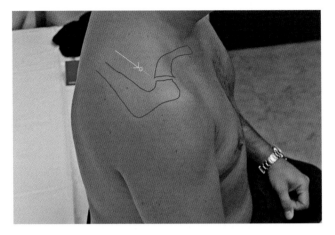

Figure 12.19 Suprascapular nerve injection.

in the presence of large osteophytes. Care must be taken not to insert the needle too deeply, not only to ensure that the sternoclavicular joint is truly injected but also to avoid accidental damage to vital structures behind this region. The amount of fluid injected typically is 1 to 2 mL.

Outcome

The therapeutic efficacy of injections with various agents in specific conditions has been investigated for certain pharmacologic agents.

Corticosteroid injections can be very successful for the treatment of acromioclavicular joint conditions, in some instances up to 5 years after the injection (29). As mentioned before, periarticular and intra-articular injections with corticosteroids seem to be equally effective for the acromioclavicular joint (24). Both corticosteroids and ketorolac have been demonstrated to provide symptomatic improvement in patients with chronic subacromial impingement (5). Finally, corticosteroid injections into the glenohumeral joint have also been reported to be beneficial in patients with adhesive capsulitis (30).

Hyaluronic acid injections have also been reported to provide approximately 1 month of symptomatic improvement in patients with cuff tear arthropathy (31). On the contrary, no benefit has been demonstrated in patients with glenohumeral osteoarthritis (32,33). Some prospective randomized studies have reported success when using hyaluronic acid injections for patients with chronic subacromial impingement (34), whereas others have found them to be inferior to corticosteroids and equal to placebo (8,10).

KEY POINTS

✓ Shoulder rehabilitation is paramount for the success of most shoulder surgical procedures, and it can be very effective, too, for the nonoperative management of certain shoulder conditions.

✓ Education of the patient and his/her support network (family, friends) contributes tremendously to the success of shoulder therapy and may allow successful rehabilitation of the shoulder without the constant supervision of a physical therapist. Home programs can be extremely effective for the shoulder.

✓ Proper use of shoulder immobilization requires selection of the immobilizer best suited for each condition, procedure and patient. A single style of immobilizer will not cover all patients.

✓ Specific therapy protocols have been developed for the management of various shoulder conditions. These protocols may need to be individualized to take into account the nature of procedure, the quality of bone or soft tissues, and observations made at the end of surgery under direct vision.

✓ Restoration of motion typically precedes strengthening. Passive motion is commonly used for the first few weeks after surgery, followed by active assisted motion with or without stretching. Strengthening is initiated with isometric exercises and completed mostly using resistance elastic bands.

✓ Scapular rehabilitation is very important for many patients and oftentimes neglected or poorly understood. So-called compass and rowing exercises can be supplemented with dedicated exercises for the serratus anterior and lower trapezius.

✓ Injections of various pharmacologic agents are very commonly used around the shoulder for diagnostic or therapeutic reasons. A combination of corticosteroids and a local anesthetic is most commonly used. Other agents explored include soluble NSAIDs, hyaluronic acid derivatives, platelet-rich plasma, growth factors, and mesenchymal cells.

✓ Corticosteroids are very effective but also known to carry the potential for adverse effects, including structural deterioration of soft tissues and bone, as well as an increased risk of surgical site infection when surgery is performed within the 3 months following the injection. Local anesthetics and corticosteroids may also be chondrotoxic in a dose-dependent manner.

✓ When injections are performed, it is important to confirm that the patient is not allergic, adhere to sterile precautions, and avoid multiple injections within a short period of time.

✓ Shoulder injections are increasingly performed under image guidance. Ultrasound-guided injections are particularly attractive, since ultrasonography also provides great diagnostic features. Some studies indicate that image guidance is more accurate than injections performed using superficial landmarks for most areas except the subacromial space.

✓ Shoulder surgeons should be trained in performing injections aimed to the subacromial space, acromioclavicular joint, biceps tendon sheath, glenohumeral joint, suprascapular nerve, and sternoclavicular joint.

REFERENCES

1. Yian EH, Dillon M, Sodl J, Dionysian E, Navarro R, Singh A. Incidence of symptomatic compressive peripheral neuropathy after shoulder replacement. Hand (N Y). 2015 Jun;10(2):243–7.

2. Thomasson BG, Matzon JL, Pepe M, Tucker B, Maltenfort M, Austin L. Distal peripheral neuropathy after open and arthroscopic shoulder surgery: an under-recognized complication. J Shoulder Elbow Surg. 2015 Jan;24(1):60–6.

3. Gulihar A, Robati S, Twaij H, Salih A, Taylor GJ. Articular cartilage and local anaesthetic: a systematic review of the current literature. J Orthop. 2015 Oct 31;12(Suppl 2):S200–10. Epub 2015 Dec.

4. Skedros JG, Hunt KJ, Pitts TC. Variations in corticosteroid/anesthetic injections for painful shoulder conditions: comparisons among orthopaedic surgeons, rheumatologists, and physical medicine and primary-care physicians. BMC Musculoskelet Disord. 2007 Jul 6;8:63.

5. Min KS, St Pierre P, Ryan PM, Marchant BG, Wilson CJ, Arrington ED. A double-blind randomized controlled trial comparing the effects of subacromial injection with corticosteroid versus NSAID in patients with shoulder impingement syndrome. J Shoulder Elbow Surg. 2013 May;22(5):595–601.

6. Itzkowitch D, Ginsberg F, Leon M, Bernard V, Appelboom T. Peri-articular injection of tenoxicam for painful shoulders: a double-blind, placebo controlled trial. Clin Rheumatol. 1996 Nov;15(6):604–9.

7. Colen S, Geervliet P, Haverkamp D, Van Den Bekerom MP. Intra-articular infiltration therapy for patients with glenohumeral osteoarthritis: a systematic review of the literature. Int J Shoulder Surg. 2014 Oct;8(4):114–21.

8. Penning LI, de Bie RA, Walenkamp GH. The effectiveness of injections of hyaluronic acid or corticosteroid in patients with subacromial impingement: a three-arm randomised controlled trial. J Bone Joint Surg Br. 2012 Sep;94(9):1246–52.

9. Osti L, Buda M, Buono AD, Osti R, Massari L. Clinical evidence in the treatment of rotator cuff tears with hyaluronic acid. Muscles Ligaments Tendons J. 2016 Feb 13;5(4):270–5. Epub 2015 Oct-Dec.

10. Penning LI, de Bie RA, Walenkamp GH. Subacromial triamcinolone acetonide, hyaluronic acid and saline injections for shoulder pain an RCT investigating the effectiveness in the first days. BMC Musculoskelet Disord. 2014 Oct 23;15:352.

11. Cunnington J, Marshall N, Hide G, Bracewell C, Isaacs J, Platt P, et al. A randomized, double-blind, controlled study of ultrasound-guided corticosteroid injection into the joint of patients with inflammatory arthritis. Arthritis Rheum. 2010 Jul;62(7):1862–9.

12. Amber KT, Landy DC, Amber I, Knopf D, Guerra J. Comparing the accuracy of ultrasound versus fluoroscopy in glenohumeral injections: a systematic review and meta-analysis. J Clin Ultrasound. 2014 Sep;42(7):411–6. Epub 2014 Mar 25.

13. Johnson TS, Mesfin A, Farmer KW, McGuigan LA, Alamo IG, Jones LC, et al. Accuracy of intra-articular glenohumeral injections: the anterosuperior technique with arthroscopic documentation. Arthroscopy. 2011 Jun;27(6):745–9.

14. Powell SE, Davis SM, Lee EH, Lee RK, Sung RM, McGroder C, et al. Accuracy of palpation-directed

intra-articular glenohumeral injection confirmed by magnetic resonance arthrography. Arthroscopy. 2015 Feb;31(2):205–8. Epub 2014 Oct 11.

15. Sidon E, Velkes S, Shemesh S, Levy J, Glaser E, Kosashvili Y. Accuracy of non assisted glenohumeral joint injection in the office setting. Eur J Radiol. 2013 Dec;82(12):e829–31. Epub 2013 Sep 7.

16. Pichler W, Weinberg AM, Grechenig S, Tesch NP, Heidari N, Grechenig W. Intra-articular injection of the acromioclavicular joint. J Bone Joint Surg Br. 2009 Dec;91(12):1638–40.

17. Peck E, Lai JK, Pawlina W, Smith J. Accuracy of ultrasound-guided versus palpation-guided acromio-clavicular joint injections: a cadaveric study. PM R. 2010 Sep;2(9):817–21.

18. Borbas P, Kraus T, Clement H, Grechenig S, Weinberg AM, Heidari N. The influence of ultrasound guidance in the rate of success of acromioclavicular joint injection: an experimental study on human cadavers. J Shoulder Elbow Surg. 2012 Dec;21(12):1694–7.

19. Pourcho AM, Sellon JL, Smith J. Sonographically guided sternoclavicular joint injection: description of technique and validation. J Ultrasound Med. 2015 Feb;34(2):325–31.

20. Dogu B, Yucel SD, Sag SY, Bankaoglu M, Kuran B. Blind or ultrasound-guided corticosteroid injections and short-term response in subacromial impingement syndrome: a randomized, double-blind, prospective study. Am J Phys Med Rehabil. 2012 Aug;91(8):658–65.

21. Aly AR, Rajasekaran S, Ashworth N. Ultrasound-guided shoulder girdle injections are more accurate and more effective than landmark-guided injections: a systematic review and meta-analysis. Br J Sports Med. 2015 Aug;49(16):1042–9. Epub 2014 Nov 17.

22. Cole BF, Peters KS, Hackett L, Murrell GA. Ultrasound-guided versus blind subacromial corticosteroid injections for subacromial impingement syndrome: a randomized, double-blind clinical trial. Am J Sports Med. 2016 Mar;44(3):702–7. Epub 2015 Dec 30.

23. Sabeti-Aschraf M, Ochsner A, Schueller-Weidekamm C, Schmidt M, Funovics PT, et al. The infiltration of the AC joint performed by one specialist: ultrasound versus palpation a prospective randomized pilot study. Eur J Radiol. 2010 Jul;75(1):e37–40. Epub 2009 Aug 3.

24. Sabeti-Aschraf M, Stotter C, Thaler C, Kristen K, Schmidt M, Krifter RM, et al. Intra-articular versus periarticular acromioclavicular joint injection: a multicenter, prospective, randomized, controlled trial. Arthroscopy. 2013 Dec;29(12):1903–10. Epub 2013 Oct 18.

25. Yoon JP, Chung SW, Kim JE, Kim HS, Lee HJ, Jeong WJ, et al. Intra-articular injection, subacromial injection, and hydrodilatation for primary frozen shoulder: a randomized clinical trial. J Shoulder Elbow Surg. 2016 Mar;25(3):376–83.

26. Werner BC, Cancienne JM, Burrus MT, Griffin JW, Gwathmey FW, Brockmeier SF. The timing of elective shoulder surgery after shoulder injection affects postoperative infection risk in Medicare patients. J Shoulder Elbow Surg. 2016 Mar;25(3):390–7.

27. Sardelli M, Burks RT. Distances to the subacromial bursa from 3 different injection sites as measured arthroscopically. Arthroscopy. 2008 Sep;24(9):992–6. Epub 2008 Jun 16.

28. Marder RA, Kim SH, Labson JD, Hunter JC. Injection of the subacromial bursa in patients with rotator cuff syndrome: a prospective, randomized study comparing the effectiveness of different routes. J Bone Joint Surg Am. 2012 Aug 15;94(16):1442–7.

29. Hossain S, Jacobs LG, Hashmi R. The long-term effectiveness of steroid injections in primary acromioclavicular joint arthritis: a five-year prospective study. J Shoulder Elbow Surg. 2008 Jul-Aug;17(4):535–8.

30. Song A, Higgins LD, Newman J, Jain NB. Glenohumeral corticosteroid injections in adhesive capsulitis: a systematic search and review. PM R. 2014 Dec;6(12):1143–56. Epub 2014 Jul 1.

31. Tagliafico A, Serafini G, Sconfienza LM, Lacelli F, Perrone N, Succio G, et al. Ultrasound-guided viscosupplementation of subacromial space in elderly patients with cuff tear arthropathy using a high weight hyaluronic acid: prospective open-label non-randomized trial. Eur Radiol. 2011 Jan;21(1):182–7. Epub 2010 Jul 25.

32. Gross C, Dhawan A, Harwood D, Gochanour E, Romeo A. Glenohumeral joint injections: a review. Sports Health. 2013 Mar;5(2):153–9.

33. Kwon YW, Eisenberg G, Zuckerman JD. Sodium hyaluronate for the treatment of chronic shoulder pain associated with glenohumeral osteoarthritis: a multicenter, randomized, double-blind, placebo-controlled trial. J Shoulder Elbow Surg. 2013 May;22(5):584–94.

34. Chou WY, Ko JY, Wang FS, Huang CC, Wong T, Wang CJ, et al. Effect of sodium hyaluronate treatment on rotator cuff lesions without complete tears: a randomized, double-blind, placebo-controlled study. J Shoulder Elbow Surg. 2010 Jun;19(4):557–63.

Index

Page references for figures are indicated by *f*, for tables by *t*, and for boxes by *b*.